KT-500-906

The Child Protection Handbook

The practitioner's guide to safeguarding children

Commissioning Editor: Ninette Premdas
Development Editor: Katrina Mather, Gillian Cloke
Project Manager: Jane Dingwall
Design Direction: Erik Bigland
Illustrator: Robert Britton

The Child Protection Handbook

The practitioner's guide to safeguarding children

Edited by

Kate Wilson BA(Oxon) DipSW DipCouns

Professor of Social Work,
University of Nottingham, Nottingham, UK

Adrian James BA MA PhD GDSA DASS

Professor of Social Work,
University of Sheffield, Sheffield, UK

THIRD EDITION

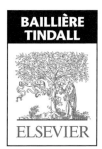

BAILLIÈRE
TINDALL

ELSEVIER

EDINBURGH LONDON NEW YORK OXFORD PHILADELPHIA ST LOUIS SYDNEY TORONTO 2007

BAILLIÈRE
TINDALL
ELSEVIER

An imprint of Elsevier Limited

First edition 1995
Second edition 2002
Third edition 2007
  Reprinted 2008

ISBN: 978 0 7020 2829 8

British Library Cataloguing in Publication Data
A catalogue record for this book is available from the British Library

Library of Congress Cataloging in Publication Data
A catalog record for this book is available from the Library of Congress

Working together to grow
libraries in developing countries

www.elsevier.com | www.bookaid.org | www.sabre.org

ELSEVIER   **BOOK AID** International   **Sabre Foundation**

ELSEVIER your source for books, journals and multimedia in the health sciences
www.elsevierhealth.com

The
Publisher's
policy is to use
**paper manufactured
from sustainable forests**

Printed in China

Contents

Editors and contributors

Editors

Kate Wilson BA(Oxon) DipSW DipCouns
Kate Wilson is Professor of Social Work and director of the Centre for Social Work at the University of Nottingham, UK. Her teaching, practice and research interests are in child welfare and therapeutic work, particularly with children and adolescents. Her writing includes two jointly authored books on non-directive play therapy and three on foster care, the latter based on a major longitudinal study on which she was co-researcher. In her previous post at the University of York, she co-founded and directed the university's programme in non-directive play therapy.

Adrian L. James BA MA PhD GDSA DASS
Adrian James trained as a social worker, practised as a probation officer, and was subsequently extensively involved in their training. After becoming an academic in 1978, he researched and published widely in the field of socio-legal studies, including the completion of two major ESRC-funded projects on aspects of social work practice in the field of child welfare and divorce. He was recently a Special Adviser to the House of Commons Select Committee on the Lord Chancellor's Department when it scrutinised the work of the Children and Family Court Advisory and Support Service (CAFCASS). Appointed as Professor of Applied Social Sciences at the University of Bradford in 1998, he became Professor of Social Work at the University of Sheffield in September 2004. He is also currently Professor II at the Norwegian Centre for Child Research at the Norwegian University of Science and Technology (NTNU) in Trondheim. His latest book, co-authored with Allison James and published by Palgrave Macmillan in June 2004, is *Constructing Childhood: Theory, Policy and Social Practice*.

Contributors

Mary Baginsky BA LLM PhD FRSA
Mary Baginsky has worked as a researcher and evaluator in universities, local and national government, independent organisations and in the voluntary sector. Until Spring 2006 she was Senior Research Officer with the National Society for the Prevention of Cruelty to Children where, amongst other work, she developed a programme of research into how the various parts of the education system were responding to their responsibilities in relation to child protection and safeguarding. She has published widely in the fields of education and social care. She now works as Senior Consultant with GHK Consultancy.

Margaret Bell BA DipSocSci MPhil CQSW DPhil
Margaret Bell is a senior lecturer in social work at the University of York. Her teaching and research interests are largely in the field of child care and protection, with a particular focus on inter-agency issues, service user involvement and working in partnership. Recent funded research projects have included empirical studies of the involvement of families, and the experiences of children, in child protection

investigations and family group conferences, and an evaluation of parenting programmes. Currently she is co-directing a national evaluation of the Integrated Children's System, funded by the DfES and WAG. Her practice experience includes work as a guardian *ad litem*, and wide experience of social work in the health field.

Arnon Bentovim MBBS FRCPsych FRCPCH BPAS DPM
Arnon Bentovim is Director of The London Child and Family Consultation Service, and Honorary Consultant Child & Adolescent Psychiatrist to Great Ormond Street Children's Hospital and the Tavistock Clinic, and is Honorary Senior Lecturer at the Institute of Child Health, University College London. Since his appointment at Great Ormond Street Children's Hospital he has been concerned with the management of child abuse from the late 1960s onwards. With colleagues he established assessment and treatment services for abused children and their families, on factors which lead to abusive behaviour in previously abused boys, family assessment approaches for children in need and their families, and has also published studies in various other aspects of child abuse including Induced Illness Syndrome – Munchausen by Proxy. He also consults to SWAAY, a residential setting for the treatment of young people who have been abused, and are abusing others.

Kevin Browne BSc MSc PhD MEd CBiol CPsychol
Kevin Browne is a Chartered Psychologist and a Chartered Biologist and is Director of The Centre for Forensic and Family Psychology for the University of Birmingham's School of Psychology. He has been researching in and publishing on family violence and child maltreatment for over 25 years; notable publications include *Child Abuse Review* from 1992 to 1999 (co-editor with Dr Margaret Lynch); *Preventing Family Violence* (with Martin Herbert, Wiley, 1997), *Early Prediction and Prevention of Child Abuse: A Handbook* (with Helga Hanks, Peter Stratton and Catherine Hamilton, Wiley, 2002) and *Community Health Approach to the Assessment of Infants and their Parents* (with Jo Douglas, Catherine Hamilton-Giachritsis and Jean Hegarty, Wiley, 2006). He is Consultant to the European Commission, UNICEF, World Health Organization and the World Bank on projects to prevent child abuse and neglect and promote child rights and protection; he held a DFID appointment of Chief Executive Officer of the High Level Group for Romanian Children (2003–2005). His research interests take a developmental perspective on forensic psychology, the influence of families on children and the causes of criminal behaviour and the prevention of crime; current research focuses on the influence of violence on children and teenagers and the childhood history of adult offenders.

Ian Butler BA(Hons) MPhil CQSW
Ian Butler is a qualified social worker with considerable practice experience. He has worked in residential and field settings, mainly with children and their families, in the statutory, voluntary and independent sectors. He is an Honorary Member of the Council of the NSPCC. He is Professor of Social Work at Bath University and a member of the Academy of Social Sciences. Currently he is on secondment to the Wales Assembly Government where he is Cabinet Advisor on Children and Young People's Policy. His main research interests include children's accounts of their social worlds, the health care of looked-after children and the practice of substitute family care. He is also interested in the development of social policy as it affects children and young people, especially young offenders.

Martin C Calder MA CQSW
Martin Calder has worked in the field of child protection and child welfare for over 20 years. He has operated as a specialist child protection social worker, child

protection coordinator and latterly as Operations Manager for the Child Protection Unit with Salford City Council, where he also has responsibility for domestic violence services. He has recently moved into Independent practice and has founded Calder Social Work Training and Consultancy (www.caldertrainingandconsultancy.co.uk) to develop further evidence-based materials for frontline practitioner use. Martin has written and published extensively around policy and procedural issues in the child protection field as well as the development of accessible, evidence-based assessment tools for frontline workers. His drive is to move beyond policy and procedural requirements to develop practice guidance that can empower rather than de-skill busy frontline practitioners from the constituent agencies of the child protection system.

Siobhan Canavan BA MSc Dip Counselling Cert Supervision BACP Accred Counsellor
Siobhan Canavan is a person-centred practitioner currently working as a Lecturer in Counselling at the Universities of Edinburgh and Abertay. She also works in private practice as a therapist and supervisor. She has worked as a planner, a tutor on social work courses, a sociologist and Lecturer in Women's Studies. Prior to her present post she worked for 8 years as the Head of the Counselling Service at the University of Aberdeen.

Rachael Clawson BA(Hons) MSW
Rachael Clawson worked as a childcare social worker in Devon, York and Nottinghamshire before taking up her current post as a Team Manager for the Disabled Children's Team in Nottinghamshire 3 years ago. She is a qualified Practice Teacher and has devised and facilitated training sessions on disabled children and child protection for Social Work qualifying programmes, Post Qualifying training and for the ACPC. Rachael is also an associate trainer for the Ann Craft Trust.

Jo Corlett BA MSc PhD RGN RNT FETC
Jo Corlett is Postgraduate Degree Scheme Co-ordinator at the School of Nursing and Midwifery at the University of Dundee. Her research interests include nurse education, family-centred care and parenting skills. She is currently the lead for the Children and Families research programme within the Early Years and Parenting research theme within the School.

Susan J Creighton BSc MSc
Susan Creighton was a Senior Research Officer at the NSPCC, where she researched for over 25 years. Her main research has been on the epidemiology of child abuse, both from cases placed on Child Protection Registers and from more general national prevalence surveys. She has also researched and written on child deaths where abuse or neglect was implicated.

Margaret Crompton BA(Hons) DipSS CertASS CQSW
Margaret Crompton is a self-employed writer/editor/lecturer/consultant. After experience as Assistant Warden in a Bethnal Green settlement, she worked in various posts for Leeds Children's/Social Services Departments and Lincolnshire SSD, as guardian *ad litem* (Lincolnshire) and as Lecturer in Social Work at Bradford and Newcastle upon Tyne Universities. Her publications since 1978 explore aspects of communicating with children/young people in a social work context. Preparing a training pack for the Central Council for Education and Training in Social Work on Children, Spirituality and Religion (1996) led her to focus her writing and teaching on developing understanding of spirituality and religion in relation to children/young people and practice in social and health care, including *Children,*

Spirituality, Religion and Social Work (Ashgate 1998) and *Who am I?* (2001) – a guide for Barnardos. She has contributed to a number of consultations, conferences, training events and publications. With her husband she also occasionally lectures and leads study groups on, and writes articles about, English literature.

Brigid Daniel MA(Hons) PhD

Brigid Daniel is Professor of Child Care and Protection, and Director of Studies for the suite of post-qualifying child care and protection courses at the University of Dundee. She is a qualified social worker and worked for some years in local authority social work in Edinburgh. She was a member of the multidisciplinary team that carried out the Ministerial Audit and Review of Child Care and Protection in Scotland which reported in 2002 in *It's Everyone's Job to Make Sure I'm Alright*. Her research interests and published books and journal articles are on child development, child neglect, work with fathers, assessment and resilience.

Brid Featherstone BA MA PhD CQSW DASS

Brid Featherstone is currently Professor of Social Work and Social Policy at the University of Bradford. Formerly the NSPCC Reader in Applied Childhood Studies at the Centre for Applied Childhood Studies, University of Huddersfield, she is a qualified social worker and has also worked as a practitioner and manager in the area of child protection. She is a founder member of the Gender and Child Welfare Network and has written widely on gender relations and child welfare. She has a particular interest in how services engage with fathers and is researching a number of projects in this area.

Donald Findlater BA MA

Donald Findlater is Deputy Director of The Lucy Faithfull Foundation, a child protection charity working in the area of child sexual abuse prevention. Following a career in the Probation Service, he joined the Foundation to establish and manage the Wolvercote Clinic, the UK's only residential assessment and treatment centre for men with allegations of, or convictions for, child sexual abuse. Donald manages the operation of the Stop it Now! UK and Ireland Helpline, and the management of Stop it Now! Surrey. He has recently been involved with the DfES in creating its *Safer Recruitment* training programme, in response to the Bichard Report, and was a member of the Nolan Committee.

Rachel Fyson BSc PhD

Rachel Fyson is currently a lecturer in Social Work at the University of Nottingham. She has previously worked as a Research Fellow for both the Ann Craft Trust at the University of Nottingham, and the Norah Fry Research Centre at the University of Bristol. Her research interests include issues around sexual abuse, learning disability, inter-agency working and policy implementation. She recently undertook the first UK study into the response of statutory education and social services to young people with learning disabilities who display sexually inappropriate or abusive behaviours.

Jo Green PGCertSystemicTherapy PGDipEthicsSocWelfare

Jo Green has worked within Local Education Authorities both as a practitioner within the Education Welfare Service and as a manager. She has a wide range of experience of working with both the voluntary and statutory sectors contributing to the development of child protection policy and practice. Most recently she has been part of the national network of Investigation and Referral Support Co-ordinators, established by the Department for Education & Skills in 2001 to support local authority education services and their ACPC partners in strengthening the procedures which safeguard children in education. She is currently seconded to the DfES and works as an Allegations Management Adviser based in the Government Office for London. She now advises Local Safeguarding Children Boards on the implementation of procedures for dealing with allegations across the whole of the children's workforce.

Liz Hall BA(Hons) PhD DipClinPsychol DipPsychotherapy
Liz Hall is a Consultant Clinical Psychologist and Psychotherapist working in private practice in Lincoln providing therapeutic work for survivors and others, supervision, training and a large number of assessment reports for the courts within the child protection services where children are at risk. She recently became the UK organiser for the Sensorimotor Psychotherapy Institute (US) and organises new training incorporating the new developments in neurobiological and attachment research and the impact of trauma on the body. She is co-author with Siobhan Canavan of *Surviving Child Sexual Abuse: A Handbook for Helping Women Challenge Their Past*, published by Falmer Press in 1989 and revised in 1993.

Catherine Hamilton-Giachritsis BSc PhD
Catherine Hamilton-Giachritsis is a Chartered Forensic Psychologist and Senior Lecturer in Forensic Psychology at the University of Birmingham. Previously she worked in Birmingham Social Services Psychology Department, undertaking assessments of families where there was considered to be a risk to children or assessing the needs of children and adolescents in such families. She is co-author of the Wiley volumes *Early Prediction and Prevention of Child Abuse: A Handbook* (2002) and *A Community Health Approach to the Assessment of Infants and their Parents*: *The C.A.R.E. Programme* (2006). In addition, Catherine has published widely on child maltreatment, family violence, the institutionalisation of infants and young children, and the links between media violence and crime.

Helga Hanks BSc MSc DipPsych AFBPsS(Chartered) UKCP registered
Helga Hanks is a Consultant Clinical Psychologist and UKCP registered Family Therapist in the Department of Community Paediatrics, St James's University Hospital, Leeds. She is also a Visiting Senior Lecturer at the Institute of Psychological Sciences, Leeds University. One of the founder members of the Leeds Family Therapy & Research Centre (LFTRC) at Leeds University which came into existence in 1979, she was Clinical Director of the Centre until late 2005. She is one of the core staff who developed the MSc in Family Therapy at the Institute of Psychological Sciences, Leeds University. Parallel to the involvement in family therapy she has become well known working in the area of child abuse within a paediatric setting, prominent for her work in sexual abuse and failure to thrive. Together with a number of colleagues she was also involved in founding the Expert Witness Group (EWG) which developed guidelines for expert witnesses in child abuse cases. She is presently involved in developing and undertaking a unique service related to supporting paediatricians emotionally and psychologically when they work in the front line of child abuse. She has published and researched widely both in the areas of family therapy and child abuse.

Ann Head MA Advanced Award in Social Work
Ann Head is a self-employed children's guardian *ad litem* in Devon and an independent social worker on the national register. She has published research on the placement of sexually abused children and has written on this subject and on the subject of sibling relationships. She has also written and lectured on the role of the

guardian *ad litem* (now children's guardian) and on the subject of children's rights. She is currently engaged in research on the subject of mediation.

Jan Horwath BA(Hons) CQSW

Jan Horwath is Professor of Child Welfare at the University of Sheffield. Jan researches and writes on the management of child welfare systems, multidisciplinary practice and assessment policy and practice. She has a social work background and was involved in the development of the English *Framework for the Assessment of Children in Need and their Families* and the accompanying training materials *The Child's World*. She has also developed, with colleagues at Trinity College Dublin, an Irish multidisciplinary framework for assessing the needs of vulnerable children and their families. Publications include *The Child's World: Assessing Children in Need and Their Families* (Jessica Kingsley, 2001) and *The Neglected Child: Identification and Assessment* (2007; Palgrave).

Deborah Kitson BA(Hons) MA CQSW

Deborah Kitson worked for Nottinghamshire as a social worker with people with learning disabilities before being appointed as Implementation Officer for Nottinghamshire Abuse Procedural Guidelines based at the University of Nottingham. She produced and revised the guidelines and is now a consultant for other agencies developing policies on the protection of vulnerable adults. Deborah was co-ordinator of the Ann Craft Trust before being appointed Director in 2002. She facilitates training on a wide range of associated issues and is author of a number of publications including *Facing the Possibility*, *Equipped to Cope* and *Training to Protect*. She was also a member of the Steering Group of 'No Secrets' and is external representative on a number of Adult Protection Committees.

Jill E Korbin PhD

Jill E Korbin is Associate Dean, Professor of Anthropology, Director of the Schubert Center for Child Development and Director of the Childhood Studies Program in the College of Arts and Sciences at Case Western Reserve University in Cleveland, Ohio, USA. Korbin received the Margaret Mead Award (1986) from the American Anthropological Association and the Society for Applied Anthropology; was awarded a Congressional Science Fellowship (1985–86) through the American Association for the Advancement of Science and the Society for Research in Child Development; and served on the National Academy of Sciences Panel on Research on Child Abuse and Neglect.

Mary Lane BA(Hons) CQSW LLB

Mary Lane began her career as a social worker in 1971 specialising in child care, adoption and fostering, and subsequently as a Children's Guardian and Reporting Officer. She qualified as a solicitor in 1994 and now has her own practice following 7 years working in local authority legal departments. She is legal adviser to two voluntary adoption agencies and to Adoption UK, and trains solicitors, social workers and CAFCASS officers in child care and adoption law. Mary is chair of the BAAF legal advisory group and the co-author of three BAAF publications: *A Summary of Child Care Law* (2006); *What happens in Court?* – a guide for children and young persons involved in care and adoption proceedings (2004); and *Fostering Now* – a pocket guide to fostering law, guidance and regulations (2004). Adoption UK published *Adoption Law for Adopters* by Mary Lane in June 2006.

Barry Luckock BA(Hons) PQCE PGDipSW

Barry Luckock is a Senior Lecturer in Social Work and Social Policy at Sussex University, where he is currently the Director of the MA in Social Work. His primary research interests are in various aspects of child care social work policy and practice. These include adoption and fostering (see Hart A, Luckock B 2004 Developing adoption support and therapy. New approaches for practice. Jessica Kingsley, London; Luckock B, Lefevre M (forthcoming 2007) Direct work with children and young people. A guide to social work practice in foster, adoptive and residential care), social work communication with children and young people (see Luckock B, Lefevre M, Orr D, Marchant R, Jones M, Tanner K 2006 Knowledge review on teaching, learning and assessing communication skills with children and young people in social work education. SCIE, London) and integrated working. He is a registered social worker.

Christina M Lyon LLB Solicitor of the Supreme Court

Christina Lyon is Queen Victoria Professor of Law and Director of the Centre for the Study of the Child, the Family and the Law at The University of Liverpool and is also a solicitor. One of only four full-time academics ever to have been appointed to sit as a Recorder (part-time judge) in Her Majesty's Courts in Family Cases and Crime, she is also Joint Editor of the *Journal of Social Welfare and Family Law*. She has written extensively in the field of children, families and the law, completed research projects for Gulbenkian, Carnegie, Barnardos, IPPR and UNICEF, and been involved in evaluative research on Children's Fund programmes. She is consulted by a range of UK organisations including BILD, the Judicial Studies Board, and the Children's Society on child protection and children's human rights. Formerly Chair of NYAS and Executive Trustee of the Liverpool Bureau for Children and Young People, she is now Independent Chair of the 0–5 Group of the Liverpool Children and Young People's Strategic Partnership Board, and the Children's Rights Advisory Forum for Alder Hey Children's Hospital. She trains a wide range of professionals working with children and young people.

Claire Mason BSc MSW

Claire Mason is currently a lecturer in the Department of Applied Social Science at Lancaster University, and prior to this was a Research Associate. She is a qualified social worker and has over 10 years' experience in the field of social care, having worked for children's charities both in the UK and South Africa. Her main research interests are child protection and family support and she has undertaken several research projects in this area. Her current research is focused around the Common Assessment Framework and its implications for social work with Children and Families.

Corinne May-Chahal BA PhD CQSW DASS

Corinne May-Chahal is currently Director of Social Work at Lancaster University, having previously been Professor of Child Care at the University of Central Lancashire and NSPCC Reader at the University of Huddersfield. She has researched and published widely in the field of child protection and has coordinated research projects for the European Commission and WHO on child maltreatment prevention. She has a particular interest in the perspective of those who have direct experience of childhood violence and disorder in family life and is the consumer representative for children on the Family Justice Council. Recent projects include protective factors for human rights violation for CAHRV (the EU Co-ordination Action on Human Rights Violation), missing children, child death and serious case reviews. Her most recent books are (with Stella Coleman) *Safeguarding Children and Young People* (Routledge, 2003) and (with Maria Herzog) *Child Sexual Abuse in Europe* (Council of Europe, 2003).

Nigel Parton BA MA PhD CQSW

Nigel Parton is NSPCC Professor in Applied Childhood Studies in the Centre for Applied Childhood Studies at the University of Huddersfield. He has researched and published widely in the areas of child protection, child welfare, social work and social theory. His books include: *The Political Dimensions of Social Work* (editor with Bill Jordan, Basil Blackwell, 1983); *The Politics of Child Abuse* (Palgrave Macmillan, 1985); *Governing the Family: Child Care, Child Protection and the State* (Palgrave Macmillan, 1991); *Social Work, the Media and Public Relations* (editor with Bob Franklin, Routledge, 1991); *Social Theory, Social Change and Social Work* (editor, Routledge, 1996); *Child Protection: Risk and the Moral Order* (with David Thorpe and Corinne Wattam, Macmillan, 1997); *Child Protection and Family Support: Tensions, Contradictions and Possibilities* (editor, Routledge, 1997); *Child Sexual Abuse: Responding to the Experiences of Children* (editor with Corinne Wattam, Wiley, 1999); *Constructive Social Work: Towards a New Practice* (with Patrick O'Byrne, Palgrave Macmillan, 2000); and *Safeguarding Childhood: Early Intervention and Surveillance in a Late Modern Society* (Palgrave Macmillan, 2006).

Stephanie Petrie BA(Hons) MSocSci DASS CQSW

Stephanie Petrie is currently a Senior Lecturer in the School of Sociology and Social Policy at the University of Liverpool. She held posts as a generic social worker and social services manager in local authorities and the voluntary sector from 1969 until 1995. She was an Honorary Fellow at the University of Hull for 11 years and, in 1995, became a full-time academic, initially at the University of Bradford and then the University of Lincolnshire and Humberside. Her research interests are in the impact of the market paradigm on policies and practices for vulnerable children, young people and their families in the community.

Melanie Phillips BA(Hons) CQSW PGDipAppSocSci

Melanie Phillips is a black social worker of Asian origin. She has 26 years of experience in social services, initially as a social worker and Senior Practitioner, working with children and families in London authorities, and subsequently providing independent training, supervision and consultancy on child care as well as undertaking research on child protection practice. Melanie has written extensively on child protection and black and minority ethnic families, was a member of the Advisory Group which developed the *Framework for the Assessment of Children in Need and their Families* (DoH 2000) and co-wrote the chapter in the *Practice Guide for the Assessment Framework on Assessing Black Families*. She has co-written a publication on the *Lessons for Practice from the Victoria Climbié Inquiry* to be published in 2007/2008 and has worked with the REU and DfES on a publication on Identity and Self Esteem of Looked after Children and contributed to the DfES research and pilots for the Integrated Children's System.

Catriona Rioch CQSW DipCPS

Catriona qualified as a social worker in 1978 and gained a Diploma in Child Protection Studies in 1995. She has worked extensively within the voluntary sector, managing projects which worked with children and young people at risk of residential care. She has also worked as a Child Protection Co-ordinator in local authority Children's Services as well as managing a therapeutic project for children and young people who had suffered trauma. She is currently Project Manager for Aberlour National Parenting Development Project (funded from Scottish Executive Youth Crime Prevention) which operates Scotland-wide and aims to assist agencies in the development and delivery of parenting programmes. The project also

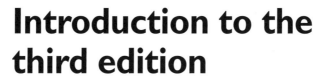

Introduction to the third edition

Since the second edition of the *Handbook* was published in 2002, the world of child protection has undergone radical changes. That an area of professional practice can alter so markedly in such a short period of time is, in itself, worthy of comment, since it underlines the challenge to which this new edition is part of the response: that of keeping up to date – with the latest theoretical perspectives, research developments, and changes in law, practice and procedures – in order to ensure that the intended beneficiaries of the efforts of those involved receive the best service possible.

It is also important to note some of the main reasons for the changes that are charted in the chapters in this new edition. Sadly, but perhaps predictably, there have been further tragedies involving the neglect and maltreatment of children since the second edition was published. Some of these have inevitably attracted more publicity than others. Most significant in this respect was the death of Victoria Climbié, an 8-year-old child from the Gold Coast who was systematically tortured and then murdered by her great aunt and the aunt's partner in North London in the year 2000. Victoria's death attracted the horrified attention of the public in Britain, partly because of the appalling circumstances surrounding her death; partly because of the fact that, yet again, a number of agencies were involved but apparently unable to identify or respond to her plight; and partly because of some of the difficult issues concerning culture and ethnicity that emerged in the course of the subsequent enquiry by Lord Laming.

This single case provided the focus for a major initiative by the government to reform services for children under the banner of the title of the Green Paper, *Every Child Matters*, which spelled out a far-reaching agenda, spreading across the entire field of services for children and families, an agenda for change that is expected to dictate changes in the field over the next 10 years. In addition to new primary legislation, we can expect a raft of supplementary regulatory guidance in the coming months, as well as what will be little short of a seismic shift in the landscape of child care practice, as the impact of the Children's Workforce Development Council begins to be felt as part of the redefinition of how this workforce is defined, of what it is comprised, and how its training needs can best be met.

It will come as no surprise, therefore, to find that the death of Victoria Climbié, *Every Child Matters*, and the provisions of the subsequent Children Act 2004 feature prominently throughout this third edition. This also, however, gives the clue to the main difficulty faced by the contributors to this volume in providing the guidance that is so important to those who practise in this demanding field: that of seeing far enough into the future to know precisely what might be the implications for practice of the wholesale changes that are to be wrought.

As editors, as well as for our contributors, it feels unsatisfactory to identify so many uncertainties when what practitioners need is clear and unequivocal guidance. It is also inevitable that the new structures, which will emerge from this process of change, will bring about extensive changes. The impact of these cannot at this stage be entirely anticipated, particularly when at their very heart are, in the case of social work, new agency structures, and in the case of other professions, new mechanisms for encouraging effective inter-professional and inter-agency collaboration. How successfully these new structures will resolve the problems identified by Laming and set out in *Every Child Matters* is a topic addressed by a number of contributors to this edition (but see especially Luckock and Stevenson). Sadly, however, it seems highly probable, on the basis of the experience of the last three decades, that these new structures and arrangements will see the emergence of as yet unanticipated weaknesses or lacunae, followed by further criticism directed at the professionals charged with the task of safeguarding children and another series of reforms generated by yet another Inquiry.

In the meantime, however, we hope that this thoroughly revised third edition will provide a valuable source of information and support for those who are struggling with the difficulties that inhere in what is, arguably, the most demanding area of all in the broad field of child welfare practice, as well as for those who are training to work in this demanding field and for those responsible for their training. Despite some real and understandable concerns over the impact of yet more changes on professionals working in the field, it has also been heartening, in putting together this edition, to recognise the progress and achievements that have been made and of which we hope the new edition will give ample evidence.

This edition retains the structure of previous editions, being divided into three sections, but to make the main issues covered in each chapter more readily accessible, each contributor has highlighted at the end of their chapter some key points and messages for practice. In addition, this new edition is being published in conjunction with a website provided by the publishers (http://evolve.elsevier.com/wilson/child/), on which can be found some of the chapters or chapter sections from both the first and second editions that we have decided to omit for reasons of space as part of the process of bringing the volume up to date but which we feel may still be of interest to those who are using the book for the first time. These include the chapter by John Simmonds from the first edition, which explores some of the personal issues for professionals involved in acknowledging and working with abuse; that by Anne Bannister on groupwork and the final anonymous chapter consisting of a detailed case account, both from the second edition. There is also an extended version of Christina Lyon's revised chapter on law, which contains more details and references to case law, which have been omitted from the third edition for reasons of length.

Nigel Parton opens Section 1, *Understanding Child Abuse*, with a critical review of recent developments and highlights the potential significance of the key changes that have been introduced in the wake of Victoria Climbié's death. Chapters by Creighton, Browne, and Hanks and Stratton from the second edition have been substantially revised, and, as new contributors to the *Handbook*, Findlater and Fyson give up-to-date perspectives on the characteristics of sexual abusers, including for the first time a discussion of young perpetrators. This new edition also sees an additional chapter by Jill Korbin, which offers a thoughtful analysis of the impact of cultural issues on child protection practice and provides a helpful discussion of the development of 'cultural competence' in practice. This is followed by a thorough revision by Melanie Phillips of her chapter on ethnicity in the light of the Laming Inquiry. A new chapter on disability by Deborah Kitson and Rachel Clawson highlights both the significant developments which have taken place in working with children with disabilities who have been abused, but also the troubling gaps which still exist in recognising abuse and intervening effectively. And finally, Ian Butler offers an up-to-date discussion of issues of institutional abuse.

Section 2, *Managing the Process of Safeguarding Children*, as before addresses aspects of the structures and processes that have been put in place in the UK to manage key stages in protecting children. A number of these chapters have been substantially updated by contributors to the previous edition. Lyon, May-Chahal (who previously wrote under the name of Wattam) and Mason, Bell, Lane, Head and Williams all highlight recent changes in their fields, identifying new research and setting out key issues in the law, policy and/or practice. New contributors in this section include Jan Horwath who, in her chapter on assessment, provides an authoritative review of a stage of the child protection process which was undergoing major changes in the months leading up to the publication of the second edition and is now, as we prepare for the third, again subject to substantial change. This is also true, as we suggest above, of issues of inter-professional and inter-agency cooperation and organisation, and Barry Luckock provides a new chapter which considers the major changes that are underway, explores some of the inherent tensions and looks ahead to the likely impact of implementation. In this section, too, we have included a chapter by Julie Taylor and Jo Corlett which takes a broader perspective than our earlier editions on issues concerning the involvement of health practitioners in child protection, again reflecting substantial rethinking about their contribution to services. Included also is a similarly thorough revision of the chapter on education, by Mary Baginsky and Jo Green.

Finally, in Section 3, *Intervention in Safeguarding Children*, we focus, broadly speaking, on those aspects of the child protection process that follow comprehensive assessment and case conference decisions and recommendations: namely the implementation of the child protection plan, through engaging with parents and providing a variety of helping services, including out-of-home care, to those who have experienced abuse – whether children, adolescents, or adults and their families. A new chapter on parenting by Brigid Daniel and Catriona Rioch brings together for the first time in the *Handbook* approaches to working with parents; their inclusion in one chapter reflects the substantial and impressive progress that has been made over the decade in focusing on understanding the needs of parents and developing ways of helping them more effectively. Although all the other chapters in this section have been updated to incorporate substantial changes, progress in two areas – those of working with families (Bentovim, Chapter 25) and policy and practice in out-of-home care (Thoburn, Chapter 27) – is perhaps particularly notable. Thoburn's chapter points out, for example, the explosion of research studies of looked-after children that has occurred during the last 7 or 8 years.

The book concludes with a chapter by Olive Stevenson entitled *Where are we now?* This, as the title suggests, takes stock of past and recent developments in child protection, and considers the implications of these for probable future changes. Written from the perspective of someone who has been closely involved in child welfare for nearly six decades, it provides a compelling overview of what has been accomplished, what has not, and what is still to be achieved. It provides a powerful conclusion to what we hope will prove to be a comprehensive and valuable source book and guide for students, practitioners, managers and academics alike.

Kate Wilson
Adrian L. James

A note on *Working Together to Safeguard Children*

In 2005, the government issued a number of draft consultation papers on *Working Together to Safeguard Children*, through the auspices of the Department for Education and Skills and HM Government. These culminated in the publication, in April 2006, of the definitive document *Working Together to Safeguard Children* which sets out how individuals and organisations should work together to safeguard and promote the welfare of children. The guidance has been updated since the previous version which was published in 1999. The new version reflects developments in legislation, policy and practice.

There were, however, significant changes between the draft versions with which readers may be familiar and the final, definitive version. These changes are outlined below.

Changes to *Working Together*

The final version of *Working Together* (HM Government 2006) has dropped chapters which were in the original 2005 drafts and there has been a renumbering of chapters in order to accommodate a new Chapter 4 entitled *Training and Development for Inter-agency Work*, which was in the draft 2005 Guidance as Chapter 7, *Inter-agency Training and Development*, and what was Chapter 4 in the 2005 HM Government draft has now become the new Chapter 5, *Managing Individual Cases*.

The old Chapter 5 in the 2005 HM Government draft entitled *Reviewing and Investigating Individual Cases: Child Death Review Processes* has now become Chapter 7, but is now simply entitled *Child Death Review Processes*.

The new Chapter 6 in the 2006 version is entitled *Supplementary Guidance on Safeguarding and Promoting the Welfare of Children* and has no counterpart in the draft HM Government 2005 guidance as it did not exist in that version at all.

The old Chapter 6 has now become Chapter 8 but with the same title as the old Chapter 6, i.e. *Reviewing and Investigating Individual Cases*.

The old Chapter 8, *Lessons from Research and Inspection*, has now become the new Chapter 9 with the same title; the old Chapter 9, *Implementing the Principles of Working with Children and their Families*, has become the new Chapter 10 with the same title; the old Chapter 10, *Safeguarding and Promoting the Welfare of Children who may be Particularly Vulnerable*, becomes the new Chapter 11 with the same title; and the old Chapter 11, *Managing Individuals Who Pose a risk of Harm to Children*, has become the new Chapter 12.

Note that the old Chapter 12 from the 2005 HM Government draft, which was entitled *Information Sharing*, has been dropped altogether, so the last chapter is Chapter 12 above on *Managing Individuals Who Pose a risk of Harm to Children*.

A number of other parts of the 2005 draft have been omitted from the final version in favour of references to specific documents such as those on *Forced Marriage* and *Female Genital Mutilation* which are now referred to in detail in the Annotated Further Reading to Chapter 11 by Professor C M Lyon, whereas some new sections have been introduced to the 2006 document which were not in the 2005 draft; for example, s.11.41 (*Children whose Behaviour Indicates a Lack of Parental Control*), s.11.53 (*Child Abuse linked to Belief in 'Possession' or 'Witchcraft' or in other ways related to Spiritual Beliefs*), s.11.76 (*Child Victims of Trafficking*) and s.11.81 (*Unaccompanied Asylum Seeking Children*). Some sections have been renamed; for example, the section in the draft entitled Child Pornography and the Internet has been renamed *Child Abuse and Information Communication Technology*.

Note also that there are six Appendices to the new document whereas there were only three in the 2005 draft. The new appendices include the three which were previously there: 1. A Statutory Framework; 2. Framework for the assessment of Children in need; 3. MOD Child Protection Contacts (which becomes Appendix 4 in the new set). The three new appendices are: 3. Use of Questionnaires and Scales to Evidence Assessment and Decision Making; 5. Procedures for Managing Allegations against People who work with Children; and finally: 6. A Guide to the Acronyms in the Document.

For those who wish to explore this area further, a downloadable copy of the 2006 version of *Working Together to Safeguard Children* is available at www.every childmatters.gov.uk/workingtogether and also appears on the website that accompanies this edition of the *Handbook* (see http://evolve.elsevier.com/wilson/child). This should be read in conjunction with Chapter 11 by Professor C M Lyon, in this volume.

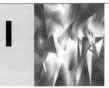 UNDERSTANDING CHILD ABUSE

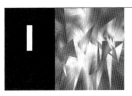

Safeguarding children: a socio-historical analysis

Nigel Parton

INTRODUCTION

The central purpose of this chapter is to demonstrate that what is now termed the 'safeguarding' of children, has a history and line of development that has been influenced by a range of social, economic and political changes over a century and a quarter, and that a knowledge of this history is crucial to explaining and understanding the current form and function of this area of practice. The focus of my analysis is changes and developments in England. While there are similar developments taking place in all the UK jurisdictions (e.g. Scottish Executive 2002) and other parts of the Western world, particularly Australia (e.g. Office for Children, Victorian Government 2005), the legislative policy and practice changes differ in detail in each case.

The changes currently being introduced in England following the publication of the Green Paper *Every Child Matters* (Chief Secretary to the Treasury 2003) and the passing of the Children Act 2004 mark a significant watershed in thinking about children's services and herald a major period of reform and change. What I will demonstrate is that while the government presented the changes as a direct response to the public inquiry into the death of Victoria Climbié (Laming Report 2003), they are much more than this.

The influences upon and the rationale for the changes have been determined only in part by concerns about preventing the deaths and abuse of children at the hands of their parents and carers. The changes have been motivated as much, if not more so, by the wish to ensure that children become skilled and productive members of the community and the *future* workforce, and do not enter into crime, as they are in protecting them from abuse and harm in the *present*. While the political momentum for the changes being introduced in England was considerably strengthened by the government being seen to be actively responding to the public inquiry into the death of Victoria Climbié, the government also took the opportunity this provided to introduce wide-ranging and radical reform which was only tangentially concerned with responding to child abuse.

The result, as I will demonstrate, is that the primary focus of official concern and intervention has broadened considerably. While in the late 1960s it was 'battered babies', in the 1970s 'non-accidental injury to children', in the 1980s 'child abuse', and for much of the 1990s 'significant harm and the likelihood of significant harm', the focus in the new millennium is 'safeguarding and promoting the welfare of the child', which is defined as:

the process of protecting children from abuse or neglect, preventing impairment of their health and development, and ensuring they are growing up in circumstances consistent with the provision of safe and effective care which is undertaken so as to enable children to have optimum life chances and enter adulthood successfully.

(DfES 2005a, p. 11)

The chapter is organised into six substantive sections: the discovery of child abuse in the nineteenth century and its subsequent disappearance in the twentieth century; the (re)discovery of child abuse in the 1960s and its initial impact on policy and practice; the growing crisis in child protection and child welfare practice more generally from the mid-1970s through to the mid-1990s; the 'refocusing' debate of the mid-1990s; and the nature of the current changes being introduced by the New Labour government following the Green Paper and the Children Act 2004. Finally, in the conclusion, I will reflect on the possible implications of these changes for professionals, parents and children themselves.

The first discovery of child abuse and its subsequent disappearance

For a phenomenon to take on the guise of a social problem requiring some form of state intervention, it first has to be defined and constituted as such, and the late nineteenth and early twentieth centuries are in many respects the period that provided the foundations and many of the central elements for what, until recently, has been termed child protection, and is now called 'the safeguarding of children'. What Linda Gordon (1989) calls the era of 'nineteenth century child-saving' (p. 20) lasted until the First World War at which point child abuse effectively disappeared as a subject of social concern, until it was 'rediscovered' by American paediatricians as the 'battered baby syndrome' nearly half a century later.

From the mid-nineteenth century there was a growing concern about child neglect and child cruelty, particularly as this was felt to contribute to delinquency or potential delinquency (May 1973). Gordon (1989) and Parker (1995) argue that child welfare only becomes an issue when women's voices are being heard strongly and in the latter half of the nineteenth century, middle-class women used their increased leisure time to engage in charitable work. Thus the welfare of children as well as the fear of delinquency emerged as a new focus for social policy, although the latter remained a major preoccupation (Hendrick 2003). In addition, a huge growth in charitable organisations followed the riots, famines and hard winters of the 1850s and 1860s which overwhelmed the Poor Law's always limited capacity to provide relief. Stedman Jones (1971) argues that 'in all known traditional societies the gift has played a central status-maintaining function' (p. 251): to give is to assert superiority, to receive without repayment is to accept an obligation to behave 'properly'. To regulate all this charitable work, the Charity Organisation Society was set up in 1869, its agents conscientiously investigating the home circumstances of the needy to ensure that they were morally deserving.

From such encounters grew a widespread concern (among the middle classes) about child cruelty and neglect (among the poor) and the first Society for the Prevention of Cruelty to Children was established in 1883, modelled on the SPCCs being established in America. The NSPCC was formed in 1889 and was hugely successful in organising the public and political campaign which produced the first legislation specifically to outlaw child cruelty and give public agencies powers to protect and remove children (Parton 1985).

The activities of the NSPCC were of great significance in this period. Ferguson (1990, 2004) has analysed cases drawn from case files of the period and shown how the new discourse of child protection was being constructed. NSPCC inspectors worked ostentatiously in the homes of poor communities describing, classifying and assigning deviancy. Here were 'social actors actively constructing the foundations of modern forms of knowledge, of therapeutic and cultural practice: in short, a professional culture that would take child protection into the twentieth century' (Ferguson 1990, p. 135). Indeed, many of the dilemmas of modern practice were here (Ferguson 1996, 1997) as inspectors advocated for clients, pondered the advisability of rehabilitating children and sought to reform and change abusing parents.

And yet, after 1918, much of this activity disappeared from view. Parker (1995) suggests a number of reasons for this: the decline of the women's movement following the granting of universal suffrage, for example, and changes in the NSPCC, to whom the government was happy to leave the responsibility for child cruelty and which became more bureaucratic and less campaigning. Ferguson (1996, 1997, 2004) has argued that the general approach of the NSPCC to publicising child deaths shifted considerably during this period. In the nineteenth and early twentieth centuries, in the early days of its existence, the NSPCC was not afraid to discuss publicly the deaths of children about whom they had direct knowledge and with whom they were working. The child death statistics were always included in its annual report. It seems that paradoxically the existence of child death was viewed as a sign that child protection was working well and was highly publicised because it meant that increasing numbers of vulnerable children were being reached by its workers and hence they were fulfilling a valuable role. By the 1920s, Ferguson argues, this approach had been transformed so that death in child protection cases ceased to be made public; not because the problem was solved but because knowledge about it was, in effect, suppressed by the NSPCC and others. Disclosure of deaths 'threatened the authority, optimism and trustworthiness of the expert system' (Ferguson 1997, p. 223).

Although the 1948 Children Act was shaped, in part, by an inquiry into the much publicised death of a child in foster care in 1945, intrafamilial abuse was still hardly on the agenda. Instead, the creation of local authority Children's Departments and the abolition of the last remnants of the hated Poor Law seemed to usher in a new, enlightened age in which families would be helped to stay together after the terrible experiences of war and evacuation. Neglect was seen as the main problem and families would be supported by preventative work from the newly professionalised social workers. As in the past, fears about child mistreatment centred on the link between neglect and delinquency and the threat to public order this would entail (Parton 1999). The earlier concerns about child abuse, as an issue in its own right, had all but been erased from public policy and professional practice.

The (re)emergence of child abuse as a socio-medical reality in the context of welfare reformism

The establishment of the local authority child care service in the post-war period can be seen as a particular instance of the growth and rationalisation of social interventions associated with the establishment of the welfare state at that time (Rose & Miller 1992). The key innovations of welfarism lay in the attempts to link the fiscal, calculative and bureaucratic capacities of the state in order to encourage national growth and well-being via the promotion of *social* responsibility and the mutuality of *social* risk, and were premised on notions of *social* solidarity (Donzelot 1988).

A number of assumptions characterised welfarism: the institutional framework of universal social services was seen as the best way of maximising welfare in modern society, whilst the nation state, working for the whole society, was the best way of progressing this. The social services were instituted for benevolent purposes, meeting social needs, compensating socially caused 'diswelfares' and promoting social justice. Their underlying functions were ameliorative, integrative and redistributive. Social progress would continue to be achieved through the agency of the state and professional intervention so that increased public expenditure, the cumulative extension of statutory welfare provision and the proliferation of government regulations, backed by expert administration, represented the main guarantee of equity, fairness and efficiency. Social scientific knowledge was given a pre-eminence in ordering the rationality of the emerging professions who were seen as making a major contribution to developing individual and social welfare and thereby operationalising increasingly sophisticated mechanisms of social regulation.

Children's Departments attempted to establish, for the first time, a professional state-sponsored child welfare service that saw the family as an object of positive social policy (Packman 1981). Heywood (1978) has argued that the legislation was passed in 'a fresh and hopeful atmosphere' and that, by the 1948 Act, 'the old paternalistic pattern of the poor law was brought to an end, and services which the individual could claim as a right were substituted' (1978, pp. 148–149): the aim was not to punish bad parents but to act in the interests of children. As the emphasis was on the strength and formative power of the natural family, this meant trying to maintain children in the family (Holman 1996). It heralded an era where families, primarily mothers, were encouraged and helped to care for their own children in their own homes and which underlined the importance of both the home and the child's own parents in their development. Where children could not live or remain at home, the priority was on placing them with foster parents rather than in the large and often impersonal institution as previously. Increasingly, the emphasis was on developing preventative services, thereby stopping children coming into local authority care in the first place; this was given legislative expression in Section 1 of the 1963 Children Act.

The practice of local authority social work with children and families during the post-war period up until the early 1970s was thus imbued with a considerable optimism for it was believed that measured and significant improvements could be made in the lives of individuals and families via judicious professional interventions. Social work operated quietly and confidently and in a relatively uncontested way, reflecting a supportive social mandate. Allowed wide professional discretion, it harmonised with a central plank of post-war reconstruction, which reflected the belief that a positive and supportive approach to the family was required and that the state and the family should work in partnership to ensure that children were provided with the appropriate conditions in which to develop.

The high point of this optimistic growth and institutionalisation of social work in the context of welfarism came with the establishment of the larger and more wide-ranging local authority Social Service Departments in 1971. It reflected the belief of the Seebohm Report (1968) that social problems could be overcome, via state intervention by professional experts with social scientific knowledge and skills in the use of relationships, and envisaged a progressive, universal service available to all and with wide community support. Interventions in the family were not conceived of as a potential source of antagonism between social workers and individual family members, whether parent(s) or child(ren). The latter were not seen as having interests or rights distinct from the unitary family itself. When a family required modification, this would be via social casework, help and advice, and if an individual did come into state care this was assumed to be in their best interests. The law was not conceptualised as constituting the nature of social work in any significant way or as significantly informing the skills required of social workers and the types of relationship deemed appropriate for work with clients. When more coercive aspects were drawn upon, these were primarily seen as a tool for fulfilling more significant therapeutic goals. It was in this context that child abuse was (re)discovered in the 1960s and 1970s.

There are two important issues to note about the modern (re)discovery of child abuse. First, it was discovered in the USA and then quickly imported into the UK, particularly via the NSPCC and a number of other social work and health professionals (see Parton 1985 for a detailed analysis of this process). As a consequence, policy and practice in the UK, and in most other English-speaking Western societies, were heavily influenced by developments and changes in knowledge, policy and practice in the USA and it is only in more recent years that policy makers, practitioners and researchers in the UK have looked to mainland Europe for different ways of thinking and different models of practice (e.g. Cooper *et al.* 1995, Harder & Pringle 1997, Hetherington *et al.* 1997, Pringle 1998).

Second, and perhaps more significantly, the initial (re)discovery took the form of the 'battered baby syndrome' following the publication of the highly influential paper by Henry Kempe and his colleagues (1962) from Denver, Colorado. Unlike the nineteenth century, it was professionals, particularly medical professionals, rather than victims, survivors, community groups and the women's movement that not only brought the issue back to public attention, but in the process also conceptualised it in certain ways. It was defined as a 'syndrome' or 'disease' and hence something in which professionals, particularly doctors, were seen as experts.

It is quite clear that the term 'battered baby syndrome' was specifically chosen, as opposed to 'physical abuse', in order to appeal to as wide an audience as possible, including conservative paediatricians. Kempe wanted no hint of legal, social or deviancy problems – the problem was *medicalised*, so that medical experts and medical technology, such as the use of the X-ray to identify old and otherwise hidden injuries, was seen as key.

The original article (Kempe *et al.* 1962) claimed that the syndrome characterised a clinical condition in young children, usually under 3 years of age, who had received serious physical abuse, usually from a parent, and that it was a significant cause of childhood disability and death. It argued that the syndrome was often misdiagnosed and that it should be considered in any child showing evidence of possible trauma or neglect, or where there was a marked discrepancy between the clinical findings and the story presented by parents. The use of X-rays to aid diagnosis was stressed, and it was argued that the prime concern of the physician was to make the correct diagnosis and to ensure that a similar event did not occur again. The authors recommended that doctors report all incidents to law enforcement or child protection agencies. It was also said that the problem was not simply concerned with poverty and that the characteristics of the parents were that: 'they are immature, impulsive, self-centred, hypersensitive and quick to react with poorly controlled aggression' (Kempe *et al.* 1962, p. 19). Such an approach was to have an enormous influence on the way child abuse was thought about for many years to come.

While the 'battered baby syndrome' proved the dominant underlying metaphor for some years, it is also clear that the category of child abuse was quickly subject to various 'mouldings' (Hacking 1988, 1991, 1992) and 'diagnostic inflation' (Dingwall 1989, p. 29). By the 1980s it included emotional abuse, neglect, sexual abuse, children at risk as well as physical abuse and was no longer focused only on children but could include young people up to 18 years old.

However, it was the public inquiry into the death of Maria Colwell that was to catapult the issue of child abuse and the practices of health and welfare professionals, particularly social workers, into the centre of public, political and media attention. This hastened the introduction of a range of new policies, practices and procedures and thereby placed the issue at the top of professional agendas (Secretary of State 1974; see Parton 1985 for a detailed analysis of the nature and impact of the Maria Colwell case).

The contemporary system of child abuse management was effectively inaugurated with the issue of a Department of Health and Social Security circular (DHSS 1974a) in April 1974 in the wake of the death of Maria Colwell. The roles of paediatricians, GPs, health visitors and social workers were seen as vital and the social services department, as the lead statutory child care agency, central. The police at this stage were not seen as crucial and it was a further circular in 1976 (DHSS 1976) which recommended that a senior police officer should be included on all area review committees and case conferences.

The collapse of the welfare consensus in child care

The optimism and confidence evident in social work and the welfarist child welfare system more generally was subject to a number of critiques from the mid-1970s onwards, and these increased further during the 1980s. Some of the anxieties emanated from within social work itself and concerned the apparent poor and even deteriorating quality of child care practice in the newly created social service departments (Parker 1980). More widely, however, a whole variety of different concerns were developing which became increasingly important in influencing the parameters of the debate. While the criticisms represented somewhat different, though overlapping, constituencies, their net effect was to undermine the optimistic welfare consensus in child welfare and to challenge the 'medicalised' conceptualisation of child abuse that had been dominant from the moment of its (re)discovery.

First, from the 1960s onwards, with the growth of the women's movement and the recognition of violence in the family, it was recognised that not only might the family not be the haven it was assumed to be but also that women and children were suffering a range of abuses at the hands of men. Much of the early campaigning was directed to improving the position of women and it was only from the mid-1970s, with the growing concerns about sexual abuse, that much of the energy was directed to the position of the children (Parton 1990). Such critiques helped to disaggregate the interests of individual family members and supported the sometimes contradictory development during the period of the Children's Rights movement (Freeman 1983, Franklin 1986, 2002).

Second was the growth from the late 1960s of a more obviously civil liberties critique which concentrated upon the apparent extent and nature of intervention in people's lives that was allowed, unchallenged, in the name of welfare (e.g. Morris *et al.* 1980, Taylor *et al.* 1980, Geach & Szwed 1983). Increasingly liberal, due-process lawyers drew attention to the way the administration of justice was unfairly and unjustly applied in various areas of child care and to the need for a greater emphasis on individual rights. However, during the mid-1980s, the parents' lobby gained its most coherent voice with the establishment of Parents Against INjustice (PAIN), which was to prove influential in ensuring that the rights of parents and of children to be left at home, free of state intervention and removal, were placed on the political and professional agendas. As a result, state intervention, via the practices of health and welfare professionals, as well as parental violence, were identified as being actively and potentially abusive.

However, it was child abuse inquiries that provided the key catalyst for venting major criticisms of policy and practice in child welfare and the competencies of social workers. While such criticisms were evident from 1973 onwards following the death of Maria Colwell (Secretary of State 1974, Parton 1985), they gained a new level of intensity during the mid-1980s as a result of the inquiries into the deaths of Jasmine Beckford (London Borough of Brent 1985), Tyra Henry (London Borough of Lambeth 1987) and Kimberley Carlile (London Borough of Greenwich 1987). It was public inquiries that provided the vehicles for political and professional debate about what to do about child abuse in a very public way and in the full glare of the media (Franklin & Parton 1991, Aldridge 1994). Not only did they provide detailed accounts of what had gone wrong in the particular cases but they also commented critically on the current state of policy and practice more generally and made recommendations as to what should be done (DHSS 1982, DoH 1991a).

Up until the mid-1980s the 30-plus inquiries had all been concerned with the deaths of children at the hands of their parents or caregivers. All the children had died as a result of physical abuse or neglect and had often suffered emotional neglect and failure to thrive. The child care professionals, particularly social workers, were perceived as having failed, with horrendous consequences, to protect the children. The deaths were viewed as particular instances of the current state of policy, practice, knowledge and skills and the way systems operated and interrelated (Hallett & Birchall 1992). Crucially, however, professionals, particularly social workers, were seen as too naïve and sentimental with parents, failing to concentrate on the interests of the children and to use their statutory powers. The emphasis in inquiry recommendations was on encouraging social workers to use their legal mandate to intervene in families to protect children, to rationalise the multidisciplinary frameworks and to improve practitioners' knowledge of the signs and symptoms of child abuse so that it could be spotted in day-to-day practice.

However, the Cleveland Inquiry (Secretary of State for Social Services 1988) provided a rather different set of concerns and interpretations of what was wrong and how we should respond. The Cleveland affair broke in the early summer of 1987 and was focused on the activities of two paediatricians and social workers in a hospital in Middlesbrough, a declining chemical and industrial town in the North East of England. During a period of a few weeks over a 100 children were removed from their families to an emergency Place of Safety (the hospital) on the basis of what was seen by the media and two local Members of Parliament as questionable diagnoses of child sexual abuse. A number of techniques for diagnosing and identifying sexual abuse developed by paediatricians and child psychiatrists were subjected to close scrutiny, particularly the anal dilation test, the use of anatomically correct dolls and 'disclosure' work. Not only was it the first scandal and public inquiry into possible over-reaction by child welfare professionals, but also the first on sexual abuse in which medical science, as well as social work, was put under scrutiny (see Parton 1991 for a detailed analysis). Unlike developments up until this point, which carried the imprint of thinking in the USA, developments in Cleveland were a very British affair and had a history and impact, both in this country and abroad, of their own (see Hacking 1991, 1992).

This time it seemed that professionals – paediatricians as well as social workers – had failed to recognise the rights of parents and had intervened prematurely in families where there were concerns about sexual abuse. While, once again, the reasons for the crisis were seen as residing primarily in inter-agency and inter-professional misunderstandings, poor coordination and communication, and the legal context and content of child abuse work, the emphasis was rather different.

Now, not only did the law itself need to be changed but there was also a need to recognise that professionals should be much more careful and accountable in identifying the 'evidence', legally framed, for what constituted sexual abuse and child abuse more generally. It was not only a question of getting the right balance between family autonomy and state intervention but also getting the right balance between the power, discretion and responsibilities of the various judicial, social and medical experts and agencies. In this respect, the judiciary was seen to be central for future decision making.

There were some other issues associated with Cleveland, however, which meant that its impact and significance were of a different order from the public inquiries which had gone before. It was about sexual abuse, and the issue of sexual abuse touched a range of sensitivities that were rarely evident in earlier concerns about physical abuse and neglect: it reached into the most intimate, hidden and private elements of family life and adult–child relations; it represented a major set of debates around patriarchy and male power and thereby opened up a range of political arguments around gender never previously evident in the official discourse; and for the first time the issue threatened middle-class and professional households. No longer could child abuse be seen as only associated with the marginalised and the disreputable sections of society: it seemed to permeate 'normal' families.

Thus, while quite different in their social location and their focus of concern, we can see a growing set of constituencies developing from the mid-1970s which criticised the post-war welfarist consensus in relation to child welfare and the medico-scientific dominance in relation to child abuse. Their concerns were most forcefully articulated in and via child abuse inquiries. What emerged were arguments for an approach where there was a greater reliance on individual rights firmly located in a reformed statutory framework and where there was a greater emphasis on legalism. Within this emphasis, the rule of law, as ultimately judged by the court, takes priority over those considerations which may be deemed, by the professional 'experts', as optimally therapeutic or 'in the best interests of the child'. Thus, by the late 1980s/early 1990s, we can see a distinct shift in the dominant discourse concerning child abuse away from the 'socio-medical' to the 'socio-legal', which had a series of implications for the way policy and practice were framed and operated.

Such developments need to be located in the context of the more wide-ranging changes that were taking place in the political environment. During the 1970s an increasing disillusion was evident about the ability of the social democratic state both to manage the economy effectively and to overcome a range of social problems through the use of wide-ranging state welfare programmes. The growth of what has been termed the New Right (Levitas 1986) proved particularly significant in shifting the nature of political discourse in the 1980s. For the New Right, the problems in the economic and social spheres were closely interrelated: they were seen to emanate from the establishment and increasing pervasiveness of the social democratic welfare state, so the prime focus for change was to be the nature, priorities and boundaries of the state itself. The strategy consisted of a coherent fusion of the economic and the social. It had its root in an individualised conception of social relations whereby the market was the key institution for the economic sphere, while the family was the key institution for the social sphere. The family was seen as an essentially private domain from which the state should be excluded but which should also be encouraged to take on its natural caring responsibilities for its members, particularly children. The role of the state should thus be reduced to: (a) ensuring that the family fulfils these responsibilities; and (b) ensuring that no one suffers at the hands of the violent and strong.

Freedom, while central, was constructed in negative terms, i.e. as freedom from unnecessary interference. Clearly, however, a fine balance had to be struck between protecting the innocent and weak and protection from unwarrantable interference – particularly from the state. In such circumstances, the law became crucial in defining and operationalising both 'natural' rights and 'natural' responsibilities. Not only did it need to provide the framework to underwrite contracts between individuals and between individuals and the state, it also needed to make the rationale for intervention by state officials into the 'natural' sphere of the family more explicit and their actions more accountable.

It is in this context that we need to understand the Children Act 1989. In many respects the Act was not consistent with other pieces of social legislation that were being introduced at the time. Many of its key principles seemed to be much more in line with the premises of social democratic welfarism than with those of the New Right. The Act took much of its inspiration from the Short Report (Social Services Committee 1984) and the Review of Child Care Law (DHSS 1985a). Consequently, the central principles of the Act encouraged an approach to child welfare based on *negotiation* with families and *involving* parents and children in *agreed* plans. The accompanying guidance and regulations encouraged professionals to work in *partnership* with parents and young people. Similarly, the Act strongly encouraged the role of the state in *supporting* families with children 'in need', and keeping the use of care proceedings and emergency interventions to a minimum.

However, the Act was centrally concerned with trying to construct a new consensus and set of balances related to the respective roles of various state agents and the family in the upbringing of children. While it would be inappropriate to see the legislation as a direct consequence of Cleveland and other child abuse inquiries, child protection was its central concern (Parton 1991). Notions of individual rights and legalism framed the legislation in ways that were not evident previously. The other key element to emerge was in terms of the *criteria* to be used for making decisions. The assessment of *high risk* was central (Parton & Parton 1989a, 1989b, Parton 1991, 1998, Parton *et al.* 1997). In the Children Act 1989, *high risk* is framed in terms of 'significant harm'. The criterion for state intervention under the Act is 'that the child concerned is suffering, or is likely to suffer significant harm' (s.31(92)(a)). Thus, for the first time, the criterion for state intervention included a prediction of what may or was likely to occur in the *future*.

Assessments of actual or potential 'high risk' would become a central concern and activity. However, in a context where the knowledge and research for assessing and identifying 'high risk' was itself contested, and where the consequences of getting that decision wrong are considerable, it is not surprising that such decisions would not be left to health and welfare experts alone. Decisions and the accountability for making them would ultimately be lodged with the court and be based on *forensic evidence*. So, while assessments of high risk were central, they were framed in terms of making judgements about what constituted actual or likely 'significant harm'. The implication was that the legal gaze and the identification and weighing of forensic evidence would cast a shadow throughout child abuse work and child welfare more generally, but it was to be subjected to a variety of checks and balances set in place via the need to work in partnership with children and families and 'working together' with a range of agencies and professionals.

By the mid-1990s we can thus characterise the nature of child protection work in England as aiming to identify 'high risk' in a context in which notions of working together were set out in increasingly complex yet specific procedural guidelines and in which the work was framed by a narrow emphasis on legalism and the need for forensic evidence.

The 'refocusing' of children's services

Despite all the changes introduced in the early 1990s, major problems continued. The number and range of public inquiries did not subside and child abuse tragedies of both under- and overprotection continued to feature in the media, including numerous inquiries into abuse in children's homes (Corby *et al.* 2001 and Butler, Chapter 10, in this volume). In particular, a major debate opened up about the future direction of policy and practice. The essential issue was how policies and practices in child protection were integrated with and supported by policies and practices concerned with family support for children 'in need'. Increasingly, it seemed, there was a major tension between the two and that this was posing major problems for politicians, policy makers, managers, practitioners and users of child welfare services (Parton 1997).

The two key catalysts for these debates were the publication of the Audit Commission Report (1994), *Seen But Not Heard: Coordinating Child Health and Social Services for Children in Need,* and the launch by the Department of Health of *Child Protection: Messages from Research* (DoH 1995a). The Audit Commission Report suggested that the aspirations and central aims of the Children Act were not being achieved and it made a number of recommendations to try to move policies and practices forward. It argued that children were not receiving the help they needed because local authority and community child health services were poorly planned and coordinated. Central to the Report's recommendations was that local authorities and the health service should produce strategic plans for children's services to target resources more effectively. The focus should be on identifying and assessing need, then producing flexible and non-stigmatising services, with a particular emphasis on the role of care managers who would coordinate provision. More emphasis should be placed on prevention and less on reactive interventions and reliance on expensive residential services. The problems in developing the family support aspirations of the Children Act 1989 were also identified in a number of research studies (Aldgate *et al.* 1992, 1994, Giller 1993, Colton *et al.* 1995, Social Services Inspectorate 1995) and explicitly identified by the Children Act Report 1993 (DoH 1994a).

The central themes and recommendations in the Audit Commission Report reflected, and were in part informed by, the findings and conclusions of a number of major Department of Health funded research projects (Birchall & Hallett 1995, Cleaver & Freeman 1995, Farmer & Owen 1995, Ghate & Spencer 1995, Gibbons *et al.* 1995a, 1995b, Hallett 1995, Thoburn *et al.* 1995) and there is no doubt that the launch of the research overview document, *Child Protection: Messages from Research* (DoH 1995a), on 21 June 1995 proved something of a watershed in thinking about child protection policy and practice in England. The decision to fund the research programme in the 1980s was a direct consequence of the fall-out from the Cleveland Inquiry (Secretary of State 1988) and the apparent paucity of knowledge in the area of child abuse, combined with the manifest confusions in the reactions of the investigative agencies. The primary focus of the research programme was the processes and outcomes of child protection interventions.

Messages from Research argued that any '*incident* has to be seen in *context* before the extent of its harm can be assessed and appropriate interventions agreed' (DoH 1995a, p. 53, original emphasis), and that the studies demonstrated that, 'with the exception of a few severe assaults and some sexual maltreatment' (p. 53), long-term difficulties for children seldom followed from a single abusive event or incident – rather they were more likely to be a consequence of living in an unfavourable environment, particularly one which was *low in warmth and high in criticism*. Only in a small proportion of cases in the research was abuse seen as extreme enough to warrant more immediate and formal child protection interventions to protect the child. It suggested that, if we put 'to one side the severe cases' (p. 19), the most deleterious situations in terms of longer-term outcomes for children were those of *emotional neglect* where the primary concern was the *parenting style* which failed to compensate for the inevitable deficiencies that become manifest in the course of the 20 years or so it takes to bring up a child. Unfortunately, the research suggested that these were just the situations where the child protection system seemed to be least successful. What seemed to be demonstrated was that there was little evidence that children referred to Social Service Departments were suffering harm unnecessarily at the hands of their parents, as implied by most child abuse inquiries, and practice was thus *successful* according to a narrow definition of child protection. This was, however, at a cost. Many children and parents felt alienated and angry and there was an overemphasis on forensic concerns, with far too much time spent on investigations, and a failure to develop longer-term coordinated treatment, counselling and preventative strategies (Cleaver & Freeman 1995, Farmer & Owen 1995).

Perhaps most crucially, valuable time and resources were seen as being wasted, particularly on investigations, with little apparent benefit. This was also a major conclusion in the Audit Commission Report. In both, the key research was the study carried out by Gibbons *et al.* (1995b) on the operation of the child protection system. This research, based in eight local authorities, over a 16-week period in 1992, identified all children referred for a new child protection investigation (1888 cases) and tracked their progress through the child protection system for up to 26 weeks via social work records and minutes of case conferences. What was seen as particularly significant was the way a series of filters operated. At the first, 25% were filtered out by social work staff at the duty stage without any direct contact with the child or family. At the second, the investigation itself, another 50% were filtered out and never reached the initial case conference. Of the remainder, just 15% were placed on the child protection register. Thus six out of every seven children who entered the child protection system at referral were filtered out without being placed on the register. In a high proportion (44% of those actually investigated) the investigation led to no further action at all: there was no intervention to protect the child nor were any services provided. In only 4% of all the cases referred were children removed from home under a statutory order at any time during the study. These findings were reflected in many of the other studies.

In light of the research, *Messages from Research* made a number of suggestions as to how 'children's safety' could be improved. It emphasised:

- the importance of sensitive and informed professional/client relationships where honesty and reliability were valued
- the need for an appropriate balance of power between participants where serious attempts were made at partnership
- a wide perspective on child protection that was concerned not only with investigating forensic evidence but also with notions of welfare, prevention and treatment
- that priority should be afforded to effective supervision and the training of social workers
- that, in the main, the most effective protection from abuse was brought about by generally enhancing children's quality of life.

More specifically, it called for a refocusing of child protection work which prioritised s.17 and Part 3 of the Children Act 1989 in terms of helping and supporting families with 'children in need', thereby keeping notions of policing, surveillance and coercive interventions to a minimum. It similarly suggested that s.47 should be read essentially as the power to *enquire* in the first instance, rather than simply being required to undertake a forensically determined investigation. While *Messages from Research* received much professional publicity, the Conservative government did not take a strong lead in attempts to 'refocus' children's services and few extra resources were made available, so that local authorities were struggling to respond to this new agenda (DoH 2001a).

Safeguarding children and childhood under New Labour

It quickly became evident, however, that the election of the New Labour government in May 1997 would take these debates and concerns forward in quite new ways and that New Labour aimed to broaden the 'refocusing' initiative beyond simply family support and child protection to embrace a much wider concern with parenting, early intervention, supporting the family and regenerating the community more generally. This was to be a key responsibility for local authorities in general, not just social service departments, and would reposition the role of health trusts, education authorities and non-government agencies, where early years and childcare services would play a key role. New Labour came to power with a quite distinctive political agenda which would not only reframe how support for parents was prioritised but would also have fundamental implications for the future of welfare policy generally (Jordan 1998).

As Paul Boateng (1999) wrote while Parliamentary Under-Secretary of State for Health:

This government is committed to ensuring that we support families, especially in their parenting role, so as to give children the best start in life. We are committed to supporting families when they seek help, and before they reach crisis point, and to making the best use of scarce public resources. It is because of that that we see the importance of early intervention. The evidence is that early intervention works. (p. 14)

The New Labour approach to the reform of children's services was prompted by concerns related to the prevention and reduction of crime and unemployment, rather than child abuse, an approach which has been further reinforced by the emphasis on the importance of social investment at the centre of policy (Hendrick 2003, Fawcett *et al.* 2004, Featherstone 2004a). With such an approach, the balance of welfare spending shifts from a concentration on services which are felt to encourage passivity to those which encourage individual responsibility and positive risk taking. The priorities thereby shift from social security benefits to services which are seen as explicitly promotional and positive, particularly health and education, and which have the effect of forestalling problems before they arise. In this scenario the section of the population that would most benefit from investment is children, particularly very young children. As Tony Blair argued in his Beveridge Lecture, when he made a commitment to abolish child poverty within 20 years, there needed to be a refocusing of the objectives and operation of the welfare state:

If the knowledge economy is an aim, then work, skill and above all investing in children, become essential aims of welfare ... we have made children our top priority because, as the Chancellor memorably said in his budget, 'they are twenty per cent of the population, but they are a hundred per cent of the future'.

(Blair 1999, p. 16)

Policies for children lie at the heart of the New Labour project to refashion the welfare state. In a context where social investment for the future becomes the prime objective, it is not surprising that it is the Treasury which has been the major driving force for introducing many of the changes in children's services. Since New Labour came to power it has introduced a plethora of new policies for parents and children and made significant changes to long-established ones (Miller & Ridge 2002, Pugh & Parton 2003, Skinner 2003, Fawcett *et al.* 2004).

Perhaps the clearest example of the New Labour approach in its first term was the introduction of the Sure Start programme which, following the success of the Head Start programme in the United States, was based on the assumption that, even when chains of causation could not be incontrovertibly established, successful efforts to reduce known risk factors and increase protection factors across a broad population could achieve a desirable preventative effect for children (Utting 1998). During the discussions which paved the way for Sure Start, Tessa Jowell, then Minister for Public Health, provided something of a mission statement for the New Labour government's reshaping of children's services:

We want services to be flexible and responsive to the needs of each child so everyone can get the best possible start to life. If Government departments work together, not only can we give best value to the children but we can also get value for money by cutting the costs of crime and unemployment which can so easily follow if children do not get help at an early age.

(HM Treasury News Release, 21 January 1998)

The Sure Start programme, designed for parents and children under 4 years of age, was announced in July 1998 as part of the government's first Comprehensive Spending Review. Not only was the programme rapidly rolled out across the country in subsequent years, it also provided an administrative model for other New Labour interventions in relation to children and families. In addition, it clearly demonstrated the importance that has been given to safeguarding and promoting children's development, the recognition of the impact of multiple disadvantages, and the important role that the state should play in combating these in a more general sense. In particular, it underlined the importance of early intervention in order to combat problems later in life. Under New Labour children and childhood have become a prime site for state intervention of a pre-emptive kind.

As part of this strategy, the Children and Young Persons Unit (CYPU) was launched in July 2000 and, while it was responsible for overseeing and administering the new £450m Children's Fund for community-based partnership projects for 5–13 year olds, its brief was much broader. Building on the work already developed in the first term of the New Labour government, and following the report of the Social Exclusion Unit (SEU) on young people (SEU 2000), it was asked to help join up policy making across government departments by removing barriers to effective working and encouraging local coordination through developing and rationalising plans and partnerships. At the same time the Prime Minister set up a dedicated Cabinet Committee for Children and Young People, chaired by the Chancellor of the Exchequer.

The two key objectives set for the Children's Fund were, first, to ensure that in each area there was an agreed programme of effective interventions that picked up on early signs of difficulty, identified needs and introduced children and young people and their families to appropriate services; and second, to ensure that children and young people who had experienced early signs of difficulties received appropriate services in order to gain maximum life-chance benefits from educational opportunities and health care and to ensure good outcomes. It was hoped that services which were described as 'universal' would have mechanisms to identify 'children at risk of social exclusion'. The Children's Fund sub-objectives give a clear insight into what it was hoped such an approach would achieve:

- to promote school attendance and improve educational performance
- to ensure that fewer young people committed crime and were victims of crime
- to reduce child health inequalities
- to ensure that children, young people and families felt that the preventative services developed were accessible
- to involve families in building the community's capacity to sustain the programme and thereby create pathways out of poverty.

The rate of change increased further when, on 25 June 2001, less than 3 weeks after the election of New Labour to its second term of office, the Chief Secretary to the Treasury, Andrew Smith, announced seven initial cross-cutting reviews that would contribute to the 2002 Spending Review, including a review into services for 'Children at Risk'. Chapter 28 of the 2002 Spending Review, entitled 'Children at Risk', set out a central plank of government activity for its second term (HM Treasury 2002). The review found that, despite extensive investment in services for children, most were not having the desired positive impact on the most disadvantaged children. The recommendations sought to ensure that support for 'children at risk' was better focused on both preventative services and the preventative elements of mainstream services.

Following the publication of the Spending Review in 2002 a whole variety of government statements were made in great rapidity, including one made on 16 August by John Denham, the Minister for Children and Young People at the Home Office, announcing that local systems to identify, refer and track (IRT) children at risk of, for example, offending, drug taking and teenage pregnancy, would be put in place across the country in the course of the following year. This would be a key focus for the Children's Fund and £600m was allocated to the CYPU in 2003–2004 from the Spending Review to carry this out. On 6 September 2002, John Denham made a further statement that, from April 2003, all local agencies responsible for delivering services to children and young people would be asked to agree a coordinated strategy for preventative services for children and young people aged 0–19. The letter to local authority chief executives also included interim guidance on the key elements of a local preventative strategy:

The aim of the preventative strategy is to promote positive outcomes and to prevent children and young people experiencing negative outcomes, both as children and young people and later in their lives as adults. By addressing the risk factors that make children and young people vulnerable to negative outcomes, such as being excluded from school, running away from home, or becoming involved in crime, the local preventative strategy will set the direction for services to reduce social exclusion.

(CYPU 2002, para. 1.2)

It is notable that all these developments were taking place precisely at the time when the Laming Report into the death of Victoria Climbié was coming to its conclusions and just prior to its publication. In the autumn the government said it was in the process of producing a Green Paper on 'children at risk', and that this would provide the framework whereby it intended to respond to the findings of the Laming Report; however, it is quite clear that concerns about child abuse were not its central focus. The primary drive for these changes had come from the Treasury and the Home Office and were much more concerned with introducing policies to prevent unemployment and crime rather than child abuse.

The Green Paper *Every Child Matters* and the Children Act 2004

When the Green Paper was eventually launched on 8 September 2003 by Tony Blair, he said that he wanted it to serve as a permanent memorial to Victoria Climbié. In his Foreword, the Prime Minister stated:

For most parents our children are everything to us, our hopes, our ambitions, our future. Our children are cherished and loved. But sadly, some children are not so fortunate. Some children's lives are different. Dreadfully different. Instead of the joy, warmth and security of normal life, these children's lives are filled with risk, fear and danger and from what most of us would regard as the worst possible source – from the people closest to them. Victoria Climbié was one of those children. At the hands of those entrusted with her eventual care she suffered appallingly and eventually died. Her case was a shocking example from a list of children terribly mistreated and abused. The names of the children involved, echoing down the years, are a standing shame to us all … responding to the enquiry headed by Lord Laming into Victoria's death we are proposing here a range of measures to reform and improve children's services.

(Chief Secretary to the Treasury 2003, p. 1)

The Green Paper was clearly presented as a response to the Laming Report and to be centrally concerned with child abuse, and it was represented as such by the media.

It was only towards the end of his Foreword that Tony Blair stated that the Green Paper was also putting forward ideas on a number of related issues, including parenting, fostering, young people's activities and youth justice. 'All these proposals are important to children's health and security' (p. 2). What is apparent is that, while the Green Paper was informed by the Laming Report, it was primarily concerned with bringing together the government's proposals for reforming children's services which it had been developing for a number of years but with a much broader remit than previously. Indeed, rather than being entitled *Children At Risk*, as originally envisaged, the Green Paper was entitled *Every Child Matters*. This was not to say the Green Paper was not centrally concerned with 'risk'; clearly it was, but this was framed in such a way that any child could, at some point in their life, be seen as vulnerable to some form of risk. The government therefore deemed it necessary that *all* children were potentially covered by its proposals. Risk was seen as a pervasive threat to all children for a variety of reasons, and it is in this context that two figures (Figs 1.1 and 1.2) included in the Green Paper are particularly helpful in understanding how the reform of children's services has been conceptualised.

Underpinning the proposals were two basic assumptions concerning the nature of recent social change and the state of current knowledge. First, the Green Paper stated that over the previous generation, children's lives had undergone 'profound change'. While children had more opportunities than ever before and had benefited from rising prosperity and better health, they also faced more uncertainties and risks. They faced earlier exposure to sexual activity, drugs and alcohol, and family patterns had changed significantly. There were more lone parents, more divorces and more women in paid employment, all of which had made family life more complex and, potentially, made the position of children more precarious.

Second, however, the Green Paper asserted that these changes had come about at a time when we now had increased knowledge and expertise and therefore were in a better position to respond to these new uncertainties and risks. In particular, 'we better understand the importance of early influences on the development of values

Figure 1.1
*Every Child Matters:
categorising children.*

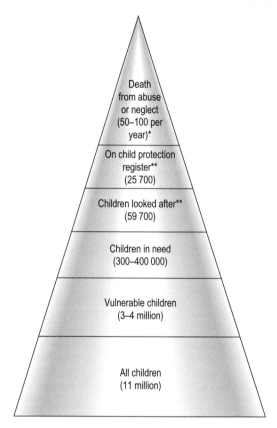

Death
from abuse
or neglect
(50–100 per
year)*

On child protection
register**
(25 700)

Children looked after**
(59 700)

Children in need
(300–400 000)

Vulnerable children
(3–4 million)

All children
(11 million)

* These children may or may not be on the child protection register,
nor looked after, nor vulnerable
** These children are included in the children in need figure, and not
all children on the child protection register are children looked after

and behaviour' (p. 15). It was thus important to ensure that this knowledge was drawn upon to inform the changes being produced, for, it argued:

we have a good idea what factors shape children's life chances. Research tells us that the risk of experiencing negative outcomes is concentrated in children with certain characteristics and experiences. (p. 17)

While research had not built up a detailed picture of the causal links, certain factors were said to be associated with poor outcomes. These included:

- low income and parental unemployment
- homelessness
- poor parenting
- poor schooling
- postnatal depression amongst mothers
- low birth weight
- substance misuse
- individual characteristics (e.g. intelligence)
- community factors (e.g. living in a disadvantaged neighbourhood).

Figure 1.2
Every Child Matters:
targeted services within a
universal context. SEN,
special educational needs.

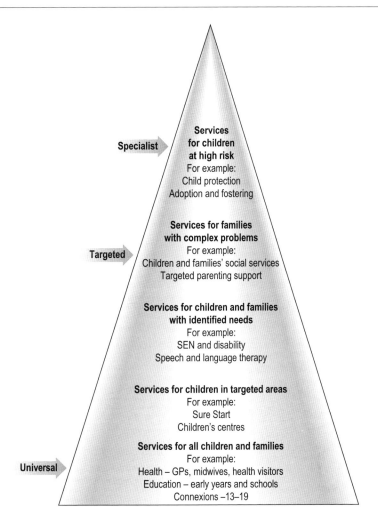

The more risk factors a child experienced, the more likely it was that they would experience negative outcomes, although the Green Paper argued that:

> research suggests that parenting appears to be the most important factor associated with educational attainment at age ten, which in turn is strongly associated with achievement later in life. Parental involvement in education seems to be a more important influence than poverty, school environment and the influence of peers. (p. 18)

Because of this increased knowledge about risk factors associated with a child's development, the Green Paper argued that it was important to intervene at an earlier stage in order to forestall problems in later life, particularly those associated with antisocial behaviour, crime and unemployment. Early intervention in childhood thus provided a major strategy both for overcoming social exclusion for children and for avoiding problems in the future.

The other area where knowledge and expertise had grown, and which was seen as vital in order to take policy and practice forward, was in relation to the major changes that had taken place to the development of new IT systems. The age of e-government was seen as having major implications for the reform and development of children's services. Not only would this provide the potential for identifying problems and enhancing attempts to intervene at an earlier stage, but it would allow different organisations and professionals to share information in order to ensure that children's problems were not missed and, crucially, children did not fall through 'the net'. The introduction of more integrated services was seen as crucially dependent on the introduction of new information technology. Following from the earlier commitment to develop IRT systems for 'children at risk', the plan was now to introduce a database for *all* children and young people via which professionals could share information whenever they had a 'cause for concern'.

In the light of these many changes, while the Children Act 1989 was seen as continuing to provide the primary legislative framework for policy and practice, the government felt it needed strengthening in certain respects. The key theme of the Children Act 2004 was to encourage partnership and sharpen accountability between a wide range of health, welfare and criminal justice agencies by:

- placing a new duty on agencies to cooperate among themselves and with other local partners to improve the well-being of children and young people so that all work to common outcomes
- a tighter focus on child protection through a duty on key agencies to safeguard children and promote their welfare through new Local Safeguarding Children Boards and a power to set up a new database containing basic information about children
- ensuring clear overall accountability through a Director of Children's Services who would be accountable for local education and children's social services and lead local change, and a Lead Council Member for Children's Services
- enabling and encouraging local authorities, primary care trusts and others to pool budgets into a Children's Trust, and share information better to support more joining up on the ground, with health, education and social care professionals working together based in the same location such as schools and children's centres
- creating an integrated inspection framework to assess how well services work together to improve outcomes for children
- taking on new powers to intervene in children's social services where an area was falling below minimum standards and intervention was seen as necessary
- the creation of a Children's Commissioner.

Section 12 of the Children Act 2004 requires Children's Services Authorities to establish Information Sharing and Assessment databases covering all children living in the area served by the authority. The government intends these databases to be tools to assist a wide range of practitioners in achieving the five outcomes for all children and young people identified in the legislation and the Green Paper, namely:

- Being healthy
- Staying safe
- Enjoying and achieving
- Making a positive contribution
- Achieving economic well-being.

The databases are not intended to be narrowly focused on child protection but aimed to improve the sharing of information between professionals, in order to improve the well-being of *all* children.

Section 12(4) sets out the information to be held on the database, which will comprise: name; address; date of birth; a unique identifying number; name and contact details of any person with parental responsibility or has day-to-day care of the child; details of any education being received, whether in an education institution or other setting; and name and contact details of a GP practice.

The subsection also provides for the inclusion of the name and contact details of any practitioner providing a specialist service (of a kind to be specified in further regulations) to a child and the fact that a practitioner has a 'cause for concern' about a child. No material relating to case notes or case history about an individual may be included on the database. If a practitioner accesses the database, it will be up to them to contact whoever flagged the 'cause for concern' to find out further details. The introduction of the new electronic databases signals the demise of the child protection registers, which have been in existence for over 30 years. In the future, where a child protection case conference concludes that a child has been abused or neglected, one or more of the categories of physical or emotional abuse or neglect will be recorded on the new electronic record, the Integrated Child System, to be developed for all children known to local authorities' children's social care services. The content of the records should be confidential and available only to legitimate enquirers.

Regulations will deal with disclosure of information to the databases, the conditions under which agencies and individuals will be granted access, the length of time that information should be held on the databases and the procedures for ensuring the accuracy of the data. There remains some doubt about how the involvement of so-called 'sensitive services' (e.g. sexual health clinics and pregnancy advice centres) should be recorded on the databases. It seems the government's preference is that information about the involvement of 'sensitive services' with a child will only be visible to 'essential practitioners'; however, this is also yet to be defined.

Conclusion

It is clear that a major impact of these changes will be to fundamentally reconfigure the relationship between the state, professionals, parents and children and that new and wide-ranging systems of surveillance are being introduced. The accumulation and exchange of information about children takes on a central and strategic role, both in assessing and monitoring the development and behaviour of children and young people and in holding a wide range of professionals to account. The role of the state will thereby broaden and become more interventive and regulatory at the same time. In effect, England is in the process of establishing a mandatory reporting system to be imposed upon professionals not based on child abuse, significant harm or the likelihood of significant harm, but on the basis of a 'cause for concern', a term which is not defined in the legislation. In the words of the then Minister for Children, Margaret Hodge, in her foreword to *Every Child Matters: Next Steps* (DfES 2004a), the vision is of 'a shift to prevention whilst strengthening protection' (p. 3). It is in this sense that the government is claiming that what we are witnessing, in England, is the most far-reaching reform of children's services for 30 years.

These changes pose particular challenges for all professionals. Some of these arise from the major organisational changes being introduced, with the establishment of new children's service authorities which are bringing together local education authorities and the child and family services of social services departments under the new Directors of Children's Services, Children's Trusts, and the replacement of Area Child Protection Committees by the new statutory Local Safeguarding Children Boards. Other challenges are posed by the need to introduce the new 'Common Assessment Framework', the integrated children system and the database under the auspices of Information Sharing and Assessment (ISA).

More particularly for our concerns in this book we need to consider two questions:

- How far does making the reporting of 'causes for concern' mandatory solve the problems in effective communication and risk assessment of abuse identified in the Laming Report and other public inquiries, and at what cost?
- Does the combining of abuse with all other concerns about a child's health and development potentially harm the quality of child protection services and therefore the safety of children?

While evidence to answer both questions is not yet available, during both the passage of the Children Bill through parliament and in much of the evidence presented to the House of Commons Education and Skills Committee which has reported on the changes, considerable alarm was expressed, particularly about the ill-defined concept of 'a cause for concern' as the criterion for information gathering and possible intervention. Many of the concerns were captured by Earl Howe in the debate in the House of Lords:

> We have here what is potentially a very large-scale system of data recording by the State on its citizens. The system is to be set up in the name of improving the welfare of all children. The names and key personal details of all 11 million children in England are to be recorded for access by professionals from a wide variety of disciplines. The vast majority of children so recorded will not be at risk of suffering significant harm or anything approaching it. The human rights aspect of that point is a question in itself which perhaps the Minister would be kind enough to comment on. But even if we set the human rights issue aside, how can we not regard this mammoth information gathering and information sharing exercise as anything other than grossly intrusive on the privacy of the family?
>
> (Earl Howe, Hansard, HL (Series 5) No 1661, Col 1154, 24 May 2004)

The changes are seen to have major implications for civil liberties, human rights, and the power and responsibilities of professionals in a wide range of social care, health and criminal justice agencies (Munro 2004, Penna 2005). The House of Commons Education and Skills Committee identified a number of problems and said that:

> We are not convinced that sufficient evidence currently exists to justify the commissioning of the proposed IT-based child indexes. We have significant reservations about whether this will represent the best use of resources and very significant concerns about critical issues such as security, confidentiality and access arrangements. We are concerned in particular that the current research evidence does not conclusively demonstrate that expenditure in this area is the best way of improving outcomes for children.
>
> (House of Commons Education and Skills Committee 2005).

The Committee felt the plans were underfunded and that key elements of the programme were not thought through.

What is evident is that the responsibilities and accountability of professionals and the various health, welfare and criminal justice agencies which employ them have become much more complex. In the process, the overall surveillance of both children and parents will, potentially, increase considerably. While the Children Act 2004 did create the post of a Children's Commissioner, who came into post in the summer of 2005, to be a voice for all children and young people, especially the most vulnerable, the post has much less independence than Commissioners in other countries, including Wales, Northern Ireland and Scotland, and has come in for considerable criticism.

The new Children's Commissioner has the weakest general function of any Children's Commissioner in the UK and Europe, and is concerned with promoting awareness of children's views and interests, rather than promoting and safeguarding their rights. There is no specific duty in relation to the rights of the child, and the independence of the Commissioner has also been subject to criticism as Ministers can 'direct' the Commissioner to undertake an inquiry (Children's Rights Alliance for England 2004). It seems that the huge increase in surveillance and potential intervention in the lives of children is not being counterbalanced by the authority and powers of the Children's Commissioner.

As I have argued elsewhere (Parton 2006), the changes currently being introduced, which attempt to safeguard and promote the welfare of children, are likely to have the effect of both increasing the regulation and surveillance of children and young people themselves, and the adults who have responsibility for them, both parents and professionals. A major problem with these changes is that because the proposed systems are so extensive, the definitions of concern so broad, and because the professionals who have responsibilities for children are held so (publicly) accountable (if things go wrong), there is a real danger that worries about children's vulnerabilities will lead to an increase in activity which only tangentially relates to the concerns of children and young people themselves. One suspects that, in the context of Figures 1.1 and 1.2 reproduced from the Green Paper, and in which there are unlikely to be sufficient resources available, an increasing amount of energy and time will be spent by professionals working in the reconfigured children's services developing and applying a whole variety of different 'threshold criteria' which aim to identify what sort of 'cause for concern' is being dealt with, what services (if any) should be allocated, who is responsible and how far they should treat information as confidential.

Such a scenario is a long way from the grand claims being made for the new services and one which is unlikely to gain the trust and confidence of the children, young people and parents who might want to use them. The overriding challenge is to ensure that the systems being introduced do not lead to a series of unintended and unanticipated consequences and are subject to human control, so that they become the vehicles for the increased safety and emancipation of children and young people, rather than the opposite.

Key points and messages for practice

- Professionals in a range of statutory, voluntary and private health, social care, education, early years and criminal justice agencies – not just local authority social workers – now have increased responsibilities to safeguard and promote the welfare of children.

- All professionals in these agencies will be required to identify and report 'causes for concern' and not just where it is felt that a child may be suffering or is likely to suffer significant harm.

- There are major organisational reconfigurations and changes taking place in relation to the new Children's Services' Trusts and Local Safeguarding Children's Boards.

- New requirements and procedures to be followed in relation to the storage, sharing, assessment and monitoring of information which aim to safeguard children but which also need to be consistent with Human Rights and Data Protection legislation.

All of the above have major implications for the role of professionals, and their relationships with each other, parents and children.

Annotated further reading

Fawcett B, Featherstone B, Goddard J 2004 Contemporary child care policy and practice. Palgrave Macmillan, Basingstoke

As the title suggests, this book analyses contemporary developments in child care policy, locating analysis both within a broad social policy context and within wider debates about the nature of childhood at the beginning of the twenty-first century. It places a particular emphasis on the importance of the idea of 'the social investment state' for understanding recent changes and has a chapter specifically addressing child abuse and child protection.

Ferguson H 2004 Protecting children in time: child abuse, child protection and the consequences of modernity. Palgrave Macmillan, Basingstoke

Drawing on an analysis of cases dating from the late nineteenth century to the present day, this book examines the development of child protection through the period and the various opportunities and challenges that have thereby been made available for both children and professionals.

Hendrick H 2003 Child welfare: historical dimensions, contemporary debates. Policy Press, Bristol

While not exclusively concerned with child protection, this book provides a comprehensive analysis and resource for anyone wishing to explore the historical contexts of childhood and child welfare policy and practice more generally. It provides an insightful analysis of the New Labour approach to these issues.

Parton N 1985 The politics of child abuse. Palgrave Macmillan, Basingstoke

The primary focus of this detailed analysis is to explain why child abuse emerged as such a significant social problem in Britain in the late 1960s and 1970s, and the way this impacted on child welfare practice more generally.

Parton N 1991 Governing the family: child care, child protection and the state. Palgrave Macmillan, Basingstoke

This takes on the story in the earlier book and pays particular attention to the social influences behind the Children Act 1989, particularly the impact of the 'Cleveland Affair'.

Parton N 2006 Safeguarding childhood: early prevention and surveillance in a late modern society. Palgrave Macmillan, Basingstoke

While in many respects the third of the trilogy, this book provides a comprehensive and detailed analysis of child protection policy and practice over the last 150 years and pays particular attention to the changes since the early 1990s, including the Green Paper Every Child Matters *and the Children Act 2004. It provides the historical detail and analysis on which this chapter is based.*

Useful websites

By far the most important website to keep abreast of the range of documents which are informing the various changes currently taking place in the wake of the Green Paper *Every Child Matters* and the Children Act 2004 is the official government website Every Child Matters: Change for Children – www.everychildmatters.gov.uk.

2

Patterns and outcomes

Susan J. Creighton

INTRODUCTION

How many children in the UK have been maltreated? What are the chances of a baby born this year being maltreated by the time she or he is 18 years old? In the average classroom how many children are recovering, or not, from past maltreatment and how many are still suffering, or not, from continuing maltreatment? Is maltreatment mainly sexual abuse, or does it include other forms of abuse as well? Are particular children more, or less, at risk of maltreatment?

Professionals working with children need to know the answers to these and other similar questions. They need to know so they can respond sensitively to individual children potentially in need, and confidently institute their local child protection procedures for those children they identify as in need of protection.

Estimates of abuse range from 'one in two girls and one in four boys will experience some form of sexual abuse before their 18th birthday' (Kelly *et al.* 1991) to 2800 children registered in the sexual abuse category in England during the year 1 April 2003 to 31 March 2004, a rate of 0.24 per 1000 population under the age of 18 years in 2003–2004 (DfES 2005b). The discrepancy between these two estimates creates confusion in the minds of the general public and professionals alike. This chapter attempts to outline the reasons behind such a discrepancy. It aims to clarify the factors that practitioners need to consider when using incidence or prevalence figures for maltreatment and how these impinge on their work with children. The main focus of this chapter is on maltreatment in the UK but draws on studies in Australia, Canada, the USA and other countries to illuminate the issues.

Review of frequency literature

Estimates of the frequency of child abuse are usually derived from either incidence or prevalence studies. Incidence refers to the number of new cases occurring in a defined population over a specified period of time – usually a year. Prevalence refers to the proportion of a defined population affected by child maltreatment during a specified time period – usually childhood.

There are five levels of professional recognition or public awareness of child maltreatment (adapted from US Department of Health and Human Services 1988):

Level 1

Those children whose maltreatment is recorded in the criminal statistics of a country and a prosecution has been mounted against the perpetrator where known.

Level 2

Those children who are officially recorded as requiring protection from child maltreatment and for whom services are provided. Examples would be the children on

Child Protection Registers in England, or substantiated cases of maltreatment in Australia and the USA.

Level 3

Those children who have been reported to child protection agencies because of concerns about maltreatment but who have not been registered. The reports may have come from members of the general public, schools, hospitals, GPs, day care facilities and mental health agencies. These children may be assessed as 'children in need' (Children Act 1989) but not as children in need of protection.

Level 4

Abused and neglected children recognised as such by neighbours, relatives or by one or both of the involved parties – the perpetrator and the child. None of these individuals, however, has reported it to a professional agency.

Level 5

Children who have not been recognised as abused or neglected by anyone. These are cases where the individuals involved do not regard their behaviours or experiences as child maltreatment and/or where the situations have not yet come to the attention of outside observers who would recognise them as such.

It is helpful to bear these five levels of awareness and/or discovery in mind when looking at the cases that are most likely to be included in incidence and prevalence studies.

Incidence studies are mainly concerned with reported and recorded cases of abuse to children – Levels 1, 2 and 3 children. Many cases of child maltreatment do not come to the notice of potential reporting authorities – Levels 4 and 5. Prevalence studies attempt to find out these hidden cases by asking a sample of adults, or young people, if they were abused during their childhood, regardless of whether or not that abuse came to light and was reported.

In the UK, the number of children placed on child protection (previously child abuse) registers (Creighton 1992, DfES 2005b) provide an annual measure of incidence. For many years the best known prevalence studies were the MORI (Baker & Duncan 1985) and Childwatch (BBC 1987) surveys of child sexual abuse. The Childwatch survey included questions on child abuse other than sexual abuse, but it concentrated on the sexual abuse cases when presenting its findings. This is interesting in view of the fact that more people reported having been emotionally or physically abused as children than sexually abused. More children are also registered annually as having been physically abused than as having been sexually abused (DfES 2005b), yet the majority of the child abuse prevalence studies conducted in the UK, and in the USA, have been on sexual abuse. This may be because of the different age distributions of the different types of abuse. Those in the youngest age group, the 0–1 year olds, are more vulnerable to physical abuse and neglect (Creighton 1992), whereas the average age of the children registered for sexual abuse was 9 years 7 months. Adults' recall of childhood experiences is very limited for the first 3–4 years of their lives, so if the physical abuse or neglect ceased before they were 4, they may well have no memory of it. The preponderance of child sexual abuse prevalence studies in the literature and the media has led to a sizeable proportion of the general public equating child abuse with child sexual abuse. Children have been murdered (e.g. in 1991 Claire McIntyre, Karin Griffin,

Angela Flaherty and Sarah Furness were all killed) following sexual abuse, but usually by strangers or acquaintances, not family members. Many more children die following physical abuse or neglect (Home Office 2005), mostly at the hands of their immediate caretakers. Abuse within the family has been, and still is, the major concern of professionals working in child protection.

Incidence studies

Level 1 incidence figures for England and Wales are available in Criminal Statistics. In the year 1 April 2003 to 31 March 2004 the Home Office (2004, 2005) recorded 70 child homicides, 6081 offences of 'cruelty to or neglect of children' and 1942 offences of 'gross indecency with a child'.

The next level of public recognition includes those cases which are officially recorded as child maltreatment – Level 2. In the UK, these are the children who are placed on child protection registers. In the USA they are those substantiated by the Child Protection Services in each State under the Child Abuse Prevention and Treatment Act (1974). In Australia they are those child protection notifications from each State or Territory that are subsequently substantiated.

Table 2.1 shows the officially recorded cases of child maltreatment in various countries.

The wide variations in rates per 1000 children and the breakdown in cases reflect a number of factors. These include the length of time the reporting system has been operating, the general level of public awareness and willingness to report, and the criteria for recording, in addition to the underlying levels of abuse and neglect in the country. Mandatory reporting was established in the USA in 1974 with the passage of the Child Abuse Prevention and Treatment Act. Non-mandatory guidance on the management of cases of non-accidental injury to children, including the establishment of registers, was issued by the Department of Health and Social Security in late 1974 (DHSS 1974a). Similar guidance was offered in Wales. Four 'confidential

Table 2.1
Official records of child maltreatment

Country	Year	Number of cases	Rate per 1000	Breakdown of cases (%)	Source
Australia	2002–2003	40 416	6.8	Emotional 34 Neglect 34 Physical 28 Sexual 10	AIHW (2004)
Canada	1998	61 000	9.7	Emotional 25 Neglect 41 Physical 25 Sexual 9	Trocme & Wolfe (2001)
England	2003–2004	31 000	2.8	Emotional 18 Mixed 14 Neglect 41 Physical 19 Sexual 9	DfES (2005b)
USA	2003	906 000	12.4	Emotional 5 Neglect 63 Physical 19 Sexual 10	US DHHS (2005)

doctors' were introduced in the Netherlands as an experiment on 1 January 1972 for 2 years. After this, a governmental institute for the prevention of child abuse and neglect was established. Official reporting appears to have started at similar times in the Netherlands, the USA and the UK. The resources made available and the public and professional awareness campaigns in the different countries varied enormously.

Officially recorded cases of child abuse and neglect are at Levels 1 and 2 of the professional recognition continuum. Not all children who are reported as abused or neglected will be officially recorded as such. In England and Wales, various studies (Association of Directors of Social Services 1987, Giller *et al.* 1992, Gibbons *et al.* 1995b) have shown that for every 10 children referred for child protection, only two will be registered. The remaining eight will be filtered out during the course of investigation and case conferencing. The Department for Education and Science now records the number of referrals to child protection registers. During the year ending 31 March 2004 there were 572 700 referrals to registers, over 18 times the number of children who were actually registered (DfES 2005b). In the USA, approximately 32% of reports of maltreatment are substantiated (Daro 1996). There have been a series of surveys conducted in the USA which attempted to ascertain cases from all professionals, i.e. Levels 1 through 3.

The US Department of Health and Human Services commissioned research surveys into the national incidence of child abuse and neglect in 1980, 1986 and 1993. The 1993 survey (US Department of Health and Human Services 1996) looked at all the cases reported to the Child Protective Services staff, as well as cases reported by a variety of professionals in other agencies who served as 'sentinels'. They were asked to be on the lookout during the study period for cases meeting the study's definitions of child maltreatment. These definitions were designed to be clear, objective and to involve demonstrable harm to the child. The research found that, in 1993, just under 1 553 800 children, a rate of 23.1 per 1000 nationwide, experienced abuse or neglect as defined by the study. Only 9% of these children were cases investigated by the Child Protective Services. Non-investigatory agencies (which included schools, hospitals, social services and mental health agencies) recognised seven times the number of child victims than investigatory agencies (police/probation service/courts and public health agencies). The overall incidence rate for neglect was 13.1 per 1000 children. Educational neglect (i.e. permitted chronic truancy or inattention to special educational needs by parents) was by far the most frequent form of neglect, with an incidence rate of 5.9 per 1000 children. This was followed by physical neglect, at a rate of 5.0, and then emotional neglect with an incidence rate of 3.2 per 1000 children. The most frequent type of abuse was physical, followed by sexual and then emotional abuse. The relative incidence rates for these were 5.7 for physical, 3.2 for sexual and 3.0 for emotional abuse per 1000 children. The overall incidence rate for abuse was 11.1 per 1000 children. These were calculated using the stringent criterion that the child had to have already experienced demonstrable harm as a result of maltreatment in order to be included. The incidence of both abuse and neglect had more than doubled since the 1980 survey.

Incidence studies which attempted to ascertain cases at Level 4, where no professional agency was involved, were those conducted in 1975, 1985 and 1995 by the Family Violence Research Program at the University of New Hampshire (Straus 1979, Straus & Gelles 1986, Straus *et al.* 1998). The 1975 and 1985 studies were of a nationally representative selection of American families with at least one child aged between 3 and 17 years living at home. One of the parents was interviewed and the studies attempted to determine whether physical abuse had occurred and at what levels of severity. Abusive violence was ascertained when the parent acknowledged that they, or their spouse, had 'punched, kicked, bitten, hit with an object, beaten up or used a knife or gun' on their child in the last year. The 1985 study obtained a rate of one in every 10 American children aged between 3 and 17 years subjected to severe physical violence each year. Compared to the rate of officially reported cases of physical abuse, Schene (1987) estimated that 'only one child in seven who is physically injured is reported'. Both these studies only included children aged between 3 and 17 years, whereas the youngest age groups, the 0–1 year olds and the 2–3 year olds, are the most vulnerable to physical abuse (DfES 2005b). Hence, the rates the authors obtained for the older age groups were likely to be underestimates of the incidence of physical abuse to all children in America. The 1995 study (Straus *et al.* 1998) included a nationally representative sample of US children under the age of 18 and a revised measure. They found a rate of severe physical assault against children of 49 per 1000, over eight times greater than that uncovered in the Third National Incidence Study (US Department of Health and Human Services 1996).

What is judged as child maltreatment changes over time within and between cultures. Creighton and Russell (1995) found that only 7% of their national sample of adults now thought it was acceptable to hit a child with an implement, whereas some 35% of them had experienced this in their own childhood. In a recent national study of parents' disciplinary strategies in the UK (Ghate *et al.* 2003), a quantitative survey of parental behaviours towards their children was followed by qualitative interviews with some of the parents and, independently, their children. The measures used in the quantitative survey were similar to those of the Family Violence Research Program in the USA, but following the qualitative interviews the definition of 'severe violence' was expanded to include 'smacking/slapping of the head or face'. Using this definition, they found a rate of severe violence to UK children of 90 per 1000 children.

Prevalence studies

Until recently, prevalence studies of child maltreatment have been almost entirely confined to child sexual abuse. Table 2.2 summarises the main prevalence studies of child sexual abuse conducted in different countries. The percentage of adults and adolescents affected varies from 6.8–20.4% of women and girls and 1–16.2% of men and boys.

The earliest prevalence studies (e.g. Finkelhor 1979) were usually conducted on samples of college students on social science courses. Social science students have the advantage of providing a captive sample but are probably not representative of the population as a whole. The studies included in Table 2.2 concentrate on samples drawn from the entire population of adults or adolescents. The wide variations among them probably reflect the differences in the methods used rather than significant geographical variation. These include items such as definitions used, how the sample was chosen and approached, the methods used to get the information from the respondents and how many refused to participate. The methodological issues involved in these studies will be discussed later in this chapter but brief details are included in Table 2.2. The factor with the greatest effect on the prevalence figures is whether or not the definition of child sexual abuse used included non-contact experiences such as exposure, in addition to contact experiences. Table 2.2 shows whether or not the definition included contact and non-contact experiences in the prevalence figures.

Table 2.2
Prevalence studies of child sexual abuse in different countries

Country	Sample	Method	Response rate (%)	Any CSA	Contact CSA	Authors
Canada	Representative population study 18+ (n = 2000+)	Hand-delivered questionnaires	94	42% women 25% men	10% girls <14	Badgley et al. (1984)
Canada	General population survey Ontario residents aged 15+ (n = 9953)	Health survey: self-administered questionnaire as part of interview	66	12.8% women 25% men	11.1% women 3.9% men	McMillan et al. (1997)
Finland	Random sample of 15–16 year olds in school	Self-administered questionnaire in school nurse's room or classroom	96	8% girls 3% boys	n.a.	Sariola & Uutela (1994)
Ireland	Random selection of adults (n = 3118)	Telephone interviews	71	30.4% women 23.6% men	20.4% women 16.2% men	McGee et al. (2003)
New Zealand	Community sample of 18 year olds	Face-to-face interviews	81	17.3% women 3.4% men	13.0% women 3.0% men	Fergusson et al. (1996)
Switzerland	Representative sample of 13–17-year-old Geneva school population (n = 1116)	Self-administered questionnaire	93.5	33.8% girls 10.9% boys	20.4% girls 33% boys	Halperin et al. (1996)
UK	Random probability sample of young adults aged 18–24 years (n = 2869)	Computer-assisted personal and self-interviewing	69	21% women 11% men	16% women 7% men	Cawson et al. (2000)
USA	Two-stage probability sample of Los Angeles adults (n = 3132)	Mental health survey Face-to-face interviews	68	n.a.	6.8% women 3.8% men	Siegal et al. (1987)
USA	Nationally representative community sample of 10–16 year olds	Telephone interviews	72	15.3% girls 5.9% boys	6.9% girls 1.0% boys	Finkelhor & Dziuba-Leatherman (1994a)

n.a., not available.

Methodological factors

The factors that need to be taken into account when planning or assessing studies of the frequency of childhood maltreatment include:

- Definitions
- Method of sampling
- Case ascertainment
- Measurement tools
- Bias
- Generalisability
- Comparability.

Definitions

The definition of childhood sexual abuse used in the MORI survey (Baker & Duncan 1985) was:

A child (anyone under 16 years) is sexually abused when another person, who is sexually mature, involves the child in any activity which the other person expects to lead to their sexual arousal. This might involve intercourse, touching, exposure of the sexual organs, showing pornographic material or talking about sexual things in an erotic way.

Ten per cent of their respondents (12% female, 8% male) reported that this had occurred to them. The definition employed by Siegal *et al.* (1987) in their mental health survey took the form of the question:

In your lifetime, has anyone ever tried to pressure or force you to have sexual contact? By sexual contact I mean their touching your sexual parts, or sexual intercourse?

Respondents who answered affirmatively were asked if they had ever been forced or pressured for sexual contact before the age of 16 years (childhood sexual assault). These specific questions, which focused on the nature of the behaviour – contact and pressured – plus the age when it happened (under 16 years), led to a prevalence figure of 5.3% (6.8% women, 3.8% men). This is one of the lowest figures for the studies but is very similar to that for the 'contact' cases in the Baker and Duncan study (derived from their Table 3, p. 461). Kelly *et al.* (1991) provide a detailed breakdown of the influence of definitions on prevalence findings in their study (see their Appendix C, p. 20). As the definitions get more 'serious' (in the sense of more intrusive and unwanted contact), so the numbers affected drop from 59% for the widest definition to 5% for the most serious.

Method of sampling

The four most commonly used methods in maltreatment studies have been: volunteer (e.g. BBC 1986), quota (e.g. Baker & Duncan 1985, BBC 1987), random (e.g. Russell 1983) and national random (e.g. Badgley *et al.* 1984). Volunteer samples are obviously going to be biased towards those with something to report. The 90% prevalence produced by the 1986 BBC Survey is what you might expect from a self-selected sample. If you produce a high-profile TV programme on a particular social problem and then invite viewers who have experienced this problem to write in and complete a questionnaire on it, you might expect a 100% prevalence of the problem among the returned questionnaires. Quota samples – in which people or households are approached until the required quota of subjects is obtained – run the same risk: that those choosing to participate will not be typical of the general population. Random samples, where each person in a population has an equal probability of being included in the sample, are preferred. Ideally, it should be a national random sample. A random sample in only one area might give the prevalence for that area but not be suitable for generalisation to other areas.

Case ascertainment

Even if a random sample of the population has been approached, the actual cases ascertained can be biased due to factors relating to: the subject, the interviewer and the measurement tool (the questionnaire). In such an emotive area as child maltreatment, it is possible that subjects either fail to recognise themselves as abused

(Berger *et al.* 1988) or repress memories of parental abuse and fail either to recall or report them. The gender, age and ethnicity of the interviewer in relation to the subject have all been shown to affect the likelihood and accuracy of the responses. Both men and women prefer to be interviewed about sexual topics by a woman, even adolescent males who have been abused by a woman (Kaplan *et al.* 1991).

The way the survey questionnaire is introduced can affect the likelihood of getting any answers. A survey presented as one on child sexual abuse is more likely to encounter a refusal than one on general health or attitudes.

Measurement tools

The wording of the questions or their position in the questionnaire (or interview) can have an impact on subject response. Questions need to be clear, simple and unambiguous. Sensitive questions which at the beginning of an interview may inhibit responses may, if placed at the end, be answered. Respondents are more likely to be engaged in the survey by a personalised approach but they may be embarrassed to answer personal questions. Surveys such as Badgley *et al.*'s (1984) study, which employed a personal approach coupled with a self-completed questionnaire, were very successful. The use of computers in surveys has also helped respondents to feel freer to divulge sensitive information (Turner *et al.* 1998). Computer-assisted personal interviewing (CAPI), where the interviewer uses a preprogrammed computer rather than a paper questionnaire, has become widely used in social surveys. Computer-assisted self-interviewing (CASI) is the computerised version of the self-completion questionnaire. The interviewer hands the computer over to the respondent for the more sensitive questions, and also demonstrates the complete confidentiality of their answers. The programme is set up to prevent the interviewers having any access to the CASI answers. The NSPCC's prevalence survey on child maltreatment (Cawson *et al.* 2000) and the national study on parental discipline (Ghate *et al.* 2003) both used CAPI and CASI technology.

It is very important to get a high response rate to the survey. Those people who refuse to answer questions are unlikely to be like those who agree, particularly in relation to child maltreatment. If only half the people you approach agree to answer the questions, then a high rate among them is misleading. The other half who refused may have done so because they were not affected. This effectively halves the prevalence estimate reported. A low response rate has the effect of turning a random sample into more of a volunteer sample. Although there is no simple acceptable response rate, rates lower than 80% are considered undesirable (Markowe 1991).

Missing data pose a similar problem. If a particular question is not answered by the majority of the respondents, the answers gained cannot be considered representative of the sample as a whole. It is important to pre-test and pilot the questionnaire or survey instrument to avoid including questions that will not be answered.

Bias

Bias is any trend in the collection, analysis, interpretation, publication or review of data that can lead to conclusions that are systematically different from the truth. Bias can be introduced in the ascertainment of cases, the design of a survey and the sample method employed. In child maltreatment reporting, it has been shown that the children of the middle and upper classes are less likely to come to the attention of the child protection agencies than those of the poor and disadvantaged. The perceived social status of the parents also affects the level of suspicion of experienced professionals about the possible non-accidental nature of an injury (O'Toole *et al.*

1983). Higher social class parents were less likely to be judged as abusive than lower class parents. Nurses and more experienced professionals were not affected by this social class bias. There are also likely to be reporting and substantiation biases in cases involving ethnic minorities, disabled children or children in out-of-home care. Hong and Hong (1991), using a sample of Californian students, found that the Chinese were more tolerant of harsh parental conduct than the Hispanics and Whites, and were less likely to ask for investigation by protective agencies in potential cases of child abuse and neglect. Nunno (1992) reported a survey of complaints of maltreatment of children in out-of-home care in the USA in 1989. Only 27% of these complaints were substantiated by child protection workers compared to 53% for familial maltreatment reports.

In addition to the characteristics of the child, the characteristics of the reporter – professional or other – has an effect on the process. In the USA, cases of child abuse reported by non-mandated sources (e.g. neighbours and schools) are less likely to be substantiated than cases reported by mandated sources (e.g. child protection services) (Eckenrode *et al.* 1988). Similarly, in the UK, Stevenson (1989) has described the relative status and perceived powers of the different agencies involved in child protection. These are all factors which can lead to bias in the recognition, reporting and registering of cases of child abuse.

Generalisability

If a prevalence or incidence study is thought to be methodologically sound, the next step is to assess how far it can be generalised. Are students in further education colleges, as in Kelly *et al.*'s (1991) sample, or students on social science courses (Finkelhor 1979) representative of all students? Are students representative of all young adults? Follow-up studies of abused children (Zimrin 1986, Finkelhor 1988, Wind & Silvern 1992, Kendall-Tackett *et al.* 1993) would seem to indicate that the loss of self-esteem, the development of behavioural problems and the inability to concentrate often found in abused children would make them less likely to go into further education than other young adults. Although the problem of generalisability is not easily satisfied, it should always be considered.

Comparability

Can we compare child abuse or maltreatment in the USA or Canada with that in the UK – or that reported in London with that in Newcastle? Most of the research has been conducted in Western countries. A number of prevalence and incidence studies have been reported recently in the literature on college students, or school children in non-English speaking eastern countries such as South Africa (Madu & Peltzer 2000), Palestine (Haj-Yahia & Tamish 2001), Hong Kong (Tang 2002) and Latvia, Macedonia, Lithuania and Moldova (Sebre *et al.* 2004). Their findings have presented a different picture to many of those from Western countries. Can the results of one study be directly compared with that of another? These are likely to be subjective judgements to some extent, but comparison of the methodological factors discussed in this section should help to provide a more objective basis for such a judgement.

Time trends

One of the most interesting areas of comparability in child maltreatment is between different times. Has child maltreatment increased or decreased over the years, or have individual types of abuse changed? Do increases or decreases in reported rates reflect actual changes in maltreatment levels or changes in professional and public awareness and willingness to report? There have been a number of studies that have looked at changes in officially reported cases and in the incidence and prevalence rates of child maltreatment over time. The next section deals with trends in reported cases in the Netherlands (Pieterse & Van Urk 1989), the USA (Daro & Mitchel 1990, McCurdy & Daro 1993) and the UK (Creighton 1992) during their first 10–15 years of operation. These demonstrate the similarities and differences in reporting, and the types of reports, in the three countries. They provide a context for examination of the changes in reported cases in the UK over the past decade.

Reported cases

In the Netherlands, Pieterse and Van Urk (1989) compared the data on reports received by the 'confidential doctor' system in its first official year, 1974, with that of 1983. They found a threefold increase in the number of verified cases over the 10 years, for both boys and girls. The incidence (number of cases per 1000 children) increased fourfold from 0.19 per 1000 children in 1974 to 0.71 in 1983. The types of abuse reported and verified had changed, from a preponderance of physical abuse cases in 1974 (64% of cases) to a preponderance of emotional abuse/neglect in 1983 (50% of cases). There were only seven cases of sexual abuse reported in 1973 compared to 189 (7% of all cases) in 1983. The increases in all types of abuse were mostly in the older age group, the 12–17 year olds, for both boys and girls. There was an increase in the detection of child fatalities but a decrease in the severity of physical abuse. No change was found in the identity of the suspected perpetrators – primarily fathers and/or mothers – or in the social conditions of the families. There was a decrease in the percentage of married parents and a corresponding increase in single mothers. There was an increase in the number of victims continuing to reside at home rather than in children's homes, which the authors attributed to the improvement in aftercare for these children.

In the USA, the rate of children reported for child abuse and neglect between 1985 and 1992 increased 50% from 30 per 1000 children in 1985 to 45 per 1000 in 1992 (McCurdy & Daro 1993). Between 1980 and 1985, there had been an average 11.4% annual increase in reports (Daro & Mitchel 1990). The rapid increase in reported cases between 1985 and 1992 was attributed to the increased economic stress caused by the recession, an increase in substance abuse and increased public awareness leading to greater reporting.

The different types of abuse reported in the USA did not show the same changes as the Netherlands data. In the USA, cases of neglect were most likely to be reported (45% in 1992), followed by physical abuse (27%), sexual abuse (17%), emotional maltreatment (7%) and other (8%). As in the Netherlands, between 1974 and 1983, the rate of confirmed child maltreatment fatalities in the USA had risen steadily between 1985 and 1992 from 1.3 per 100 000 children in 1985 to 1.94 per 100 000 in 1992. As McCurdy and Daro (1993) reported: 'This means that more than three children die each day in the US as a result of maltreatment' (p. 13).

By contrast, in the UK in 1992 one to two children were victims of homicide each week (HMSO 1995). This was still the case in 2003 (Home Office 2005). As with deaths, the reporting or registration rates for child maltreatment are much lower in the UK than in the USA, although they have also shown increases over the years. The registration rate trebled over 7 years from 1.16 per 1000 children in 1984 to 3.40 per 1000 children in 1990 (Creighton 1992). This was largely due to the change from Child Abuse Registers to Child Protection Registers in 1988 following the DHSS guidance *Working Together* (DHSS 1988). This led to a massive increase in registrations in the 'grave concern' category, i.e. children who had not been abused but were thought to be at significant risk of abuse. In the UK, registers were initially 'Non-Accidental Injury Registers' between 1975, when most were established, and 1980 when they became Child Abuse Registers. Cases of physical abuse were the only type of abuse to have been reported since 1975. Between 1976 and 1979, the registration rate for cases of physical abuse remained steady but increased gradually from 1979 to 1984. There was a marked increase between 1984 and 1985, and between 1985 and 1990 the rate fluctuated from year to year. The physical abuse rate ranged from 0.44 in 1976 to 1.02 per 1000 children under 15 years in 1989 (Creighton 1992).

Among the abused children placed on UK registers between 1980 and 1990, cases of physical abuse predominated, followed by sexual abuse, neglect and emotional abuse. Given the historical evolvement of registers from non-accidental injury, through child abuse to child protection registers it is not surprising that registrations for physical abuse predominated until 1997. The rate of registrations for sexual abuse increased most between 1985 and 1986, reaching a peak of 0.65 per 1000 children under 17 years in 1987 (Creighton & Noyes 1989), after which it declined. The sudden increase in reported cases of sexual abuse in Cleveland (Butler-Sloss 1988) was in 1987. Whether the decline in registered cases of sexual abuse following 1987 was due to fewer cases being recognised, or greater caution in reporting and registering them, could not be determined. The NSPCC register data (Creighton 1992) showed evidence of increased caution in cases of sexual abuse with regard to assessing severity and the suspected perpetrator after 1988. It failed to show any evidence of workers assigning cases they would have registered as sexual abuse in the past to the grave concern category instead. It is unfortunate that the changes in registration criteria introduced by the guidance *Working Together under the Children Act 1989* (Home Office *et al.* 1991) mean that the registrations for sexual abuse from 1991 are not comparable with those from 1988 to 1990. The 1991 guidance excluded the grave concern category as a separate reason for registration. Children who were thought 'likely' to be physically, sexually or emotionally abused or neglected were to be registered in the appropriate category. This means that the registrations for sexual abuse from 1991 includes both children who have been sexually abused and children thought likely to be sexually abused. It is not possible to see if the decline in registrations for actual child sexual abuse between 1987 and 1990 continued or reversed. As in the Netherlands, there was a decline in the rate of serious and fatal injuries in the early years (1975–1976) of the registers (Creighton 1992). From 1976 to 1984 the rate remained fairly stable but there was a marked increase between 1984 and 1985. From 1985 to 1990, the rate of serious and fatal injuries fluctuated but at a higher rate than that between 1976 and 1984 (Creighton 1992). The DfES and its predecessor, the DOH, does not collect information on the severity of the injuries inflicted on children registered in the physical injury category so there are no comparative data for the last decade.

As registers became established, more older children were placed on them, particularly for sexual abuse but also for physical injury. The Netherlands data showed an increase in older children being reported to the confidential doctors between 1974 and 1983. In the UK, the average age of the children registered for physical abuse increased from 3 years 8 months in 1975 to 7 years 1 month in 1990 (Creighton 1992). Boys were consistently over-represented amongst the children registered for physical abuse, whilst the overwhelming majority of children registered for sexual abuse were girls. More boys than girls were registered for neglect.

The family situation of the children registered in the UK changed over the years from 1975 to 1990, with fewer children living with both their natural parents and more living with their natural mother alone and with their natural mother and a father substitute. The Netherlands data showed a similar decrease over the years in children living with both their natural parents and an increase in mothers alone, but they do not include information on father substitutes. In the UK generally, there were major demographic changes over the period of the NSPCC register research (Central Statistical Office (CSO) 1993), with increases in divorces and the number of single mothers. In spite of these changes, and some of the more lurid headlines in the tabloid press, the majority of UK children continue to live with both their birth parents. This was not the case for the children placed on Child Protection Registers in England. By 1990, just over a third of the registered children were living with both their birth parents (Creighton 1992). The registered children were eight times more likely to be living with a father substitute than children nationally from similar social classes.

The three studies on the officially reported cases of child maltreatment in the three countries (the Netherlands, the USA and the UK) show some differences but more similarities. Over the different time periods covered by each they all show increases in the number of children officially reported as having been maltreated.

Over the period 1994–2004 the number of new registrations in England showed only a slight increase from 2.6 per 1000 children in 1994 to 2.8 in 2004 (DfES 2005b). The breakdown by type of abuse has also changed. In 1994 registrations for physical abuse still predominated, followed by neglect, sexual abuse and emotional abuse. By 2004 registrations for neglect were more than double any other category whilst registrations for emotional abuse almost equalled those for physical abuse. Registrations in the sexual abuse category had declined gradually. From 2002 they constituted the smallest number of new registrations. A multiple category of abuse, comprising children registered for more than one type of abuse, was introduced from 1 April 2001 to avoid double counting in other categories. Prior to this the separate combinations of abuse, except for emotional abuse (e.g. neglect and physical abuse) had been detailed. From 2002 there were more registrations in this mixed category than for sexual abuse. There were more boys than girls registered from 1997 to 2004, but since there are more boys born each year, the relative registration rates have been similar and were the same in 2004 at 2.7 per 1000 children under 18 (DfES 2005b). Table 2.1 demonstrates the current similarity of the breakdown of officially recorded cases of child maltreatment in the different countries.

Incidence and prevalence changes

There have been two major studies looking at incidence rates of child maltreatment at different times, both conducted in the USA. The first, the three National Incidence Studies (NIS-1, NIS-2 and NIS-3) (US Department of Health and Human Services 1988, 1996, Sedlak 1990) were conducted in 1980, 1986 and 1993. They collected all cases of child maltreatment recognised and reported to the study by 'community professionals' in a national probability sample of 29 states throughout the USA. The child had to have experienced demonstrable harm as a result of the maltreatment. The data included all the cases reported to the Child Protection Services (CPS) staff during the study period, plus cases coming to the notice of other non-CPS agencies (e.g. hospitals, schools, etc.) who were acting as 'sentinels' on the lookout for such cases during the study. The data coming to light here would cover Levels 1 through 3 of public awareness outlined at the beginning of this chapter. The second study, from the Family Violence Research Program (Straus 1979, Gelles & Straus 1987, Straus *et al.* 1988), attempted to assess the physical abuse conducted at public awareness Level 4 by asking a nationally representative sample of parents with a child aged 3 through 17 years (0–17 in the 1995 survey) at home about their behaviour towards a randomly selected child in the last year. They conducted national surveys in 1975, 1985 and 1995. The two sets of studies produced very different findings.

The three National Incidence Studies showed a considerable increase in the incidence of maltreatment cases coming to light in each survey. The maltreatment rate per 1000 children more than doubled between 1980 and 1993 whilst the physical abuse rate increased by 84%.

By contrast, the three national surveys conducted by the Family Violence Research Program in 1975, 1985 and 1995 showed a 65% decrease in the rate of child physical abuse between 1975 and 1995. The disparity between these two sets of findings for the physical abuse of children can be explained if we look at the definitions employed and the actual rates in the two studies.

The National Incidence Studies used a definition of physical abuse which specified that the child must be live-born and under 18 years of age at the time of the abuse, the abusive behaviour must have been non-accidental and avoidable, the perpetrator had to be either a parent or adult caretaker (over 18) and the child must have suffered demonstrable harm. The incidence rates they discovered were 3.1 per 1000 children in the population in 1980 and 4.3 per 1000 in 1986. By 1993 this had increased to 5.7 per 1000 children.

The Family Violence Research Program surveys used a definition of physical child abuse which included acts of behaviour by a parent to a child between the ages of 3 and 17 years (0–17 in 1995) which had a relatively high probability of causing an injury. These included: kicking, biting, punching, hitting with an object, beating up and threatening or using a knife or gun on the child. The incidence rates they found for these types of behaviour were 140 per 1000 children in 1975, 107 per 1000 in 1985 and 49 per 1000 in 1995. Although this 1995 figure represents a considerable decrease compared with the 1975 figure, it is still nearly 10 times greater than the 1993 incidence figure found in the National Incidence Study.

The severe violence inflicted on children uncovered by the Family Violence Research Program surveys may not have caused any noticeable injuries or demonstrable harm. Very few of the children so affected would have been reported, or recognised, as abused to either child protection or other agencies. Schene (1987) estimated that, on the basis of the 1985 national survey incidence rate and the official reported rate for that year, only one physically abused child in seven was reported.

Changes in childhood sexual abuse prevalence rates over the years have been assessed by comparing a number of studies conducted in the 1970s and 1980s with that of Kinsey and his co-workers in the 1940s (Kinsey *et al.* 1953). Feldman *et al.* (1991) reviewed the Kinsey report and 19 prevalence studies reported since 1979 using predetermined criteria for quality of information, commonality of definitions of childhood sexual abuse and research design. They found that the more recent studies, with the strongest methodology and where definitions of childhood sexual abuse were similar, reported prevalence figures similar to those of Kinsey in the 1940s, in spite of differences in study design and populations surveyed. Using a definition close to Kinsey's, i.e. girls younger than 14 years of age having sexual contact with an adult male at least 5 years older, and the studies with the best research design gave three studies, including Kinsey's. The other two were reported in 1984 (Badgley *et al.*) and 1987 (Siegal *et al.*), and all three produced prevalence figures of between 10 and 12% for girls younger than 14 years of age. Prevalence studies conducted more recently (see Table.2.2 for details) have found similar figures. Feldman *et al.* (1991) concluded that the increased number of reports of child sexual abuse was not due to a true increase in prevalence but to changes in legislation and public awareness. They stressed that this should not deter child protection professionals from continuing to provide treatment and preventative services to sexually abused children.

Implications for practice

There are a number of implications for practitioners to be drawn from the review of the literature in the previous section. The most important of these is probably the fact that, in spite of the varying estimates produced by the different studies, there can be no doubt that there is a large base group of children who have been, or are being, maltreated. What is also clear is that only a fraction of them are being reported to child protection practitioners. Before feeling overwhelmed by the size of the problem confronting them, practitioners should also bear in mind that the majority of children are not abused or maltreated. The importance of incidence and prevalence studies on child maltreatment is in giving practitioners a sense of the base underlying rate of the problem and the characteristics of that population. It is against that background of knowledge that they can look at the individual cases referred to them and assess the likelihood that they are cases of maltreatment.

The finding that, even with vastly increased reporting rates, only one American child in seven who was physically injured was reported (Schene 1987, commenting on the Gelles & Straus 1985 survey) has implications for intervention. Are practitioners concerned only about the cases which come to light or the abusive behaviour *per se*? Gelles and Straus (1987) quote Erikson's theory that 'the number of acts of deviance that come to community attention is a function of the size and complexity of the community's social control apparatus – in this case, the child protection system'. There has been increasing concern (Dingwall 1989, Parton & Parton 1989a) that social control has taken over from social support in the child welfare services. Child protection has taken priority over child care. As more and more resources are put into increasing the size and complexity of the child protection system, and hence identifying more 'cases', there seem to be fewer resources available for the treatment and monitoring of these identified cases. There is a worrying dearth of research and evaluation studies into the effectiveness of the various forms of intervention in child maltreatment cases both in the UK and the USA. As Starr (1990) argued: 'Without such studies we cannot determine the effectiveness of treatment and prevention efforts that, while well intended, may have no effects on the participating parents and children, or, worse still, may have unintended negative consequences.'

Child protection practitioners are compelled to intervene in identified cases of child abuse and neglect for largely negative reasons. These include the social control system within which they work, the fear that if they do not intervene the child will die or be seriously damaged, and the longer-term adverse effects on the abused child deprived of treatment.

These are powerful motivators for action, though contrary to the general ethos of help and support that brought many practitioners into the child welfare services. The available evidence from the prevalence, incidence and other studies is not encouraging. It implies that the more the child protection system is expanded, the more cases of child abuse and neglect will come to official recognition. Intervention, tragically (e.g. Jasmine Beckford, Tyra Henry), does not always save a child's life. The findings on the long-term effects of child abuse and neglect are equivocal. Prevalence studies on general populations reveal large numbers of adults, abused as children, who appear not to have suffered long-term adverse consequences. Similarly, follow-up studies of abused children (Toro 1982, Finkelhor 1988, Kendall-Tackett *et al.* 1993) have found that about a third of the victims show no symptoms of abuse in the short term, and larger numbers show none in the longer term. Socio-economic status and related factors may be more important than abuse in determining the course of a child's development. More research needs to be conducted into those factors which protect individual children, and which are the cases of maltreated children and their families where practitioners can most usefully intervene. Practitioners should also be lobbying for regular re-appraisals of the child protection system, to assess whether it provides the most effective use of human and financial resources – for example, the programme of research funded by the Department of Health and summarised in their publication *Child Protection: Messages from Research* (DoH 1995a). Gelles and Straus (1987), speculating about the reasons behind the decrease in incidence rates over the 10 years 1975–1985, suggested that changes in attitudes and cultural norms regarding the social acceptability of family violence may have led to changes in overt behaviour. Public education campaigns play a vital role in attempting to change such attitudes.

The wide differences between the reported rates and types of abuse in the different countries also have implications for practitioners. Is the USA intrinsically more abusive to its children than such European countries as the UK and the Netherlands, as the relative reporting rates would suggest? Or does mandatory reporting, a massive public education programme and nationally available treatment programmes lead to a narrowing of the gap between actual and reported incidence? Pieterse and Van Urk (1989) advocated mandatory reporting in the Netherlands in an attempt to reduce the discrepancy between the two countries' reported rates. Would mandatory reporting in the UK lead to more reports than the present non-mandatory inter-agency collaboration? Although UK professionals are not statutorily required to report cases of child abuse, most of them have some reporting duty written into their codes of ethics. Not to report a case would be an exception in the UK. In the USA, with mandatory reporting, the National Committee for Prevention of Child Abuse found a 40% substantiation rate for reports in 1992 (McCurdy & Daro 1993). In the UK, with a non-statutory system of referring, only 15% of child protection referrals in eight local authority social services departments in 1991 were subsequently registered (Gibbons *et al.* 1995b). A non-statutory system does not seem to lead to a decrease in initial referrals in relation to final registration.

The UK differed from the USA in the 1980s and early 1990s in registering so few cases of neglect, and from the Netherlands in the small number of cases of emotional abuse registered. The fact that Child Protection Registers were initially Non-Accidental Injury Registers until 1980 may have led to a professional bias towards physical abuse in the UK at the expense of other forms of abuse. Gibbons *et al.* (1995b) found that only 7% of the cases initially referred for neglect reached the register and most were screened out of the system at an early stage, usually without the offer of other services. Very few cases of emotional abuse were referred at all. The child protection system in the UK was initially designed to rescue children in immediate danger and, as such, was unsuited to the more insidious effects of neglect or emotional abuse. Neglected and emotionally abused children may not be in immediate need of protection but they are nevertheless 'in need'. Practitioners should be aware of, and be responsive to, those needs. The recent increases in registrations for both neglect and emotional abuse (DfES 2005b) could be indicative of such responsiveness.

Finally, practitioners need to be aware of the methodological factors underlying the various published studies of child abuse and neglect incidence and prevalence.

In child protection, practitioners walk a tightrope between either too much (e.g. Cleveland) or too little (e.g. Kimberley Carlile) intervention in the public's mind. In choosing either to intervene or not to intervene in a particular case, they need to be able to speak authoritatively about the population base they are drawing from:

- How rare is this particular type and severity of abuse in the general population?
- Does this case share any of the characteristics of cases identified in the most rigorous studies?
- Might various biases be operating in the reporting or ascertainment of this case?

The more aware practitioners are of these factors, the more likely they are to make a convincing case for either intervention or non-intervention.

Summary

This chapter has looked at the five levels of public and professional awareness of child abuse and neglect on which any estimate of the frequency of the problem will be based. As the public and professionals in a country become more aware of the problem of child maltreatment the reported incidence increases.

The incidence and prevalence studies reviewed have shown wide variations, both between and within countries, in the rates of child maltreatment reported and the different types of child abuse. A large part of these differences may be due to the methods employed in the studies, in particular the definitions used and possible sources of bias. A broad definition of abuse – say sexual abuse not involving contact – will ascertain many more cases than one involving only contact or penetrative acts. With any socially deviant act, particularly one that attracts the moral opprobrium that child maltreatment does, the possible sources of bias increase. Social class, ethnicity, perceived status, experience and the characteristics of the children themselves are all factors that can lead to bias in the recognition, reporting and registering, or substantiation, of cases of child maltreatment.

The methodological factors of generalisability and comparability of prevalence and incidence studies are particularly important for practitioners. It is against these that they have to weigh up their own individual referrals and decide whether, or to what extent, they should intervene.

Examination of the changes in incidence and prevalence rates of child maltreatment over time have shown increases in reported cases, decreases in the incidence of physical abuse and no change in the prevalence of child sexual abuse. Possible reasons for the discrepancies between these findings are discussed. The role of public education in changing public attitudes towards violence within families, and their effect on reducing the incidence of physical abuse of children, is stressed.

The gap between actual and reported cases has important implications for practitioners, as has the somewhat negative controlling ethos of child protection practices. Practitioners can feel helpless in the face of an ever-increasing number of child maltreatment referrals and the possible consequences of not intervening. Incidence and prevalence studies provide a picture of the underlying base rate of maltreatment and the characteristics of the abused population. Research is needed into identifying those children and families where intervention is vital and those which can be diverted into less controlling and more supportive systems.

Conclusions

Child maltreatment is a culturally defined phenomenon. In the UK the death of Maria Colwell at the hands of her stepfather led to the establishment of multidisciplinary child protection procedures. Initially these focused on the physical abuse (non-accidental injury) of children. In contrast, the media, and through them the general public, have focused on the sexual abuse of children. The television companies – the BBC's Childwatch and Channel 4's MORI poll – were the agencies first concerned with finding out how many children nationally had been abused (the prevalence rate). The prevalence they were concerned with was that of child sexual abuse.

This professional focus on the physical abuse of children and the public one on their sexual abuse led to neglected and emotionally abused children disproportionally being filtered out of the child protection system. Increasing numbers of referrals and limited resources getting into the system meant children and families were not receiving badly needed services. The Children Act 1989, with its emphasis on providing services for all children in need, attempted to rectify this. There has been continuous growth in the number of child protection registrations in the neglect and emotional abuse categories since the introduction of that Act. This is testament to UK child protection practitioners' commitment to tackling all forms of child maltreatment.

Key points and messages for practice

- Large numbers of children are being maltreated and only a fraction of these are coming to the attention of child protection practitioners.

- If practitioners can intervene in only a fraction of cases they need to feel confident that their intervention will have a positive outcome for the child. More research is needed into the effectiveness of different treatment methods.

- Child protection practitioners need to be vigilant to ensure that the child protection system serves children and families rather than itself.

- Public education plays a vital role in changing attitudes towards the acceptability of family violence and hence behaviour.

Annotated further reading

Creighton S J 1992 Child abuse trends in England and Wales 1988–1990 and an overview from 1973–1990. NSPCC, London
Provides an overview of the trends in registered cases of child abuse and neglect in the UK over 18 years. It also examines the characteristics of the different types of abuse, the children, their parents, suspected perpetrators and families in addition to the management of the cases.

Cawson P, Wattam C, Brooker S, Kelly G 2000 Child maltreatment in the United Kingdom: a study of the prevalence of child abuse and neglect. NSPCC, London
Provides data on a nationally representative sample of young adults' childhood experiences of all forms of maltreatment including implications for policy and practice arising from the findings.

Department of Health 1995 Child protection: messages from research. HMSO, London
Provides an overview of research on the child protection system in England including summaries of the individual projects.

Finkelhor D 1994 The international epidemiology of child sexual abuse. Child Abuse and Neglect 18(5):409–417
Provides an overview of child sexual abuse surveys in 21 countries.

Kelly L, Regan L, Burton S 1991 An exploratory study of the prevalence of sexual abuse in a sample of 16–21-year-olds. PNL: Child Abuse Studies Unit, London
   Provides an extremely useful breakdown of prevalence rates by different definitions of sexual abuse.

Markowe H 1988 The frequency of child sexual abuse in the UK. Health Trends 20(1):2–6
   Provides a concise survey of UK sexual abuse frequency studies and detailed consideration of their methodological weaknesses.

Pilkington B, Kremer J 1995 A review of the epidemiological research on child sexual abuse: community and college student samples. Child Abuse Review 4(2):84–98
   Provides a summary of prevalence studies on child sexual abuse in community samples from the 1920s to 1990.

Useful websites

Australian child maltreatment data: www.aihw.gov.au/publications/cws/cpa02-03/cpa02-03.pdf
Child Welfare Information Gateway (formerly the USA National Clearinghouse on Child Abuse and Neglect Information and the National Adoption Information Clearinghouse): www.childwelfare.gov
Information on forthcoming 4th National Incidence Study in the USA: www.nis4.org/nishome.asp

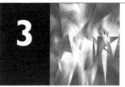

3

Child abuse: defining, understanding and intervening

Kevin Browne and Catherine Hamilton-Giachritsis

INTRODUCTION

The most serious consequence of child maltreatment is death and the most telling indicator of the need for early prevention is the high rates of child murder and manslaughter in the youngest age group of children (Wilczynski 1997). Indeed, child maltreatment is one of the most common causes of death in young children in the UK today. The occurrence of child death because of abuse in the UK is estimated to be nine per one million children, but as high as 24 per one million children in the USA (UNICEF 2003). Notably, four in every five child abusers are the biological parents, with the risk of death greatest for children less than 5 years and particularly babies under 1 year of age (Browne & Lynch 1995, UNICEF 2003). Therefore, prediction, prevention and protection must occur from birth, with implementation of strategies identified from previous reviews on child deaths (Axford & Bullock 2005) and the assessment of children and their families (DoH *et al.* 2000, Browne *et al.* 2006).

The extent and definition of child abuse

In the book *Early Prediction and Prevention of Child Abuse* (Browne *et al.* 2002a), three major forms of child abuse and/or neglect are identified: physical, sexual and emotional. Each type of maltreatment is characterised into 'active' (abuse) and 'passive' (neglect) forms (Table 3.1). Active abuse involves violent acts that represent the exercise of physical force to cause injury or forcibly interfere with personal freedom. Passive abuse refers to neglect, which can only be considered violent in the metaphorical sense, as it does not involve physical force. Nevertheless, it can cause both physical and emotional injury, such as non-organic failure to thrive in young children (Browne 1993, Iwaniec 2004). However, victims of child maltreatment are unlikely to be subjected to only one type of abuse. For example, sexual abuse and physical abuse are usually accompanied by emotional abuse, which includes verbal

Table 3.1
Forms of maltreatment

	Physical violence	**Psychological violence**	**Sexual violence**
Active abuse	Non-accidental injury Forced coercion and restraint	Intimidation Emotional abuse Material abuse	Incest Sexual assault and rape
Passive neglect	Poor health care Physical neglect	Lack of affection Emotional neglect Material neglect	Failure to protect Prostitution

(From Browne & Herbert 1997, Preventing family violence. Wiley, Chichester, with kind permission from John Wiley & Sons Limited.)

assault, threats of sexual or physical abuse, close confinement (such as locking a child in a room), withholding food and other aversive treatment. Within each type of maltreatment, there is a continuum of severity ranging from mild to life threatening (Browne & Herbert 1997, Browne 2002).

The definitions currently used in England and Wales for children placed on child protection registers, as outlined in *Working Together to Safeguard Children* (DoH *et al.* 1999, pp. 5–6), include the following categories:

- Physical abuse may involve hitting, shaking, throwing, poisoning, burning or scalding, drowning, suffocating, or otherwise causing physical harm to a child. Physical harm may also be caused when a parent or carer feigns the symptoms of, or deliberately causes ill health to a child that they are looking after. This situation is commonly described using terms such as factitious illness by proxy or Munchausen syndrome by proxy.
- Emotional abuse is the persistent emotional ill-treatment of a child such as to cause severe and persistent adverse effects on the child's emotional development. It may involve conveying to children that they are worthless or unloved, inadequate, or valued only insofar as they meet the needs of another person. It may feature age or developmentally inappropriate expectations being imposed on children. It may involve causing children frequently to feel frightened or in danger, or the exploitation or corruption of children. Some level of emotional abuse is involved in all types of maltreatment of a child, though it may occur alone.
- Sexual abuse involves forcing or enticing a child or young person to take part in sexual activities whether or not the child is aware of what is happening. The activities may involve physical contact including penetrative (e.g. rape or buggery) or non-penetrative acts. They may include non-contact activities, such as involving children in looking at, or in the production of, pornographic material or watching sexual activities, or encouraging children to behave in sexually inappropriate ways.
- Neglect is the persistent failure to meet a child's basic physical and/or psychological needs, likely to result in the serious impairment of the child's health or development (including non-organic failure to thrive). It may involve a parent or carer failing to provide adequate food, shelter and clothing, failing to protect a child from physical harm or danger, or the failure to ensure access to appropriate medical care or treatment. It may also include neglect of, or unresponsiveness to, a child's basic emotional needs.

All the above categories are used for both intrafamilial and extrafamilial abuse and neglect, perpetuated by someone inside or outside the child's home. Mixed categories, which register more than one type of abuse and/or neglect occurring to a child, are also recorded. This is especially important when considering 'organised abuse', which is defined as: 'Abuse which may involve a number of abusers, a number of abused children and young people and often encompasses different forms of abuse.' It involves an 'element of organisation' to a greater or lesser extent (Home Office *et al.* 1991, p. 38). For further discussion on the definition of and response to organised abuse, see Department of Health (1994b), Bibby (1996a) and Gallagher (1998).

Since 1989, the Department of Health has accurately assessed each year the number of children and young persons on child protection registers in England. The estimates are based on annual statistical returns from 150 Local Government Authorities. Figure 3.1 shows the rate per 10 000 children for those on the register at 31 March 2005 by age (DfES 2006). The overall rate was 25 900 children under 18 years of age (23 per 10 000). Of these, 43% were registered for neglect, 18% for physical abuse, 19% for emotional abuse, 9% for sexual abuse and 12% were mixed categories for registration. The highest rates were found in very young children under 1 year (51 per 10 000, 12% of the total). The likelihood of being on the registers then decreases with age, with 69.6% of children on registers aged 9 years or younger (DfES 2006).

Overall, 12 500 girls and 13 000 boys in England were considered to require protection from maltreatment on 31 March 2005, together with 310 unborn children. Allowing for population, rates for boys and girls were the same (23 per 10 000). Girls have higher rates of sexual abuse (11% of girls compared to 8% of boys); however, although more boys are physically abused, in percentage terms it is equal for boys and girls at 15% (Table 3.2). NSPCC figures show that over 80% of the physical abuse most likely to cause death or handicap (i.e. head injury) occurs to children aged younger than 5, with an over-representation of boys. Over half of all head injuries occur to infants aged less than 1 year (Creighton & Noyes 1989, Creighton 1992).

Figure 3.1
Rate of registration per 10 000 children by age at 31 March 2005 (produced from Department for Education and Skills 2006, Table 4c, with kind permission).

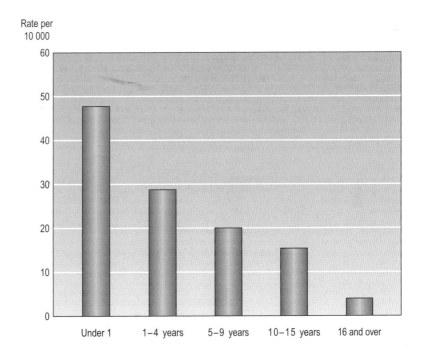

Table 3.2
Approximate number, percentages and rates of registrations (children up to the age of 18 years) by categories of child maltreatment at 31 March 2005 (n = 25 600*)

Category	Boys			Girls		
	n	%	Rate per 10 000[+]	*N*	%	Rate per 10 000[+]
Neglect	5800	45	10	5300	43	10
Emotional abuse	2700	21	5	2500	20	5
Physical injury	2000	15	4	1900	15	3
Sexual abuse	1000	8	2	1300	11	2
Multiple	1500	11	3	1500	12	3
Total	13 000	100	23	12 500	100	23

(Adapted from Department for Education and Skills 2006, Tables 4a–c, with kind permission.)
* Excluding 310 unborn children, [+]figures rounded to nearest whole number.

Incidence figures on child maltreatment should be contrasted with prevalence figures. Prevalence rates based on English young adults (18–24 years) retrospective self-reports show that 7% were assessed as experiencing serious physical abuse, 6% as having suffered serious absence of physical care (neglect), 6% as having experienced serious psychological/emotional maltreatment and 4% had reported sexual abuse by a family member with a further 15% by a non-family member or stranger (Cawson *et al.* 2000). However, a further 14% of respondents were assessed as having experienced intermediate levels of physical abuse and a further 9% as having experienced intermediate levels of physical neglect (Cawson *et al.* 2000). Young women reported more sexual and emotional abuse than young men (Cawson *et al.* 2000).

Thus, it is not surprising that a report of a particularly nasty incident of sexual abuse or cruelty to an infant or a child murder often makes its way onto the front pages of our daily newspapers, to a special inquiry and back again to the media. After much painful analysis and discussion, an attempt is made to discover where 'procedures' for managing cases have broken down (Axford & Bullock 2005).

There is a need to recognise the fact that it is not necessarily the 'procedures', but that parents' social circumstances, attitudes and behaviour need to be changed in order to prevent children being attacked. If these facts were faced honestly, education and training could be offered to parents who are unable to cope. This might actually prevent the recurrence, if not occurrence, of child maltreatment. Approximately one in eight children registered in 2005 had previously been on the child protection register (13%, DfES 2006). Prevalence figures have shown that 27% of cases of child abuse referred to police child protection units were already known to the police authorities on account of previous injury to the child under review (Hamilton & Browne 1999). Repeat victimisation is a common finding throughout the child abuse literature, yet it is apparently little appreciated by those who intervene in child-abusing families (Hamilton & Browne 1998). Nevertheless, the prevention of child maltreatment must be based on a comprehensive understanding of the causes of child abuse and neglect.

Causes of child abuse and neglect

In seeking to understand the many causal factors involved in child abuse and neglect, several theoretical models have been proposed. However, some researchers distinguish between acts of physical violence and other forms of abuse because the causes and their potential solutions are different (see Frude 1989, 1991). While all harmful acts have some causes in common, other factors are unique to physical abuse and neglect. Therefore, it might be suggested that the following outline is more related to physical maltreatment. However, poverty, social isolation, family breakdown and poor parent–child relationships are associated with all forms of child abuse and neglect (Straus & Smith 1990, Brown J *et al.* 1998, 2006, Putallaz *et al.* 1998, Hampton 1999, Dixon *et al.* 2005b) and have been cited as risk factors for child sexual abuse (Finkelhor 1980, Bergner *et al.* 1994). Furthermore, a third of sexually abused children have been previously physically abused (Finkelhor & Baron 1986), indicating that a number of common factors are involved (Hamilton & Browne 1998, 1999).

Social and cultural perspectives

Studies of abusing families (e.g. Garbarino 1977, Krugman 1986, Browne & Saqi 1988a, Straus & Smith 1990, Gelles & Cornell 1997, Brown J *et al.* 1998,

Hampton *et al.* 1998) have shown that social factors such as low wages, unemployment, poor housing, overcrowding, isolation and alienating work conditions are associated with child maltreatment. Such factors are seen by Gelles (1987) and Gelles and Cornell (1997) as causing frustration and stress at the individual level, which in turn may lead to violence in the home. Notably, it is relative poverty (where parents feel that they are economically disadvantaged within their community) that creates stress and may increase the risk of aggression (Wilkinson 1994, Murray *et al.* 1999). However, since physical abuse of children is not confined to families in the lower socio-economic groups but is spread across the entire class spectrum, this interpretation may be questioned. Nevertheless, it is suggested that social and environmental stress factors may have a greater influence on child maltreatment in lower class families than in middle-class families (Browne 2002). All socio-economic groups may be susceptible to individual factors that influence child abuse and neglect, such as psychological disturbance, alcohol and drug abuse (Browne 2002). For all social classes, Gelles' (1983) 'exchange theory' proposes that the private nature of the family home reduces the 'costs' of behaving aggressively, in terms of official sanction. This results in a higher probability of violence in the home, where there are fewer social constraints on aggressive emotional expression. Thus, family 'privacy' makes child abuse less detectable and easier to commit (Browne 1988, Straus *et al.* 1988, Browne & Herbert 1997).

An alternative approach, but one that is also couched in terms of the social position of the people involved, can be referred to as the micropolitical view. This holds that individual violence is a microcosm of the power relations in the wider society. For example, a common feminist explanation of violence towards women and children is to view it as a function of their generally oppressed position in society. Within this framework, the purpose of male violence is seen as to control other family members and ensure that women remain subordinate (Gilbert 1994). This perspective suggests that violence from women in the family is a consequence of their victimisation by men, either as self-defence or as re-directed aggression towards their children (Dobash & Dobash 2004). Hence, it is suggested that interventions must focus on stopping the violence by removing or treating the violent man. It is proposed that violence from the woman would then cease. However, researchers have pointed out that aggression occurs in same sex relationships (Island & Letellier 1991, Renzetti 1992), as well as female to male (Straus 1997, 1999, Archer 2000, 2002). Patterns of family violence are more complex than the feminists would suggest, sometimes involving female perpetrators of child maltreatment in the absence of male violence (Browne *et al.* 2002b).

The broadest sociological perspective (Gil 1970, 1978, Straus 1980, Goldstein 1986, Levine 1986) holds that cultural values, the availability of weapons and the exposure to unpunished models of aggression affect personal attitudes towards violent behaviour. These, in turn, influence an individual's acceptance and learning of aggression as a form of emotional expression and as a method of control over others. This process may begin early in life through children witnessing violence in the home and/or through the media by being allowed access to age-inappropriate images on TV, video/DVD, computer games and the internet (Browne & Hamilton-Giachritsis 2005).

Within British and American societies, it would appear that violence in the family home is considered less reprehensible than violence outside it. There is a general acceptance of physical punishment as an appropriate method of child control, with 9 out of 10 children being disciplined in this way in the UK and USA (Gelles & Cornell 1997, Nobes & Smith 2000). By contrast, 16 countries in Europe have now outlawed smacking and corporal punishment of children by their parents and guardians, which clearly defends the rights of the child (UN 1989, 2005).

Biological and psychological perspectives

In contrast to the social and cultural approach, biological and psychological perspectives concentrate on individual personality characteristics, often of a deviant nature. The biological perspective highlights the individual rather than society as the main focus of responsibility for violence. High levels of testosterone have been linked to high levels of aggression, dominance and antisocial behaviour, whilst low serotonin has been linked to impulsive aggression (Holtzworth-Munroe *et al.* 1997). Other researchers have focused on the role of head injury in the causation of family violence. However, whilst some research has found a relationship between partner violence and head injury (Rosenbaum *et al.* 1994, Warnken *et al.* 1994), most domestically violent men do not have known head injuries and therefore it cannot explain the majority of family violence.

The links between spouse abuse and child maltreatment has recently been recognised, highlighting that child physical and/or sexual abuse occurs in approximately half of the families where there is spouse violence (Goddard & Hiller 1993, Browne & Hamilton 1999). Where both spouse abuse and child maltreatment are occurring in the family, mental health problems, alcohol and drug dependency appears to be the most significant risk factors for violence (Browne & Hamilton 1999). Indeed, there is increasing evidence of a relationship between parental mental health problems, especially substance misuse, and severe child maltreatment (Browne & Saqi 1988a, Falkov 1996, 1998, Wilczynski 1997, Cleaver *et al.* 1999, Sanders *et al.* 1999).

In the USA, early surveys of battered women showed that 60% of their partners had an alcohol problem and 21% had a drug problem (Roberts 1987), with the majority of female victims suffering from mental health problems as a result. Some authors propose that these are the major causes of family violence (Pernanen 1991). However, it is more likely that alcohol and drug dependency typically relieves the offender of the responsibility of his behaviour and gives the victims a justification for remaining in the family in the hope that he will control his addiction and end his aggression. Furthermore, the majority of individuals who abuse drugs and alcohol admit they have been violent to their dependants while not under the influence of alcohol and drugs (Sonkin *et al.* 1985). Nevertheless, adult mental health services are considered by Reder and Duncan (1999) as the missing link in the child protection system.

Traditionally, it was assumed that all parents who maltreated their children had mental health difficulties, when in fact only a minority of child abusers have mental health and addiction problems (Browne & Herbert 1997, Falkov 1998). Other psychological predispositions of abusive individuals have been acknowledged, including a tendency to have distorted perceptions of their children (Rosenberg & Reppucci 1983), and difficulty dealing with anger, self-centred and an external locus of control over their lives (Browne *et al.* 2002b). Some of these factors may be related to their own childhood and the increased likelihood of having been a victim of abuse, neglect or witnessing violence in the family (Dixon *et al.* 2005a).

Attachment theory

A combination of the biological and psychological approaches was realised by John Bowlby's attachment theory (Bowlby 1969, 1980), which was influenced by studies of instinct and imprinting (Lorenz 1965, 1966) and the evolutionary determinants of social behaviour (Harlow 1959), and formulated within a psychodynamic framework following Freud (1964). Attachment theory claims that there is a critical period of human social development around 6 months of age when infants develop an attachment to their primary caregiver, usually the mother. A sensitive mother is the basis of a secure attachment which gives the infant confidence to explore their physical and social environment. By contrast, insensitive mothers are more likely to have infants with insecure/anxious attachments, who may be ambivalent and pre-occupied with showing attachment behaviours (e.g. clinging, crying) at the expense of exploration. They may also be avoidant of the attachment figure after learning that their attachment behaviours meet with unresponsive parenting.

Children develop a model of themselves and others, based on prior experiences with caregivers, and these influence the development of later relationships (Morton & Browne 1998). Children use these models to base their expectations about future interactions (Bowlby 1980, Cassidy & Shaver 1999). Maltreated children may form a representation of their caregivers as unresponsive, rejecting and unavailable, and have problems adapting to major developmental tasks, such as development of an autonomous self and forming relations with their peers (Cicchetti & Lynch 1993). Therefore maltreated children are at risk of not learning the skills necessary for forming healthy relationships with future children or partners (Bartholomew *et al.* 2001).

Social learning perspective

More than 40 years ago, Schultz (1960) claimed that the source of violence in a family context lies in unfulfilled childhood experiences. This approach is based on the assumption that people learn violent behaviour from observing aggressive role models (Bandura 1973). In support of this argument, Roy (1982) has stated that four out of five abusive men were reported by their partners as either observing their fathers abusing their mothers and/or being a victim of child abuse themselves. In comparison, only a third of the abused partners had witnessed or had been victims of parental violence as a child.

There is evidence that violence between parents affects the children in a family (Jaffe *et al.* 1990, Browne 1993, Carroll 1994). The behaviour and psychiatric problems discovered in children of violent marriages include truancy, aggressive behaviour at home and at school, and anxiety disorders (Jaffe *et al.* 1986, Davis & Carlson 1987). It is suggested that such children learn aversive behaviour as a general style for controlling their social and physical environments, and this style continues into adulthood (Gully & Dengerink 1983, Browne & Herbert 1997). This perspective provides one explanation for why a large percentage of individuals who maltreat their partner or child have witnessed violence between their parents or been abused and/or neglected themselves as children, which has been reported in many studies (Holtzworth-Munroe *et al.* 2000, Newcomb & Locke 2001, Egeland *et al.* 2002, Dixon *et al.* 2005a). However, not all perpetrators of family violence have experienced or witnessed maltreatment in the home during childhood. Indeed, Kaufman and Zigler (1987) propose an intergenerational rate of child maltreatment of only 25–30%.

The special victim perspective

Some authors suggest that characteristics of the victims may increase the likelihood of maltreatment. Thirty years ago, Friedrich and Boroskin (1976) reviewed the complex reasons why a child may not fulfil the parent's expectations or demands, with the child in some way regarded as 'special'. For example, studies have found prematurity, low birth weight, illness and handicap to be associated with child abuse (Lynch & Roberts 1977, Browne & Saqi 1988a, Starr 1988). Indeed, it has been pointed out that the physical unattractiveness of these children may be an important factor for child abuse (Berkowitz 1989). Furthermore, the extra stress associated with caring for a sick child or a child with growth difficulties has also been associated with maltreatment (Iwaniec 2004, 2006). However, in a study of children and siblings within an abusive household, little evidence was found for child characteristics contributing to scapegoating a particular child (Hamilton-Giachritsis & Browne 2005).

Interaction focused models

Some researchers have advocated a more interactive approach that includes the social relationships of the participants and their environmental setting, rather than seeking to isolate the person or situation. This entails a move from the individual psychological level to a study of social interactions between members of the family.

Interpersonal interactive perspective

Toch (1969) looked not only at the characteristics of violent men but also at the context of their violence and the characteristics of their victims. He concluded that aggressive behaviour was associated with 'machismo' and the maintenance of a particular personal identity in relation to others. The family systems perspective (Minuchin 1974) denotes that each member of the family exerts an effect on the violence. Thus, individuals in the family are not viewed as simply passive recipients of abuse, rather they are part of a dynamic process and contribute to the chances of aggression occurring in the family (Hughes & Fantuzzo 1994). However, it is important to note that holistic approaches to family violence do not aim to place blame with the victims of family violence, or shroud the seriousness of physical abuse endured by women. Rather this perspective is adopted to explore the violent family as a whole, considering all members of the unit, in order to understand why maltreatment is fostered and continues.

The person–environment interactive perspective

Frude (1980) puts forward the notion of a causal chain leading to 'critical incidence' of child abuse. This is a function of complex interactions between the individual and their social and physical environments. The 'critical incidence model' of child abuse is presented in Figure 3.2 and can be described as follows:

- Environmental stress situations, which are usually long term (e.g. poverty), influence domestic abusers to assess their personal situations differently from non-abusing family members (i.e. as threatening).
- They perceive a discrepancy between their expectations for life and social interactions and what they actually see happening. This often results in feelings of frustration for the person.
- Anger and emotional distress are likely as a response to these situations rather than problem-solving strategies for change.
- Lack of inhibitions with regard to violent expression, together with a lower threshold of tolerance, increases the possibility for violence. This is, of course, enhanced by disinhibitors such as alcohol or drugs.
- Under the above conditions, even a facial expression (perceived as a dirty look) can lead to, or trigger, an incidence of violence.

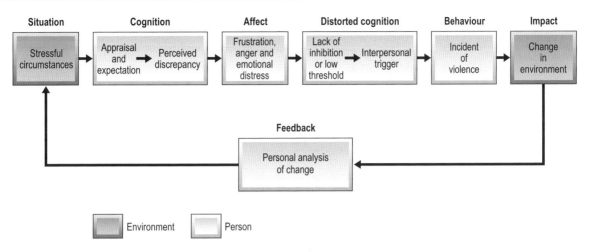

Figure 3.2
The cognitive–behavioural model of critical incidence (adapted and modified from Frude 1980, 1989 and Hollin 1993 by Browne & Herbert 1997, Preventing family violence. Wiley, Chichester. With kind permission from John Wiley & Sons Limited).

These causal links result in the caregiver being more easily provoked to take violent action. Frude (1991) challenges the assumption that 'abusers' differ from 'non-abusers' and suggested that they might be more usefully considered as points on a continuum. For this reason, he argued that studies of interactions in the family may have much to contribute towards our understanding of domestic violence and child abuse and neglect. Frude's causal chain model demonstrates the need to assess a violent person's understanding of the environment. Their perceptions, attitudes and attributions will all influence the possibility of overt aggressive behaviour. In relation to violent behaviour, Browne and Howells (1996) have developed the work of Novaco (1978) on anger arousal. This work emphasises the role played by cognitive processes, such as appraisal and expectations of external events, in evoking an aggressive response.

Integrated models

Recently, there has been a move away from accounting for violence in the family purely in terms of individual psychopathology. Instead, models are proposed that attempt to integrate the characteristics of abusing parents, their children and the situation in which they live. Child abuse and neglect cannot be explained by a single factor: it is a consequence of complex interactions between individual, social and environmental influences (see Belsky 1980, Browne 1989, Browne & Herbert 1997, Belsky & Stratton 2002).

The inadequacies of single factor explanations have led to a psychosocial approach which integrates sociological and psychological explanations for family violence and child abuse. Originally proposed by American researchers (e.g. Gelles 1973), this perspective suggests that certain stress factors and adverse background influences may serve to predispose individuals to violence.

It has been claimed that 'predisposing' factors may form a basis for identification of families 'at risk' of violence (e.g. Browne & Herbert 1997, Dixon *et al.* 2005a). However, a more pertinent question is why the majority of families under stress do not abuse their children. It may be that stress will only lead to violence when adverse family interactions exist. Browne *et al.* (2006) have recently taken this approach for community health interventions to prevent child maltreatment. They conceptualise child maltreatment as a social–psychological phenomenon that is 'multiply determined by forces at work in the individual, the family, as well as in the community and the culture in which both the individual and the family are embedded' (Belsky 1980). Given a particular combination of factors, an interactional style develops within the family, and it is in the context of this interaction that child abuse occurs. This approach may be equally adopted to explain other forms of family violence.

Multifactor perspective

The study of social interactions and relationships can be seen as occupying a central and potentially integrating place in explaining the causes of aggression in the family. In relation to child abuse and neglect, Browne and Herbert (1997) present a simplified version of the multifactor model (Browne 1988). Stress factors and background influences are mediated through the interpersonal relationships within the family (Fig. 3.3).

The model refers to 'situational stressors', which may include the following four components:

- *Relations between caregivers*: intermarriage, marital disputes, step-parent/cohabitee or separated/single parent
- *Relations to children*: spacing between births, size of family, caregivers' attachments to and expectations of their dependants
- *Structural stress*: poor housing, unemployment, social isolation, threats to the caregiver's authority, values and self-esteem
- *Stress generated by the child*: e.g. an unwanted child, one who is incontinent, difficult to discipline, often ill, physically or mentally disabled, one who is temperamental, frequently emotional or very demanding.

The chances of these situational stressors resulting in maltreatment are mediated by (and depend on) the interactive relationships within the family. A secure relationship between family members will 'buffer' any effects of stress and facilitate coping strategies on behalf of the family. By contrast, insecure or anxious relationships will not 'buffer' the family under stress and 'episodic overload' – such as an argument or a child misbehaving – may result in a physical or emotional attack. It is suggested that overall this will have a negative effect on the existing interpersonal

Figure 3.3
The causes of family violence and child maltreatment (from Browne & Herbert 1997, Preventing family violence. Wiley, Chichester. With kind permission from J Wiley & Sons Limited).

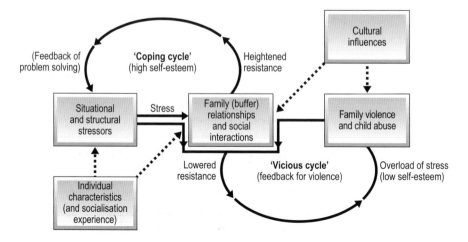

relationships and reduce any 'buffering' effects still further, making it easier for stressors to overload the system once again. Hence, a positive feedback ('vicious cycle') is set up which eventually leads to 'systematic overload', where constant stress results in repeated physical and emotional assaults. This situation becomes progressively worse without intervention and could be termed 'the spiral of violence'. In some cases, violent parents will cope with their aggressive feelings towards their child by physical or emotional neglect, to avoid causing a deliberate injury (Iwaniec 2006).

As indicated earlier, culture and community values may also affect attitudes and styles of interaction in family relationships which, in turn, will be influenced by the social position of individuals in terms of their age, sex, education, socio-economic status, ethnic group and social class background.

According to Rutter (1985), aggression is a social behaviour within everyone's repertoire, and he suggests that it is under control when the individual has high self-esteem, good relationships and stress is appropriately managed. However, the quality of relationships and responses to stress in the family will depend on the participant's personality and character traits and their pathology, such as low self-esteem, poor temperament control and psychological disorders. These may be a result of early social experiences, which may indirectly affect behavioural investment in the family. Two main features of violent families are a lack of skill in handling conflict and discipline and high rates of aversive behaviour. These coercive family interactions have been previously described by Patterson (1982) and are seen as the primary focus for intervention.

In conclusion, it is suggested that stress factors and background influences are mediated through the interpersonal relationships within the family. Indeed, these relationships should be the focus of work on prevention, treatment and management of family violence and child maltreatment. It is at this level that health and social service professionals can make a significant contribution.

Implications for assessment and intervention

Services for children in need are rarely offered until they have been placed on a child protection register and, typically, this happens after maltreatment has already occurred. However, there is the potential for prevention as good family relationships and parent–child interactions can act as protective factors and provide some resilience to social and environmental stress impinging on the family and increasing the possibility of violence (Browne & Herbert 1997). It is important to consider maltreatment in the light of these family dynamics. Hence, intervention needs to be aimed at any negative interaction or lack of interaction between a child and their caregiver which results in harm to the child's physical and psychological development (e.g. Sanders & Cann 2002).

Levels of prevention

It is important to distinguish between prevention at the primary, secondary and tertiary levels (Hamilton & Browne 2002):

- *Primary prevention* aims to prevent the problem of child maltreatment before it occurs in the general population. Therefore, primary prevention is achieved via media campaigns and with universal services offered to the whole population on a routine basis (e.g. maternity services, health visits following the birth of a child, etc.)

■ *Secondary prevention* focuses on targeting families identified on the basis of risk factors associated with the prediction of child maltreatment. Thus, secondary prevention targets services at selected 'high risk groups' of families in need of more support, offering intervention before maltreatment occurs. The selection process can be simply based on one or two risk factors (e.g. young mothers with socio-economic problems, Olds *et al.* 2002) or an actuarial approach where a risk factor checklist is used and scored to identify families who score over a threshold (Browne *et al.* 2006).

■ *Tertiary prevention* measures attempt to minimise the consequences of victimisation in those families detected to be maltreating their children. This may include predicting and prioritising those parents (already known to child protection services) who are likely to go on to seriously harm or fatally abuse their child(ren). In addition, those children who are likely to be the victims of recurrent maltreatment by the same or different perpetrators are identified (Hamilton & Browne 1998, 1999). Therefore, tertiary prevention is achieved via specialist services for the treatment of maltreating families. Intervention is offered only after 'significant harm' has occurred.

Examples of strategies for prevention at each of the above levels are listed in Table 3.3. However, the primary care of children and their families is usually limited by resources allocated to the health sector. In practice, most countries offer child protection services only to those families most at risk of maltreating their children. This is due in part to the social and professional concern about children dying who were already known to child protection agencies, despite the fact that the majority of child deaths occur in families who are not previously known to child protection agencies (Reder & Duncan 2002).

To counteract the focus on tertiary intervention, a body of research has considered the costs of implementing primary and/or secondary forms of prevention compared to the costs associated with the consequences of child maltreatment. It

Table 3.3
Strategies for prevention

Primary	Secondary	Tertiary
■ Prenatal, perinatal and early childhood health care that improves pregnancy outcomes and strengthens early attachment ■ Promoting good parenting practices ■ Public awareness activities (i.e. through media and campaigns) ■ Community education programmes on UNCRC ■ Availability and accessibility of social services, supports and networks ■ School-based activities towards non-violence	■ Perinatal and ongoing identification of at-risk children and families ■ Family support such as home visiting ■ Clearly established referral system of support services ■ Substance abuse treatment programmes ■ Community-based, family-centred support, assistance and networks ■ Information available about community resources and safety planning ■ Schools-based social services for high stress environment	■ Early diagnosis ■ Proper interdisciplinary services to ensure medical treatment, care, counselling, management and support of victims/families ■ Reintegration in a child-friendly community/school ■ Adequate child protection laws and child-friendly courts

(Adapted from WHO 1999)
UNCRC, United Nations Convention on the Rights of the Child.

has been estimated that the use of an intervention such as the Positive Parenting Programme (Sanders 1999) can cost only €26 per child to implement yet can reduce the prevalence of childhood behaviour problems by 26% (Mihalopoulos *et al.* in submission). Thus, based on the estimated £735 m per annum spent in the UK on the consequences of child maltreatment (National Commission of Inquiry into the Prevention of Child Abuse 1996), a potential saving of €286 650 000 could be made if the programme were implemented across the UK. Similarly, research in the USA of a nurse home-visiting programme targeted to disadvantaged first-time mothers, who were under 21 years of age, single parents and with serious financial problems, showed an overall saving of US$180 per family in the 1980s (Olds *et al.* 1993), when taking into account family aid, food stamps, medical aid and costs of other services, such as child protection agencies.

Thus, it appears that the cost–benefit of providing earlier interventions is a powerful argument to local and national government, particularly when considered alongside the emotional and physical harm done to children and their families when maltreatment occurs. It should also be recognised, however, that the training of general practitioners, community psychiatric nurses, health visitors and midwives requires a greater focus on child protection. Without this refocusing, there will be a reliance on tertiary prevention at greater financial and human cost. One way of achieving this is to bring child protection into the wider arena of child welfare, which is seen as the remit for all professionals working with children in any capacity. The health sector is a key agency in the early prediction and prevention of child adversity. Indeed, health professionals are the front line in promoting children's optimal health and development.

Public health approach to prevent child abuse and neglect

These realisations have led to the development of a public health approach to child protection. This may be defined as follows (Browne & Hamilton-Giachritsis 2003):

- Child abuse and neglect is considered within the broader context of child welfare, families and communities.
- Children's developmental needs are assessed in general rather than specifically in relation to child protection.
- The parent's capacity to respond appropriately to their child(ren)'s needs is evaluated.
- Consideration is paid to the impact of wider family and environmental factors on the capacity to parent.
- Child protection is integrated within health and social services to families, while promoting positive parenting and enhancing parental capacity to meet the needs of children.

In the UK, the role of health professionals tends to be limited to inter-agency collaboration on health and medical issues. However, a more positive development has been the move for child protection professionals towards a more family-based approach to assessment, seeing child maltreatment in the wider context of the family.

Framework for the assessment of children and families

In England, this move towards a family context began with the *Framework for the Assessment of Children in Need and their Families* (DoH *et al.* 2000). The framework guidelines were primarily aimed at social workers to encourage them to take

Figure 3.4
*Framework for the assess-
ment of children and their
families (reproduced with
permission from
Department of Health,
Department of Education
and Employment and the
Home Office 2000).*

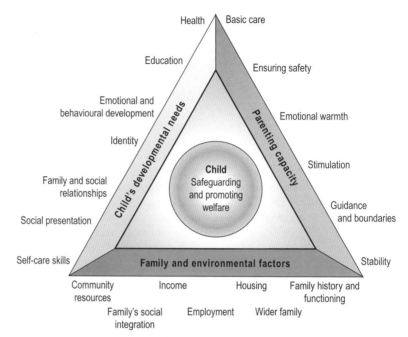

a broader approach to child protection, including a holistic view of family assessment, considering the wider environment and its influence on family functioning.
Specifically, three family components are assessed (Fig. 3.4):

- developmental needs of the child
- parents' capacity to meet the child's needs
- social and environmental factors that impinge upon the parents' capacity to
  meet the child's needs.

Nevertheless, it can be argued that this more holistic assessment of the family
arrives too late, as social workers will only be involved once a child has been suspected of significant harm. A public health approach would dictate that this form of
assessment be carried out on all newborns during the first year of the child's life.
Although any community professional could be involved in this process, in the UK
such a preventative approach would be the responsibility of primary health care
teams and community-nurse home visitors in particular. It is unfortunate that social
workers are so overwhelmed with reactive child protective work that there is little
opportunity or resources for them to be used, perhaps more effectively, in a proactive and preventative way (as many social workers would prefer). As the causes of
family violence are now better understood, preventative social work is both possible and desirable.

Assessing violent families: how safe is the child? the use of home health visiting

In keeping with recommendations for practice (Hall & Elliman 2003) and the
Children Act 1989, a Child Assessment Rating and Evaluation (CARE) Screening
Programme was introduced into the Southend Community Care Services for the

identification of 'need' in all families with newborns in that area for three years (Browne *et al.* 2000, 2006). This is achieved in partnership with parents. The CARE programme is designed for community-based primary health care professionals to:

- offer a child- and family-centred assessment of need that covers the child's first year of life, rather than being a one-off judgement
- offer an objective assessment of parenting capacity and family difficulties as a basis for referrals and joint work with other agencies
- offer, for the first time, the means for parents to identify their own situation and perceptions of parenting
- offer reliable behavioural indicators (such as parental sensitivity and infant-to-parent attachment) to distinguish between priority families and the remainder of the population.

Following the four home visits during the first year, the community nurse is required to indicate the plan for the period up to 5 years of age when their involvement traditionally ceases. There are two options: 'routine surveillance' where the community nurse is reactive to the family's requests and needs, and 'prolonged active management' where the community nurse is proactive and continues to make regular visits to the family because the child is in 'need' or is of 'concern'. All children on the child protection register would fall into the latter category. Either at this time or at any during the first 12 months, referrals can be made to other agencies for additional support. These include home visiting services (e.g. postnatal depression, infant sleep), voluntary groups (e.g. mother and toddler, counselling), health services (e.g. paediatricians, psychologists) and social services (e.g. nursery placements, family support). In some instances, child protection procedures may have to be implemented.

The theoretical basis, guidelines and implementation of the CARE programme can be found in Browne *et al.* (2006). In summary, early use of screening checklists (e.g. Lynch & Roberts 1977, Browne & Saqi 1988a) demonstrated the need for the inclusion of additional forms of assessment (Browne 1995b, Dixon *et al.* 2005a). Therefore, the purpose of the programme is to assess risk factors through a checklist, but also parental perceptions, attributions and sensitivity over four visits. The development of the child's attachment behaviours is also monitored, as a potential protective factor.

The CARE programme is based on work showing that there are five important aspects to consider when assessing violent parent–child relationships (Browne 1995a, Browne *et al.* 2006):

- Caregiver's knowledge and attitudes towards child rearing
- Parental perceptions of the child's behaviour
- Parental emotions and responses to stress
- Parent–child interaction and behaviour
- Quality of parenting and infant attachment.

Knowledge and attitudes towards child rearing

Research suggests that abusing and non-abusing families have different attitudes about child development. Starr (1982) found that one of the differences between abusing and non-abusing parents is that the abusing group sees child rearing as a simple rather than a complex task. Many of them show a lack of awareness of their child's abilities and needs (Hyman & Mitchell 1975). For example, parents with much higher expectations of their children may attempt to force their child to behave in a manner that is developmentally beyond them.

Parental perceptions of child behaviour

It has been shown that abusing parents have more negative perceptions of their children's behaviour than non-abusing parents. They perceive their children to be more irritable and demanding (Browne & Saqi 1987, Crittenden 2002). This may be related to the fact that abused children are more likely to have health problems and eating or sleeping disturbances. Alternatively, it may be a direct result of the unrealistic expectations often reported for abusing parents (Martin & Rodeheffer 1976, Rosenberg & Reppucci 1983, Putallaz *et al.* 1998). In addition, parental attributions have been related to how and whether a child will be abused (Stratton & Swaffer 1988) because they attribute more negative intentions to their child's behaviour in comparison to other parents (Zeanah & Zeanah 1989). Maltreating parents may interpret certain age-appropriate behaviours as deliberate or intentional non-compliance, concluding that this behaviour is an indication of the child's inherent 'bad' disposition. Thus, abusive parents may see their child's behaviour as a threat to their own self-esteem, which then elicits a punitive attitude and an insensitive approach to parenting.

Parental emotions and responses to stress

The majority of incidents of physical abuse which come to the notice of the authorities arise from emotionally stressful situations where parents are attempting to control or discipline their children (Patterson 1982). Abusive parents are significantly harsher to their children on a day-to-day basis and are less appropriate in their choice of disciplinary methods compared to non-abusive parents. It is the ineffectiveness of the abusive parent's child-management styles that contributes to the abuse. If the parent's initial command is ineffective and is ignored by the child, the situation will escalate and become more and more stressful until the only way the abusive parent feels they can regain control is by resorting to violence. Patterson (1986) described rejecting parents as very unclear on how to discipline their children. They punish for significant transgressions, whereas serious transgressions such as stealing go unpunished. Where threats are given, they are carried through unpredictably. Neglectful parents show very low rates of positive physical contact, touching and hugging, and high levels of coercive, aversive interactions.

A factor common to many child abusers is a heightened rate of arousal in stressful situations. In a study conducted by Wolfe *et al.* (1983), abusive and non-abusive parents were presented with scenes of videotaped parent–child interactions, some of which were highly stressful (e.g. children screaming and refusing to comply with their parents) and some of which were non-stressful (e.g. a child watching television quietly). The abusive parents responded with greater negative psycho-physiological arousal than did the non-abusive comparison groups. Thus, it may be suggested that poor responses to stress and emotional arousal play a crucial role in the manifestation of child abuse and neglect (Webster-Stratton 1990). The extra stress associated with caring for a sick child or a child with growth difficulties has also been associated with an increased likelihood of maltreatment (Iwaniec 2004).

Parent–child interaction and behaviour

Effective parenting is characterised by a flexible attitude, with parents responding to the needs of the child and the situation. House rules are enforced in a consistent and firm manner, using commands or sanctions where necessary. In most situations, the child will comply with the wishes of the parent and conflict will not arise. In recent years, there has been a rise in the number of positive parenting programmes aimed at assisting parents to develop these skills (e.g. Daro 2002, Sanders & Cann 2002, Webster-Stratton & Herbert 1994).

Interaction assessments demonstrate that abused infants and their mothers have interactions that are less reciprocal and fewer in number than their matched controls, whether in the presence or absence of a stranger (Hyman *et al.* 1979, Browne 1986, Browne & Saqi 1987, 1988b). Observational studies provide evidence that social behaviours and interaction patterns within abusing and non-abusing families are different. Abusing parents have been described as being aversive, negative and controlling, with less pro-social behaviour (Wolfe 1985, Crittenden 2002). They also show less interactive behaviour, both in terms of sensitivity and responsiveness towards their children. This may result in infants developing an insecure attachment to their abusive caregivers, which in turn produces marked changes in the abused children's socio-emotional behaviour, in accordance with the predictions of attachment theory (Browne & Saqi 1988b). Nevertheless, the consequences of maltreatment are not the same for all children. Findings suggest that there are more behaviour problems in children who are both abused and neglected (Crittenden 1985, 1988). Abusing and neglectful parents, together with their children, suffer from pervasive confusion and ambivalence in their relations with each other. This is not the same as simple parental rejection. It reflects rather an uncertainty in the relationship which leaves the child vulnerable and perplexed as to what is expected.

Quality of parenting and infant attachment

Ainsworth *et al.* (1978) examined the relationship between the infant's attachment (as measured by the infant's responses to separation and reunion) and the behaviour of the mother in the home environment. Their findings suggested that maternal sensitivity is most influential in affecting the child's reactions. In the homes of the securely attached infants, the mother was sensitive to the infant's behaviour and interactions, while insecurely attached, avoidant infants were found to be rejected by the mothers in terms of interaction. It was suggested that the enhanced exploratory behaviours shown by these infants were an attempt to block attachment behaviours which had been rejected in the past. In the home environments of the insecurely attached, ambivalent infants, a disharmonious mother–infant relationship was evident, and the ambivalent behaviours shown were seen as a result of inconsistent parenting. Since these original observations, children have also been observed to be disorganised (D) in their attachment style to the primary caregiver (Main & Solomon 1986, 1990). These children could not be easily classified into Ainsworth's original categories of avoidant (A), secure (B) and ambivalent (C) (see Cassidy & Shaver 1999, Solomon & George 1999).

It has been suggested that, in some cases, the link between experiences of abuse as a child and abusing as a parent is likely to be the result of an unsatisfactory early relationship with the principal caregiver and a failure to form a secure attachment (Bowlby 1984, Bartholomew *et al.* 2001, Newcomb & Locke 2001, Egeland *et al.* 2002). For many years it was considered that there were four important dimensions to caregiving style (Maccoby 1980): sensitivity/insensitivity, acceptance/rejection, cooperation/interference, accessibility/ignoring. These four dimensions may be heavily influenced by parental attitudes, emotions and perceptions of the child. Van Ijzendoorn (1995) and De Wolff and van Ijzendoorn (1997) analysed previous research involving a total of 5000 parent–infant dyads. They noted a three-way association between the mother's internal working model of relationships

Figure 3.5
Path model for the relations among the mother's internal working model, maternal sensitivity and infant attachment (adapted with permission from Cassidy et al 2005).

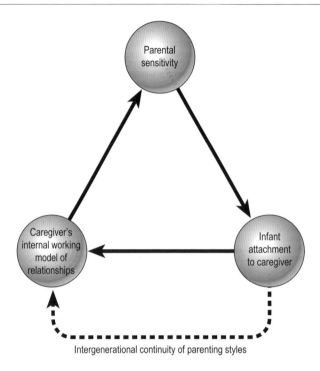

Intergenerational continuity of parenting styles

(derived from her own early attachments), her current parenting behaviours and the quality of infant to mother attachment (Fig. 3.5). However, recent research has begun to consider why the children of some insensitive mothers still develop a secure attachment, whereas other children do not. Early findings indicate that it may be the extent to which the mother provides a 'secure base' for the child that is instrumental in this outcome (Cassidy *et al.* 2005).

Conclusion and recommended intervention strategies

It follows that the parent–child relationship should be the focus of work on the prevention, treatment and management of child maltreatment, and that interventions to achieve these goals are most effectively carried out in the homes of families (Sanders 1999, Sutton 2000, Herbert & Harper-Dorton 2002, Iwaniec 2004, 2006). The ultimate aim is to engage parents in the process of working with professionals. Indeed, some programmes have developed self-directed parenting programmes for families with children at risk of emotional-behavioural problems who otherwise choose not to engage with services (Connell *et al.* 1997, Markie-Dadds & Sanders 2006). Those involved in the treatment of abusive families should be concerned with the development of a 'secure' relationship between parent and child (see Berlin *et al.* 2005). It is not sufficient to evaluate treatment programmes on the basis of the occurrence or non-occurrence of subsequent abuse. Helping parents to inhibit violence towards their children may still leave the harmful context in which the initial abuse occurred quite unchanged.

However, maltreating parents are often socially isolated and may be less likely to seek help from outside agencies who could provide assistance or emotional support (Miller-Perrin & Perrin 1999). If they do interact with other people, abusive or neglecting parents are most likely to choose people in similar situations to themselves, so they gain no experience of alternative parental styles or coping strategies and continue to be ineffective in controlling their children. Effective intervention strategies to control and prevent child abuse and neglect have recently been reviewed (Little & Mount 1999, Dubowitz & DePanfilis 2000, Browne *et al.* 2002a). Therefore it follows that home visitation as an early intervention strategy is essential to engage those families most at risk of child maltreatment. Community nurses are best placed to assess the needs of infants, the parents' capacity to meet those needs and social–environmental factors that may impinge on this capacity. If they identify infants and their families in need, then appropriate referrals can be made to relevant state and voluntary agencies.

Whilst there are many examples of primary and secondary prevention approaches involving the health sector (see Browne *et al.* 2006), the majority of social work intervention techniques operate at the third level of prevention (intervention and treatment after violence to the child has occurred). Some children are removed from their family home and placed in local authority care when it is considered unsafe for them to be helped and supported at home with their parents. For example, in England, approximately 12% (3000) of those on the child protection register on 31 March 2005 were 'looked after' by local authorities (5% of all children in public care; DfES 2006). Of these, according to official data (which does not round up to 100%), 79% were placed with foster parents, 4% were living in children's homes or secure units, 13% were placed with parents and 3% were placed for adoption, living independently, missing from placement or other residential settings (DfES 2006).

Future strategies for intervention should place more emphasis on working with violent adults in the family, insisting that the offender leaves the home rather than the child. The treatment of offenders is perhaps the most effective way of protecting children in the long term; without treatment, offenders are likely to reoffend and place the same family or other families at risk (Hamilton 2002). There is an urgent need to develop community treatment programmes for violent men and women, some of whom acknowledge the need for support prior to committing an offence. Prison treatment programmes and court diversion schemes for convicted or cautioned offenders, respectively, reach just the tip of the iceberg.

Key points and messages for practice

- Active abuse involves violent acts that represent the exercise of physical force to cause injury or forcibly interfere with personal freedom. Passive abuse refers to neglect, which can only be considered violent in the metaphorical sense, as it does not involve physical force. Nevertheless, it can cause both physical and emotional injury, such as non-organic failure to thrive in young children.

- The chances of situational stressors resulting in maltreatment are mediated by (and depend on) the interactive relationships within the family. A secure relationship between family members will 'buffer' any effects of stress and facilitate coping strategies on behalf of the family.

- The parent–child relationship should be the focus of work on the prevention, treatment and management of child maltreatment, and that interventions to achieve these goals are most effectively carried out in the homes of families.

- Child maltreatment is one of the most common causes of death in young children in the UK today.

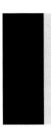

- The study of social interactions and relationships can be seen as occupying a central and potentially integrating place in explaining the causes of aggression in the family.

- Future strategies for intervention should place more emphasis on working with violent adults in the family, insisting that the offender leaves the home rather than the child. The treatment of offenders is perhaps the most effective way of protecting children in the long term.

Annotated further reading

Browne K, Hanks H, Stratton P, Hamilton C 2002 Early prediction and prevention of child abuse: a handbook. Wiley, Chichester

This is an update of an earlier volume and provides an excellent guide to the prediction of various forms of abuse, including fatal child abuse and neglect, physical maltreatment, emotional child abuse and neglect and sexual abuse and neglect. The account of primary and secondary prevention using an ecological analysis, focuses on positive parenting and prevention through prenatal and infancy and home visiting. There is also a useful outline of tertiary prevention, helping children and families affected by abuse by examining the impact of abusive experiences, a focus on intergenerational transmission, the role of family therapy, focusing on emotionally abused and neglected children, and working with offenders including a chapter on preventing the victim-to-offender cycle. This text is written by leading American and UK authors.

Browne K, Douglas J, Hamilton-Giachritsis C, Hegarty J 2006 A community health approach to the assessment of infants and their parents: the CARE programme. Wiley, Chichester

This book describes a method of assessment and intervention for infants and their families entitled the Child Assessment Rating and Evaluation (CARE) programme. The aim of the programme is the early prediction and prevention of problems for child health, development and protection.

All aspects of the programme are discussed in full, including assessing the emotional development of infants and their parents, observation of parent–infant interaction and child protection issues. The evidence-based research behind the programme is discussed and a detailed evaluation of the programme's effectiveness is provided. This practical volume also includes:

- *assessment tools and guidelines on how to use them (including the Index of Need)*
- *guidance on working with parents*
- *detailed case illustrations*
- *tips on managing workloads*
- *advice on caseload management*
- *discussion of the cost effectiveness of home visiting.*

A Community Health Approach to the Assessment of Infants and their Parents *aims to inform policy and practice. It is an invaluable tool for all primary care health workers, including health visitors, social workers and paediatricians.*

Useful websites

The assessment tools described in A Community Health Approach to the Assessment of Infants and their Parents *are available to download online at www.wiley.com/go/care*

4

Child sexual abuse: who are the perpetrators?

Donald Findlater and Rachel Fyson

INTRODUCTION

If we are to intervene, effectively, in problems concerning actual or suspected child sexual abuse, it is imperative that the phenomenon of abuse, the identity, behaviour patterns and motivations of victims, offenders and other parties and the wealth of research (with its many limitations) are well understood. Without such understanding, risk – with its various meanings – will be poorly considered and assessed, children may not be well protected and the suspected or known abuser, their partner and others involved may not receive fair or just treatment.

Myths about sexual abuse and abusers abound, with stereotypes of abusers too often distracting professionals and public alike. Common beliefs include:

- sex offenders are an isolated group of sick men
- sexual abuse is restricted to single incidents of uncharacteristic aberrant behaviour by otherwise ordinary men
- all sex offenders are wholly bad and remain profoundly dangerous to all children across their life spans
- children often make up stories of sexual abuse
- sexual abuse is a consequence of family problems
- abusers are distinctly adult and male
- child sexual abuse is a modern phenomenon and a feature of 'western civilized societies'.

The reality is, mostly, very different. Accurate knowledge about offenders helps all in society to both protect children and provide effective interventions for victims, abusers and their families.

The research reviewed here challenges some deeply held beliefs about those who abuse children, for in reality there is no single 'type' of abuser. Sexually abusive behaviour occurs across all socio-economic, cultural, racial and religious groups. Those concerned with child protection need to know that diversity is the main factor characterising those who sexually abuse, that most sexual offending takes place within the context of a relationship which the offender makes with the child in order to gain compliance and prevent disclosure, and that physical and emotional abuse may be concurrent features. They must also not fall into the trap of assuming that the family itself is at fault when a child is sexually abused by a family member, especially where the abuser is an adult. Offenders create or exacerbate family dysfunction in order to abuse undetected. Those responding to family members affected by sexual abuse need to recognise this.

Over the years, repeated studies have found that at least one in 10 children across the world experience sexual abuse. In their UK survey of some 3000 young adults, the NSPCC discovered that 16% had experienced unwanted sexual contact (Cawson *et al.* 2000). McGee and colleagues report that 20% of women and 16% of men reported contact sexual abuse during childhood (McGee *et al.* 2003). Freyd *et al.* suggest that 20% of women and 5–10% of men *worldwide* experienced child sexual abuse (Freyd *et al.* 2005). There is a consensus amongst researchers that 'under reporting … is consistent and universal' (Watkins & Bentovim 1992, p. 201).

Research findings have varied in their conclusions about the relative proportions of intrafamilial and extrafamilial child sexual abuse. Finkelhor found that 44% of reported sexual abuse of girls was committed by family members. The equivalent figure for boys was 17% (Finkelhor 1979). However, Kelly and colleagues found a much lower rate of intrafamilial abuse, concluding that although most children are abused by adults and peers they know, these are not always – or even in the majority of cases – family or household members (Kelly *et al.* 2000). Whatever the nature of the relationship, Grubin concludes that 'the majority of child molesters sexually assault children known to them … with up to 80% of offences taking place in either the home of the offender or the home of the victim' (Grubin 1998, p. 16).

The vast majority of child sexual abuse remains undisclosed, this despite the increasing public awareness and concern about such behaviour and an evident wish, across society, to protect children. As the NSPCC reported: 'Only a quarter of respondents with sexual experience, unwanted or with a person five or more years older, had told anyone about it at the time. When they had, their confidant was usually a friend, less often a family member, and very rarely police or other professionals' (Cawson *et al.* 2000, p. 90). In her USA study, Russell discovered that only 6% of extrafamilial and 2% of intrafamilial abuse was reported to the police (Russell 1983). In the UK, Kelly *et al.* reported that only 5% of child sexual abuse was reported to anyone, only 2% was reported to an official agency and only 1% was prosecuted (Kelly *et al.* 1991). As we know, the vast majority of reported sexual offences are not convicted in a criminal court.

The short- and long-term consequences of child abuse are reported elsewhere in this volume (see especially Chapter 5 by Hanks and Stratton). One particularly tragic outcome for *some* child victims of sexual abuse is an increased propensity to sexually abuse in their own right – some refer to this as the 'cycle of sexual abuse' (Pritchard 2004). We return to this issue later in the chapter.

However hard pressed our child and public protection agencies may be, we have to recognise that we continue to deal with only the 'tip of the iceberg' of both victims and abusers. Despite this, the sex offender register had risen to some 28 500 in England and Wales by March 2005, and is estimated to top 100 000 individuals by 2015 (Batty 2006). Fortunately, not all these individuals present an immediate, grave risk to children. But some do. Many will live in households that include children and it is clearly important that competent assessments are undertaken to gauge and help manage risk – an activity that crucially involves the offender and other adults, as well as any professional involvement. However, in the face of the scale of the 'epidemic' of child sexual abuse, most being unreported, it is imperative that the wider public is informed and involved in extending appropriate community child protection.

Adult sexual abusers

Who sexually abuses?

Individuals who sexually abuse children are an extremely diverse group. Up to one-third of all reported sexual offences are committed by children and young people (Grubin 1998, Fisher & Beech 2004), an issue which we address in detail in the second part of this chapter.

Whilst female sex offenders comprise only 0.5% of the imprisoned sex offender population of England and Wales (Home Office 2001), the actual proportion of sexual offences against children committed by women is much higher. Grubin reports that less than 5% of sexual offences against children are known to have been committed by women, 'often in association with men' (Grubin 1998, p. vi). However, Finkelhor and Russell (1984) concluded from a survey of data then available, that some 20% of male victims and 5% of female victims were sexually abused by an older female. Ford notes that 12% of children calling ChildLine about sexual abuse in 2002/3 were calling about a female abuser, with mothers featuring in half of these calls from girls, and 19% of the calls from boys (Ford 2006).

It is often assumed that most female perpetrators are coerced by males, but studies of this population have 'male coerced' as only one of at least three typologies; the other typologies most frequently discussed in the literature are the 'intergenerationally predisposed group' who abuse their own young children, often regarded as replicating their own childhood abuse, and the 'teacher-lover' who sees herself as such and abuses adolescents with whom she believes she is having an 'affair' (Eldridge 2000, p. 315). Societal denial frequently accompanies female sex offending, leading to inadequate assessment of and intervention with both the women abusers themselves and also their victims.

It is nonetheless beyond doubt that the majority of child sexual abuse is carried out by males, most of them adult, and for this reason – unless the context suggests otherwise – offenders will be referred to as 'he' throughout the remainder of the chapter. What follows then, is based upon what is known and reported about this population. These men are a heterogeneous group: their motivations, personalities, victim choices, social functioning and reoffending risks are profoundly varied. Some have a clear sexual preference for children, but the majority do not, and hence cannot properly be described as paedophiles (Grubin 1998). Myers concludes that sex offenders are:

a heterogeneous group with few shared characteristics apart from a predilection for deviant sexual behaviour. Furthermore, there is no psychological test or device that reliably detects persons who have or will sexually abuse children ... there is no profile of a typical child molester.

(Myers et al. 1989, p. 142)

In the same vein, Salter concludes that:

these men are characterised by their diversity. An offender could as well have been a professor as a pauper, a minister as an atheist, a teetotaller as an alcoholic, a teenager as a septuagenarian ... moreover, an offender might as well have had an extensive history of arrests as none at all ... these patients did not seem to share any definable demographic or personality traits to render them distinctive.

(Salter 1995, p. 16)

In fact 'the most striking characteristic of sex offenders ... is their apparent normality' (Salter 1995, p. 180).

It is generally believed that the vast majority of sex offenders are not mentally ill in the sense of having a diagnosable mental illness (Grubin 1991). In her review of opinion on sex offending and mental illness, Knopp concludes that fewer than 8%, perhaps as few as 1%, of men charged with sexual offences have an underlying psychiatric illness and in few cases did this mental illness 'cause' the sex offending (Knopp & Stevenson 1990).

Choice of victim and crossover Issues

In recognising the heterogeneity of sex offenders, it is also important to recognise that some repeat offenders appear consistently to target the same victim type, whereas others have more diverse interests, and their risk needs to be assessed accordingly. Confidential self-report studies show that multiple paraphilias (i.e. more than one type of deviant sexual interest) are commonplace. Weinrott and Saylor (1991) asked a group of 'sexual psychopaths' about their previous unreported sexual offending:

- 32% of the rapists of adults admitted abusing children
- 12% of child abusers admitted at least one attempt at forced sex against an adult female
- 34% of extrafamilial child molesters had sexually offended against their own children
- 50% of known incest offenders admitted to child abuse outside the home.

Other confidential self-report studies from the USA (Abel *et al.* 1988, Abel & Rouleau 1990, Faller 1990) report a range of crossover statistics that evidence the caution needed in assessing both size and direction of risk, with multiple paraphilias often the norm rather than the exception in those with sexual convictions. What is not clear is whether these sampled populations are in any way typical of sex offenders more broadly to allow generalisations to be based upon them. Recent crossover data from a UK sample, but based on reconviction rather than self-report, suggest that offenders with male victims present more future risk to female children than offenders with female victims present to males. There is little gender crossover involving post-pubescent children, though offenders with younger child victims appear less concerned with the gender of any future victim (Friendship & Thornton 2002).

In assessing offenders, we need to entertain the possibility of crossover whilst not assuming it. We must also recognise that the likelihood of crossover relates to both motivation and opportunity. Crossover may not have occurred because the offender has no interest. Equally, it may not have occurred because the opportunity was not evident or the risk of detection or reporting was judged by the offender to be too great. Should opportunity arise or risk of detection recede, then abuse may become more likely. Those assessing risk to potential future victims must also recognise that, especially in a family setting, significant harm may be caused to a child as much through exposure to abusive attitudes and behaviour towards women and children as through any direct sexual abuse (Eldridge 2000).

Patterns of sexual offending

When they initially come to public attention, as well as subsequently, offenders often engage in denial at a number of levels. This can include absolute denial of any wrongdoing, minimising the extent and likely impact of the abuse, or denial of sexual motivation. They minimise, justify, excuse or blame others in much the same way as most human beings do when guilty of reprehensible behaviour. They often state that it 'just happened', 'it was an accident', or that drink, drugs, depression, stress or relationship problems were to blame. In reality we know that, in most cases, offenders' actions were premeditated: they imagined what they wanted to do, targeted and manipulated a child, whilst also manipulating others who might have protected the child. The extent of conscious planning varies between offenders (Eldridge 2000).

Over the past quarter-century and more, a number of theoretical models have been developed to explain, in part, 'why', but mostly 'how', sex offenders operate. Whilst no single model is without its shortcomings, their use, often in combination, can significantly help child protection and criminal justice workers, the offenders, their victims and their families to make sense of past behaviour, allocate responsibility appropriately and begin to address issues of treatment need and future risk management. Before exploring two such models in some detail, it is important to acknowledge the insights and perspectives offered from other sources. For a fuller exposition and critique of the various models and theories, the reader is referred to the work of Ward, Beech and colleagues (Ward *et al.* 2006).

Organic explanations for sexual offending have suggested that temporal lobe abnormalities or an unusually strong sex drive account for sexual aggression (Lanyon 1991). Such explanations seem only relevant to a small minority of offenders where evidence of such problems exists. Developmental theorists, building on the work of Freud, posit a distinction between fixated and regressed offenders, with the former having a consistent primary sexual interest in children and the latter, having developed an appropriate sexual interest in adults, 'regressing' into sexual contact with children in stressful circumstances (Lanyon 1991). Such theorists also often explain incestuous child molestation as the fault of the dysfunctional family as opposed to the responsibility of the abuser. However, as more has been understood about the tactics of abusers, it seems more logical to see any family dysfunction as an *effect* of the manipulation of the abuser rather than as a cause of the abuse. As Salter concludes:

The family, however, may wittingly or unwittingly provide the opportunity ... They do not provide the motivation or the willingness to offend. Rather, a sick or absent mother, a helpless or depressed one, an alienated child who is unlikely to tell or to be believed if she does, each allows the offender the opportunity to offend.

(Salter 1988, p. 53)

Social learning theorists propose imitation of modelled behaviour as a mechanism for learning, with children taking their parents as their model for appropriate sex roles. Where offenders have been the victims, directly or otherwise, of sexual abuse, one can see the potential imitation of modelled behaviour. For those without such victimisation as children, we might need to look beyond immediate family, to peers and media, for the relevant learning. We must also recognise that many victims of abuse do not become abusers – there is evidently no direct causal link between being a victim and becoming an abuser. As noted by Grubin, 'a history of sexual abuse as a child is neither necessary nor sufficient to lead to adult sex offending (Grubin 1998, p. vi).

Of course we must also recognise the social context in which sexual abuse takes place in Western society. The fact that the majority of abusers are male, and the majority of victims female or children, is taken by feminists as evidence that sexual abuse is the result of patriarchy, with males maintaining control over females and children due to an evident power differential. Sexual abuse, then, is as much about power as it is about sex. Such conclusions have much to contribute to any serious consideration of prevention of sexual abuse at a community or societal level (Itzin 2000).

Marshall and Barbaree bring together evidence on biological, behavioural, cultural and sociological factors into an 'integrated approach' to sexual abuse. They posit that 'the task for human males (in normal development) is to acquire inhibitory controls over a biologically-endowed propensity for self-interest associated with a tendency to fuse sex and aggression' (Marshall & Barbaree 1990, p. 257). They summarise their approach as follows:

Biological inheritance confers upon males a ready capacity to sexually aggress, which must be overcome by appropriate training to instil social inhibitions towards such behaviour. Variations in hormonal functioning make their task more or less difficult. Poor parenting, particularly the use of harsh or inconsistent discipline in the absence of love, typically fails to instil these constraints and may even serve to facilitate the fusion of sex and aggression, rather than separate these two tendencies. Socio-cultural attitudes may negatively interact with poor parenting to enhance the likelihood of sexual offending, if these cultural beliefs express traditional patriarchal views.

(Marshall & Barbaree 1990, p. 272)

As stated previously, these explanations for sexual abuse contribute much to our understanding but may not be of great assistance in assessing and responding to risk. In our multi-agency child protection context, models are required that inform all aspects of work with families and offenders. We now turn to the two models that have influenced professional practice for over 20 years, each of which identifies the primary role of the abuser at all stages of the abuse process.

Finkelhor's 'four preconditions' – a model

Following a review of all the factors which, in the early 1980s, were believed to contribute to sexual offending by adolescents and adults, Finkelhor (1984, p. 54) concluded that four preconditions needed to be met before sexual abuse could occur, specifically:

1. A potential offender needed to have the *motivation* to abuse a child sexually.
2. The potential offender had to *overcome internal inhibitors* against acting on that motivation.
3. The potential offender had to *overcome external inhibitors* to committing sexual abuse.
4. The potential offender or some other factor had to undermine or *overcome a child's possible resistance* to the sexual abuse.

Motivation

Finkelhor suggests three components combine to generate a motivation to have sexual contact with a child: intimacy with children satisfies profound emotional needs in the offender (emotional congruence); men who offend are sexually aroused to children (sexual arousal); and men have sex with children because they are unable to meet their sexual needs in socially appropriate ways (blockage). The varying 'mixture' of these components between different individuals or at different stages may help to explain variations regarding victim choice, and the strength and persistence of motivation.

Overcoming internal inhibitors

We do not know how many people have a motivation to abuse but are inhibited from acting on it. But for those who have abused, we know most will have had to quieten their consciences in order to perpetrate their abuse. This internal dialogue will vary between offenders and victim choice. Some will persuade themselves that children (at the relevant age) are interested in and benefit from sexual activity with a loving adult or parent; or that the children were so young they wouldn't remember; or that it was a wholesome part of their sexual education; or that 'all men think about sex with children' and 'if it was so wrong, why does the internet have so many naked images of children'. Some will have used alcohol or drugs to assist in their own disinhibition.

Post abuse, the offender may resolve not to repeat the behaviour but over time such resolve may weaken. In the absence, often, of the child reporting the abuse, the offender may convince himself that this was because the child approved of the behaviour and wishes to repeat it.

With the passing of time and repetition of abuse, internal inhibitors are likely to erode, potentially to the point of seeming non-existence. Of course a small proportion of offenders are psychopathic or sadistic, when a social conscience and a concern for others are largely absent. In addition, due to their own family background and social learning, some individuals will believe that sexual contact between an adult and a child is fine. Such individuals may not go on to abuse out of a fear of the consequences of detection, rather than out of concern for the harm caused.

Overcoming external inhibitors

In order to abuse, the motivated and disinhibited offender must manipulate or exploit third parties who might prevent the abuse. Typically within a family situation such third parties include mothers, siblings, other relatives and neighbours. These otherwise protective factors in a child's life may be incapacitated due to sickness, bereavement, learning difficulties, mental ill-health or other factors. Mothers may themselves be intimidated or abused by the abuser, so that even if they witness the sexual abuse of their child, they are afraid to intervene or report, or they may be unable to acknowledge what is happening due to their own abusive experiences in childhood. In addition, many abusers are seen as kind and caring individuals by those around them. Perhaps as much as anything, the media portrayal of paedophiles as 'monsters' disables potential protectors as they cannot equate such portrayals with a loved or trusted adult within a family environment – they can't, then, accurately interpret the concerning behaviours that may go on around them.

Overcoming the resistance of the child

Whilst it should not simply be left to children to be their own protectors, it must not be denied that most children have some capacity to avoid or resist abuse. Some, of course, grow up in an environment in which there are few appropriate sexual boundaries, so the child may not learn at home about what is 'normal' and what is not. This is not to blame them when they have suffered abuse, but rather to remind us all that children need appropriate information as well as the confidence to know that 'saying no' and reporting unwanted sexual contact is the right thing to do.

Abusers undoubtedly sense that some children are not good targets for abuse, due to their likely resistance or their likely reporting. Children who are emotionally insecure, needy or unsupported are particularly vulnerable. The offender can offer attention, affection or bribes; he or she can corrupt (e.g. through exposure to pornography), confuse, intimidate and threaten. Whilst most abusers will manipulate their child victims at a number of levels, others will simply use brute force and threats to gain compliance and silence.

We know that children very often feel they are to blame for the abuse, and may be additionally distressed at the fact of any physiological arousal or pleasure they experienced. However, despite how any professional audience may regard the behaviour, we must remember that, in the minds and words of the abuser and

Figure 4.1
Four preconditions to sexual abuse (adapted from Finkelhor 1984).

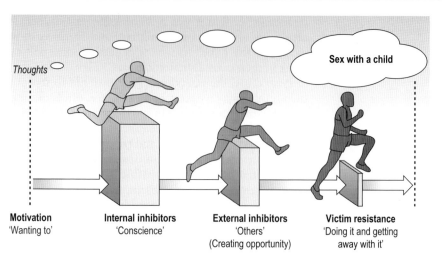

Thoughts

Sex with a child

Motivation
'Wanting to'

Internal inhibitors
'Conscience'

External inhibitors
'Others'
(Creating opportunity)

Victim resistance
'Doing it and getting away with it'

victim, the 'abuse' word may never figure. The abuser may see the behaviour as an expression of 'love' and may have manipulated and confused the child to see it in the same light. In view of this, and of the dependence created and the fear of the consequences of telling, it is little surprise that so few child victims are able to report what is happening to them.

Figure 4.1 illustrates a representation of Finkelhor's model developed by therapists with the Lucy Faithfull Foundation in their work at the Wolvercote Clinic, who found it helpful to share this model with all parties involved – abusers, victims, family members, professionals – using the 'hurdles' image and the notion of a journey or 'race'. All the parties could then help construct the detail of each part of this journey to help make sense of the process of abuse: to help them see how they manipulated or were manipulated; to help them take appropriate responsibility for their parts in the past but, more critically, their parts in a safer future.

Wolf's 'cycle of sexual abuse'

The cyclical, self-reinforcing, addictive nature of sexual offending was usefully illustrated by Wolf in his 'multifactor model of deviant sexuality' (Wolf 1985). Whilst developed little by Wolf himself, his work has been taken by others, typically practitioners, to aid a more extensive understanding of the different patterns of offending seen in different offenders and in different contexts (Eldridge 1998, Sullivan 2002, Carich & Calder 2003). The components he acknowledges in his model include:

- motivation (or pro-offending thinking and behaviour)
- sexual fantasy, rehearsal and masturbation
- targeting of a child
- grooming of victims, others and environment
- abuse
- guilt and fear
- cognitive distortions.

To attain some sense of the process suggested by Wolf, see Figure 4.2. Wolf's explanation is as follows.

An early history of physical and emotional abuse, sexualisation or neglect, leads to the development of deviant sexual interests. The child learns inappropriate behaviours and develops a poor self-image, alongside a belief that men have the

Figure 4.2
The developing cycle of sexual abuse (adapted from Wolf 1985).

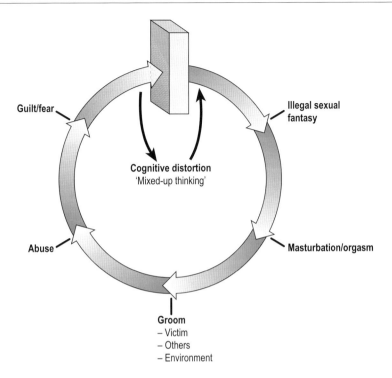

power to control the lives of weaker individuals. A second factor in Wolf's model is the presence of disinhibitors, which disrupt the normal social control against sexual deviance. These disinhibitors might be drugs or alcohol, or perhaps less obviously pornography and media messages that normalise sexual deviance. A third necessary factor is deviant sexual fantasy – the offender learns that sexual fantasy feels good and offers an escape from uncomfortable feelings of powerlessness and vulnerability. Masturbation to deviant fantasies positively reinforces associations with deviant sexual behaviour, increasing its attractiveness.

At this point the individual is a potential rather than an actual offender. Wolf suggests that some triggering event prompts feelings of inadequacy and powerlessness, causing the individual to withdraw into deviant sexual fantasy where he is in control and can feel good. The fantasy often incorporates an actual available, potential victim, who is targeted for abuse. The potential offender plans the abuse in fantasy, implementing this plan in reality through the grooming and manipulation of the victim as well those in a position to protect the victim or prevent the abuse. This also involves creating the opportunity for abuse – the time and the place. The offence is then carried out.

At various points around this cycle the individual is likely to experience guilt or fear, both whilst anticipating the abuse and following its commission. Wolf states that 'cognitive distortions' (mixed-up or twisted thinking) were present or developed by the offender to facilitate the whole process and, indeed, to reduce guilt. Such distortions are referred to as 'learned assumptions, sets of beliefs and self-statements about deviant sexual behaviours ... which serve to deny, justify, minimise and rationalise an offender's actions' (Calder 1999a, p. 122). Calder (1999a) also states that common cognitive distortions include the notions that:

- children want and benefit from sexual contact with adults
- children consent to such contact

- children are under no pressure to have sex with an adult
- sexual contact between an adult and a child is not harmful
- children are sexually seductive
- adult men are entitled to satisfy their sexual needs, no matter what cost to others.

The perpetrator is left with an underlying awareness that he has done something shameful, which further damages self-esteem, making further deviant sexual fantasising and offending more likely. Over time, and after a number of offences, the cycle is developed and maintained by increasingly distorted thinking and positive feelings associated with sexual release. Thus the sexual abuse serves both sexual and non-sexual needs, especially the need for power and control.

With its cyclical, self-reinforcing components, it is easy to understand why Wolf's model has proved attractive to assessors and treatment providers alike. While not without its limitations (Ward & Stewart 2003), it fits well into an understanding of addictive behaviours and, alongside Finkelhor's model, assists in the application of relapse prevention techniques (Laws 1989, Pithers 1990). In treatment, offenders identify their own patterns of offending. Once these are articulated, they can be explored in detail, with the offenders identifying ways in which these cycles can be broken. As in areas such as substance misuse, such work involves anticipating risky situations based on past behaviours, and planning/implementing strategies to avoid these risks, or manage them without relapsing (abusing). Ideally, such strategies involve the offender himself operating with the support of other individuals working in a personal or professional capacity (Mann 2004, Brown 2005).

How risky are sex offenders?

'A risk is a hazard that is incompletely understood, and whose occurrence therefore can be forecast only with uncertainty' (Hart *et al.* 2003, p. 207). When considering risk, it is critical that we define our terms. Risk of reconviction is very different from risk of reoffending, or indeed risk of causing harm. Low risk of reconviction in an incest offender does not, necessarily, translate into low risk to children in a family environment. Some high-risk offenders may not be regarded as particularly dangerous; for example, those who indecently expose have a high likelihood of repetition, but, typically, cause less harm than those who commit contact sexual offences. So what do we know of sex offenders' risk? How can we measure and express it, and what can we do to reduce or extinguish it?

Whatever the public belief, it is important to acknowledge that only some 20% of those convicted of sexual offences against children are reconvicted for similar offences (Grubin 1998, Hanson & Bussiere 1998). There are subgroups of offenders that can be identified with much higher reconviction rates, and it is one task of risk assessment instruments or protocols to identify individuals in such groups. Whilst accepting that risk of reconviction across the population of sex offenders is low, it is also persistent, i.e. some will reconvict many years after their initial conviction. In the recent study by Cann and colleagues of 419 sex offenders released from prisons in England and Wales, 10% reoffended within 2 years, 16% within 5 years, 20% within 10 years and 25% within 21 years. Thus 5% were reconvicted for the first time more than 10 years after release from prison (Cann *et al.* 2004).

Studies consistently show that exhibitionists have the highest recidivism rates, followed by extrafamilial offenders (with most studies suggesting that those who offend against boys *and* girls, or those who exclusively offend against boys, have higher recidivism rates than extrafamilial offenders who exclusively abuse girls), with the lowest reconviction rates being found in intrafamilial offenders (Brown

2005). For example, Marshall and Barbaree report recidivism rates of between 41 and 71% for exhibitionists, 13–40% for extrafamilial offenders against boys, 10–29% for extrafamilial offenders against girls and 4–10% for incest offenders (Marshall & Barbaree 1990).

Given the acknowledged low rate of reporting and of conviction, we must recognise the limitations of reconviction rates as evidence of risk of reoffence. For example, if the victims of incest appear least likely to report of all victims (Russell 1983), then may the low reconviction rates of such offenders be more a consequence of lower reporting rates than of less reoffending? Attempts have been made to assess *reoffending* rates as opposed to reconviction rates through the use of records held by police and child protection agencies. Marshall and Barbaree concluded that there were 2.4 reoffences for every official reconviction (Marshall & Barbaree 1988). Taking a broader definition of recidivism – one that includes all 'offence-related sexual behaviour' – Falshaw and colleagues suggest that the official reconviction rate must be multiplied by a factor of 5.3 to achieve a fair view of recidivism (Falshaw *et al.* 2003). Whatever cautions these studies suggest in our judgement about convicted offenders' risk, we must not assume that these 'multipliers' can be applied *uniformly* across all groups of offenders.

Some features in groups of offenders and types of offending are shown, through research, to relate to elevated risk. The single strongest predictor of risk is deviant sexual preference, i.e. where deviant sexual interest is greater than any non-deviant sexual interest. Number and type of prior sexual convictions are also strong predictors: those with more previous convictions are higher risk, as are those with male victims, stranger victims and non-contact offences. Young adults (18–24 years) tend to reconvict more than older adults, as do those diagnosed with antisocial personality disorder. Those who started, but failed to complete treatment, are also shown to be at increased risk (Hanson & Bussiere 1998).

It is important that child protection workers are aware of the current debate, particularly within criminal justice circles, about the respective merits of two different approaches to risk assessment: actuarial and clinical. Actuarial techniques currently focus on a small number of factors known from research to be associated with the reconviction of sex offenders. In allocating the assessed offender into a category – low, medium, high, very high risk – probability of reconviction is established. Reconviction rates for those categories are 10%, 20%, 40% and 60%, respectively, using Risk Matrix 2000, the actuarial instrument used in public protection agencies across the UK and applied to adult male offenders (Grubin 2004). Such instruments are highly effective at identifying the small group of offenders who will reconvict at a high rate. However, they tend to underestimate risk in first-time offenders (e.g. intrafamilial offenders with female victims). Currently, such instruments can only be used with convicted populations, as they are validated on samples drawn from this population.

Clinical risk assessments focus on the pathology of the individual being assessed and, unlike actuarial techniques, can accommodate all features the assessor considers relevant. Critics of clinical risk assessment emphasise a lack of structure and consistency and the potential biases they incorporate. However, they can and do often incorporate idiosyncratic features that may be especially relevant to the particular case being assessed, including context of risk (e.g. family home with specific children), allowing risk management and intervention strategies to be more readily identified (Hart *et al.* 2003, Grubin 2004). As Kemshall concludes, regarding convicted offenders, the ideal is a 'comprehensive risk assessment' combining the features of both actuarial and clinical approaches (Kemshall 2001).

What then, of internet child pornography offenders? This particular field is changing rapidly and our understanding remains only partial. Research from across the world provides evidence of great variations in contact sex offending by those found in possession of child pornography (Calder 2004a, Quayle *et al.* 2006), though it is the case that children are sexually abused in order to satisfy the demand for such images. The process of obtaining child pornography has undergone a huge transformation with the arrival of the internet, and the motivation of the viewer *may* be different – less well formed, potentially more a curiosity than an established sexual interest – than we would expect of an individual who sought out print or video material at personal cost and risk.

Questions are yet to be answered about the relationship between the nature of the child pornography and the likelihood of contact sex offending against children by the viewer. Whilst courts currently sentence more severely those with larger collections of images of the most abusive nature (i.e. younger children, with portrayals of sexual activity or violence involving adults), practitioners are finding that those viewing less extreme material (e.g. posed, naked pictures of lone adolescents) may represent a more immediate risk of acting out their sexual interests in such children. The internal inhibitors may be fewer and the opportunities greater.

The practitioner is encouraged to engage with the most current research evidence in this particular area before arriving at conclusions, recognising that information placed in the public domain is often partial at best.

Sex offender treatment

Given the potentially devastating consequences of sexual offending on victims and their families, implementing effective approaches to sex offender treatment is critical in order to reduce future risk of reoffending. Treatment programmes have proliferated over the years and have undergone considerable expansion in response to the development of new models, as well as research findings about sex offenders themselves and about treatment effectiveness (Carich & Calder 2003, Ward & Stewart 2003, Kemshall & McIvor 2004, Brown 2005). They are referred to here because many of the sex offenders being considered by child protection professionals will have had access to one or more of these programmes, or may be referred to one. Those professionals involved need to understand something of the content of such programmes, the evidence of their effectiveness and the research evidence on their impact upon risk of reoffence.

Sex offender treatment programmes for adult males in England and Wales are almost exclusively provided for currently convicted sex offenders by prison and probation services. In some areas of the country programmes may additionally be made available by health providers or by non-governmental organisations (e.g. NSPCC). However, such provision is patchy and small in scale. Whoever is the provider, no-one claims that sex offender treatment is a 'cure' but rather assists in the development of self-management.

Groupwork is seen as the most effective means of programme delivery (Mandeville-Norden & Beech 2004), with programmes typically running for between 100 and 240 hours in total, depending on perceived treatment need. Such need is determined by assessment, which would normally include the use of actuarial measures as well as psychometric (self-report) tests.

A primary goal of these cognitive–behavioural programmes (i.e. they target the thinking errors and their associated behaviours) is the reduction of cognitive distortions and other distorted attitudes (Marshall *et al.* 1999). As well as addressing such patterns of dysfunctional thinking, programmes consistently target the 'offence-specific problems' of lack of victim empathy as well as deviant sexual arousal. Some offenders have additional 'socio-affective problems' (e.g. low self-esteem and poor assertiveness and relationship skills). The latter often relate to a sense of isolation and subsequent gravitation towards children as a source of comfort and intimacy. Learning from these aspects is undertaken alongside an increasing understanding of the offender's personal pattern of offending through the use of the Finkelhor, Wolf and similar models. Relapse prevention techniques are then taught, assisting the offender to acknowledge situations or feelings that might precipitate risk, developing strategies and techniques to manage or avoid such risks. As well as focussing on such *avoidant* activity, current programmes are more actively exploring the use of the 'good lives model' of sex offender intervention.

> This [model] requires clinicians to offer concrete possibilities for living good or worthwhile lives that take into account each individual's abilities, circumstances, interests and opportunities … we should be clear about what are reasonable possibilities and help them acquire the requisite skills and capabilities to increase their chances of living such lives. An enhancement model, not a harm avoidance one, should drive the rehabilitation of offenders.
>
> (Ward & Stewart 2003, p. 27)

For some (perhaps many) offenders, family life with children may be one aspiration. The question for professionals is whether such an aspiration is 'reasonable' with regard to offender motivation and, particularly, child protection.

As for the evidence of effectiveness of sex offender treatment programmes, the literature is not fully conclusive, though it is broadly optimistic. Part of the difficulty is in variance in programme design, delivery and treatment populations; part is in the low base rate for reconvictions of sex offenders, requiring long-term studies to allow confidence in results. However, Hanson's recent meta-analysis of 43 treatment outcome studies found that sex offenders who participated in cognitive–behavioural treatment had significantly lower rates of sexual recidivism than those who did not undertake such treatment. Untreated sex offenders recidivated at a rate of 17% compared with a rate of 10% for those who had completed treatment programmes (Hanson *et al.* 2002).

Regarding family contact and reconstruction

Where, following abuse, contact with the family is being considered and, indeed, where family reconstruction is a possibility, the satisfactory completion of treatment, as outlined above, would normally be a prerequisite. But it should not, in itself, be sufficient reassurance to professionals about the future safety of the children. Eldridge and Still (1998) have considered a complex range of issues that need attention.

Invariably, the offender's own progress in treatment is one factor, including his acceptance of full responsibility for his offending, his development of empathy for his victims, his recognition of the needs of his children as paramount, his development of a comprehensive relapse prevention plan and his recognition both of his own responsibility for future self-management and of the role of significant adults (professional, family and other) in such future risk management. In addition, his partner will need to have undertaken her own work to have come to an understanding of the offender's responsibility for past offending, to have gained insight into the offender's patterns of behaviour and relapse prevention plan, and to recognise her children's needs as paramount. She also needs to be judged to be making her own free choice about family reconstruction, rather than being pressured into it.

In addition to the foregoing, the child victim and other children of the family need to have undertaken their own therapy. They, too, must be able to make a free choice regarding contact with the offender and family reconstruction. It is important that they recognise that responsibility for past offending is entirely that of the offender; they must be securely attached to their non-abusing parent, as well as having access to one or more adults outside the immediate family who they can confide in should concerns arise. Eldridge and Still also consider aspects relating to extended family and others (Eldridge & Still 1998).

Clearly, family reconstruction is a complex business if it is undertaken responsibly. It is attempted in rather more cases than it is achieved, but sometimes the attempt facilitates more informed decision making by the non-offending partner. Even if family reconstruction is not achieved, the attempt has a positive effect. Professionals need an awareness of the various components, many of which have application where past offenders are commencing a relationship with a new partner with children, or where children are in prospect.

Young people who sexually abuse

In contrast to adult sexual abusers, whom child welfare professionals largely relate to in terms of risk, children and young people who sexually abuse present a more complex set of dilemmas. They are children, but they may pose a danger to other children. They are sexual abusers, but they may also be victims of abuse. They have abused, but they may or may not continue to do so into adulthood.

This section will not attempt to provide answers as to what is 'normal' sexual behaviour for children and young people, or to give definitive explanations for the myriad causes of the inappropriate or abusive sexual behaviours that some children and young people may display. However, what it *will* attempt to do is to give readers a broad overview of the issues associated with children and young people who sexually abuse, briefly outline current policy and practice, and tentatively suggest some factors which professionals should bear in mind if they notice that a child or young person in their care is behaving in a sexually inappropriate or abusive manner.

In reflecting upon child maltreatment in general, and child sexual abuse in particular, there is an understandable tendency to think in terms of adult perpetrators and child victims. However, the truth of the matter is that some children and young people sexually abuse, and that this abuse may include serious acts such as rape. The exact extent to which young people are involved in the sexual abuse of others can never be known, but there is strong and consistent evidence which demonstrates beyond doubt that the sexual abuse perpetrated by young people is a significant element in the overall levels of abuse suffered by children and young people.

The most comprehensive recent study into the prevalence of child abuse and neglect in the UK (Cawson *et al.* 2000) found that:

The typical [sexual] abuser was likely to be someone close in age to the victim: most commonly identified as a boyfriend or girlfriend, but for many a fellow pupil or student, a brother's or sister's friend or 'someone recently met', which would include young people met at parties, 'raves' and other places where the young congregate. (p. 95)

This is an important finding, but one which many parents and professionals may find hard to accept, since it challenges the notion of childhood as a time of innocence and requires us to ask uncomfortable questions about why some children and young people might come to behave in such a manner. Hackett (2004) highlights the way in which Cawson *et al.*'s report was greeted with shock and disbelief in some parts of the media – a response which, he argues, is a demonstration of an ongoing climate of 'denial and disbelief' (Hackett 2004, p. 9) in relation to children and young people who sexually abuse others.

However hard it is to acknowledge the existence of this problem, an awareness of the possibility that some children and young people may sexually abuse *must* be incorporated into the mindset of all those who work with children. A failure to do so will inevitably impede efforts to safeguard children from abuse. What muddies the water, however, is that professionals need not only to acknowledge the possibility that children and young people may sexually harm or offend, but also to accept that not every act between children which could be construed as sexual in nature is necessarily abusive. Younger children in particular may engage in quasi-sexual experimentation – such as looking at, or even touching one another's genitals – as part of a natural curiosity about their bodies (Johnson 1999, quoted in Calder 2005a). This kind of behaviour must not be labelled as abusive if it occurs between children who participate voluntarily in this 'play' and are of similar age and ability. Recent reports from the United States suggest that, as awareness of the phenomenon of juvenile sexual abuse has risen, incidents in which very young children are inappropriately labelled as sexual abusers are also increasingly being identified (Johnson & Doonan 2005). This is clearly neither helpful nor just, particularly when the social and legal consequences of being labelled as a sexual abuser have the potential to permanently damage a young person's life chances (see Longo & Calder 2005 for a detailed discussion of the use of sex offender registration with young people who sexually abuse).

Before going further it is helpful to define what is meant by the term 'young people who sexually abuse', not least because many commentators (Masson 1995, Hoghughi 1997, Hackett 2004, Calder 2005a) have remarked upon the confusing and sometimes contradictory language that may be used in respect of this troubled and troubling group. Here, the term 'young person who sexually abuses' will be used in preference to the more concise but less forgiving term 'juvenile abuser'. This is in recognition of the fact that, as Hackett (2004) asserts, the latter phrase allows no space for the young person to be anything other than an abuser, neither permitting the possibility for change nor providing encouragement to do so. The term juvenile sexual offender will, however, be used when discussing those young people who have been judged by the criminal justice system to have committed a sexual offence.

The size and nature of the problem

Recent UK crime statistics support the estimate that somewhere between one-fifth and one-quarter of all sexual crimes in the United Kingdom are committed by juvenile offenders (Home Office 2005b). Whilst this provides a useful indicator of the proportion of sexual crimes perpetrated by juvenile, rather than adult, offenders, the absolute number of sexual crimes recorded in official youth crime statistics is low. In 2003/04, the most recent year for which figures are available, 1796 sexual offences are recorded as having been perpetrated by juvenile offenders, representing just 0.6% of total youth offending (Youth Justice Board 2005). However, these figures must be regarded with caution, since sexual crimes of all kinds are notoriously under-reported and most acts of sexual abuse by young people never come to the attention of any statutory authority (Vizard *et al.* 1995). Moreover, even those incidents that do come to the attention of social services, Youth Offending Teams or the police may not appear in official statistics, since it is common practice to divert alleged juvenile abusers away from the criminal justice system whenever possible (Vizard *et al.* 1995, Hoghughi 1997, Lovell 2002). To put this in some kind of perspective, Hoghughi (1997) estimated that only 10–15% of all cases where adolescents are *known* to have behaved in a sexually harmful or abusive manner ever become 'cases' in statutory services of any kind.

Crime statistics do not provide details regarding the nature of the sexual offences perpetrated, but research evidence supports the belief that many juvenile abusers have committed serious acts, including a high proportion of rapes or attempted rapes (Vizard *et al.* 1995, Dolan *et al.* 1996, James & Neil 1996, Manocha & Mezey 1998, Fyson 2005).

Moving away from statistics to examine the issue from a practice perspective, the type of act that practitioners and researchers include within the umbrella term 'sexual abuse' varies, but is most often divided into 'contact' and 'non-contact' abuse. The former may include actual or attempted anal or vaginal penetration, oral–genital contact or other forced contact of a sexual nature. The latter may include genital exposure/'flashing', watching others engaging in sexual activity, watching pornography or obscene telephone calls. Although all abuse impacts negatively on victims, contact abuse is likely to have more profound and damaging consequences. The high proportion of rape and attempted rape amongst the acts perpetrated by young people who sexually abuse is therefore of great concern.

The majority of victims of young people who sexually abuse are other children, typically known to the perpetrator and younger by an average of 3–5 years (Vizard *et al.* 1995, Dolan *et al.* 1996, James & Neil 1996, Hackett 2004). This is congruent with other findings (Cawson *et al.* 2000) that indicate the extent to which children and young people are responsible for child sexual abuse. It has been suggested that the preponderance of adolescents who sexually abuse other, younger, children is in part a consequence of the social space that adolescents inhabit, thus giving them access to younger children in a manner not available to potential adult abusers (Taylor 2003).

Characteristics of children and young people who sexually abuse

Crime statistics indicate that the vast majority of recorded juvenile sexual offending is perpetrated by males. The figures in Table 4.1 would suggest that juvenile sexual offending is an overwhelmingly male behaviour. Current research findings would also support the idea that the majority of young people who sexually abuse are male, although several recent studies indicate that the proportion of females involved may be higher than offender statistics indicate, at around 8–10% (James & Neil 1996, Blues *et al.* 1999, Taylor 2003). This suggests that there are differences in the way that statutory services, including education, social services and the police, respond to male and female juvenile abusers, with the former more likely than the latter to be criminalised.

The peak age for sex offending amongst males is consistently found to be between the ages of 12 and 16 (Glasgow *et al.* 1994, Vizard *et al.* 1995, Hoghughi 1997, Hackett 2004). This finding is constant across prevalence studies, incidence studies and offender statistics. Individuals aged 12–16 are more than twice as likely to perpetrate acts of sexual abuse than children or adults of any other age. It has been suggested that one of the contributory factors in sexually abusive behaviour, which may account for the peak in sexually abusive behaviour at this age, is the surge of testosterone that accompanies the onset of puberty for males (Glasgow *et al.* 1994, Hackett 2004).

Table 4.1
Sexual offences by gender
2003/04

	Male	Female	Total
Number	1766	30	1796
Percentage	98%	2%	100%

(From Youth Justice Board 2005.)

A number of other characteristics are consistently reported as evident at higher rates amongst samples of young people who sexually abuse in comparison to their non-abusing peers. These are:

- prior experiences as victims of abuse and neglect
- educational underachievement and/or learning disabilities
- problems with empathy and attachment.

Each of these will be addressed in turn, but it is important to remember that these *average* similarities mask a broad span of *individual* differences. There are currently no known predictive factors that make it possible to determine, prior to an abusive act being committed, whether any particular young person will sexually abuse others.

Similarly, although it has long been understood that many, or even most, adult male sex offenders may have begun their careers of sexual abuse as adolescents (Longo & Groth 1982), for the majority of young people it is a behaviour which they outgrow. However, based on current knowledge, it is not possible to predict which young people who sexually abuse will simply grow out of such behaviours and which will develop into adult sex offenders. The implications of this for professional practice are that it is never safe to ignore sexually inappropriate or abusive behaviour amongst young people.

Prior experiences as victims of abuse and neglect are common amongst populations of young people who sexually abuse others. Studies report high rates of sexual abuse, ranging from 25% (Dolan *et al.* 1996) to 29% (Manocha & Mezey 1998), or even 35% (James & Neil 1996). This has led to the use of the term 'victim-abuser' which encourages professionals to recognise the dual needs of these young people. The same studies, as quoted above, also demonstrate a strong correlation between young people who sexually abuse and childhood experiences of physical abuse, with reported rates of 30%, 24% and 42%, respectively. Other studies have also noted a positive relationship between young people witnessing domestic violence and their engaging in sexually abusive behaviour (Bailey & Boswell 2002). However, there is no direct or linear relationship between experiencing childhood abuse and perpetrating acts of sexual abuse (Freidrich 1998), and the majority of children who are victims of abuse will never harm others.

High rates of *educational underachievement and/or learning disabilities* are also noted in many studies of young people who sexually abuse (Bagley 1992, Vizard *et al.* 1995, Manocha & Mezey 1998). However, as studies of adult males who sexually abuse do not indicate any over-representation of men with learning disabilities (Hayes 1991), this finding may be a consequence of the fact that most studies of young people who sexually abuse are based upon clinical populations (i.e. young people who have been referred for treatment). There are many reasons why young people with learning disabilities might be over-represented in a clinical sample (O'Callaghan 1999), including a lack of confidence amongst non-specialist social workers or Youth Offending Team workers in their ability to work effectively with these young people (Fyson 2005), resulting in a tendency to refer on to clinical services.

Problems with empathy and attachment are a common finding in those studies which have examined the psychological well-being and/or dysfunction of young people who sexually abuse. Barbaree *et al.* (1998) identify intimacy deficits and severe emotional loneliness as being amongst the key causative factors associated with sexually abusive behaviours; others have highlighted attachment insecurity as another predisposing factor (Smallbone 2005). However, it must be borne in mind that these are explanations for behaviours rather than predictive factors.

UK policy and practice

As the above summary indicates, much of the available information regarding young people who sexually abuse is drawn from either clinical samples or criminal statistics and, as such, may be of more use to professionals as background information, rather than directly supporting their practice. This rather medicalised and academic approach to a social and very concrete problem is arguably reflected in current UK policy: despite the relatively high public profile of child sexual abuse, the government response to the challenges posed by children and young people who sexually abuse others remains muted and lacking in coherence (Lovell 2002). The *Working Together* guidance on inter-agency working to safeguard children (DoH *et al.* 1999) states that 'such children are likely to be children in need' (p. 70), and appears to discourage the use of child protection conferences for young people identified as having sexually abused others. The extent to which this guidance is adhered to by practitioners remains uncertain, but it is known that at least some local authorities are explicitly rejecting the approach prescribed by government in favour of their own procedures (Fyson *et al.* 2003) which emphasise the need for ongoing supportive intervention and regular opportunities for risk assessment.

The impossibility of predicting which young people who sexually abuse others are likely, without effective interventions, to continue their abusive patterns of behaviour into adulthood provides professionals with an imperative to intervene early and effectively. However, it is apparent that in many cases this does not happen. Generic social workers and other professionals who work closely with young people may feel that they lack the skills necessary to work with young people who sexually abuse (Ladwa-Thomas & Sanders 1999). Referring on for therapeutic help would appear to be the obvious solution, but provision of such specialist services remains at best patchy (Masson & Hackett, 2003). Furthermore, there is evidence that the scarcity of therapeutic services has led to some young people with learning disabilities who sexually abuse being denied therapy because it may take them longer than other young people to fully engage with, and benefit from, talking therapies (Fyson 2005).

As a consequence of this lack of specialised therapeutic services, many young people who sexually abuse will remain the responsibility of social services' child protection teams or, where the criminal justice system has become involved, the Youth Offending Team. It is therefore important that these teams develop ways of working that acknowledge the danger which young people who sexually abuse may pose to other children; for example, if the young person can no longer live with their own family they should not be placed in a foster home where there are vulnerable younger children.

In working with young people who sexually abuse, the development of an effective risk management framework is essential. Such frameworks facilitate the systematic assessment of the risk which the young person may continue to pose to others and balance these against any existing protective factors. This approach can help to clarify the decision-making process and ensure that *all* relevant factors are taken into consideration (Calder 2001a). An understanding of risk as a dynamic construct is central to a good risk management framework, as is the principle that young people can and should be encouraged to take responsibility for managing their own risk (McCarlie & Brady 2005). The risk that a young person who sexually abuses presents will vary over time and be influenced by a variety of factors, including their home environment, their family, their school and their social influences, as well as the effectiveness of input from professionals. It is therefore important to work not only with the young person, but also with other 'risk factors' – particularly the young person's family (Hackett *et al.* 2002) – in order to minimise risk most effectively.

Professionals' responses

In the face of current deficiencies in the provision of specialist services, what action should frontline child welfare professionals take in response young people who display sexually harmful or abusive behaviours?

First, it is important simply that professionals acknowledge that children and young people can and do sexually abuse others. This is especially important for teachers, youth workers and other professionals who have regular, direct contact with children and young people, since they are best placed to spot inappropriate sexual behaviour before it develops into more serious acts of abuse.

Second, all relevant information must be systematically recorded and shared with other professionals as necessary. The *Every Child Matters* Green Paper (Chief Secretary to the Treasury 2003) and the Children Act 2004 together provide a framework for the provision of holistic children's services, but they must now be put into effective practice.

Finally, whilst working to safeguard children and young people from abuse, professionals must also remember that young people who sexually abuse others are still children, often children who have themselves suffered abuse, and children with a great need for support and understanding in order to enable them to change.

Conclusion

To summarise, we have come to know a great deal about sex offenders and the process of offending, but the more we learn the more we realise how much is still to know.

What is beyond doubt is that child sexual abuse has been present across the lifespan of mankind and it continues to cause tremendous harm to a large proportion of our population. The statutory agencies are involved in only a small proportion. Whilst such agencies and their workers must undertake their roles armed with the knowledge and skills that the latest research and practice can offer, it is imperative that all adults in our communities be given sufficient and sound information to feel empowered to recognise abuse or its potential and to take action to prevent it – child protection has to be 'everybody's business'.

Key points and messages for practice

- Wolf and Finkelhor gave us some highly useable models to understand the behaviour of sex offenders and the process whereby others are manipulated, including victims and potential protectors. Practitioners need to keep these models in their 'back pocket' and use them to make sense of situations where child sexual abuse is known or suspected. They not only help to unravel the past but also give crucial frameworks for helping create a safer future.

- Given that so many children are sexually abused, so few offences are reported and so few of these reported offences achieve a conviction, the professional community must recognise its limited 'reach'. Crucially, it must work to ensure that all adults, including potential offenders, their friends and families, and the parents and carers of young people with sexually worrying behaviour are aware of the extent of abuse and the role all can play in prevention. We must recognise that prevention is better than cure, and, with the necessary knowledge and support, child protection can be everybody's business.

■ Although many adult sexual abusers begin their offending careers during adolescence, most juvenile sexual abusers will not continue to offend as they grow older. A useful analogy to help remember this is to think that although many professional footballers began playing as children, most children who play football do not grow up to become professional football players.

■ It is not possible to predict which children and young people displaying inappropriate sexual behaviours will develop into young people who sexually abuse, nor which young people who sexually abuse will continue abusing and become adult paedophiles. It is therefore important to identify, and respond to, sexually inappropriate or abusive behaviours in all children and young people as soon as they are noticed.

Annotated further reading

Calder M 2001 Juveniles and children who sexually abuse: frameworks for assessment, 2nd edn. Russell House, Lyme Regis

Aimed at practitioners, this volume outlines the key variables which must be taken into account when assessing the ongoing risk posed by young people who sexually abuse and provides a framework for the management of cases.

Calder M (ed) 2002 Young people who sexually abuse: building the evidence base for your practice. Russell House, Lyme Regis; Calder M (ed) 2005 Children and young people who sexually abuse: new theory, research and practice developments. Russell House, Lyme Regis

Two edited volumes which gather together the latest research and practice evidence from across the English-speaking world. They provide a wealth of information regarding the causes, consequences and (risk) management of young people who sexually abuse.

Calder M (ed) 2004 Child sexual abuse and the internet: tackling the new frontier. Russell House, Lyme Regis

A recent collection of (almost) current understanding about the internet, child pornography and its relationship to child sexual abuse. In a rapidly changing technological context, a very useful insight into the range of ways in which the internet is used by those with a sexual interest in children, how we might approach assessment and treatment in this familiar and not so familiar population and how the internet may be promoting an increase in the sexual abuse of children.

Finkelhor D 1984 Child sexual abuse: new theory and research. Free Press, New York

The first highly readable exposition of Finkelhor's 'four preconditions to child sexual abuse' theory, with examples of its application. Whilst perhaps not as sophisticated or extensive as some more recent theoretical offerings, it provides a clear and robust framework for thinking about sex offending and its management, especially within a family context.

Hackett S 2001 Facing the future – a guide for parents of young people who have sexually abused. Russell House, Lyme Regis

One of few publications addressed directly to the parents of children and young people with sexually problematic behaviour. Highly readable and practical, including content on 'normal' sexual behaviour, as well as on the development of problematic sexual behaviour, the setting of boundaries, the partnership between professionals and parents and a way forward. A realistic and hopeful perspective.

Hackett S 2004 What works for children and young people with harmful sexual behaviours? Barnardos, Ilford

A readable and succinct review of the current literature, including evidence concerning the association between victimisation and abusive behaviour, the causes of sexually abusive behaviours in young people and indicators of best practice in relation to assessment, intervention, reoffence risk and case management.

Itzin C (ed) 2000 Home truths about child sexual abuse. Routledge, London

A remarkable, broad-ranging 'reader', with content including the excruciating detail of individuals' victim experiences and the details and limitations of research, the wisdom of those who assess and treat offenders, victims and families, and the insights of those who influence policy. A really useful source book and touchstone to remind practitioners of the many issues and perspectives that need addressing if we are to combat child sexual abuse.

Lovell E 2002 'I think I might need some more help with this problem ...'. Responding to children and young people who display sexually harmful behaviour. NSPCC, London

Provides a solid overview of the research base and complements this with a thorough analysis of UK law, policy and guidance relating to this issue.

Ward T, Laws D R, Hudson S (eds) 2003 Sexual deviance: issues and controversies. Sage, Thousand Oaks, CA

For those who want a good overview of the 'journey so far' in our understanding of sex offender assessment and treatment. It includes the debate over the best means to assess risk, the experience of technological insight gained through the measurement of deviant sexual arousal, the use of chemicals to suppress arousal, the distortions of offenders and how to combat these, a review of the theories developed over the last quarter century, with an exposition of the 'good lives' model, modern sex offender management strategies and policy and a plea for a public health approach to prevention. All in bite-sized pieces.

Useful websites

The Lucy Faithfull Foundation: www.lucyfaithfull.co.uk

This charity works to safeguard children from sexual abuse by assessing and treating people who have perpetrated, or are affected by, child sexual abuse. They also contribute to legislation, policy and procedure reviews concerned with safeguarding children in faith communities, in schools, in leisure facilities, on the internet and living away from home.

Respond: www.respond.org.uk

Respond works with adults and children with learning disabilities who have either perpetrated an act of sexual abuse and/or have been victims of abuse. Freephone helpline: 0808 808 0700

Stop It Now!: www.stopitnow.org.uk

This organisation aims to prevent child sexual abuse by encouraging abusers and potential abusers, their family and friends, to seek help. It provides information intended to help adults recognise worrying behaviour in themselves or others, and aims to give them the confidence to take responsible action when they suspect that something is wrong. Freephone helpline: 0808 1000 900

NOTA (National Organisation for the Treatment of Abusers): www.nota.co.uk

NOTA is the only professional multidisciplinary organisation in the UK dedicated to work with sexual abusers. It aims to enhance public protection by enabling practitioners to develop and share best practice via its conferences, training, newsletters and publication of the *Journal of Sexual Aggression*.

5 Common forms and consequences of child abuse

Helga Hanks and Peter Stratton

INTRODUCTION

Progress in the protection of children from maltreatment requires a full recognition of the range of forms that abuse may take, of the indicators that a child may be being abused, and of the consequences of abuse. At present, despite recent contributions such as those by Browne *et al.* (2002a), Reece (2001) and a section on child abuse in *Forfar & Arneil's Textbook of Paediatrics* by Hobbs *et al.* (2003), we cannot claim to have advanced as far in any area as we might have hoped. It is therefore necessary to interpret the theory and evidence that we do have available in order to achieve as clear a picture as possible. In individual cases it is essential to be able to judge the level of risk the child is exposed to by being left in the abusive family, what aspects of abuse are most damaging and therefore are the most urgent targets for protection, and what consequences, both short and long term, the child may need professional help to overcome. In addition, much diagnosis and detection depends on working back from signs (physical and behavioural) in the child to forms of abuse known to produce these signs. At a service level, an estimate of the effects of abuse is needed to plan services, and to specify the training needed by workers. Nationally and internationally, a realistic understanding of the widespread and serious consequences of abuse would indicate the scale of need, the urgency of the problem, and the resources needed to tackle it.

There are many factors that work against being able to make even an approximate evaluation of the effects of abuse. This is true both for individual cases and in the general context. The history of child abuse has been one in which clear medical evidence has been the first, and necessary, indicator before the problem was accepted. Even in physical abuse more than 40 years after Kempe's seminal paper (Kempe *et al.* 1962) medical consequences of abuse are still regarded as more tangible evidence (Hobbs *et al.* 2003) and are better understood than the psychological consequences. But the resistance to recognising the full range and severity of the effects of abuse goes much deeper. Abuse is a painful reality and everybody, given the chance, would prefer to avoid the pain of recognising it. Maybe our own relative terrors as children, or our inadequacies as parents, are brought closer to awareness as we encounter obvious examples of abuse. And of course, many professionals and policy makers who work in this field have been victims of earlier maltreatment in their own lives. Finally, by confronting maltreatment we risk becoming aware of our own capacity to abuse and also risk being overwhelmed by the scale and horror of the problem.

Because of the variety of factors working against a clear recognition of the effects of maltreatment, we start this chapter with a consideration of two sources of difficulty: myths about children, and the power of denial. Next we provide a framework for understanding the consequences of maltreatment which is designed to give full weight to psychological as well as physical effects. The core of the chapter uses representative examples from the great volume of published research and clinical experience to map out the major consequences in different areas of child maltreatment.

Perceptions of children: what really creates a 'spoilt child'

During the twentieth century, Western society gave considerable thought and discussion to the issue of how children should be brought up. We entered the so-called 'child centred' era. With hindsight we can easily detect deficiencies in earlier views, and with insight we may even criticise our current beliefs. Two themes that apply both to the past and the present relate to the idea that if children get their way they will become too powerful and the rather contradictory image of the child as a helpless recipient of influence. What seems to unite the two positions is an assumption of conflict between what children want and what parents want. Giving children what they want is assumed to be at the expense of parents and, indeed, many parents place themselves under financial and other stresses in order to provide material goods or an endless stream of events for their children. With such a limited and materialistic definition of the duties of good parents, it is not surprising that children are first seen as passive consumers of parental resources, and then become resented for having such power to demand what they do not appreciate.

The 4-hour feeding schedule is an example of a demand for compliance, sameness and the teaching of obedience. Here the rules are that the child that cries at night must not be picked up and comforted, the child who has not eaten their dinner must not have a pudding, there must be no talking during mealtimes, etc. These are just a few examples of what people generally think might spoil a child.

Though it is not an original idea, we would like to draw attention to what we consider to be the true meaning of a 'spoilt' child. Something being spoilt is defined in the dictionary as being damaged or injured, something made useless, valueless … destroyed. The paradoxical juxtaposition of the meaning of 'the spoilt child' in the English language alerts us to a fundamental ambivalence about the rights of children. When attempting to help maltreated children, professionals and parents alike have to take into consideration that these are the children that someone has tried to spoil, in the 'real' (dictionary) sense. Abused, maltreated children are the children that are at risk of being spoilt.

This issue is important for another reason. Many children, adolescents and adults who have been maltreated have, over the years, described how they feel. The cry from those who have been abused that they feel and are treated as 'damaged goods' is a stark reminder of what being spoilt really means.

The other myth, which can damage professional attempts to care for maltreated children, is of the child as a passive recipient of influence. Our whole approach to child rearing, and to education, reflects this assumption. We are very ready to talk of the effects of education, of child care practices and of maltreatment on the child. It is much more difficult to recognise that children are active participants in creating their worlds. Perhaps we are afraid of blaming the victim; perhaps it is just easier to see things from an adult's point of view. But damage is not primarily something that can be put into a child to be carried around, invisible inside them. Damaging environments are places in which children nevertheless have to function and grow. The ways they function and the form of their growth will be affected and that is what we need to understand. It may be helpful to think in terms of the child adapting to the environment. The important effects of abuse are at least as likely to be in the kinds of adaptations the child comes to make as in simple direct consequences. This is an idea we return to after considering the second issue that obstructs the clear recognition of the effects of abuse.

Denial

> In every eye there is a spot that is incapable of sight. The optic disc exists as a black hole right next to the central point of clearest vision. Yet anyone who has not learned the trick of finding it would swear that there is no such void.
>
> (Summit 1988, p. 51)

Kempe and Kempe (1984) pointed to the stages that society needs to go through in its progressive recognition of the reality of child abuse. These stages are progressive defences of denial to keep out a recognition of something that is unacceptable and at odds with the view we want to have of ourselves and our society. Equally we know very well that abused children may take refuge in denial to avoid the destructive effects of recognising what is being done to them. But, in our experience, even committed professionals still have to use denial in self-protection (Summit 1988).

Denial and the effects of abuse are intricately linked. The reader is referred particularly to Summit (1988) and Furniss (1991). The material that follows about the forms, function and areas of denial of child sexual abuse (CSA) has been taken from Furniss (1991).

Forms of denial

These can be seen in the context of the abuse being denied by the abuser, the non-abusing care giver, the child or other family members, as well as by professionals, the law and society as a whole. But focussing on the family system, each person might deny different aspects of the abuse. It may be total denial that any abuse has taken place or it may be partial denial of:

- abusive circumstances
- damaging effects, both on the child and family
- the addictive and repetitive nature of CSA by the perpetrator
- the abuser's responsibility.

The functions of denial

Denial is used because it is, in the short term, effective in reducing anxieties, which may relate to:

- the legal consequences
- consequences for family and relatives
- psychological consequences for both abused and abuser
- social consequences
- financial/work/career consequences.

There are several forms of denial by which to disclaim responsibility for abuse; for example:

- primary denial of any abuse
- denial of severity of acts
- denial of knowledge of abuse (perpetrators may say they were drunk, asleep, depressed, tired, etc.)
- denial that the maltreatment was abusive (this may involve pretending that the abuse was, for instance, a normal/educational activity)
- denial of the harmful effects of the abuse (the abusive act is said not to have harmed the child or only harmed them a little)

■ denial of responsibility (the perpetrator makes the child responsible for the abuse, saying that the child triggered the abuse by their behaviour).

Child maltreatment is linked to denial because the pain, helplessness, worthlessness and rejection that children feel when they are maltreated have to be hidden in some way. We have many examples in Western society which indicate that child abuse is much easier to blame on professionals who identify the children and the problem, than on an acknowledgement that all is not well in society and particularly in the family where unfortunately, but undeniably, most abuse takes place.

Case example 1

Keely, who is 9 years old, was in therapy because she had been severely maltreated all her life. She had been in care in a stable foster home for a number of months and recently began not only to disclose further specific incidences of her abuse but also to behave in a way that made it difficult to contain and look after her. She began hitting adults and children alike, ran away (the foster parents thought she was with older youngsters and experiencing sex), lied, stole and then felt terribly sorry, sobbing and pleading with the foster parents not to send her away. The discussions between the professionals and foster parents centred on the fact that Keely was going through a very difficult time in coming to terms with her previous abuse. One way of explaining what was happening is outlined below.

When children are maltreated consistently and severely (though what children can take varies from one to another), they have to build up some defences in order to bear what is happening to them. When there is no help to deal with the psychic pain, the pain becomes encapsulated, as if put into a sealed space. This idea comes from psychoanalytic literature and is called encapsulation (Ferenczy 1949). The sealed space might be thought of as a nut with a shell that has become harder over time and all the painful, angry, desperate feelings are contained within this nut.

However, when children like Keely have the chance to 'open up', so to speak, and feel secure to let the feelings come out (through a crack in the nut's shell if you like), the situation described above might occur.

During one therapy session, when Keely talked about what had been happening in the previous few weeks, the therapist told her the story of the nut and said: 'It feels as if nobody knows the strength of the feelings that are in this nut. It is such a surprise to you to discover some of the terrible feelings of revenge and anger you might have inside that nut. So much so that you feel that you could kill someone. (Keely had taken a broom and tried to hit her foster mother with it during the last week. She had also said afterwards that it was a terrible feeling because at that moment she could have killed her.) The feelings are so strong that at that moment of discovery they are difficult to control.' Keely, who had been sitting very still and listening, burst into tears and wept bitterly.

Becoming very sad is one reaction to abuse that needs to be worked through/tackled in therapy; being angry is another. But these children with their strong feelings also need some very practical input. In Keely's case, the therapist had a meeting with the child, the foster mother and the social worker and discussed with them the fact that Keely needed some help in managing her angry feelings. After this meeting the issues about setting boundaries, what could be done and what could not be done by Keely were discussed, particularly when she felt hopeless and out of control. It was suggested that she should try not to hurt either herself or others, should work out who to involve, ask for help and talk to at such times, and other specific actions. What Keely might do to minimise and avoid these difficult situations was discussed. The foster carers were asked to see Keely through these difficult times and not be afraid to call for help if they needed it from the social worker or others.

The concept of 'denial' has changed over the years and researchers and clinicians have been preoccupied with issues related to minimisation, how decisions and attitudes are formed and how child abuse can be missed or even ignored both in the public and professional setting. An important example can be found in the research carried out by Hetherton and Beardsall (1998) when they examined the reporting of females as perpetrators of sexual abuse. They discovered that female sexual abuse of children remains so rarely recognised because it seems to deviate both from cultural norms as well as the ideal of women as mother or caregiver and therefore not thought to be capable of such an act. An equally important example relating to the 'backlash' that has reverberated throughout the world in cases of child abuse is the discovery of children being sexually abused in the Dutch town of Oude Pekela which provoked a significant '… backlash in the Dutch nation. Sceptical people immediately labelled the case as mass hysteria' (Jonker & Jonker-Bakker 1997, p. 552).

Denial is also touched on in Arnold and Cloke's (1988) paper. Importantly, they talk of the reasons why abuse can keep its momentum to such an extent and see the cause in the fact that society keeps abuse hidden for all manner of reasons: personal, political and religious. 'Societal denial' of abuse, they recommend, can be lessened by creating child-friendly communities in which there is a climate where children can be heard, respected appropriately and listened to.

The earlier writings about denial and the clear naming of the phenomenon are still an important guide today. Calder *et al.* (2001, pp. 212–218) discuss the issues around denial when dealing with juveniles and children who sexually abuse. Bentovim (2002) spells out some of the issues in relation to the outcome research undertaken and reported by Monck *et al.* (1996) which, as Bentovim points out, demonstrated that: '… denial that abuse had occurred was the most frequent response by perpetrators in a series of 99 children' (see also Findlater and Fyson, Chapter 4, in this volume, on young perpetrators).

Considering and assessing the impact of denial and disbelief on the abused children, both in the short and long term, is central in thinking about consequences. This is particularly pertinent when parents, professionals and courts give messages that they do not believe the child and thereby compound the effects on the child. The impact that denial has on the '…mental health status [of the children] was also significantly related to whether the child was believed and supported by their mother, or whether they felt criticised and therefore felt a negative sense of self esteem' (Bentovim 2002, p. 290).

At a recent (2005) ISPCAN Conference in Berlin, Goddard reported his research into how children described their experience of abuse and how this affected them. He talked about the children being candid and very clear in their descriptions, telling the researchers how disempowered and vulnerable they felt. The title of the talk and a forthcoming book is *The Truth is Longer than a Lie*, the words of a 12-year-old girl who tried to explain to them that it was easier, and took much less time to deny, retracting her story of abuse and saying that it did not happen than telling the detail of the continuous abuse she suffered (Mudaly & Goddard 2006).

Once it is possible to recognise the range of factors which might make us underestimate the effects of abuse, we are better able to confront the huge amount of evidence on particular aspects of these effects.

Severity of abuse

The subject of severity has been a difficult one and has preoccupied different professional groups in various ways. The demand in the legal field for clarity and proof of the extent of the abuse is one requirement. The measurement of emotional and psychological consequences, the medical consequences of injuries and the social issues that are brought into the open about standards of care are other concerns. Horwath, in her chapter on assessment (see Chapter 13, in this volume) guides us through many of these issues and we will here briefly concentrate only on the subject of severity and how it might be measured. An 'invited commentary' by Hobbs (2005) highlights some important considerations. This comment raises the issues of how to measure severity: whether we should think of the length of time over which children have been hit, and therefore becoming chronic, or whether the frequency is more important. How to measure the force and associated violence with which children are physically abused is a part of the jigsaw of measuring severity. Hobbs made an important observation when he said that: 'The level of violence may be the same, the consequences vastly different' (p. 950). May-Chahal and Cawson (2005) reported on 2869 young adults in their important study to investigate the prevalence of child abuse and neglect in the UK. Without going further into this study the conclusions are a sad reflection of how far, or not, we have come in caring for our children. The authors state that: 'the maltreatment of children in the UK today remains an extensive social problem' (p. 969). (For further discussion of this issue, see May-Chahal and Mason, Chapter 12, in this volume.)

So far it has been difficult to quantify 'severity' of abuse and particularly the emotional and psychological consequences of child maltreatment. We know from the literature and research into some of the forms of abuse (i.e. emotional and sexual) that when a child is repeatedly abused over a long time the consequences are more severe. However, a caution is raised by research carried out by Barnett *et al.* (1993) who developed a system for measuring severity. They discovered that when they assessed 'mild' abuse of children it nevertheless turned out to have a powerful effect on the children's adjustment. This raised the concern that those children who come out of an assessment as having been abused 'mildly' in comparison to others would be excluded from treatment, their response to what happened not recognised and the psychological consequences ignored. If we follow this line of thinking, we might influence child care and parenting issues negatively by ignoring the extent to which the individual child in their particular circumstances may be affected detrimentally by child-rearing practices.

On the other hand, Hobbs (2005) points out that because as a society we rely heavily on controlling children by physical means we could fall into a pattern of assessing parental physical control of their children as abusive when it is not. May-Chahal and Cawson (2005) worked with newly developed definitions when examining the prevalence of physical abuse and lack of care. These are:

- serious/continuous physical abuse
- intermediate/intermittent physical abuse
- cause for concern.

Hobbs *et al.* (2003) divide the injuries received by the children into bruises, burns, fractures, etc. and then concentrate on describing the presentation and patterns of the physical injuries in exact terms and locations on the child's body. While this way of recording does not put the injuries into broader categories, it does give a graphic description and a sense of what the children have endured.

Brassard and Hardy (1997) discuss a range of assessment scales and techniques and recognise that a definition of severity in the legal arena is highly complicated.

They recommend the *Guidelines for the Psychosocial Evaluation of Suspected Psychological Maltreatment in Children and Adolescents* (APSAC 1995), which can determine both 'acts' of maltreatment and demonstrate the 'harm' that has either occurred or could occur in the future. However, in many American states, professionals are not permitted to make such a determination until after the evidence has been collected for court.

So there is a beginning of assessing the extent and severity of harm done. Certain scales can be useful but do not stand undisputed. Sanders and Becker-Lausen (1995) developed the Child Abuse and Trauma Scales (CATS), which measures three subscales – sexual abuse, punishment and neglect. Because the scale seemed to be robust, Kent and Waller (1998) added an emotional subscale to the CATS and had positive results, while admitting that further validation was essential.

Briere (1992) talks of the 'symptoms' of abuse and uses them as a guide or indicator to measure the impact of the abuse on the individual. However, this is not an assessment tool of severity but a tool to recognise what has happened to the person. The literature on resilience (Hawley & DeHaan 1996, Walsh 1996, Rutter 1999) may also give us some indication of the ways in which children react differentially to a variety of stressors, including abuse. Rutter (1999) usefully and importantly reviews the issues on resilience and the implications for when family therapy could be a preferred way of helping.

When a child has been physically abused, bruised, burnt and/or their bones broken (Hobbs *et al.* 1999, 2003, Reece & Ludwig 2001), an element of severity can be assessed. Is it a 40% burn? Is there one fracture or several? But even here the severity of the injury and the resulting emotional impact are difficult to assess. When we move to psychological consequences such as the trauma of physical and sexual abuse, the whole area of emotional and psychological abuse, and the consequences for attachments of being attacked in any way by someone close, the potential consequences now and in the future become even harder to judge.

Read (1998) links child abuse and severity of disturbance in an adult psychiatric population and comes to the conclusion that: '... child abuse may have a causative role in the most severe psychiatric conditions, including those currently thought to be primarily biological in aetiology' (p. 366).

The *Journal of Child Abuse and Neglect* devoted an entire Special Issue (English, DJ (ed) 2005) to the topics of definition, severity, chronicity and other dimensions which connect to the impact that abuse has on child development. Eight papers are based on the 'LONGSCAN' study of 545 maltreated children who are being followed up throughout their childhood. Although the articles are oriented to research, they are also an essential resource for practitioners who want to take classification beyond legal and administrative formats.

We now turn to review the kinds of effects that different forms of abuse may create. In order not to be overwhelmed by the complexity, we offer three sets of concepts to help coordinate the material: abuse as trauma; the child's adaptation to abuse; and the central issue of attachment.

Fundamental concepts in abuse

Trauma and neurobiological effects of abuse

Recent research on victims (often adult) of a variety of catastrophes has given us an understanding of the effects of trauma which is also helpful in making sense of events surrounding abuse. Briere (1992) gives a very clear account of the theory, practice and effects. Joseph (1999) has given an insight into the neurology of traumatic dissociative amnesia. He is critical of those denying the damage to certain structures in the brain and the functional integrity of the brain when trauma has occurred. His review of the literature is a helpful guide. He comes to the conclusion that trauma does affect the brain and has consequences which indicate that memory loss is only too common, particularly after repeated traumatic events. Glaser's (2000) review described the then new research and work looking at child abuse and neglect and the influences abuse has on the brain. Glaser (2005 and personal contact) developed her and colleagues' work on the subject. She pointed out that the physical, behavioural, cognitive and emotional consequences now have counterparts to the psychological consequences known so far and recognised in how these children's brain structure, chemistry and brain function are affected. The research into the neurobiological effects of child abuse is showing how particularly early abuse has consequences on the brain which are profound in their effects on abused children's later adjustment. Glaser (2005) said that: 'While the sequence of development within the brain is genetically determined, the nature of this development is determined to a considerable extent by the young child's experiences.' She continues by saying that some functions may not develop if the children have been abused and that negative behaviours and actions will affect the brain's connectivity. The important message this kind of research seems to highlight is that while we '… can add new learning and experiences throughout life into our brain structures and functioning, previous patterns cannot be erased, only added onto and more slowly'. Glaser concluded that: 'A further aspect of child maltreatment which has a profound effect on brain development is the significant neurobiological stress which the young child experiences.' She pointed out that it is the experience of a secure attachment which can protect the brain 'from the worst effects of stress'.

However, returning to the traumatic effects that children who have been abused may suffer, Bentovim (1992, p. 24) points out that:

Trauma comes from the Greek word meaning to 'pierce'. In the context of physical injury it implies that the 'skin is broken', that something intact has been breached. It implies a certain intensity of violence, with long-standing consequences for the organism. From the physical notion of trauma, the notion of psychological trauma arises: an event that in a similar intense or violent way ruptures the protective layers surrounding the mind with equally long-lasting consequences for psychic well-being. Helplessness overwhelms, mastery is undermined, defences fail, there is a sense of failure of protection, disintegration, acute mental pain as the memory of the event intrudes and replays itself repeatedly.

The traumatic stress response thus imperceptibly becomes the 'post-traumatic stress disorder'. This type of consequence might be seen in any victim of a traumatic event. A car accident, floods, fires, earthquakes and more personal tragedies will all be included.

The physical pain is closely linked to the psychological experience and pain of the individual. However, there is a difference between an adult's experience of trauma and that of a child. Something additional happens to children because they, by virtue of their age, are in a developmental stage in which they lack the perspectives by which adults can distinguish and make sense of the traumatic event in which they have been involved. Because trauma, and what it means to human beings, is so complex, it is helpful to differentiate two kinds of issue when considering the consequences of such an event:

- Short-term consequences
- Long-term consequences.

It must also be recognised that the effects of child abuse are dynamic and interact with each other; that the experiences and adaptations interweave and become part of the child's developmental process, shaping their view of the world and most importantly themselves.

Childhood trauma is thus likely to affect the child immediately – during and after the abuse – and this can cause post-traumatic stress, resulting in painful (physical and emotional) effects, and contributing to cognitive distortions (see Bowlby 1988, Briere 1992, Berliner 2002) of all kinds. Abuse will often influence the child's developmental stage and will show itself in arresting or slowing down development, while the child's resources go into coping with the abusive situation.

Many children, sometimes after only a brief period of protest, start developing ways of 'coping', as one might describe it, and keeping as safe as possible. Summit (1988) called this 'accommodation'. (Summit's thinking helps us to understand how children adapt, maintain the secret, take the responsibility, feel the guilt, begin very reluctantly and slowly to tell of their experiences, and then retract, particularly if put under any pressure or if the child's story is not believed.) Others also describe an important developmental process called 'adaptation' (see below). Both these processes are like psychological survival mechanisms and help the child and adult to cope with the continuing maltreatment. Children may develop behaviours they think can keep them safe or lessen the immediate physical and emotional pain. It is as well to note here that children who have been abused by a stranger once and then made safe, will not have to engage in this accommodation to the abusive situation.

Trauma may also affect the child and adult in the long term. The long-term consequences that will encompass the above two notions set adaptation and accommodation firmly into a defensive pattern from which some victims never emerge. These patterns become a more intrinsic part of the individual's functioning and are likely to generalise to other aspects of their psychological development throughout life.

Case example 2

Zake, a 5-year-old boy, had witnessed the brutal murder of his father, and had developed a way of existing in the world by abandoning speech and only humming tunes. He said later that he thought that if he only hummed tunes he could stop thinking of what he witnessed around his father's death, and if he could stop thinking about it then he would not feel so terrible.

Thinking of the unthinkable, experiencing and then re-experiencing painful and humiliating episodes is what the children attempt to avoid, both in the short and the long term. But such psychological manoeuvres are not accomplished without a price. In order to repress such events, considerable psychic energy has to be expended.

The developmental stage may be influenced in such a way that the child is arrested in their development at the time of the abuse. For instance, many small children, though not all, who have been maltreated have very little language. Cognitive distortions as a consequence of trauma – misunderstandings, memory loss, blocking and dissociation – may also occur. Any such cognitive distortion carries a cost through distorting subsequent learning, understanding and adjustment.

Berliner (2002) stresses that treatment has to be designed to fit the individual child and family. Assessments related to the abuse, the attachment relationships, the trauma and post-traumatic stress experienced by the children are all guiding factors in what kind of treatment might be most beneficial. In the study by Kolko *et al.*

(2002) it was shown to be helpful for older children to distinguish their role in the escalation of their physical abuse. Children often feel the abuse is their fault and in this study ways of helping some children to identify the 'risk factor' vis-à-vis their own behaviour were demonstrated. For some children it will include being a little more in control of the situation.

There is, of course, so much more to say about trauma, but chapters in this book, especially that by Ryan (Chapter 23), and other references will guide the reader to more detailed descriptions on this subject.

Adaptations

It is often useful to take behaviour that we might describe as 'symptomatic' and instead see it as an adaptation the person has made. With adults, if we think of, say, depression as a symptom, there is a certain range of things we can think of doing to cure it. If we think of depression as the best adaptation that a person could manage to the circumstances they are in, we can have different ideas about how to help them; for instance, whether they could achieve the same with some alternative adaptation or whether they could change the demands they have felt obliged to meet. We might even consider whether depression was the safest route for them to take at the time, and not automatically presume we should try to change it. The shift is not towards blaming them but to seeing people as having made the best response they could manage at the time, while opening up the possibility of helping them to make a more useful response in the future. Adaptation is a broader version of the ideas contained in the concept of accommodation.

To a large extent the emotional and behavioural effects we see are the attempts of maltreated children to adapt to the environment surrounding them, including their caregivers (Stratton & Hanks 1991). From this point of view the behaviour of the child is not a 'symptom' but the best response they could make for their own protection. Think of a child who flinches every time someone moves suddenly anywhere near them. Classifying this as a symptom of twitchiness, or as a neurotic behaviour, is not only unhelpful, it also disparages the child. Seeing flinching as an adaptive response to an environment in which you might be suddenly assaulted without warning makes more sense and also opens up ideas of what might be done about it.

Adaptations to abuse may unduly focus the resources of the child: 'We might best regard the children in such families as having acquired a specialism in coping with the particular demand, but thereby risking limiting other potentials.' (Stratton 2003, p. 351).

Further limitations may come from the reaction of others to the adaptation. Here we enter the concept of transactional adaptation described by Stratton (2003). For example, a child's withdrawal and isolation from peers may be the result of parental rules that wish for a quiet and unassuming child. Other parents may be irritated by a timid, withdrawn child and respond angrily to such a child, who may adapt by putting on displays of aggressive behaviour. Some children find mealtimes traumatic because of emotional tension surrounding eating, or at a more extreme level because they have had burning hot food forced into their mouths. They may adapt by using every way possible to avoid meals (and become labelled as 'poor feeders' as a result). Children who have been sexually exploited may adapt by using the sexual behaviour they have been 'taught' in order to obtain much needed cuddles from adults. Or they may provide the sexual behaviour to avoid punishment. Either way they may be further maltreated by having their adaptation labelled as a symptom of sexual promiscuity. Each of these examples demonstrates that adaptation is not usefully regarded as a unidirectional process in which abusive behaviour by an adult creates an effect in the child. Desperate adaptations made by the child to survive physically and emotionally in the family may be operated in the world outside and create transactional cycles that are themselves abusive. Within the family the child's initial adaptations feed into the transactional process with the abusive parent in ways that can escalate to a stable pattern of abuse (Belsky & Stratton 2002). In fact, parents are themselves adapting to wider systems:

It is doubtful that maltreatment can be eliminated so long as parents rear their offspring in a society in which violence is rampant, corporal punishment is condoned as a child-rearing technique, and parenthood itself is construed in terms of ownership.

(Belsky & Stratton 2002, p. 103)

The ways in which cycles of adaptation to abuse build up, and the implications of these cycles for treatment, have been described in detail by Stratton and Hanks (1991). Because abuse has multiple determinants, treatment should, if possible, be directed at least to the whole family system, but in ways that take account of the wider systems within which the family is functioning (Randall & Henggeller 1999, Dallos & Draper 2005).

For the purposes of this chapter we would ask the reader to keep in mind that *all* of the identified consequences of abuse should be thought of as adaptations by the child. The outcomes of abuse can then be seen more clearly as following from the adaptation the child is forced into, and not just as a deficit built into the child by the abuse itself.

Attachment relationships of maltreated children

Attachment is a specific relationship and human beings are quite unable to exist without it. For the infant and child it provides a base from which to explore the world and works in a way to ensure that the child's needs are met (Bowlby 1988).

This exploration of the world is recognised as being vital for the infant's development and shows optimal effects when a parent figure is available to provide a secure base. A baby can attach to about five people who are close to the infant and develops the initial most important steps of attachment during its first year of life. The role of the attachment figure(s) is to reduce anxiety in stressful situations and provide the infant and child with the confidence to explore and experience unknown and new situations. Attachment to significant adults in infancy is also the foundation for lasting relationships throughout life; for instance, anxious attachment is often the consequence when a child has to take responsibility for keeping close to an attachment figure (most often the mother).

Infants and young children attach to figures who are their caregivers even when these caregivers are reluctant, neglectful and maltreating towards the child. What it encourages the child to do, in these circumstances, is to try harder, and stay closer, in their effort to make the situation more tolerable (Crittenden & Ainsworth 1989). It also seems that the children often believe that if only they behaved in a different way, or engaged in more of the same behaviours, the adults would stop being maltreating. This issue of the children thinking and believing that somehow this abusive relationship is their fault feeds into the adaptational cycle of trapped attachments. Adults who have been maltreated as children, in later life often puzzle over why and how it was that they would run towards the caregiver or close adult and greet them warmly even though they were fully aware of the painful relationship and afraid of it.

Poor relationships may also occur because of the loss of a primary figure, especially if this happens while the infant is between 6 months and 3 years. In addition, multiple breaks and separations can have considerable consequences and cause more long-term distress to the child. It needs to be acknowledged that some separations are inevitable and will not harm the child. In a 'good enough' environment, separations can in fact give a child the experience that they are safe even when, say, mother is not there, and also that she will return. However, longer-term separations repeated over this sensitive period between 6 months and 3 years can lead to the child becoming very withdrawn, uncommunicative, agitated and anxious. Alternatively, the child may show in their behaviour that they cannot discriminate and are therefore inappropriately friendly and/or overfriendly to any adult, even someone strange to the child. For professionals this may become quickly obvious when a child on a first visit to a clinic for instance offers kisses and demands cuddles from people they have never met before.

The early attachment patterns are the foundation for future development. The pattern is a dynamic one, changes over time throughout the child's growth and development, and depends on the experiences the child has. It is a powerful process and has strong links to the development of how the child and later adult perceive themselves. Children model on their significant caregivers and will react to many situations with the model in their minds. This is particularly relevant when it comes to the maltreated child as an adult in a parenting position, when their experience becomes a model for their own parenting. Early attachment patterns influence the adult's way of behaving and form part of a cyclic pattern which has intergenerational consequences.

Morton and Browne (1998) reviewed what is known about attachment in relation to child abuse. They emphasise that patterns of attachment that have been found useful for assessment can also be utilised when children and families are in treatment and for interventions to the family or professional system. They also make an important point about the intergenerational patterns of attachment, and state that: '...insensitive parenting (maltreatment can be seen as an extreme form of insensitivity) will produce an insecure attachment relationship in the infant. This will lead to a poor representational model of the self, which in turn will influence the formation of future relationships' (p. 1100). Thus the abuse can continue from one generation to the next.

Crittenden (2002) analysed her work in the attachment field, framing her own experience of fostering children around questions which consider what treatment can achieve, how to understand abuse in terms of attachment theories, and what the issues around danger and attachment are. She presents her dynamic-maturational model of patterns of attachment in adulthood. One aspect in particular interested us and that is her curiosity around 'Why do professionals do what they do?' From a systemic family therapy point of view it is important to see 'helper and helped' as part of a system and promote a more equal way of working in therapeutic settings. Equally, becoming aware of the different attachment strategies each of us uses in our decision making and behaviour when dealing with child abuse cases is essential in engaging with clients, whether child or adult.

Crittenden and Claussen (2003) gathered important new research studies. Authors writing in this book formulate new theories of attachment and extend their existing theories. Attention has been paid to attachment and how it works in different cultures and how attachment in older age groups can be conceptualised.

With the three broad potential consequences of abuse (trauma, adaptation and disrupted attachment) in mind, we now consider specific forms of abuse in turn.

Physical maltreatment and its consequences

Physical abuse, like all other forms of abuse, has a strong emotional component/counterpart, and disentangling the specific consequences of the physical and emotional aspect is not easily done. Physical abuse can vary from moderate to severe and, in a considerable number of cases, it can be fatal (Hobbs *et al.* 1999). The review of the child abuse inquiries presented by Reder and colleagues (Reder *et al.* 1993, Reder & Duncan 1999) describes the devastating end of the continuum of all forms of child abuse and gives us some insight into the seriousness of the maltreatment of children. Wissow (1990, p. 172) states that:

homicide is among the leading causes of death for American children ages 1–14 … Most of the deaths among children under the age of 3 represent fatal child abuse … A consequence so grave … our actions if there were any were too late, thoughts about prevention were either not there or so hesitantly formed they came too late and there is nothing we can make good about it.

Speight (1989) pointed out that diagnosing physical abuse or non-accidental injury is important, not least because the maltreatment can be so severe that the child dies, or that brain damage persists and handicap is the consequence.

Detailed descriptions of the issues can be found in Wissow (1990) and Hobbs *et al.* (1999), and in Helfer *et al.* (1997), Reece and Ludwig (2001) and Hobbs *et al.* (2003) who address the medical issues and link them to psychological and emotional factors.

Bruises are the most commonly encountered injury, followed by fractures and brain injury (Hobbs *et al.* 1999). They also point out (p. 78) that 'abusive fractures usually result from the more extreme forms of violence and represent serious injury. They may co-exist with other signs of trauma: external (e.g. bruises, scratches) or internal injuries. The internal injuries may result in subdural haematoma, retinal haemorrhage or internal injuries to the abdomen.'

Physical abuse results in the physical injuries which leave wounds to heal and scars visible. Such scars can occur from bruises, cuts, bites, kicks, marks from beatings with objects, burns and scalds. The outwardly invisible/internal injuries, as in bone fractures, breaks and other internal injuries can also be present. Powerful as these images of physical damage are, it is essential also to consider our three concepts: the trauma for the children in experiencing such assaults; the kinds of adaptations they will have had to make simply to try to survive; and the effects on attachment processes when their parents have maltreated them or failed to protect them. Psychological interventions need to go alongside the physical treatment for any of these injuries.

All professionals have to be vigilant in order to detect the physical injuries children present with, either in hospital and medical centres or in social services offices, nurseries and schools. Denial can occur when children are brought with obvious physical injuries just as much as with less visible or detectable signs in emotional abuse, sexual abuse or forms of neglect.

The effects of physical abuse are influenced by several factors that can either stand alone or arise in combination. These factors are:

- the relationship of abuser to child
- the nature of the abuse
- the severity of the assault
- the child's age
- the child's development

- how long the traumatic event lasted
- how often the traumatic event was repeated.

With the research and clinical work undertaken in the area of neurobiological effects of abuse (see above), it is now clearer that the stress caused by repeated abusive situations is very likely to cause adverse effects in successive stages of development. Glaser (2005) states that for small infants the consequences are particularly stark in that certain functions of the brain may simply not develop when they are stressed through experiences of abuse. In slightly older children the effects of abuse can either be disruptive to the developmental process of the child or halt it in a certain phase. This is often called being 'stuck', or fixated at a certain developmental stage.

Case example 3

One of the children presenting for a medical absolutely and resolutely refused to take off his T-shirt to have his chest listened to. The doctor tried to persuade the child and eventually became firm, telling the child that he would not be hurt but that they had at least to lift his shirt and put the stethoscope to his chest. When they lifted the garment the child let out a piercing yell as if he was very badly hurt. What the doctor saw was a chest full of scars from a burn which had occurred 2 years previously. The child became inconsolable and wept for a long time, kicking anyone who tried to come near him. A little later he told his mother that when the doctor lifted his shirt he felt as if he was back in the time and place when he was burnt 2 years ago. He said this happened every time he had to take his shirt off and that he had learned to keep it on. If he could keep a shirt on always, day and night he said, he would not see the scars, not be reminded of what had happened, and therefore not feel the pain over and over again. This phenomenon is called 'flashback'.

'Flashbacks' (see Case 3) are not only caused by visible stimuli: for children with physical injuries such as burns or badly healed breaks, the injury is a constant reminder of what happened. As Bentovim (1992, p. 25) pointed out, when any human being has to 'cope with the uncopeable' the individual devises strategies, often quite unique and individual, to avoid the stress which is caused. Bentovim said:

'The basic response is the replaying and re-enactment of the event thrust into experience, e.g. through flashbacks triggered by reminders, spontaneously, or during play, through dreams or nightmares. There are struggles to overcome these experiences by 'avoidance' or attempts to delete reminders, avoiding places, people, situations that trigger memories; or through dissociation – a form of self-hypnotism which blanks the experience out, creating a hole in the mind. Finally the overwhelming traumatic experience can induce a state of arousal and irritability, and can affect sleep and the ability to relax.'

Major psychological signs of physical maltreatment

Children who have been subjected to deliberate, and sometimes planned, harm have a very different experience of their treatment than children who may have been smacked or even hit hard by their caregivers but have been given explanations, ways of changing the cause which led to them being chastised, and possibly even an apology.

The well-known facial expression of frozen watchfulness which can be seen in many maltreated children is there for a very long time, if not for life. It relates to the mistrust of others, of feelings about being unsafe in an unpredictable position and the likelihood of being harmed at any time. Threats to the child's basic sense of security can trigger adaptations in the form of emotional responses ranging from anxiety and being withdrawn, to angry and uncontrollable acting-out behaviour.

Children respond to physical maltreatment often in the way they behave. There is no doubt that individuals will develop their way of doing this and most often this happens in an unconscious way and the resulting behaviours are not necessarily something the children can be in control of. We have tried to put together a list of behaviours and symptoms which may alert those in charge of the children and help to make some assessment of what might have happened to children. Thinking like this can help in providing a basis for estimating the potential consequences of maltreatment and can also be used as indicators that a child may have suffered maltreatment. In the bulleted list, common consequences are listed against ■, while those that are strong indicators of abuse when exhibited by an individual child are listed with →.

Children who have been physically maltreated may experience:

- ■ stress-related symptoms (tension, headaches, psychosomatic symptoms)
- → being very alert and aroused as if in a constant state of readiness of an attack, sudden fear of being injured
- ■ intrusive thoughts appearing as if from nowhere
- → sudden intrusive thoughts and consequent action of being violent, often perceived by others as uncontrollable aggressive impulses (see Case 1)
- ■ flinching as if for no specific reason
- → avoiding any thought or talk of the abusive event(s)
- → dreams and nightmares of the traumatic abusive events.

Simultaneously, delays can include:

- ■ developmental delays
- ■ delayed gross or fine motor development (gross: walking, jumping, climbing; fine: holding a pencil, picking things up, holding feeding implements, etc.).

As the children get older the consequences can manifest themselves in:

- ■ angry behaviour
- ■ depression
- ■ anxiety
- ■ dissociation, which includes detachment and numbing effects
- ■ repression (developing a way of not consciously remembering the abusive event).

Unpredictableness of maltreatment and its consequences

The unpredictable nature of maltreatment is often an added strain on the child which precludes having the time or energy to concentrate, learn, play and form relationships. Instead it leaves the child with a need to be watchful, careful, predict when an attack might occur, pretend that nothing is worrying them, etc. This pattern of alertness can be seen in adults who have been maltreated as children, and – as in childhood – it still prevents the adult from concentrating, learning and forming relationships. An interesting study (Wright *et al.* 2005) about the resilience in mothers who are child sexual abuse survivors highlights how unpredictableness amongst other aspects, hinders the development of protective strategies and may lead the person abused into avoidance and denial, self-destructive coping methods and psychological distress.

Engel (1998) provides a useful guide by taking the reader through the stages experienced by adults who have been abused as children. We are presented with descriptions of people's behaviour and feelings and also with the clinical signs so often present when an adult begins to cope with these issues. There is also the issue of parental models. Children who have been maltreated often say as adults that hitting and punishing is the right way to bring up children, as if there is no other way.

Emotional abuse and its consequences

'Rather than casting psychological maltreatment as an ancillary issue, subordinate to other forms of abuse and neglect, we should place it as the centrepiece of efforts to understand family functioning and to protect children' (Garbarino *et al.* 1986, p. 7).

The definition used in the *Working Together to Safeguard Children** document states that:

Emotional abuse is the persistent emotional ill-treatment of a child such as to cause severe and persistent adverse effects on the child's emotional development. It may involve conveying to children that they are worthless or unloved, inadequate or valued only insofar as they meet the needs of another person. It may feature age or developmentally inappropriate expectations being imposed on children. It may involve causing children frequently to feel frightened or in danger, or the exploitation or corruption of children. Some level of emotional abuse is involved in all types of ill-treatment of a child, though it may occur alone.

(DoH *et al.* 1999, pp. 5–6)

Iwaniec (1996) also includes 'the crippling overprotection of a child', something that has possibly been overlooked so far.

Although society's response overall to this form of maltreatment has been slow, Creighton (Chapter 2, in this volume) provides a discussion of increasing proportions of registrations under this category.

Wissow (1990) quite rightly reminds us that though it is now much more accepted that parents should pay more attention to their children in every respect, how they should relate to their children remains a controversial issue. He said that: 'While a warm and loving parent–child relationship is widely advocated as essential, significant minorities still feel that strict discipline and a certain detachment (especially from fathers) are important elements of child-rearing' (p. 158). This is one area in which cultural differences in definitions of appropriate care must be taken into account (Stratton & Hanks 1991). The debate about the definition of emotional abuse is still not settled, not least because there are different opinions of whether the emphasis should be on the abuse of the child or the behaviour of the parent. Brassard and Hardy (1997) offer a useful account of the issues involved in the assessment of emotional abuse. Glaser and Prior (2002) almost deconstructed what we know so far about emotional abuse and neglect and developed some very helpful categories around the area of prediction and early recognition.

It is not fully understood why children react differently in the face of maltreatment and why some show more severe consequences than others when they have had abusive experiences. Attention has been paid to the phenomenon of 'resilience'

---

* The most up-to-date version of this document was published by HM Government in 2006. For a full discussion of this, see Chapter 11.

in human beings. How do some children and adults who have been abused manage to lead a less disturbed life despite their abusive childhood experiences? Heller *et al.* (1999) point out that while there are no clear answers at present, there are better understood indicators which link to the abusive situation and how the children are treated during that time. Kagan *et al.* (1978) showed that how children perceive themselves, and how their inner self develops, are of crucial importance. The self is influenced by both adults and peers and if children receive persistently negative feedback then their view of themselves will be affected.

There is no such thing as a perfect parent or a perfect child. Every parent will at some time or other behave towards a child in such a way that the child will be upset, may be frightened or feel rejected, and suffer a loss of self-esteem etc. What happens after this event of commission (an active or cruel behaviour towards the child) or omission (behaviour which neglects or ignores the child, even when they are in unsafe or dangerous situations) in the adult's behaviour towards the child is what matters. The parents may manage to acknowledge and 'make good' the situation, giving the child appropriate alternative options for behaving. If reparation is made, the child learns that people/parents/caregivers can make mistakes but that they can recognise them as such. However, even the 'making good' of a poor/hurtful situation to the child is not going to be helpful if the situation occurs repeatedly. When the caregiving is constantly changing (doing hurtful things then making good), it becomes inconsistent and potentially damaging.

Garbarino *et al.* (1986) provided us with a helpful model which distinguishes between the different forms of emotional maltreatment. This model is still a useful guideline as to how to understand emotional maltreatment and has led to other definitions:

- rejecting
- isolating
- terrorising
- ignoring
- corrupting.

These are the categories essential in order to recognise children who are maltreated emotionally. Childhood inevitably includes experiencing some of these patterns at sometime or other, but our capacity to cope with such treatment in an environment where it is repeated over and over again is fairly limited. Such behaviour delivered consistently towards a child is damaging.

Egeland *et al.* (1988) claim from their longitudinal study that emotional abuse has the most serious consequences for a child's social and intellectual development. These researchers showed, for instance, that verbal abuse and psychological unavailability, as well as physical abuse and neglect, produced children who presented with anxious rather than secure attachments and that they showed frustration, hostility and anger. Developmental skills also declined for the group of children having to live with verbal abuse and the unavailability of their parents. The children in this group were quickly frustrated when attempting tasks and approached new tasks feeling negative towards them and anxious. From this study, it seemed that children who were emotionally maltreated suffered more severe setbacks in their performance skills than those children who were physically abused or neglected. This is particularly important to recognise and gives an insight into the possibility that emotional abuse can be more damaging than physical abuse. The research indicated that this may be because the children who are physically harmed may receive this treatment more sporadically than those children who are emotionally abused, whose maltreatment is much more likely to be a constant feature in their and their parents' lives.

Glaser (1993) developed a model that has enhanced our understanding further. She proposed six dimensions of emotionally abusive or inappropriate relationships, as follows:

- persistent negative attitudes (negative attributions and attitudes, harsh discipline and over-control)
- promoting of insecure attachments (through conditional parenting)
- inappropriate developmental expectations and considerations
- emotional unavailability
- failure to recognise a child's individuality and psychological boundaries
- cognitive distortions and inconsistencies.

She and colleagues (Glaser & Prior 2002) developed this further and produced a classification and a model to help predict emotional abuse and neglect.

Crittenden (1988) described different family patterns in maltreating families. For instance, the neglecting families had a pattern of ignoring the children, and these children – who were practically invisible to their caregivers – were passive and cognitively delayed before they reached year 1. As they grew older, their behaviours altered and they became 'uncontrolled and seekers of novel experiences'. At that stage, these children need a great deal of looking after and fall into the category of being abused by 'omission' as much as by 'commission'. Claussen and Crittenden (1991) showed that much psychological abuse intercorrelates with physical abuse and other forms of abuse of children and that when this happens the developmental risks increase accordingly. Both Wissow (1990) and Hobbs *et al.* (1999) would endorse these findings.

Non-organic failure to thrive (NO-FTT) and its consequences

Taylor and Taylor (1976) stated what is in essence still accepted today when they said:

The period between the start of weaning and the fifth birthday is nutritionally the most vulnerable segment of the human life cycle. Rapid growth, loss of passive immunity and as yet undeveloped acquired immunity against infection produce dietary needs more specific and inflexible than at later periods. (p. 820)

We would add that special attention is necessary to the infant's needs in the feeding situation from birth onwards. It is recognised that many children (e.g. 5% of an inner city population) fail to thrive before the weaning period (Skuse 1985, Hobbs *et al.* 1999, 2003). Drewett's (2005) paper highlights the importance of slow weight gain in the first 2 month of life in identifying children who fail to thrive.

The consequences for children who fail to thrive for non-organic reasons are better understood now, and detailed discussions can be found in Frank and Zeisel (1988), Hanks and Hobbs (1993), Boddy and Skuse (1994) and Hobbs *et al.* (1999). The overall consequences of FTT relate to developmental retardation and include motor, language, intellectual, social and behavioural components.

A definition of FTT needs to encompass a wide range – from the child not growing fully to their potential at one end, and the situation being life threatening for the child at the other end of the continuum (Table 5.1). Psychological aspects of development can be delayed, sometimes irreversibly, with emotional and cognitive deficits (Table 5.2).

It is interesting to note where different definitions put their emphasis. Is it something that the child is to be responsible for? 'The feeding interaction in FTT appears

Table 5.1
The physical consequences of failure to thrive (after Hanks & Hobbs 1993, Hobbs et al. 1999)

Overall body shape	Thin and wasted, little fat
Feet and hands	May be swollen, red and cold
Arms	Thin, mid-upper arm circumference (Hobbs *et al.* 1999)
Stomach	Large and swollen
Hair	No shine, looks wispy, thin, is falling out
Brain	Can be retarded particularly in early months (Illingworth 1983, Frank & Zeisel 1988)
Physical growth	Can be permanently damaged including a poor posture

Table 5.2
Developmental consequences of non-organic failure to thrive

- Developmental delay
- Delayed motor development
- Delayed language development
- Delayed intellectual development
- Delayed social development
- Delayed behavioural development

to be unsuccessful, because the child does not achieve an adequate nutritional intake' (Boddy & Skuse 1994, p. 407); is it that 'the child refuses to gain weight in an appropriate manner' (Illingworth 1983); or is it that FTT results from caregivers feeding an infant inadequate calories – not enough food or an inappropriate diet? It is important for practitioners to carefully review their assumptions and decide where to put their energies in terms of interventions. FTT in small children is a potentially life-threatening situation and needs clear thinking which will not be helped by concentrating on deciding who is to blame.

Recently, an important addition to the field of failure to thrive has come from one of the foremost authorities on this subject. Iwaniec (2004) combined 20 years of follow-up research with her in-depth knowledge and experience of children who are failing to thrive and their parents, and produced a text which no one working in child protection should be without.

Both parents and professionals alike find it difficult and emotionally taxing to recognise and acknowledge when a child fails to thrive, let alone realise that if nothing is done to remedy this state of affairs the consequences can be severe and at times result in death. Iwaniec *et al.* (1985, p. 251) pointed out that children who fail to thrive can show consequences that can lead to the child having a 'pattern of unmalleable behaviour, resistance to new routines' and that their 'general volatility of mood and behaviour, appeared to make them difficult to rear from early life. Feeding routines, and other training tasks, were made into fraught enterprises for many parents'.

This leads to a further complication in intergenerational terms and warrants detailed research. Understanding how mothers perceive the causes is crucial to any intervention in this relationship and to aiding the ultimate growth of the child. FTT is one situation in which the child's adaptation to mistreatment or mishandling may easily be misconstrued by a parent. The child's avoidance of the (possibly traumatic) mealtime may be interpreted as the child's wilfulness, or just lack of interest in food on the child's part, and so the underfeeding continues.

McCann *et al.* (1994) researched the eating habits and attitudes concerning body shape and weight of 26 mothers who had children who were failing to thrive nonorganically. These mothers, none of whom was either bulimic or anorexic, restrained their NO-FTT children from eating, for instance, 'sweet' foods. Thirty per cent of these mothers restricted their children in the consumption of foods they considered fattening or not healthy. Despite the objective measurements of weight and height which were low in the NO-FTT children, 50% of these mothers believed that their NO-FTT children had 'normal' weights and 38% were convinced that their children's shape was the same as that of other ordinary children who did not fail to thrive. They did not seem to be able, for whatever reason, to perceive their children's position. This coincides with our clinical experience (Hobbs *et al.* 1999).

Parents, grandparents and professionals have made the following comments to us while we were working with children who were severely failing to thrive. Such children are well below the third centile in weight, look thin and are visibly much smaller than most children of the same age:

> 'Not to worry, we are all small in our family.'
> 'He runs around too much to put on weight, that is why he is thin and little.'
> 'His dad says he will catch up when he's older.'
> Grandmother said in the clinic: 'all my children were small when they were young, he will catch up, just leave him alone.'
> 'I will not have you think I don't feed him; he is to blame, he won't eat.'
> 'I think you [doctor, psychologist] are fussy, there are much thinner children on the estate where I work, you should see them and not worry his mother.'

Such statements indicate the difficulties caregivers can have while trying to protect themselves from the psychological distress of a child who does not eat. However, such interpretations have considerable consequences for the child, particularly when the lack of food intake continues because of such beliefs and makes it difficult to achieve change.

Observations of children eating

In an attempt to understand the mutual adaptations of parent and NO-FTT child, we have been observing, or if possible filming, children during a main meal-time. Their eating behaviour and the families' rules about eating have often provided us with the information we needed in order to come up with adequate interventions.

The video recordings have also enabled us to detect some of the interactions that have become established in the pattern of poor feeding and how this has made itself felt in the child's behaviour and development.

Children can become frightened and stop eating when:

- the food is too hot and the child's mouth is burnt during feeding
- the pieces of food are too large and the child cannot chew them adequately
- they are fed roughly and injured during feeding
- they are left alone to eat the food and have no social contact or model of a positive attitude to eating
- food is consistently delayed until the child is desperate, so they are too distressed to be able to eat by the time it is offered.

Recognising the emotional consequences in NO-FTT

The emotional consequences of NO-FTT need to be assessed for each individual child. We have recognised that a checklist is helpful in determining how the child is behaving emotionally and what the carer's experience is in looking after the child.

Hobbs *et al.* (1999) compiled such a checklist of opposite reactions (Table 5.3). This checklist is a guideline only. It is not a diagnostic tool but may help the professional and parent to recognise that behaviours such as those listed in Table 5.3 are often present in children who fail to thrive. Further, it may help those involved to be more able to help the child in these areas rather than to ignore them.

Table 5.3 *Possible behaviours by children with failure to thrive*	Still		Confused
	Expressionless		Insecure
	Unresponsive		Anxious
	Sad		Demanding
	Depressed		Frustrated
	Not inquisitive		Frantically searching
	Minimal or no smiling		Tearful
	Little vocalisation		Angry
	Detached		Rejecting

Iwaniec *et al.* (2002) concentrated on issues of failure to thrive linked to emotional abuse and neglect, and described a particular path for interventions with regard to this form of abuse and to parenting.

Neglect and its consequences

Neglect of children is one of the most obvious aspects of maltreatment where not only are the caregivers of the children responsible, but also where the issue has to be widened to include society as a whole and a global view has to be adopted. As an example, the neglect of children in the Developing World is the responsibility of the individual country, as well as that of the industrialised nations who may exploit a Third World country's natural resources. Poor health care, poor education, drug addiction, crime and starvation are often the consequences on one level in society.

Helfer (1990) stated that it is within the grasp of all of us to understand the consequences of a neglected childhood and how this permeates from one generation to the next. Hobbs *et al.* (1999, p. 126) take this further and point out that: 'Childhood is a vulnerable time and needs which are not met during the child's period of growth and development may have irreversible consequences.'

Neglect is defined in *Working Together to Safeguard Children* (DoH *et al.* 1999, p. 6) as:

the persistent failure to meet a child's basic physical and/or psychological needs likely to result in the serious impairment of the child's health or development. It may involve a parent or carer failing to provide adequate food, shelter and clothing, failing to protect a child from physical harm or danger, or the failure to ensure access to appropriate medical care or treatment. It may also include neglect of, or unresponsiveness to, a child's basic emotional needs.

Kempe and Goldbloom (1987) defined neglect as: 'a very insidious form of maltreatment. It implies failure of the parents to act properly in safeguarding the health, safety and well-being of the child'. Stevenson (1998a) has a unique understanding of the issues of neglect in society and emphasises particularly that small children do not have time to wait for interventions to be successful. The children's developmental stages are progressing and will be shaped by the abuse. Interventions may either be too late or the children have grown up and adapted into ways of being which make it hard to address the changes.

The consequences of neglect, as in physical abuse, can range from death of a child through neglect (death from cold, starvation, lack of medical and daily care) to children who are dirty and unkempt, not stimulated to learn and left to their own devices. Iwaniec's (1996) description of children and their circumstances when there has been neglect and failure to thrive are recognised as giving the practitioner both practical and theoretical insight into the problem.

Cantwell (1997) and Hobbs *et al.* (1999) describe the various patterns of neglect, including lack of car seat belts, helmets when cycling, lack of medical care, lack of hygiene in the home, clean food, drink and water, physical and emotional care and adequate supervision appropriate to the developmental stage of the child and teenager. Six per cent of UK children under 12 years of age are known to lack the most basic care (Cawson *et al.* 2000). This included often going without food, not having any clean clothes, not getting medical care even when they were ill, being left alone, and generally having to care for themselves. Hobbs *et al.* (2003) advocate that the jigsaw approach of gathering information from a number of contacts who know the child would build up a picture and distinguish between the different maltreatments a child may experience. It is important to consider that neglected children come not only from poor but also from well-off families.

As with FTT, there are cases in which the needs of the child are clearly not being met, but which it would not necessarily be appropriate to label as abuse; for example, if the parents fail to provide the kinds of interaction needed for the child to form attachments. We have suggested that the important task is to decide upon the child's requirements for healthy growth, and not be so concerned about apportioning blame (Stratton & Hanks 1991). To some extent the decision will vary between cultures, and the decision about whose responsibility it is to provide these requirements will also vary. It is appropriate that we should have a progressive debate, and a progressive raising of the level of what we regard as essential requirements. In the year 2006 we would, for example, claim that there is clear evidence about the negative consequences for a child of having inadequate models of attachment relationships. The disruption to both childhood and long-term development seems to be serious enough to justify a claim that the child who is not given the basics of social development is suffering neglect.

Children have a right to expect to be cared for, have a roof over their heads, clothes for all seasons and food and drink given to them. Children also have the right to expect to be nurtured, taught what they need to live in their society and to be kept safe from harm. Adults – and particularly parents – have a duty to provide these basic needs for their children and a duty to ask for help if they cannot manage the task.

Neglect is closely linked to emotional abuse in that, as a result of their neglect, the children often:

- are very passive in infancy
- are sometimes very active, but totally unfocused when older
- have a limited ability to attend to the behaviour of others
- show significant developmental delay
- have poor speech and learning ability
- have poor ability to interact socially
- are accident prone because they are not properly protected
- may have stunted growth.

Neglect is an important factor when it comes to child death. The Victoria Climbié Inquiry (Laming Report 2003) highlighted these issues most clearly. Reder and Duncan (1999) add to our understanding about how neglect contributes to cases when maltreated children die.

Neglect is not well researched, if only because it is difficult to define where the boundaries of neglectful behaviour towards children lie.

Sexual abuse and its consequences

Sexual maltreatment of children is the subject most written about, particularly since 1987 and the Cleveland Inquiry. It is in this area that more distinct categories of effects can be recognised. There is no doubt that children (boys and girls) who are abused in childhood are harmed, and often considerably. The ordinary, more normal path of child development is disrupted by the sexual abuse and the short- and long-term consequences are sadly inescapable. CSA is an aversive and damaging experience for children, with harmful effects often present throughout life. Extensive documentation and research can be found in Glaser and Frosh 1988, Bentovim 1992, Briere 1992, Hobbs *et al.* 1999, Reece and Ludwig 2001, Browne *et al.* 2002a and Hobbs *et al.* 2003, to mention just a few of the available resources.

Physical consequences

Paediatricians, starting with Henry Kemp, have taken a lead in working in the area of abuse and sexual maltreatment. We recommend that readers make themselves familiar with the physical aspects of this form of abuse so that they can cooperate with medical staff in such situations. Texts to consult include Wissow (1990), Hobbs and Wynne (1993), Meadow (1993), Helfer *et al.* (1997) and Hobbs *et al.* (2003). What is striking in CSA is that the physical injuries exist along a continuum from severe injury and death to no physical injuries at all.

Psychological consequences

Effects of CSA may be short or long term, and usually the child experiences both forms. Further division may be useful:

1. emotional and behavioural effects
2. education and learning
3. all forms of interpersonal relationships.

The *short-term effects* of CSA can show in terms of fear, anxiety, aggressive behaviours, angry outbursts, hostility and feeling 'got at' (persecuted), and developmentally inappropriate sexual behaviour.

The *long-term effects* of CSA have been found in terms of anxiety, depression, feeling isolated, lack of trust, poor self-esteem, self-harming behaviours (including eating disorders), dissociation and the range of traumatic and post-traumatic effects. Guilt and shame are invariably present.

It is sobering to reflect on the fact that potentially the list of effects on the child in both the short and long term can be overwhelming. We give some indication of the consequences below, dividing the most salient effects into three age groups. These effects may stand singly or present in clusters of behaviours, depending on each child's environment and specific situation.

Common consequences, which may also occur following other types of abuse or childhood disturbance, are listed against ■; those that are strong indicators of sexual abuse when exhibited by an individual child are listed with →.

For the preschool child, the effects may show in:

→ sexually explicit play and behaviour
■ wetting and soiling
■ delayed language and development
■ eating and sleeping problems
■ dysfunctional attachment behaviour

- withdrawn or overactive states
- aggressive behaviours (to self and others)
- clinging behaviour and becoming mute.

For children between the ages of 6 and 12 years, the above effects may be recognisable, with further elaborations:

- poor learning and concentration
→ heightened sexual behaviour and arousal
- truanting and self-neglecting
- depression and anxiety
- psychosomatic illnesses
- physical risk-taking
- poor social skills
- as if out of control at times
→ avoidance of men or women (depending on gender of abuser).

For the older child, the effects include any of the above-mentioned patterns with further escalations:

→ sexually precocious behaviour, sibling abuse, prostitution
- solvent/alcohol/drug abuse
- self-harming and suicide attempts
- anorexia and bulimia
- changes in school performance
- isolation from peers
→ starting to sexually abuse other children.

Overall, one may view the child's position in the following way. The difficulties of sexually abused children are:

- lack of individuation
- poor interpersonal relationships
- communication problems
→ inappropriate sexual behaviour and confusion about it
- low self-esteem, feelings of depression and anxiety
- feelings of shame, guilt and powerlessness
- feelings of dissociation
→ experiencing something akin to the 'damaged goods syndrome'
- trauma and post-traumatic stress syndrome.

The behaviours can have both a delayed and an immediate impact on a child. What we have witnessed is that it can take a long time before certain behaviours emerge. Some consequences can emerge quickly, some emerge over time and then fade, and yet others can be triggered by events such as having a baby, the death of the perpetrator, the death of a non-abusing parent, or a child of the previously abused adult approaching puberty and potential sexual activity.

Vizard (1993) highlighted another dimension when she stated that: 'sexually abused children often behave in a confusing way in relation to the abuse experience. This may be because their experience of sexual abuse was itself confusing.'

She proposes three levels of experience:

1. bodily experience
2. external world experience
3. inner world experience.

She also postulates that many children who have been subjected to CSA experience physiological arousal at the time of abuse and this results in a body memory. The memory is then lodged both as a thought and as a feeling, sexual and exciting in nature, which can give rise to a memory of sounds or visual images connected to the abusive situation. This feeling memory, so to speak, stands instead of the psychic memory of the actual event. So the intense experience of the act of CSA may have switched off the mind memory but activated the body memory. In children who have been chronically sexually abused, this body memory can function quite independently. It also includes passive and active modes. The active body memory can present in physical arousal. The passive body memory may appear like a psychosomatic conversion (headaches, stomach aches, wetting and soiling, being mute). The stress factors related to this dimension are discussed further below.

Most professionals working in this area recognise that CSA has consequences that are difficult to overcome and usually leave the person with lifelong problems. The degree to which these problems rule a person's life can, as with all forms of maltreatment, vary. We have begun to talk to a very small group of people who experienced CSA as children but who feel they are leading a life not dominated by the consequences of this experience. What has made it possible for these people to be different is not quite clear. One of the recognisable factors is that they have been able to tell a trusted adult and that they have been believed and protected from that moment on. Another important factor seems to be that they have not been blamed for the event.

There is considerable evidence that CSA is an aversive experience for children. It has also been recognised that very young children often go through periods when they are not aware that the sexual contact imposed on them is abusive. As the children get older, they do become aware of the fact that they are involved in a relationship(s) which is wrong or disapproved of. Often, this awareness comes about when the child has been given an injunction to secrecy. The issue of secrecy in itself leads to considerable difficulties both for the children and those around them. Should the children attempt to disclose, they often enter into a world of denial, described above, and then into internal confusion.

Even if they have not been warned by the perpetrator, the children are often painfully aware of the consequences of releasing their secret. Not only will they be disapproved of in many cases, but also the turmoil created within their family or institution will be extremely painful to them and often result in the children themselves being blamed. This recognition is often built into the perpetrator repertoire of both 'grooming' the child and maintaining the abusive situation. The use of threats to silence children in intrafamilial CSA is common and includes the threat of loss of love, separation or physical harm.

Another important distinction has to be drawn between children who have been sexually abused within the family, and thus experienced incest, and those children who have been abused by someone outside the immediate family.

Incest at any age seems to leave considerable consequences, particularly in the areas of relationships, trust, closeness and dependency. If the incest started early in life and continued over time, the child is shaped into sexualised behaviours which are observable but difficult to overcome. Summit's (1988) 'accommodation syndrome' (a seminal paper) describes the position of the child and leaves no doubt about the consequences of incest and the breaking of the incest taboo. Hobbs *et al.* (2003) described what happens to children when they either break the silence and report the sexual abuse or, as is far more common, keep the secret, accommodate to the abuse and try to protect themselves from the perpetrator. Whatever relationship the perpetrator has to the child, we have to remember that child sexual abuse is always the adult's responsibility, not the child's. Hobbs *et al.* (2003, p. 75) state: 'The cost the child pays for the abandonment of active resistance [against the abuse] is insecurity, victimisation and a loss of psychological well-being and self-esteem.' From helplessness and secrets, to entrapment and accommodation, the children feel powerless to resist the sexual abuse. Children often are put in the position of having to bargain with perpetrators and feeling that they have to protect siblings or friends by continuing to endure the abuse:

> Secondly, there is the need to protect the other parent, the family home and integrity of the family. Seemingly the child has the power to destroy the family, but the responsibility to keep it together. Parent and child roles have been subtly reversed. The child has accommodated to the situation at the expense of herself and her needs.
>
> (Hobbs *et al.* 2003, p. 75)

In respect of the sexualised behaviour, so often witnessed when children have been abused over a considerable time, as long ago as 1984 Kempe and Kempe (p. 190) realised that these children are 'trained to be a sexual object'. They also highlighted how, in such circumstances, the children (assumed at that time to be almost invariably girls abused by men) 'try to make each contact with any adult male an overt sexual event'. It is interesting that, in 1985, sexual abuse by women was not discussed, in public at least. However, we now know that women do abuse children sexually, and the same behaviour occurs for boys and girls abused by men and women (Mathews *et al.* 1989, Hanks & Saradjian 1991, Elliott 1993, Saradjian 1996, Hanks & Wynne 2001). A recent study (Tardif *et al.* 2005) investigated sexual abuse perpetrated by adult and juvenile females and concluded that problematic and conflict-ridden relationships with their parents, developmental disturbances, physical and sexual victimisation where just some of the characteristics related to the abusive behaviour.

The effects of post-traumatic stress preoccupied those working in the child abuse field for a long time (Finkelhor 1986, Wyatt & Powell 1988, Bentovim 1992, Briere 1992, Hobbs *et al.* 1999, 2003, Browne *et al.* 2002a, Myers *et al.* 2002, Vetere & Cooper 2005). Children and adults who experience traumatic responses to their abuse are often in the grip of their experience in a manner that is well outside their control. They may re-enact the events, engage in inappropriate sexual behaviours (hence the often-witnessed sexualised behaviour), have visualisations of the event(s), and have actual flashbacks and triggering memories which obscure any concentration on ordinary aspects of their lives. The effects may lead to avoiding places, things and people that may in turn trigger memories of the event, and it can also lead to dissociation and sometimes multiple personality and deletion of memories, which further leads to irritability or distractedness.

For the adult, the long-term difficulties can include problems in sexual adjustment or aversion to appropriate sexual contact. Equally, consequences can occur when the abused child grows up and has their own child. As parents, they may become overprotective (thinking 'I will never leave my child with any person because they may be abused'), or they may be neglectful, not having had any experience themselves of being adequately cared for. Boundaries may be blurred and crossed, and closeness may be difficult to achieve. Once again, our increasing understanding of attachment is relevant here, but in sexual abuse in particular it is essential to think in terms of adaptation rather than deprivation. The child who experiences sexual abuse will have to adapt in ways that preserve their psychological and physical integrity as much as possible. Most adaptations will be in a form that leaves them resistant to forming trusting, emotionally close relationships. Such adaptations, however sad, are entirely understandable and, in some contexts, quite functional. The challenge to the professional, and to society more generally, is to provide contexts in which the child can begin to explore alternative adaptations and so start to undo some of the harm that has been done to them.

One further point we wish to emphasise is that there is an important distinction relating to the intergenerational patterns of abuse. What we know about the repeating cycle of abuse is that many of the adults who sexually abuse have been abused sexually as children themselves. This connection is sometimes taken to mean that a sexually abused person automatically abuses sexually when they grow up. Many adult survivors voice this concern and feel as if they are doomed to repeat the pattern. What has to be added to the equation is that most adults who have been sexually abused will not become a perpetrator of abuse. Furthermore, we know of specific factors that can be protective, as discussed above and by Egeland (1988). The findings of Crouch *et al.* (2001) make a similar point for physical abuse. Experience of childhood abuse was indeed a predictor that the adult would abuse, but a perception that they had received support at the time, leading to a recognition of current social support, significantly reduced the risk that they would abuse. What we can say is that while the abused do not inevitably become abusers, when the history of abusing children and adults is examined, it almost always shows that they have been abused as children themselves

Conclusion

It is the issue of protective factors on which we wish to conclude. Much of the value of knowing about the consequences of abuse is that the knowledge is a first step towards effective protection of children. Facing up to the many different forms that abuse takes, and knowing the common consequences, alerts us to the possibility that abuse has occurred when we see children showing these signs. It indicates the tasks that treatment must undertake. Hopefully, it will also make sense to those in the child protection system who investigate cases and when cases come to court. It also enables us to identify maltreated individuals who have managed to avoid these consequences, and to discover what has been protective, or ameliorative, for them. Recognising the full extent of the forms and consequences of abuse may look like a dispiriting exercise. But when the positive potential of this knowledge is recognised, there is every good reason to continue to try to understand the significance of the harm that abuse does to children.

Acknowledgements

To our patients – all the people who have entrusted us with their difficulties. The cases quoted in this chapter are composite cases so as not to break confidentiality of any specific individual and to respect people's trust. We would also like to thank Dr Chris Hobbs and Dr Jane Wynne for their continued support and wisdom.

Key points and messages for practice

- To further reduce the incidence and prevalence of all forms of child abuse and neglect and to recognise and effectively counteract the ways that society contributes to the continuation of abuse of its children. The cycle of abuse has to be broken at a societal level.

- Not to ignore certain forms of abuse such as failure to thrive in infants and young children.

- To rethink, restructure, research and determine what is necessary for many children in terms of treatment, the type of treatment and particularly the length of treatment.

- Short-term interventions are not adequate for children who have been abused, particularly to alleviate long-term consequences of abuse.

- Protecting maltreated children is more difficult if it is undertaken in a context of resistance and obstruction. It is therefore important to understand the forms and origins of denial so that we can work to progressively change our own forms of resistance and those of the public, politicians, journalists and judges, alike.

- Recognising the consequences of abuse has significance for both identification and treatment. While the research is complex, it provides both extensive data and ways of understanding what effects known abuse is likely to have on the child in the short and longer term, and also of judging when the behaviour of children that is giving rise to concern should give rise to suspicions of abuse.

- High quality training for professionals must be given priority.

- We need to continually develop our understanding of the factors that protect children from long-term deficits, and particularly from continuing the cycle of abuse into the next generation.

Annotated further reading

Adcock M, White R, Hollows A (eds) 1998 Significant harm. Significant Publications, Croydon
This book centres on the 1989 Children Act which has had a profound influence on everyone's practice. It covers all forms of abuse. A must for every practitioner.

Bell M 1999 Child protection: families and the conference process. Ashgate, Aldershot
This is an interesting book for those wishing to undertake evaluative research. Though written specifically with social workers in mind, it describes research and how it can be used when working with families and children in need.

Bentovim A 1992 Trauma-organised systems. Physical and sexual abuse in families. Karnac, London
Another important book by Bentovim discussing all forms of abuse and relating it to trauma-organised systems and what that might entail for the child, family and professional involved.

Briere J N 1992 Child abuse trauma. Sage, Newbury Park, CA
This book describes the theory and treatment of the lasting effects of child abuse, and examines the interrelationship between the different forms of abuse and neglect with an emphasis on the trauma that such experiences have on the victim of abuse.

Browne K, Hanks H, Stratton P, Hamilton C 2002 Early prediction and prevention of child abuse. Wiley, Chichester
Authors with international reputations contribute to this book, which is arranged in four sections. Prevalence, prediction and prevention are the main themes.

Ceci S J, Hembrooke H 1998 Expert witness in child abuse cases. American Psychological Association, Washington, DC
Though the topic of expert witness has not been described in the chapter, this book will help professionals and guide them through the often incomprehensible legal system when they are to appear as expert witnesses. The book is written from an American perspective but has valuable advice for the British reader.

Hobbs C J, Hanks H G I, Wynne J M 1999 Child abuse and neglect – a clinician's handbook, 2nd edn. Churchill Livingstone, Edinburgh
A textbook written with both the medical and therapeutic practitioner in mind. It has been described by reviewers as 'a landmark textbook in the field of child abuse and neglect'. The many tables, diagrams, drawings and the photography make the material accessible to the reader in a way that is quite unique. The 2nd edition of this book includes not only updated references but also a considerable amount of new material.

Hobbs C J, Wynne J M (eds) 1993 Baillière's clinical paediatrics, Vol. 1, Child abuse. Baillière Tindall, London
This is an important collection by some of the most experienced writers in the field. It covers aspects of ritual abuse, the handicapped child and maltreatment, recent advances in radiology with reference to

child abuse, as well as interviewing children, emotional abuse, the cycle of abuse in adolescents and many other contributions. The 14 chapters are all very well written and relevant to the practitioner.

Iwaniec D 2004 Children who fail to thrive. Wiley, Chichester

Dorota Iwaniec is an expert in this field and has produced follow-up research with children who fail to thrive over a period of 20 years. The book is fascinating, filled with incredible insights into the children and families for whom FTT is an issue. No-one else has done a follow-up study stretching over this length of time. Iwaniec is a rigorous researcher and yet makes her subject very readable. We recommend this book to anyone working in the area of child maltreatment – in fact, it is a must.

Wissow L S 1990 Child advocacy for the clinician – an approach to child abuse and neglect. Williams & Wilkins, Baltimore

Another important textbook combining physical issues of child maltreatment and psychological issues. A powerful and thorough piece of work combining the medical and psychological.

Wyatt G E, Powell G J 1988 Lasting effects of child sexual abuse. Sage, Newbury Park, CA

Despite the fact that this book was written in 1988, it is an outstanding contribution, focusing on the effects of child sexual abuse.

6

Issues of gender

Brid Featherstone

INTRODUCTION

This chapter will provide a brief summary of themes from the literature on gender and offer an outline of the key issues which have emerged in relation to child abuse. It has two main purposes: to offer a gendered analysis of the current policy context and to reflect on the practice implications of contemporary policies.

Gender and gender relations: some background themes from the literature

The term gender was central to the political and academic project which emerged from second wave feminists in the late 1960s. As women started to challenge their confinement to the maternal and the 'private', it was judged necessary to challenge the assumptions that dominated within the wider culture and the sciences, including the social sciences, about what was considered 'right' or 'natural' for women and indeed men to *do* or *be*. Thus the project had an affinity with the development of social constructionist perspectives generally within the social sciences (Featherstone 2006). It emphasised the importance of interrogating how women were socially constructed, although over time there have been and continue to be debates about the appropriateness of a clear distinction between biology, culture and the role, if any, played by the psyche in constructing or resisting gendered identities (Flax 1990).

Feminists also challenged the specific model of the family that had achieved the status post-war of being both universal and normatively privileged – that of the male breadwinner with an economically dependent wife who took on caring responsibilities for him and their biological children. They also deconstructed 'the family', identifying it as the site of power relations, thus challenging the then dominant construction which was that of a consensual unity of complementary interests. Moreover, activities that had previously been hidden within the family, such as violent and abusive behaviour by men to women and children, were publicly named and challenged. Furthermore, activities such as women's caring were named as unpaid labour. This does not mean, however, that there was unanimity among feminists, particularly in relation to what should be campaigned for in relation to family life (see Bryson 2002).

From an initial focus on offering a voice to women and rendering visible their experiences and desires, there was a shift towards exploring and challenging *gender relations*.

Gender both as an analytic category and social process is relational. That is, gender relations are complex and unstable processes … constituted by and through interrelated parts. These parts are interdependent, that is, each part can have no meaning or existence without the others.

(Flax 1990, p. 44)

Putting this simply, a notion of 'man' does not make sense without having a notion of 'woman', and vice versa. Consequently, shifts in the meanings attached to being a woman have complex and wide-ranging implications for the meanings attached to being a man.

The recognition of gender as relational had a number of important implications. It obliged attention to be given to the constructed and unstable nature of categories such as masculinity and femininity and the necessity to engage with how these shifted relationally over time. This underscored the continued links between the theoretical and the empirical as women's and men's lives changed in complex ways over the decades in many of the countries from where feminism emerged. From the earliest days, however, although there was an acceptance that gender relations were power relations, there have been continuing debates about the nature and extent of such power relations. Such debates received urgent impetus from the recognition that the categories 'women' and 'men' were internally differentiated in terms of ethnicity, class, sexuality and disability (e.g. Segal 1987, 1997).

Alongside and partly interrelated with a range of other conceptual moves within the social sciences, feminists have seen language as a key site for battle in relation to contested meanings and gaps. This has been of prime importance in relation to naming and understanding violent and abusive behaviour.

Contemporary developments in gender-informed scholarship

It is beyond the scope of this chapter to summarise the wealth of work going on in this area. I want to draw attention to that which I consider particularly pertinent for practitioners engaging with families. Early feminist critiques of the family as a site or even *the* site of women's subordination have evolved and, according to Smart and Neale (1999), the term 'family practices' sums up the shifts that have occurred in feminist theoretical and empirical work (see also Morgan 1996). This challenges the notion of the family as a thing or an institution, reflecting the influence of theoretical currents such as post-modernism, the continued emergence of diverse family forms and the evidence of a dispersal of family practices across a range of households, often involving complex mixes of blood, kin and non-kin relationships.

The term 'practices' emphasises fluidity. More than this the term 'practices' allows us to conceptualize how family 'practices' overlap with other social practices (for example, gendering practices, economic practices and so on). Moreover, while 'practices' are historically and culturally located, they allow us to imagine the social actor who engages in these practices and may choose to modify them.

(Smart & Neale 1999, p. 121)

An example of work from within this approach is that of Smart and Neale's own research into men, women and children's accounts of 'family practices' post-divorce. It is very clearly not simply about offering a voice to women which was a key concern of early feminist work. It forms part of a wider academic project around rethinking care and caring responsibilities more generally, which has found academic expression in the funding of research projects such as CAVA based at the University of Leeds and the work on rethinking citizenship by Lister (1997, 2003a). CAVA has provided the umbrella for a number of inter-related research projects such as:

- Who looks after children when parents work?
- How do mothers and fathers negotiate caring responsibility after divorce?
- Who do single people go to for support?

It has attempted to develop what Williams (1999, p. 675) has called a 'moral grammar' from below. Thus it focuses not only on what people do but also what values and moral frameworks are being used to engage with ongoing dilemmas in a changing landscape where a particular model of family life – that of male breadwinner, economically dependent wife looking after the care needs of the family – does not dominate at either the level of policy or practice. Studies such as that by Duncan and Edwards (1999) of lone mothers' understandings of the notion of responsibility, and Lewis's (2001) work on the meanings attached by married and cohabiting couples to commitment and responsibility, all appear influenced by a concern to explore views from the 'bottom up'. Children from a range of ethnicities have explored their views on differing family forms (Brannen *et al.* 2000) and children's views on post-divorce family life have been explored by Smart *et al.* (2001). Much of this work appears indebted to the earlier work of Finch (1989), who explored family obligations among adults in the context of a particular policy climate in relation to community care, which sought to prescribe who should support whom.

Discussion

Why is the above scholarship relevant to those practising in the areas of child welfare and protection? According to Ferguson (2004), in contrast to the period of simple modernity, which was characterised by men, women and children knowing their place within a context of fixed meanings attached to masculinity and femininity, and socially sanctioned conventions around marriage, we are now in a 'new era'. Welfare practitioners are operating within fluid landscapes where gendered contracts are being rethought and recast, as well as attempting to be reinforced. Changes in family form and processes cannot be simply ascribed to changes in gender relations, nor can they be understood simply using a gendered lens; however, ignoring the complexities of shifting gender relations is also deeply problematic.

Nonetheless, the dangers of using a gendered analysis also need to be kept in mind, particularly in the area of sexual violence where there continues to be a need to remain alert to the dangers of assuming that gender is the end of an analysis rather than the beginning. As I have argued elsewhere:

By signposting the reality and consequences of male violence to women and children, feminists started a process which continues to be necessary. *Which* men and *why* are questions which require ongoing explorations at a range of interlocking levels in relation to gendering, economic, social and cultural processes. To signpost the responsibility of men for much of the violences practitioners encounter in family life is to begin rather than end that process.

(Featherstone 2004a, p. 11)

This chapter will, therefore, argue for the importance of continuing to develop gendered analyses whilst remaining alert to the dangers of finality and closure. As argued in Ferguson (2004), engaging with the fluid world of family relationships and the practices of welfare practitioners obliges caution about theories/analyses which seek to solidify or cast in stone profoundly mobile or 'liquid' processes.

Gender and child abuse: locating contemporary developments

The aim of this section is to offer a broad historical overview of developments. Some historians have argued that child welfare only becomes an issue when women's voices are being heard strongly and indeed the origins of 'modern' child protection systems are often traced back to a particular historical period when women began to engage in charitable work (Parton 2002). This period coincided with what became known as first-wave feminism. Gordon (1986), an American historian, argued that first wave feminism in the nineteenth century was actively involved in social work and child protection work. Organised feminism at that time was part of a liberal reform programme, a programme for the adaptation of the family and civil society to new economic conditions. She argued that, consciously or not, feminists felt that these conditions provided important possibilities for the freedom and empowerment of women and were to be embraced as part of a move away from an era where men held unquestioned property rights over women and children: 'child protection work was an integral part of the feminist as well as the bourgeois programme for modernising the family' (p. 75).

Gordon, writing in the 1980s, noted that, historically, 'feminists have been important advocates of modern social control. Yet contemporary feminist theoreticians have tended also exclusively to condemn social control' (p. 62). Certainly when the feminist influence in social work became apparent in the 1970s (see Featherstone 2004b), it was located within a wider uneasiness by feminists about the desirability of demanding, and/or the ability of the State to deliver, emancipatory possibilities for women. Feminists within social work, particularly in the UK where much social work occurred within the statutory sector, were therefore positioned uneasily. Some argued, however, for the importance of working in and against the State (Birmingham Women and Social Work Group 1985) whilst others were more pessimistic about the ability of the State to deliver (Wilson 1980). The welfare state, for example, was argued to be based upon gendered assumptions about the normative roles of men and women.

In general, feminists working on issues such as domestic violence and rape developed women-run services outside the statutory sector (e.g. refuges and helplines such as Women's Aid and Rape Crisis). Services such as refuges were also provided for children. Whilst State controls were sought in relation to punishing violent and abusive men, there was a considerable degree of suspicion about invoking the State to support women. Moreover, given its historical association with disciplining women, initially little attention was paid to whether State supports were necessary to discipline women in the interests of children.

However, the increased recognition of harms to children, such as child sexual abuse, obliged an active engagement with existing child welfare and protection services. Moreover, a pragmatic recognition emerged that domestic violence was not likely to be taken seriously by statutory social workers unless the harms to children were emphasised (Mullender & Morley 1994). It is important to note that the seeking of State control to discipline black men was questioned by black feminists in the context of racism (Featherstone 2004a).

Feminist engagement with child abuse in the 1980s and much of the 1990s centred largely on emphasising the harms to women and children from violent and abusive men. They were particularly active in highlighting the prevalence of child sexual abuse and its links with other forms of male violence. The notion of a continuum was coined by Kelly in 1988 to underscore the linkages between a range of activities from pornography, rape, domestic violence and child sexual abuse and the continuities between what had often been treated as discrete activities. An underlying analysis sought to situate the evidence of men's disproportionate involvement in such activities within an understanding of the underlying rationale for such behaviour – that of men's desire to maintain power over women and children.

Feminists also questioned intervention strategies. Hooper (1992) pointed out how often interventions in relation to child sexual abuse left women responsible for the protection of children but without adequate resources. Milner (1996) noted both that men resisted intervention and social workers colluded through a focus on mothers.

There was some recognition of complexities and of the need to disrupt binary analyses of peaceful women/violent men. For example, there was a recognition that women could abuse their children. Furthermore, the conflation of women and children's interests which seemed to flow from earlier analyses of domestic violence was challenged by feminists such as Hooper and Humphreys (1997). They argued that the complexities of mother–child relationship issues, which may have pre-dated the child sexual abuse and/or domestic violence, needed to be understood. Moreover, they argued that it was important to engage with the complexities of women and children's relationships because otherwise the effects of men's abuse on such relationships could be missed.

Many of these critiques fed into a developing analysis of the complexities of mothering as a set of practices and motherhood as an institution. For example, it was argued that feminists had often colluded in and promoted a fantasy of the 'perfect mother', thus obscuring the complexities and difficulties of actual mothers' feelings and experiences and/or rendering any difficulties attributable to the impact of men's behaviour or patriarchal institutions generally (Featherstone 1997).

However, whilst there was feminist attention paid to the complexities of mothering, feminist writings on men and masculinities in relation to child abuse were less well developed. There was a debate about the desirability of invoking State powers against black men, although there was also a counter-argument about the importance of not silencing women and children and recognising their rights to live lives free from violence or harm (Featherstone 2004a).

A sense of orthodoxy or closure around analysing why men predominated as perpetrators of domestic violence was evident in much of the feminist literature according to some writers (Featherstone & Trinder 1997). Men were constructed as a unitary category, consciously engaged in rational behaviour to maintain power over women and children. A key aspect of the critique was that differentiation within the category 'men' – on the basis of class, ethnicity, sexuality and so on – was not seen as legitimate by many feminists researching in the area of domestic violence: indeed, a single set of meanings was attached to men's behaviour. Whilst their focus was on analysing the discourses circulating within the feminist research literature aimed at policy makers and professionals, Featherstone and Trinder did argue that social workers appeared receptive to this literature. Humphreys (1999) disputed this, arguing that there was often little evidence of feminist-influenced analyses on social work practice with domestic violence (see also Scourfield 2003). However, it is important to note Featherstone and Trinder's overall point was that research and analyses were dominated by a particular feminist discourse. Featherstone and Lancaster (1997) advanced compatible arguments in relation to both theory and practice with men who sexually abuse. Scourfield (2003), from his research into the occupational culture of social workers, agreed with this analysis, which was that men were constructed as a unitary category whose behaviour carried singular meanings.

The context for feminist-inspired interrogations in the 1980s and much of the 1990s was that provided by successive Conservative administrations. The demographic, social and economic contours of this period have been well documented (e.g. Fox Harding 1997). There was a dramatic increase in child poverty (Bradshaw 2002) and considerable changes in family life with a growth in divorce rates (which started to level off in the mid-1990s) and in lone parenthood (mainly lone motherhood). Moreover, whilst there was a substantial growth in the number of women, including mothers, entering the paid labour force, child care provision remained poor. There was little support from the State in relation to developing an infrastructure which would enable the balancing of family and work responsibilities, and Benn's (1998) research with mothers in the mid-1990s noted that many felt they were trying to survive in two worlds with opposing priorities.

Men's positions in the workforce also changed in complex ways with the decline in many traditional industries, and there were particular issues for men in areas where heavy industries all but disappeared. Ruxton (2002) argued that the impact of economic restructuring in the 1980s and 1990s led to some groups of men clearly increasing their power, whilst others experienced downsizing and unemployment. At the end of the 1990s, the number of 'economically inactive' men (i.e. not employed or recorded as unemployed) outnumbered the recorded unemployed by two to one. Whilst this reflected government policies for claimants to move off the employment register and onto disability and sickness benefits, and tighter approaches to staff selection by employers, Ruxton speculates that some men may have retreated from increasingly difficult circumstances into incapacity.

Practice developments in this era in relation to child abuse have been well documented in the literature (Fox Harding 1991, Parton 2002) and it is beyond the remit of this chapter to outline these. Suffice to say that the publication of *Messages from Research* (DoH 1995) seemed to signal the need for a shift from an incident-focused reactive practice towards one that was more contextually located and that examined the emotional ecology within which the child(ren) were being brought up (see Parton 1996 for a discussion of this approach and the limitations of the analysis; see also Featherstone 2004a for a gendered analysis of *Messages from Research*).

Based on her research into domestic violence, Humphreys (1999) expressed a range of concerns which had both specific and general currency in relation to practice in the 1990s. The allocation of resources to investigating incidents at the expense of prevention or support programmes had particular consequences for women experiencing domestic violence: there was a tendency to focus on mothers, with little attention being paid to men. Minority ethnic families often experienced a particularly poor service due to a lack of sensitivity and racism. Women were expected to separate or remain separated from violent men whilst often not being offered the necessary resources, either materially or in terms of therapeutic services. This had resonance with Hooper's (1992) earlier work on the issues for women whose children had been sexually abused (often by a partner). She found that they ended up taking on prime responsibility for children's protection and healing whilst being offered little concrete help by agencies, including statutory social services departments (see also Farmer & Owen 1995). Indeed it could be argued that women undertook the child protection task of managing the ongoing risks to the child, particularly in a context of low conviction rates for perpetrators and often their continued geographical proximity.

New Labour and gender: the broad picture

Feminism has often appeared to be a dirty word in New Labour circles, appearing to reflect a desire in the early days particularly to build 'a big tent' and move away from an identification with what were seen as sectional interests (Franks 1999). However, New Labour has engaged with longstanding feminist concerns, particularly in relation to childcare support for working parents and the balancing of work and family responsibilities. As Bryson (2002) notes, 'these are no longer seen as feminist luxuries but central political demands' (p. 147).

Lister (2003b) argues that much of what has developed under New Labour in relation to family policy and children's services needs to be understood within an overall project of building a 'social investment state'. This term appears to have emerged from Giddens (1998), who argued that the welfare state needed to be replaced by a social investment state whose key guideline should be investment in human capital wherever possible, rather than the direct provision of economic maintenance. Analysts, such as Jenson and Saint-Martin (2001) from Canada and Lister (2003b) in the UK, have developed this further in relation to understanding the rationale behind the policies that have emerged.

It is argued that the social investment state has become central to a project seeking to link social and economic concerns in the context of the challenges posed by globalisation. Whilst the old welfare state sought to offer protection from the market, a social investment state recognises this is neither possible nor desirable – people need integrating into the market. In a globalised world, people's security comes from their ability constantly to adapt to new challenges; thus the State will enable this in a variety of ways. The State invests in cautious and highly targeted ways to ensure that people, men and women alike, are best placed to participate in the global economy.

The notion of *time*, which underpins the social investment state, is of interest here. The results produced by an investment are located in the future whereas consumption is something that occurs in the present. For State spending to be effective and worthwhile, it must not be directed towards the present but rather seen as an investment that is geared towards producing rewards in the future. Thus spending may legitimately be directed to:

- supporting and educating children because they hold the promise of the future
- promoting health and healthy populations because they pay off in terms of future costs
- reducing the probability of future costs of school failure and crime with a heavy emphasis on children
- fostering employability so as to increase future labour force participation rates.

Spending on children, particularly in the early years of their lives, is thus strongly legitimated. Remedial policies for adults are a poor (and costly) substitute for interventions in childhood (e.g. Esping-Andersen's edited collection 2002). It is in this context that the emergence of initiatives such as *Sure Start* can be understood (see Jeffery 2003 for an outline of this programme).

There are many criticisms to be made of the instrumental approach to children, which is promoted by the social investment approach, not least that it is not located within more holistic approaches to children to be found within the UN Convention on the Rights of the Child (Lister 2003b). Moreover, this instrumental approach coexists with the increased demonisation of children, particularly in the context of their rights to occupy public space (e.g. James & James 2001).

However, in the context of the concerns of this chapter, a key criticism must be the way in which policies for the abolition of children's poverty have been pursued in isolation from any acknowledgement of the links between their poverty and that of their caretakers, who are often women (Lister 2003b). The strategy therefore obscures the need to pay attention to gendered inequalities in the labour market. Whilst this has implications for all children, there may be particular issues for those who come to the attention of services because of concerns about neglect. Whilst there have been ongoing debates about the precise nature of the links between poverty and neglect, there is a recognition that there are links and, moreover, that neglect is also a gendered issue. For example, as Turney (2005) argues, a construction of the 'neglectful mother' has underpinned much of social work practice but there is an absence of discussion about what constitutes 'neglectful fathering' (Daniel & Taylor 2005).

The ambivalence on the part of the State, historically, towards mothers entering the paid labour force has all but disappeared (Land 1999). This valorisation of the paid worker identity has been strongly challenged by feminists who argue for the need for a 'political ethics of care' to underpin policy. Williams (2001), for example, challenges the values underpinning the welfare settlement being developed by New Labour and argues for a shift away from the normative assumption that independence through paid work is the desired goal for all. By contrast she argues for a recognition of our interdependence and calls for a more rounded conception of citizenship with which to underpin policy, which would acknowledge the importance of care as an expression of citizenship responsibilities. We are all interdependent and need care as well as needing to give it: care involves a complex set of practices, which are meaningful in their own right and can promote the civic duties of responsibility, trust, tolerance for human limitations and frailty, and acceptance of diversity.

This perspective is of considerable importance in a policy climate where the promotion of paid work coexists with increasing responsibilities being placed upon parents. Lister (2003b) has noted more generally that, in return for the promise of investment in economic opportunity by the State, increased emphasis is being placed upon the responsibilities of citizens in a number of respects:

- to equip themselves to respond to the challenges of economic globalisation through improving their employability
- to invest in their own pensions
- to accept responsibility for their children.

The last responsibility found expression in key pieces of legislation introduced by the Conservatives, such as the Children Act 1989 and the Child Support Act 1991, and has been continued under New Labour and inserted into a broader project. As has been documented, this project has gendered implications in the context of an ongoing gender division of labour in relation to parenting. Thus, it is more likely that mothers will carry the weight of responsibilities for truanting children and antisocial behaviour (see Featherstone 2004a for an analysis of parenting orders under the Crime and Disorder Act 1998, and Lister 2003b for a discussion of the gendered implication of antisocial behaviour legislation more generally).

The gendered implications for those who are involved with services because of child protection concerns are less well rehearsed in the policy literature in the UK. In the US there have been ongoing concerns about the promotion of a worker identity for mothers by the State and the tensions this can pose for those who are also expected to be responsible for supervising and protecting their children in cases of domestic violence and child sexual abuse (Brandwein 1999, Featherstone 2004a).

There have been some attempts to recognise fathers as parents and in particular to begin to address the balancing of work and care responsibilities. Developments in relation to concrete material changes in working practices have been patchy, however, and need to be understood within an overall context where British fathers work the longest hours in Europe. Therefore, the focus of change efforts has been more often twofold: targeting specific groups of fathers through time-limited service initiatives, and encouraging service providers in health and social care to be more responsive to fathers. The difficulties of this focus will be addressed more fully below.

New Labour, gender and 'child abuse'

As indicated, the predominant concerns of New Labour have been to abolish poverty and foster early intervention initiatives such as *Sure Start* programmes in order to facilitate children's life chances. This could be seen to fit with the longstanding concerns of child welfare advocates, such as Holman (1988) and Tunstill (1997), about the deleterious impact of poverty on the ability of parents to offer children what they need to flourish in their own families, but also with the interlinked concern that those children who were removed from their families and placed in State care were overwhelmingly from poor backgrounds. However, it is of interest to note that Tunstill (1999) has expressed concern about the policy emphasis on parental employment as the key means of abolishing children's poverty.

Initially, New Labour sought to construct child abuse within language which seemed directly borrowed from *Messages from Research* (DoH 1995). For example, in their report submitted to the UN Committee on the Rights of the Child in 1999 (there is a requirement that a report is submitted every 5 years) it was argued that physical and sexual abuse in the home is often triggered by pressure on families and that 'real benefits could arise if there was a focus on the wider needs of children and families, rather than a narrow concentration on the alleged incident of abuse' (quoted in Roberts 2001, p. 59).

At times, the language of 'stress' has emerged to provide an underpinning rationale for why difficulties occur and for related policy and practice initiatives (Parton 2002). For example:

Many of the families who become the subject of child protection suffer from multiple disadvantages. Providing services and support to children and families under stress may strengthen the capacity of parents to respond to the needs of their children before problems develop into abuse.

(DoH *et al.* 1999, p. 2)

However, the mobilisation of the language of stress may obscure as much as it illuminates. Busfield (1996), in her exploration of gender and mental health issues, argues that stress is a notoriously imprecise and slippery term. There is a need to distinguish between the way the concept of stress is used to refer to certain features of an individual's social situation (stressful situations or stressors) and to the physical or psychological responses to stress (stress responses). Busfield argues that even if we only use the term to refer to situations rather than responses, we still have to identify the domain of the stressful – the features that are considered likely to prove stressful. 'Potentially the domain is infinite; in practice researchers limit the range quite considerably, incorporating varying assumptions as to what is stressful in their research' (p. 191). Divorce and unemployment are usually included but not war or sexual abuse.

Exclusion of issues such as childhood sexual abuse from the list is not only a matter of the presumed exceptional nature of the occurrence, according to Busfield, but also because of another common limitation on the domain of the stressful: it is usually restricted to recent occurrences – usually the previous year or 6 months – rather than to more distant events. Furthermore, the domain of stressful situations tends to focus on events rather than ongoing difficulties. When the focus is only on events, then becoming unemployed during the period in question is included while being unemployed is not. This distinction is relevant to many features of women's situations such as 'the possible ongoing stresses of domestic labour and child care or managing household tasks alongside full-time work outside the home. It also applies to the quality of relations within the home … and to the experience of discrimination' (Busfield 1996, p. 192).

There are important issues, therefore, in what counts as a stressor. Moreover, it is important to think through very carefully what is a source and what is a response. How can we understand domestic violence in particular situations? For example, there is evidence to suggest that violence by men to women can emerge as a result of unemployment (Ruxton 2002) and during pregnancy (Daniel & Taylor 2005). It is therefore important to deconstruct terms such as stress and domestic violence, and to think through how these may be related in particular circumstances to men's particular investments in particular discourses of masculinity and their structural positions in relation to class, ethnicity and so on (Segal 1997).

Busfield does accept that there is empirical support for the existence of a link between stressful events and psychological distress but argues for complex models which account for the ways in which individuals express inner tension and distress. Moreover, such models need to have a gendered dimension to engage with the complexities of how men and women handle psychological distress.

Overall, the discourse of stress and pressure upon parents not only obscures gendered differences between parents, but also legitimates wider strategies that fail to pay attention to uncomfortable questions such as 'What causes sexual abuse?' and 'Do dominant constructions of fathering and mothering reproduce generational power relations and oppressive behaviour between men, women and children?'

Every Child Matters: A Consultation Process (DfES 2003a) (hereafter referred to as ECM) has been a key document in pulling together the diverse range of initiatives that have proliferated since 1997 and advancing an overarching vision. Whilst this document raises a host of concerns at conceptual, policy and practice levels, the purpose of the discussion here is to explore its gendered implications rather than more general concerns.

Daniel *et al.* (2005) identify a range of issues which are neglected within ECM, including the failure to recognise children as gendered and to use a gendered perspective to engage adequately with the causes and consequences of maltreatment. Furthermore, there is no attention paid to the possible gendered implications of particular initiatives in relation to intervention and prevention.

Children as gendered

The failure to recognise children as gendered means that there is an inadequate appreciation of the implications of research evidence that would suggest that boys and girls often have different patterns of help-seeking, although both share a reluctance to engage with formal sources of support. Whilst girls appear better equipped to use their friendship network as sources of support than boys (Fuller *et al.* 2000), boys can police each other in relation to dominant constructions of masculinity (Frosh *et al.* 2001). Moreover, there continue to be gendered differences in parents' abilities to act as sources of support. Mothers emerge more often as sources of support for children than fathers (Featherstone & Evans 2004).

Boys and girls also appear to have different levels of vulnerability in relation to abuse and the consequences can be different. For example, girls appear more vulnerable to sexually abusive behaviour and sexualised bullying (Featherstone & Evans 2004) whilst boys, when sexually abused, can struggle with constructions of masculinity that censor or invalidate their experiences of victimisation.

Gender and maltreatment

In relation to sexual abuse the vast majority of perpetrators are male (Frosh 2002). Furthermore, much sexual abuse either occurs outside the family or from family members other than parents. The pattern of abusive behaviour amongst adults who sexually abuse children can often be traced back to adolescence (Daniel *et al.* 2005).

Whilst causation in relation to engaging with sexually abusive behaviour is complex, a key issue must be to tackle male socialisation processes, wider cultural tendencies to sexually objectify women and children, and the complexities of power relationships between men, women and children. There may also be a need for approaches to sex and relationship education that address gender issues with boys and girls and promote equal and consensual relationships. Government strategies, certainly within ECM, do not address this but seem to suggest that the primary route for intervention is fostering supportive and secure family relationships (Daniel *et al.* 2005). Whilst this will be important on a number of levels, it cannot be enough.

The gendered implications of support and intervention

In relation to the wide range of intervention strategies proposed from early intervention onwards, there is a failure to engage with what is already known about the gendered nature of implications of service intervention. For example, women are often the sole focus of intervention, even when the source of the difficulties is a man (Scourfield 2003). As indicated previously, they are expected to carry considerable responsibility for protection when the child has been sexually abused, and there is little evidence from recent research (Featherstone 2004a) to suggest that this has changed from the picture painted by Hooper over a decade ago (1992).

The introduction of domestic violence as a child protection issue in countries such as Canada would suggest that the consequences for women and children have not been positive in many respects (Davies & Krane 2006). In particular it would appear that it is becoming increasingly common to hold women responsible for 'failing to protect' children because they are being subject to domestic violence. Within a frame that privileges the child, the woman's own pain and suffering can disappear or be seen as a less valid area for intervention. Men disappear from interventions and the onus once more remains on the mother to separate from the perpetrator within a specific time frame or face losing her children.

With the mainstreaming of domestic violence as a child protection issue in the UK, primarily as a result of the Adoption and Children Act 2002, we are in uncertain times. Whilst it is early days, there is anecdotal evidence to suggest that rates of notification by the police to social services departments are proving overwhelming and that responses to mothers are either non-existent or over-punitive, whilst men are not being engaged with by services (Featherstone & Peckover forthcoming).

Whilst ECM and later developments such as the *National Service Framework for Children, Young People and Maternity Services* (DoH/DfES 2004) do acknowledge the need to 'engage fathers', this is almost completely tokenistic (certainly in ECM), and inadequately rooted in an understanding of broader gender issues. Whilst the premises upon which the call to engage fathers are not spelt out adequately in either document, they would appear to be twofold: fathers need to be involved in order to foster better outcomes for children; and/or fathers are eager to be involved with services but are being thwarted unfairly by discriminatory service providers.

In relation to the first premise, the research evidence from longstanding academic researchers such as Lamb and Lewis (2004) would suggest that the familial context in which father involvement occurs is crucial. Basically, the quality of adult relationships matters greatly: father involvement which exacerbates or causes conflict, hostility and/or violence between the adults concerned will not foster good outcomes for children. In relation to the second premise, the picture is rather more complex than that of eager fathers being thwarted by discriminatory service providers. Whilst there remains an urgent need for good quality research evidence in this area, it would appear that whilst some fathers can indeed be ignored by practitioners, others are resistant to becoming involved with service providers. This can lead to their needs going unmet (Ferguson 2004) or can be even more problematic in terms of their actual or threatened behaviour. Fathers do not form a homogeneous category. Most crucially, whilst those who have come to the attention of child protection services often share commonalities at a structural level in terms of being poor and/or unemployed (Ryan 2000), they often differ, not only in terms of the subject positions they invest in, but also in terms of specific biographical experiences (e.g. experiences of abuse, mental and physical ill health, substance misuse).

A range of services to 'engage fathers' have emerged in more recent years through a variety of funding mechanisms. For example, the Home Office funded some 3-year projects aimed at specific groups of fathers judged hard to engage (Featherstone 2003). *Sure Start* programmes have been encouraged to develop initiatives in relation to engaging fathers and, indeed, the proposed Children's Centres will be obliged to develop services in this area. However, there is a paucity of community resources for men, including fathers who are violent. Moreover, as yet little in the way of guidance has emerged for workers in statutory services, where it is probable the men who cause most difficulties for women and children are to be found, and there is no consideration of the training and support needs for those (predominantly female workers) involved in working with such men. Moreover, the failure to incorporate an understanding of gender relations means that no attention is paid to the possible implications of introducing men into what have been women-only services. The complexities of men and women's lives are obscured with little recognition of the possibility that whilst many men may wish to engage and cooperate, others will be resistant and/or violent and thus require specialist and contextually appropriate interventions.

Discussion

We are in complex times, gender wise. Overall, there has been a shift towards 'explicit' family policies under New Labour, which marks a historical change in social policy, given the previous invisibility of the family in terms of social policy. After an uncertain start, such family policies do not promote a particular model of family to be adhered to and there have been and continue to be important shifts towards recognising the validity of diverse family forms. In terms of gender, women's (including mothers') aspirations to be workers have been fully recognised, although there remain concerns about such a blanket approach. The issues for those fleeing violence and/or coping with the consequences of abusive behaviour towards children have not been addressed in terms of developing policies which can balance work and care, however, and although there have been some moves towards recognising men as 'fathers', these remain limited and tentative.

Unlike under previous Conservative administrations, children's poverty has been recognised as a serious social problem and ambitious targets set for its abolition.

However, there are real concerns about how sustainable New Labour's approach is in a context in which many adults are only able to access flexible low-wage jobs in a gender-stratified labour market (Toynbee 2003).

In terms of specific service developments, however, new sites of practice have emerged post-1997 which lend a patchy and piecemeal character to the contemporary landscape. In some areas, where targeted services such as *Sure Start* operate, a range of sources of support for men and women, boys and girls have emerged. As Children's Centres come on line, there will also be a geographical expansion of support services, although there is considerable concern about the lower levels of funding being attached to these Centres, particularly in the context of their prioritisation of employment, child care and early years education over family support (Featherstone 2005).

Once again, statutory services are undergoing a complex process of structural reform, addressing fundamental questions such as the integration of services and their reorientation towards early intervention and prevention. However, it is hard, within the welter of policy documents on structure and function, to get any sense of the messy, everyday realities of an enterprise which is concerned with women (usually) visiting other women (and occasionally men) in their homes and assessing how they care for their children. In this context, remarkably little attention continues to be paid to issues such as 'psychological and emotional experience or expressiveness' (Ferguson 2004, p. 164) and yet the reality of such work involves engaging with intimate relationships in intimate spaces such as people's homes.

As an educator trying to engage with students around the practice implications of implementing the *Framework for the Assessment of Children in Need and their Families* (DoH *et al.* 2000), I am often uncomfortably aware that I cannot advocate certainty in relation to what should be done and what 'truths' govern what should or is allowed to be seen. Whilst such uncertainty can result in a retreat into defensiveness, it can also mean that many workers operate in a confused and messy hinterland. The complexity of gendered relationship is only part of this landscape but it is an important part and, moreover, a part which is worked out in the context of class and ethnic divisions.

There has been a broader recognition that many women and men are involved in everyday experiments in living and in ongoing negotiations about their roles and responsibilities, which attest at the very least to a 'democratic possibility', if not reality (Lewis 2001). However, as Ferguson (2004) notes, it is often assumed that those who come to the attention of, or ask for help from, child welfare professionals are stuck in an antidemocratic time warp and/or are uninterested in the new possibilities that are open to men and women in their relationships with each other and their children. He argues, on the basis of his research in the Republic of Ireland, that this is inaccurate and points out the paradox of such judgements being made by those who, in their own lives, are trying out new possibilities for themselves. A process of 'othering' may operate to distance workers from service users, but this is neither always a conscious process nor, of course, completely unrooted in the material realities of some service users' lives and their relationships with services, which can be hostile and disengaged.

Whilst in an earlier section I located some of the difficulties attached to a project to 'engage fathers', it is this project that actually holds out some of the best opportunities for opening up discussion about contemporary gender relations, particularly in the context of anxieties about class and ethnicity. From my experience of evaluating a number of services and of seeking to engage students with this agenda, it has become very obvious that it obliges important questions to be asked, not only about what men and women service users want or do not want from each other, but also how men and women workers feel and engage with such issues. It often obliges engagement with gendered anxieties about men, and uncomfortable issues such as how men from different classes and 'races', such as African–Caribbean men, can become marked as 'dangerous', or how men from South Asian backgrounds can be marked as straightforwardly 'patriarchal'.

Finally, I want to signpost an important area that requires ongoing thoughtful interrogation. Any examination of key feminist demands on 'the State' in the last few decades would suggest that problematic and unintended consequences have ensued. Whilst these are currently very sharply posed in relation to the linkages that have increasingly been made between domestic violence and child protection in law, policy and practice, they are not unique to this arena. For example, a key feminist demand of the 1980s was that the focus of intervention in child sexual abuse work should be to remove the perpetrator rather than the child. In practice, as outlined previously, once the risk was judged by workers to be removed, ongoing support was not offered, often leaving mothers to cope as single parents, with little financial and material support. Currently, such is the scale of the difficulties posed for mothers in certain countries where domestic violence has been recognised as a child protection issue (another feminist demand) that some have called for a 'moratorium' on further legislation (Jaffe *et al.* 2003).

I am not counselling here that we return to the early days of feminist pessimism about the role of the State (although I would suggest that being aware of the issues that were raised then continues to be important). I am also sympathetic to Ferguson's (2004) arguments that social workers can offer possibilities for 'life planning' to abused women and their children, although these are often local accomplishments and, in my experience, undertaken against the odds of time and resource constraints in statutory agencies. My own research would suggest that possibilities such as these have more obviously been available in well-funded *Sure Start* programmes, where staff have had a clear understanding of the importance of engaging with the impact of violent and abusive behaviour, as well as the time and resources to deal with it carefully and sensitively (Featherstone 2005).

It is beyond the scope of this chapter to attempt to conceptualise 'the State' today. There needs, however, to be an engagement by those concerned with gender to engage with debates in this area. If we continue to make demands on policy makers, it is essential that we are alert to the need for, and try to build in the possibility of, auditing and feeding back the unintended consequences of such demands. One strand in this is the need to engage those who are at the receiving end of such policies in their formulation; however, whilst this is important, it too is limited as there will be competing demands and interests.

Conclusion

This chapter has traced the contours of a literature on gender and the ways in which it has informed thinking, policy and practice in relation to child abuse. It has been concerned to offer a gendered analysis of the policy context under New Labour, both in relation to more general policies in child welfare but also in relation to child protection. Whilst it recognises some of the progressive possibilities that have opened up under New Labour, it also counsels caution. It argues for a reflective approach to making demands on policy makers and locates this within a particular reading of the difficulties and unintended consequences of practice in relation to child sexual abuse and domestic violence.

- There is a need to monitor and audit the gendered implications of policies in relation to whether they reinforce women's sole responsibility for the care and protection of their children, particularly in a context where women are expected to assume a paid worker identity.

- There is a need to challenge practices that focus on mothers' behaviour and abilities if it is the men in their lives who are causing the difficulties.

- Language is important. When we design interventions for parents are we really planning for mothers *and* fathers?

- Boys and girls can have different patterns of help-seeking and different responses to maltreatment.

Annotated further reading

Featherstone B 2004 Family life and family support: a feminist analysis. Palgrave, Basingstoke
This is useful because it explores how men's, women's, boys' and girls' lives are changing within a rethinking of family practices and the meanings attached to family. It analyses how family support policies under New Labour are engaging with such changes and, based upon the author's own research in a variety of family support projects, outlines the possibilities and the obstacles for developing practices which challenge oppressive constructions of masculinity and femininity.

Ferguson H 2004 Protecting children in time: child abuse, child protection and the consequences of modernity. Palgrave Macmillan, Basingstoke
This combines a historical analysis with an interrogation of contemporary state practices with vulnerable families. It offers evidence from the author's own research in the Republic of Ireland that social workers can contribute towards opening up democratic possibilities for family members, possibilities which can counter gendered and generational violence and abuse.

Scourfield J 2003 Gender and child protection. Palgrave, Basingstoke
This is based upon an ethnographic study of the occupational culture within social work in a region in the UK and analyses how social workers constructed the men and women with whom they worked in relation to a range of discourses around masculinity and femininity. It would suggest that there continue to be powerful imperatives in statutory social work towards focusing on mothers and ignoring fathers and men, even when it is the men's behaviour which is causing many of the family difficulties.

Taylor J, Daniel B 2005 Child neglect: practice issues for health and social care. Jessica Kingsley, London
This is an edited collection which brings together up-to-date research and thinking about neglect. It has very useful chapters on mothers and fathers. The chapter on fathers is particularly helpful as this is such a poorly theorised and understood area.

Useful addresses

Gender and Child Welfare Network: Professor Brid Featherstone, Department of Social Sciences and Humanities, University of Bradford BD7 1DP

Useful websites

CAVA: Centre for Research on the Politics, Practices and Ethics of Care: www.leeds.ac.uk/cava
Families, Lifecourse and Generations (FLaG) Research Centre: www.leeds.ac.uk/family
Fathers Direct: www.fathersdirect.com
National Family and Parenting Institute: www.nfpi.org.uk

7 | Issues of culture
Jill E. Korbin

INTRODUCTION

The relationships between child maltreatment and culture are complex, politically charged and fraught with unresolved issues. The fundamental challenge in fully incorporating culture into child maltreatment work is to respect diversity while ensuring equitable standards of care for all children, regardless of background. The incorporation of culture into child maltreatment work has implications for general principles of child protection and for effective intervention with individual families.

A recent review of the child development literature by a panel of experts in the United States identified culture as the second of ten core concepts, noting that 'Culture influences every aspect of human development and is reflected in child-rearing beliefs and practices designed to promote healthy adaptation' (Shonkoff & Phillips 2000, p. 3). Important efforts are underway to examine how best to serve diverse populations (e.g. Brophy et al. 2005).

Cultural competence

The term cultural or ethnic competence was introduced to child protection by anthropologist James Green (1978, 1982) to refer to acquired abilities to transcend cultural boundaries. The term, used more widely in the US than in the UK, has come to be regarded as indispensable in effective child protection and other human services work (e.g. Korbin 1987a, 1997, Cross et al. 1989, Abney 1996, Korbin & Spilsbury 1999). Cultural competence is grounded in the ability to stand in other people's shoes and to view the world through their eyes. Cultural competence moves beyond an individual's untrained abilities to be sensitive to other cultures; rather, cultural competence must be acquired as a repertoire of knowledge and skills.

Two conceptual frameworks are key to culturally competent knowledge. First, cultural competence requires knowledge not only about culture broadly conceptualised, but also about variability both within and between cultures. This knowledge facilitates the ability to 'unpack' culture. Second, cultural competence requires an understanding of the balance between ethnocentrism and cultural relativism. These key components of cultural competence assist in the assessment of which aspects of a family's difficulties are 'cultural', which are 'abusive' or 'neglectful', and which are a combination of factors.

'Unpacking' culture: between and within cultural variability

Hundreds of definitions have been offered for the concept of culture, most centring on the ideas of culture as learned and shared, and as the interpretive force that guides interactions among people. Culture is not monolithic or static, but variable and dynamic: culture is not uniformly distributed and is experienced differently, varying, for example, by age, gender and social roles, and by individual differences in experience, personality or temperament.

Broad categorisations of peoples on the basis of physical characteristics (e.g. skin colour) do not necessarily reflect cultural reality (Korbin 1981, 1997, Abney 1996, Fontes 2001): white British do not form a homogeneous group any more than do black groups. Designations such African and African–Caribbean show a wide range of variation based, for example, on tribal or religious affiliations. While it may seem obvious, referring to people who come from Uganda and Cote d'Ivoire simply as 'African' makes as much sense as expecting commonalities between all the peoples in France and Germany. In the United States, designations such as Latino/Hispanic, Asian/Pacific Islander, Native American Indian, African or African–American similarly group peoples in ways that may mask rather than illuminate culture.

Diversity among European–Americans is less frequently the subject of comment, but this diversity is equally powerful. Geographic considerations also are less frequently noted; for example, Puerto Ricans living in New York may be quite different from Puerto Ricans living in Cleveland, Ohio, and Pakistanis living in Leicester may be quite different from those living in Bradford. Because variability within the group can, and often does, exceed variability between groups, it becomes critical to 'unpack' culture to understand how it works in all of its complexity. In addition to concerns about intracultural variability, when culture or ethnicity is identified on the basis of characteristics such as skin colour, these groupings may not represent culture at all, but be a proxy for socio-economic advantage or disadvantage.

Ethnocentrism and cultural relativism

A second key component of culturally competent knowledge is the balance between ethnocentrism and cultural relativism. Ethnocentrism is the belief that one's own cultural beliefs and practices are not only preferable, but also superior, to all others. In contrast, cultural relativism is the belief that each and every culture must be viewed in its own right as equal to all others, and that culturally sanctioned behaviours cannot be judged by the standards of another culture. An exclusive reliance on either position has serious implications for practice.

As illustrated in Figure 7.1, an unmoderated ethnocentric position disregards cultural differences and imposes a single standard for child care practices: it is counterproductive for effective child protection because it attempts to impose the beliefs and behaviours of one group, the dominant culture, on all populations. The end result of unmoderated ethnocentrism is the risk of false positives, or misidentification of cultural practices as child maltreatment. Conversely, an unmoderated relativist position suspends all standards and runs the risk of false negatives, or misidentification of maltreatment as culture.

Figure 7.1
Cultural competence in child protection.

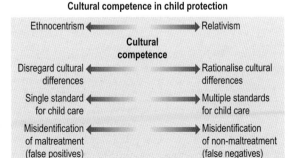

Cultural competence in child protection

Culturally competent definitions of child maltreatment

Child care practices must be viewed from the perspectives of both insiders and outsiders to the culture in question. Examples of practices that would be differentially defined as abusive or neglectful by different cultural groups abound in the cross-cultural record (e.g. Korbin 1981) and cross-cultural research has not yielded a universally accepted set of parenting guidelines. Further, debates about 'good enough' parenting suggest that, even within one society, what constitutes proper child rearing is highly contested. The plethora of child care books in the United States and the UK points to controversies about such basic tasks of child rearing as feeding practices, sleeping patterns and disciplinary approaches. The anthropologist Margaret Mead commented that one of the rare regularities of American childrearing is the commitment of one generation to do things differently from their parents.

Cultural conflict in defining child maltreatment generally arises because of differences in child care beliefs and practices. Seriously abused and neglected children look sadly similar across cultural contexts, however, and consensus is growing about these types of maltreatment (e.g. Daro *et al*. 1996). Nevertheless, child maltreatment encompasses so many grey areas that, in practice, what constitutes abuse or neglect is often highly contested across cultures. As illustrated in Figure 7.2, the greater the divergence in child care practices and beliefs, the greater the potential for cultural conflict in definitions of maltreatment (Korbin 1997).

Examinations of child maltreatment cross-culturally involve three levels of definition (Korbin 1981, 1987a, 1997), which will be considered in more detail below:

1. cultural differences in child care and childrearing practices
2. idiosyncratic or individual deviance from cultural norms
3. societal abuse or neglect of children.

Child maltreatment can be further identified across cultures as those acts that are preventable, proximate and proscribed, terms that differentiate child maltreatment from other harms to children. 'Preventable' and 'proximate' distinguish child maltreatment from other circumstances that have detrimental consequences for children (such as natural disasters) and tie the behaviour more closely to parent or caregiver, rather than to larger societal harms such as warfare. In contrast, 'proscribed' puts the act into a cultural context in that the behaviour should be prohibited by the culture in question (Finkelhor & Korbin 1988). These criteria make the definition of child maltreatment flexible enough to encompass a range of cultural contexts.

Figure 7.2
Cultural conflict in defining child abuse and neglect (reproduced with permission from Korbin 1997).

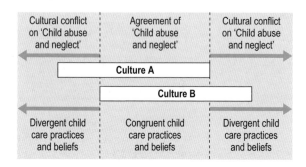

Cultural differences

At the first definitional level, the cross-cultural literature provides a wealth of examples of differential definitions of what constitutes child maltreatment (e.g. Korbin, 1981, 1987a, 1997, Ima & Hohm 1991, Fontes 2005). Although it is one thing to assemble a list of behaviours from other cultures that seem abusive or neglectful, it is equally, if not more instructive to view one's own culture through the eyes of others. The ability to understand one's own culture is the stepping stone to being able to understand other cultures. For example, in Eurocentric nations, common paediatric advice is that it is developmentally important for infants and young children to sleep independently. This does not, however, preclude debate about the advantages and disadvantages of co-sleeping versus letting children cry at night, with both sides of the debate viewing the other as improperly raising their children.

Independent infant and young child sleep arrangements, however, are unusual cross-culturally. A classic anthropological study of co-sleeping in traditional Japanese culture found that two generation co-sleeping was viewed as preferable and expected throughout the life cycle (Caudill & Plath 1966). Among rural Hawai'ian–American-Polynesians, a young child sleeping alone is considered at best unkind, and at worst, dangerous (Korbin 1990). Leaving an infant to cry itself to sleep was difficult to comprehend among the Bena, a traditional highland New Guinea society, in which it was believed that a crying infant's spirit could escape through the open fontanelle causing death (Langness 1981). Viewing human behaviour from an evolutionary perspective, McKenna and colleagues (1990) have hypothesised that co-sleeping may be advantageous because parents and children may coordinate breathing and sleep cycles, thereby preventing apnoea spells possibly related to sudden infant death syndrome (SIDS).

At this first definitional level of cultural differences rooted in variation in child-rearing beliefs and practices, cultural competence assumes an orientation of cultural and ethnic *difference* rather than *deficiency*. A deficiency approach is ethnocentric in the insistence that one cultural standard is superior to others, while a difference approach allows a more circumspect and contextual perspective without compromising child well-being. Nevertheless, as discussed below, an unmoderated difference orientation has its dangers.

Cultural conflicts in health care settings provide examples of the difficulties in sorting out what is abusive. Following a *difference* orientation, health care practices that are firmly grounded in a cultural tradition generally are not reported as abusive. A dramatic example is 'coin rubbing' as a medical practice among the Vietnamese. This practice involves forcefully pressing metal coins on the body of an ill child to force out or push out the illness. This results in a striking linear pattern of bruises. When first observed in United States' medical facilities, the impulse was to report these families for abuse. However, 'coin rubbing' is a cultural curing practice administered with good intentions, without anger or rage, and usual medical practice is not to report these families for abuse (Yeatman *et al.* 1976).

However, as noted above, just because a practice or behaviour is 'cultural' does not mean that it is also good for all members of the society (Edgerton 1992). Keeping in mind that unmoderated relativism is also potentially misleading and dangerous, two subcategories of cultural differences should also be considered:

1. Cultural practices may cause harm.
2. Cultural practices need to be viewed in the context of socio-cultural and environmental change.

Cultural practices may cause harm

Culturally based practices may cause injury or be harmful to children. Some practices are physically challenging and painful. For example, there has been wide-ranging debate about the harms and benefits to children in the course of harsh initiation rites (e.g. Langness 1981). Culturally based practices may have only good intentions, but nevertheless cause harm. In the southwest of the United States, for example, lead poisoning in young children was linked to indigenous medications – 'azarcon' and 'greta' used to cure 'empacho' ('empacho' is an illness defined by many Hispanic populations as a bolus, or lump, in the stomach that must be purged). In some localities, indigenous medications had high concentrations of lead (Trotter *et al.* 1983). Educational and community awareness efforts were successful in decreasing the use of ingredients found to be harmful, and substituting alternative ingredients and remedies. The incidence of lead poisoning was thus addressed without denigrating the culturally based need for and approach to curing 'empacho'. This example illustrates how a *difference* orientation allows greater flexibility in solutions and is more suited to cultural competence than is a *deficiency* orientation that seeks to change cultural practices and beliefs.

Socio-cultural and environmental change

Because culture is not static but constantly changing, cultural competence must take into account circumstances surrounding culture change. A child care strategy well suited to one situation may not be suited to another. For example, Polynesian (primarily Maori) children, who comprised approximately 10% of the child population of New Zealand, constituted over half of the children reported as not being properly supervised (Fergusson *et al.* 1972). This over-representation results, in part, from cultural conflict in the definition of child maltreatment related to misunderstandings of Polynesian patterns of sibling caretaking. In the indigenous setting, sibling caretaking is highly valued by both children and adults and is central to Polynesian socialisation patterns (Gallimore *et al.* 1974, Korbin 1990). Polynesian adults do not view children being left alone with siblings as neglectful or dangerous.

Ritchie and Ritchie (1981) point out that it is not merely cultural misunderstanding or cultural conflict that accounts for the disparity in reporting statistics. They argue that, in changing circumstances, cultural practices that are valued and adaptive in one setting may indeed be dangerous to children in another. In the move to urban settings, Maoris often found themselves living in the city's poorest sections, in substandard housing that more easily catches fire, on streets with fast-moving cars, and isolated from a larger supportive network of kin. Sibling caretaking in this changed setting may indeed pose increased risk to children of accident and injury. However, it is not sibling caretaking *per se* that is of concern, but sibling caretaking in its new context.

Intracultural variability

Thus far we have been exploring differences between cultures. Cultural competence also demands an understanding of the range of variability within any given cultural context. As noted earlier, diversity exists within any culture or ethnic group along the lines of generation, acculturation, education, income, gender, age, temperament and past experience. Intracultural diversity, and the continuum of acceptable and unacceptable behaviour within any culture, must therefore be understood, since this is the level at which cultural practices can best be differentiated from maltreatment.

At this second level of definition, unmoderated cultural relativism comes particularly into play with the potential for misrepresentation of culture or use of culture as a justification for abusive or neglectful acts. Indeed, this second definitional level is the most likely point of entry for cultural considerations. If a child has suffered a consequence and the parents or caregivers claim that the harm results from a culturally acceptable behaviour, the worker has little way to assess the veracity of such claims without knowledge of the culture and the range of acceptable behaviours: maltreating parents often try to explain or justify their behaviours and the overlay of culture increases the complexity of assessments. A practice or behaviour, particularly if it carries the potential or actuality of harm, cannot be accepted as a cultural difference simply because the parent says so. However, because culture is so politically charged, workers may hesitate to challenge parental or caregiver explanations for fear of appearing racist or ignorant (Brophy *et al.* 2005).

Distinguishing cultural differences from child maltreatment at this second level of definition has been hampered in child protection in large part because child protection workers are usually restricted in their community contacts to problematic individuals and families. Child protection workers thereby are much more likely to be exposed to problematic behaviours than to the full continuum of acceptable and unacceptable behaviours. Proposals for neighbourhood or community-based services could help to ameliorate this problem by increasing familiarity with the larger community.

An additional complexity at this level of definition is that children are not equally protected from harm within the same cultural context (Korbin 1987b). Some categories of children, such as children with diminished social supports (e.g. orphans) or demographic profiles (e.g. girls in some cultures) may receive a lesser standard of care and protection than their cultural peers. An example of this complexity can be seen in recent cases and concerns about witchcraft and child deaths in the UK. On the one hand, there is concern that child deaths can be attributed to 'culture' in the melding of traditional beliefs with fundamentalist religious groups. On the other hand, only some children seem to be at risk.

Societally based harm to children

The third level of concern in culturally competent definitions of child maltreatment is not strictly cultural. Nevertheless, it can be mistaken for or confounded with culture. This third definitional level reflects the level of harm or deprivation that the larger society is willing to tolerate or permit, either actively or passively, for some or all children. Examples include exploitative child labour (i.e. labour outside of a family or apprenticeship context), high rates of child poverty, disparities in health, and so on. It is important to consider this level in culturally competent formulations because ethnic minority families are too frequently over-represented in these categories of health disparities and poverty. Culture, then, should not be confused with structural conditions detrimental to children and families.

Linking culture and child maltreatment

The reasons for the differential distribution of child maltreatment rates, both within and between populations, are rarely specified. These differences have variously been attributed to racism or cultural misunderstandings, to the increased scrutiny of poor families by child welfare agencies, or to the increased stresses of poverty experienced by minority families. Such differences in incidence or prevalence are sometimes assumed to reflect cultural patterns, but these patterns are rarely specified or measured. An early study by Dubanoski and Snyder (1980) found that

Samoan–Americans were over-represented and Japanese–Americans under-represented in abuse reports in Hawai'i. They suggested that this finding was explained by Samoan beliefs that children should be physically disciplined, and that this discipline spilled over into abuse. This work took an important step in trying to elucidate the differences between cultural groups that may increase the risk of abuse. However, because culture is not monolithic, as discussed above, intracultural variability must also be considered. Actual physical punishment was not measured within each population, leaving the assumption that the value on physical discipline is causally linked to actual physical discipline and abuse.

In a subsequent publication, Dubanoski (1981) addressed both inter- and intra-cultural variability, comparing Hawai'ian–American and European–American child maltreatment reports. Hawai'ian–Americans were over-represented while European–Americans were under-represented in the State of Hawaii's child abuse reports. Hawai'ian–American families were low on *'ohana'* (extended family) involvement (Dubanoski 1981). More recently, Coohey (2001) in a sophisticated study examined the complexities of the concept of *familism* among Latinos and Anglos. *Familism,* while more characteristic of Latinos, nevertheless differentiated between abusive and non-abusive mothers in both groups.

While a review of culturally competent intervention and treatment is beyond the scope of this chapter (see Tharp 1991, McGoldrick *et al.* 1996, Cohen *et al.* 2001, Fontes 2005), such an approach should focus not only on pathological behaviours that can be labelled maltreatment, but equally importantly on cultural strengths that can mitigate risk. As in the example above, if family involvement differentiates abusive and non-abusive families within a single culture, this can be used to counter other adverse circumstances. Before adopting too facile a reliance on extended networks, however, explorations need to be made as to whether the network for that particular family is a positive network (Thompson 1995, Korbin 1998).

Concluding remarks: incorporating culture in child maltreatment

This chapter has focused on culturally competent work in child protection, in particular how we conceptualise diversity between and within cultural contexts. Although culturally competent child protection should have as its first priority the child's well-being, it must also consider the child within a cultural context, since this provides both risk and protective factors. Culture is best viewed in an ecological framework that focuses on the concentric spheres or inter-relationships within and between different levels of social systems. Originally formulated by Bronfenbrenner (1979) and elaborated by subsequent researchers (e.g. Cicchetti & Lynch 1993, National Research Council 1993), the ecological approach has become particularly influential in child care assessment practice in the UK because it acknowledges the complexity of social situations. In so doing, it requires those making assessments to take account of a wide range of factors, including children's cultural, socio-economic and ethnic characteristics, as well as the parent–child relationship, the composition of the extended family, and the degree of neighbourhood and community support available to a parent or caregiver, as well as factors such as the child's age, development, functioning and behaviour, and the interaction between all of these factors.

The importance of cultural context, within-culture variability and the need to specify what is significant about a particular cultural context precludes a library-like card catalogue of strategies for working with specific cultural groups. While knowledge of general cultural patterns provides an important starting point, each individual and family must be assessed on their merits by viewing the child as nested in the ecological levels of the family, the community, socio-economic conditions and the larger cultural context.

- Cultural competence involves acquired knowledge and skills about cultural diversity that extends beyond individual qualities of cultural sensitivity.

- Practitioners should understand the range of both between- and within-cultural diversity.

- Both unmoderated ethnocentrism (the belief that one's own culture is superior) and unmoderated cultural relativism (the belief that all cultures must be seen in their own right without judgement) will lead to misidentification of child maltreatment.

- Cultural competence is important both as a general approach to child protection and for practice and intervention with individuals and families.

Annotated further reading

Brophy J, Jhutti-Johal Y, McDonald E 2005 Minority ethnic parents, their solicitors and child protection litigation. Oxford Centre for Family Law and Policy, Oxford
This report to the Department of Constitutional Affairs concerns efforts to work with culturally diverse families in the legal system.

Cicchetti D, Lynch M 1993 Toward an ecological/transactional model of community violence and child maltreatment: consequences for children's development. Psychiatry 56:96–118
This paper presents an ecological model that includes risk and protective factors and the dimension of time across ecological levels.

Korbin J (ed) 1981 Child abuse and neglect: cross-cultural perspectives. University of California Press, Berkeley
This edited volume presents ethnographic accounts of child maltreatment across a range of cultures from China, East Africa, India, Latin America, Polynesia, Taiwan and Turkey.

National Research Council 1993 Understanding child abuse and neglect. National Academy Press, Washington, DC
This volume reports on findings of an expert panel on the state of child maltreatment research. It is based on an ecological–developmental perspective.

Shonkoff J, Phillips D (eds) 2000 National Research Council and Institute of Medicine. Neurons to neighborhoods: the science of early childhood development. National Academy Press, Washington, DC
This volume reports on the findings of an expert panel on the current state of scientific research on child development. Culture is the second of ten core concepts.

Thompson R 1995 Preventing child maltreatment through social support: a crucial analysis. Sage, Thousand Oaks, CA
This volume presents an analysis of the relationship of social networks to child maltreatment. Thompson critically evaluates the types of social support that can increase or decrease the risk of child maltreatment.

McGoldrick M, Giordano J, Pearce J (eds) 1996 Ethnicity and family therapy, 2nd edn. Guilford Press, New York
This volume discusses a range of issues in treating ethnically diverse families, including ethnic matching of therapist and client and cultural appropriateness of various interventions.

Scheper-Hughes N (ed) 1987 Child survival. Anthropological perspectives on the treatment and maltreatment of children. Reidel, Dordrecht
This edited volume considers aspects of child maltreatment across a range of diverse cultures.

Useful websites

International Society for Prevention of Child Abuse and Neglect: www.ispcan.org

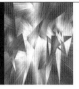

8

Issues of ethnicity

Melanie Phillips

INTRODUCTION

Understandably, the agencies with whom Victoria came into contact have asked the question: 'If Victoria had been a white child, would she have been treated differently?' Having listened to the evidence before me, it is, even at this stage, impossible to answer this question with any confidence. Much has been made outside this inquiry of the fact that two black people murdered Victoria, and a high proportion of the staff who had contact with her were also black. But to dismiss the possibility of racism on the basis of this superficial analysis of the circumstances is to misunderstand the destructive effect that racism has on our society and its institutions.

(Laming Report 2003)

The Inquiry Reports into the deaths of Jasmine Beckford on 5 July 1984, Tyra Henry on 1 September 1984, Sukina Hammond on 6 December 1988 and Victoria Climbié on 25 February 2000 highlighted to differing degrees the fact that race, culture and ethnicity were relevant to an understanding of the circumstances leading to their deaths but left many unanswered questions as to where, when and how these issues should be more effectively addressed in the future.

Safeguarding children presents difficult dilemmas for the public and professionals to address in balancing the rights of individuals with the safety of children. In considering issues of race, ethnicity, language and culture, there are particular challenges to be overcome:

- How can cultural beliefs be respected whilst ensuring that children in all communities are protected?
- Should the effects of racism and disadvantage be understood and accounted for in a child protection context?
- All children deserve to be protected from significant harm, but how should issues of race, ethnicity and culture be considered in decisions about child welfare?

This chapter attempts to address these questions by identifying the extent of, and limits on, our current knowledge and identifies the implications for policy and practice with black and minority ethnic children and their families.

For the purposes of this chapter, 'black' refers to children and families of African, African–Caribbean and Asian descent; 'race' refers to the social categorisation of people defined by skin colour and physical characteristics; 'culture' represents the shared behaviours, attitudes and traditions of a group of people characterised by similar language, symbols, food, dress, history, etc., and 'ethnicity' describes geographic origin and heritage that are acquired by birth.

Review of recent literature and research

Bulmer defines an ethnic group as:

a collectivity within a larger population having real or putative common ancestry, memories of a shared past, and a cultural focus of one or more symbolic elements which define the group's identity, such as kinship, religion, language, shared territory, nationality or physical appearance.

(Bulmer 1996, in HMSO 2003, p. 7)

Although in recent years the term 'ethnic minority' has acquired a pejorative meaning, it is more accurately used to describe the proportion of a particular ethnic group within a specified country. Within the UK population there are both white and black minority ethnic groups, with the largest white minority ethnic group being Irish. Under the census categorisation used in 2001, statistical data are organised into 'white' and 'minority ethnic' categorisations, which masks differences within the white population. Within England the population of 'white' people (National Census Categorisation 2001: National Statistics Online 2005) is the majority ethnic group, comprising 92% of the population.

In the last 50 years, the black minority ethnic population of England has grown from 0.5% in 1951 (Skellington & Morris 1992) to 8% in the 2001 census (National Statistics Online 2005). However, the national picture hides a great deal of regional variation in that minority ethnic populations are concentrated in urban areas, with nearly half of the total minority ethnic population (45%) being concentrated in London (where they comprised 29% of all residents) and 13% in the West Midlands. In the North East and South West they made up only 2% of each region's population (National Statistics Online 2005). The largest minority ethnic group nationally is Indian, at 22% of the minority ethnic population, followed by Pakistanis at 16%, those of mixed ethnicity at 15%, black Caribbeans at 12%, black Africans at 10% and Bangladeshis at 6%. In some local authorities the black population is the majority ethnic group and the white population is in the minority (Skellington 1996, p. 52).

The statistical information on ethnicity provides an important overview of the context in which communities live and work, and helps to inform us about the similarities and differences in their experience of life in this country. Whilst there are differences between minority ethnic groups, the salient factor that emerges from the data about the black minority ethnic population is their experience of physical and material disadvantage. In the Annual Local Area Labour Force Survey 2001 (National Statistics Online 2005), Bangladeshi men had the highest unemployment rate at 40%, while Bangladeshi women had the highest unemployment rate at 24%, six times greater than that of white women. Young black African men, Pakistanis, black Caribbeans and those belonging to the mixed group also had very high unemployment rates, ranging between 25 and 31%.

People from black minority ethnic groups were much more likely to live in low income households. Pakistanis and Bangladeshis were much more likely than other groups to be living on low incomes – almost 68% living in low income households. Forty-nine per cent of black non-Caribbean families also lived on low incomes as compared to 21% of white families (Department for Work and Pensions 2000/2001).

The current Indices of Deprivation (DETR 2000) also show that black communities live in areas of high social deprivation, and most black people live in authorities that fall within the category of 'most deprived', using six 'domains' of deprivation: income, employment, health deprivation and disability, education skills and training, housing, and geographical access to services. It is within this context that the collective term 'black' becomes particularly significant:

There is a value to the focus on ethnicity. The disaggregation of 'black' into its historical, geographic and cultural components ... enables the different outcomes of different groups ... enabling, if practice follows research, resources to be appropriately targeted. But this focus also normalises divisions by ethnicity rather than the solidarity of racialised groupings and experiences. Yet the National Statistics Online of 2004 reveals that while the black ethnic groups have a broad range of experiences in employment, income and education, it is their experience of racism that there is the most common ground.

(Prevatt-Goldstein, in Thoburn *et al.* 2005, p. 14)

The Race Relations Act 1976 (as amended by the Race Relations Amendment Act 2000) gives public authorities a general duty to promote race equality and the Children Act 1989 places a duty on local authorities:

to safeguard and promote the welfare of children in need; and so far as is consistent with that duty, to promote the upbringing of such children by their families, by providing a range and level of services appropriate to those children's needs.

(s.17 Children Act 1989)

Given the socio-economic circumstances of many black minority ethnic communities, it would seem likely that black families from the most disadvantaged communities would be over-represented in family support provision. The evidence shows a somewhat different picture: in the *Children in Need* Census of 2001, only 3% of Pakistani children and 2% of Bangladeshi children were categorised as 'in need' as a result of 'low income' compared to 8% for white families and 16% for black and mixed families:

Whilst mixed race children and black children are considerably more likely to be known to social services, their pattern of needs and services received are similar to white children in need ... however, children of Indian, Pakistani or Bangladeshi [origin] follow a different pattern. Disability is much more likely to be the reason why services are needed.

(Bebbington & Beecham 2003, p. 1)

From current data, however, the ethnic groups most likely to be in receipt of family support services under the category of family dysfunction, abuse, neglect or parenting problems are African and African–Caribbean families and mixed heritage families (Thoburn *et al.* 2005).

The explanation for this is far from straightforward, but indicators are that social and community stigma in using formal services, the availability of family and community support and a lower level of evident drug, alcohol and mental health problems may be factors which influence the referral to, and take up of, formal and informal family support services (Thoburn *et al.* 2005).

It would be easy to infer from these data that despite social and economic hardship, some black communities are managing their family and social problems without the support of family support services. This may be true, but we do not yet have a detailed enough picture of the needs of the diverse ethnic communities to know whether this is the result of self-sufficiency or unmet need.

Evidence from elsewhere indicates that the use of family support services by black communities is dependent upon how that service is offered. In their survey of family centres undertaken in 1998, Butt and Box found:

Only a small number of (family) centres ... worked regularly with black families. It is possible to identify some of the distinguishing features of these centres: the centres were more likely to have black staff, as well as having on average more black staff. These centres were also likely to have organised specific services for black users as well as having undertaken outreach work. The centres were also more likely to provide day care.

(Butt & Box 1998, p. 106)

Section 17 of the Children Act places the duty of 'safeguarding' children on local authorities alongside promoting their welfare through family support. 'Safeguarding' defines a broad responsibility, which is further extended in the Children Act 2004, but it embraces the protection of children from harm as well as providing support for children in need. All children who are suffering or likely to suffer harm are children in need but not all children in need are in of protection.

There are no accurate figures for the exact number of children who experience harm as a result of parental behaviour, and the extent to which ethnicity may be a variable in the prevalence of harm is not nationally established. Attempts to quantify this are beset with difficulties as statutory services do not screen all children to identify those who may be in need of protection, but rely upon public and professional notification of abuse. When social services receive information that a child may be suffering or is likely to suffer harm as a result of physical, sexual or emotional abuse or neglect, they are obliged to make enquiries to investigate these concerns under s.47 of the Children Act 1989.

In 2004, 572 200 referrals were made to social services departments (National Statistics Online 2005). It is not clear how many of these referrals resulted in s.47 enquiries, but 11% of these resulted in core assessments (s.47 enquiries would normally instigate a core assessment). There is no ethnic breakdown of these figures, but earlier research indicates differential patterns of referral for black minority families:

Although black parents (primarily African Caribbean) were equally likely as white parents to refer themselves, there were differences in referrals from statutory agencies. For example the police and schools were much more likely to refer black youngsters for reasons of delinquency than white youngsters. Similarly black mothers were much more likely to be referred for reasons of mental health by the police and the health service than white mothers.
(Barn 1993, p. 102)

In 1997, Barn and colleagues found that while white parents made self-referrals to social services for help and support, black families were more likely to be referred by a statutory agency such as the police, health or education. Families of mixed parentage were the most likely to seek social services' help, the majority of these referrals coming from white mothers (Barn *et al.* 1997).

Barn *et al.* also found that Asian families were more likely to be referred for physical abuse of children (75% of referrals compared to 39% for white children, 29% for African–Caribbean and 38% for mixed parentage children) and less likely to be referred for neglect (11% for Asian children as compared to 32% for white children and 26% for mixed parentage and African–Caribbean children) and for sexual abuse (16% for white children as compared to 8% for other groups).

Gibbons *et al.* (1995b) also found disparities in referral rates:

Black and Asian families were over-represented among referrals for physical injury (58%v42%) and under-represented among referrals for sexual abuse (20%v31%) compared to white families ... Black and Asian families were more often referred for using an implement to inflict physical injury. (p. 40)

The explanations for these differences vary. Barn *et al.* (1997) suggest:

Although issues of 'race' and ethnicity have been given some attention within social services in the last two decades, understanding and appreciation of different norms, values and traditions are still at an embryonic stage and often located within a Eurocentric framework. (p. 39)

Gibbons *et al.* (1995b) also cite cultural differences but give a different explanation as to how these should be interpreted:

This illustrates cultural differences in child rearing, and the difficulty of deciding what forms of physical punishment are 'acceptable' in Britain. (p. 40)

Barn *et al.* (1997) locate an understanding of cultural difference within a context of 'cultural racism' in which the lifestyles and traditions of different cultural groups are ascribed positive or negative significance by professionals and organisations as a consequence of racism, whereas Gibbons *et al.* (1995b) link the referral statistics to intrinsic cultural differences whose origins lie within the communities themselves.

The statistical information from referral rates informs us about which families become subject to a referral to social services as a result of professional or public concern and are not accurate reflections of the actual rate of abuse within a given community. Research indicates that there are broad similarities between ethnic groups in their experience of abuse.

Cawson *et al.* (2000, quoted in Thoburn *et al.* 2005) interviewed a sample of 2869 young people born in the UK from a range of ethnic groups aged 18–24 about their past experiences of family life and found that most had experienced verbal ill-treatment and some form of physical punishment such as being slapped on the bottom, hand or leg.

A quarter of the sample reported more serious violence, including being hit with implements, punched, kicked, burned or scalded, knocked down and choked with most of this occurring at the hands of parents, especially mothers ... A sizeable minority (38%) grew up in families where there was 'a lot of stress' and this was broadly similar across ethnic groups.

(Thoburn *et al.* 2005, p. 73)

If professionals assume that there are high rates of physical chastisement and low rates of sexual abuse in black communities, they are less likely to identify sexual abuse and more likely to make assumptions about discipline in those communities, particularly when 'cultural differences' are identified as the cause of these disparities. Such assumptions can have dangerous consequences for the protection of black minority ethnic children. This issue will be covered in more detail later in the chapter.

Working Together to Safeguard Children (DfES 2006) states that a child should be subject to a child protection plan when the child is at risk of continuing significant harm because they have suffered ill treatment or impairment of health or development as a result of physical, emotional or sexual abuse or neglect and that safeguarding the child requires inter-agency help delivered through a formal child protection plan. This replaces earlier guidance issued in 1999 (*Working Together* 1999, DoH *et al.*) which stated that children who needed a child protection plan to ensure their protection from significant harm should be placed on a child protection register. As the 2006 guidance has yet to be fully implemented at the time of writing this chapter, there is no available data as to which children will be subject to child protection plans. The most reliable sources of data on child protection and ethnicity currently remain the numbers of children subject to s.47 Inquiries, and the number of children placed on the child protection register.

From the evidence currently available, it is not possible to establish how many s.47 Inquiries under the Children Act 1989 result in child protection conferences and whether there are differences in this respect between different ethnic groups. Indications from earlier research (Gibbons *et al.* 1995b) are that 73% of cases referred for investigation resulted in no protective action at all and that 'the child's racial background' was not a factor in influencing which referrals were selected for conference and registration.

Establishing a direct link between the likelihood of registration and ethnic origin would be hard to achieve, but the registration figures for different ethnic groups do not correlate with the population statistics for ethnicity in many local authorities or in the national picture.

The number of black minority ethnic children on the child protection register is 17% compared to 13% of the general population of black minority ethnic children

(Thoburn *et al.* 2005), which suggests an over-representation of this aggregated group. Within this there are interesting differences between ethnic groups in that children of mixed parentage are over-represented at 6% as compared to 3% within the population whilst Asian or Asian British are under-represented at 4% as compared to 6.4% within the population. The population of black or black British on the register is the same as that in the general population at 4%.

The DfES figures for ethnicity are not broken down into registration categories, but earlier research (Barn *et al.* 1997) showed that, in all groups, black children were over-represented on the child protection register under the category of physical abuse compared to white children, with 71% of Asian children placed on the register registered under this category, compared with 64% of African–Caribbean and mixed parentage children and 56% of white children.

In terms of neglect, there was also an over-representation of some groups of black children compared to white children, with 27% of African–Caribbean and 21% of mixed parentage children registered under this category, compared with 15% of white children. Only 10% of Asian children were registered under this category. For sexual abuse there was an under-representation of black children compared to white children, with 9% of African–Caribbean and 10% of Asian and mixed parentage children registered under this category, compared with 17% of white children. For emotional abuse, 5% of Asian, mixed parentage and white children were registered under this category. No African–Caribbean children were registered under this category.

Some of Barn's findings echo those of other researchers in that black children tended to be over-represented in cases of physical abuse and under-represented for sexual abuse. However, smaller and more localised studies cannot indicate national trends and there are still gaps in our knowledge and understanding of the relationship between ethnicity and registration. What is evident is that single factor explanations such as 'cultural variations' are insufficient in encompassing the complex dynamics that influence decision making throughout the child protection process.

Race, culture and ethnicity not only have an impact on the number of children known to family support and child protection social services, they are also significant in terms of the population of children looked after by local authorities.

It was in the 1960s that concerns were first raised about the number of black children in the care system, and studies conducted in the 1960s and 1970s (Soul Kids Campaign 1977, Batta *et al.* 1979) identified an over-representation of African–Caribbean and Asian children in care compared to white children, with particular concerns being expressed about the number of children of mixed parentage coming into care.

Two studies in the 1980s (Adams 1981, Wilkinson 1982) reflected the high proportion of black children in the care of local authorities. In their 1989 study, Rowe *et al.* also state that:

> Black children were over-represented in admissions to care of all six project authorities, although the extent to which this was happening varied considerably.
>
> (Rowe *et al.* 1989, in HMSO 1991, p. 14)

There are slightly different messages in respect of Asian communities. In Rowe's study (Rowe *et al.* 1989) Asian children made up 8% of the care population, whereas in Barn's study (Barn 1993) Asian children made up only 2% of the population of black children in care. However, in later research (Barn *et al.* 1997) Asian children made up 14% of the care population. Relative to the local Asian child care population, this revealed an over-representation of Asian children in the care system.

This study also highlighted an over-representation of children of African–Caribbean origin, as well as an over-representation of children of dual heritage.

Although these studies gave strong indications that race, colour and ethnicity were significant in care admissions, there were no nationally available figures on children looked after until the introduction of the *Quality Protects* initiative in 1998. This initiative was set up by the Department of Health to deliver its agenda for modernising social services and improving outcomes for children. *Quality Protects* required local authorities to collect and collate data on a range of outcomes for children and submit these to the Department of Health on a yearly basis relative to a number of predetermined performance indicators. With the publication of these figures it became possible to have a more comprehensive picture of the looked-after population and to have much more detail about ethnicity than was previously possible.

In the most recently published data, black children collectively continue to be over-represented in care, comprising 18.5% of the care population as compared to 13% in the general population (National Statistics/DoH 2003) and that children of dual heritage (particularly where one parent is African–Caribbean and the other is white European) are over-represented in the care population, whilst Asian children continue to be under-represented. These findings reflect the predominant messages from research studies.

It is already evident from family support and child protection research that our knowledge about ethnicity and child protection is primarily located in the statistics detailing which children and families are in receipt of which services. There is as yet a paucity of information that 'tracks' decision making to help us understand the narratives behind the statistics, and to identify whether these narratives are different for black compared to white children. The exceptions to this are Barn's studies in 1993 and 1997 which provide a comparative commentary on the paths into care for black as compared to white children.

Barn (1993) found a link between race and rapidity of admission into care:

The Wenford research was able to ascertain that black children came into care much more quickly than white children. For example, in the first 4 weeks of referral, 28% of black children were admitted into care compared to 15% of white children.

(Barn 1990, p. 236)

She also found that:

black children were much more likely than white children to come from higher socio-economic groups. For example, 47% of the black children's mothers were in white collar and skilled manual occupations compared to 22% of white children.

(Barn 1990, p. 233)

Whilst economic and social factors are significant contributory factors in admission rates to care, and black families are economically disadvantaged through racism, it is also apparent from this that an explanation of the statistics based purely on economic and social disadvantage is inadequate, as was seen in family support research.

This is substantiated by Barn's examination of case files and interviews with social workers and natural parents, where 'preventative work … was less likely to be done with black families and children' (Barn 1990, p. 243). She also found that although the majority of black children entered care via the voluntary route, they were as likely as white children to be made subject to compulsory care and that they were much more likely to be made subject to parental rights resolutions than white children.

In her follow-up study of looked-after children in 1997, Barn found that the rate of entry into care was still significantly different for black children compared to white:

Higher numbers of African Caribbean children became 'looked after' within two weeks than any other ethnic group (68% compared with 59% of mixed parentage, 50% of Asian and 49% of white).

(Barn *et al.* 1997, p. 63)

The research tells us that race, culture and ethnicity are variables that affect outcomes for children, but more information is needed for us to understand how these outcomes are achieved, and the extent to which differential judgements and decision making operate for black children as compared to white children. Research can highlight anomalies and raise questions about causation, but a better understanding of causation has to be located within an analysis of practice.

Implications for practice

The first public statement that professional decision making about a black child at risk of harm might have been influenced by racial, cultural and gender-based stereotyping was voiced publicly in 1987, in the Inquiry Report into the death of Tyra Henry. The Inquiry Panel identified the lack of family support provision for Tyra's grandmother Beatrice Henry that led to Tyra's return to her parents, where she was subsequently killed by her stepfather.

There is a positive, but nevertheless, false stereotype in white British society of the African Caribbean mother figure as endlessly resourceful, able to cope in great adversity, essentially unsinkable. We do think that it may have been an unarticulated and unconscious sense that a woman like Beatrice Henry would find a way of coping, no matter what, that underlay the neglect of ... social services to make adequate provision for her taking responsibility for Tyra.
(London Borough of Lambeth 1987, p. 108)

A subsequent Inquiry (Bridge Child Care Consultancy Service 1991) into the death of Sukina Hammond, a black child of dual Caribbean and white parentage, also linked professionals' views and values about race and culture with their responses to Sukina and her family:

We know that agencies that are moving towards trying to be more sensitive and understanding towards the racial and cultural needs of their client group, do risk failing to recognise the particular needs of an individual child. In addition, white professionals who have undergone anti-racist training can sometimes over-compensate out of fear of being accused of racism.
(Bridge Child Care Consultancy Service 1991, p. 84)

The Laming Report into the death of Victoria Climbié also raised concerns that race and culture influenced professional decision making:

There can be no excuse or justification for failing to take adequate steps to protect a vulnerable child, simply because that child's cultural background would make the necessary action somehow inappropriate.
(Laming Report 2003, p. 346)

Inquiry Reports into the deaths of children represent the most extreme end of the child protection spectrum, as most children do not die as a result of child abuse. However, inquiries do provide us with opportunities to reflect on professional practice and to identify the factors which contribute to the constellation of circumstances that leave the most vulnerable children at risk of serious harm.

It has already been demonstrated that black children are over-represented in the referral figures for physical abuse, as summed up by Thoburn *et al.* (1995):

Disagreements about the appropriateness of physical punishment feature in a disproportionate number of cases involving black families. (p. 200)

A pervading assumption that underpins responses to the protection of black children is that physical punishment of black children is intrinsic to the cultures of black minority ethnic groups. In fact physical punishment of children is common across all cultural groups (Cawson *et al.* 2000). There is a distinction, however, between physical punishment of children, which includes smacking children, and using implements or a level of force likely to result in injury to the child. Although views differ in this country as to whether smacking children is an acceptable form of discipline, the use of physical forms of chastisement is not culturally specific. The same is true of physical abuse, which occurs in all communities:

Physical injury to children occurs in black families just as it does within white families, but it is no more or less a part of black culture than of white culture. Physical abuse is unacceptable whatever the context. If physical abuse was a part of black culture then all black children would be unsafe within black communities.

(Dutt & Phillips 2000, p. 56)

Given that the overwhelming majority of black minority ethnic children are not physically abused by their parents, culture cannot be an explanation for the causation of abuse to the minority who do experience physical injury. The question to be addressed, therefore, is what causes some parents to physically injure their children: is this the same for all families, regardless of ethnic origin, and what is the place of culture in an assessment of likely or future harm?

After the death of Jasmine Beckford in 1984, Louis Blom-Cooper, chairing the London Borough of Brent Panel of Inquiry into her death, highlighted the lack of research aimed at predicting which children were 'high risk' in terms of parental dangerousness:

Research designed to refine the techniques for predicting accurately those children who will continue to be at risk are urgently required and we recommend that such research should be undertaken.

(London Borough of Brent 1985, p. 289)

In the years that followed, a significant proportion of the research on families who physically abused children focused on the characteristics of abusive families in order to attempt to establish which families would pose a greater risk to their children. Checklists, such as those used in *Protecting Children: A Guide to Social Workers Undertaking a Comprehensive Assessment of Children* (DoH 1988a) were developed to assist professionals in making judgements about which children in which families would be more vulnerable to harm.

As assessment tools, however, lists of 'dangerous factors' are of limited value in predicting abuse:

No single characteristic (and indeed no combination of characteristics) can be used as a 'marker' to differentiate between abusive and non-abusive families and we need to avoid the tendency to caricature abusive families by overstating the degree to which they are similar to one another or different to other families.

(Frude 2003, p. 195)

Many of the factors identified in the checklists, such as being a single parent, having been in care or prison, having an inadequate education or being unemployed (DoH 1988a, Stone 1993), were factors that reflected the social and economic circumstances of families, and would be much more likely to be present in disad-vantaged communities. Given the social and economic circumstances of many black minority ethnic families outlined earlier in the chapter, the use of this set of criteria to predict abuse would be likely to result in a disproportionate number of black families being factored into any 'risk assessment'.

Frude (2003) argues against such an approach, and suggests that the aetiology of physical abuse has to be understood in terms of the interaction between parent and child in which abuse is an act of aggression committed by an angry parent in response to a trigger event, usually, although not always, precipitated by a child's behaviour.

All parents experience difficulties in dealing with children's behaviour. However, when tired, normal child behaviour will cause frustration and anger to a parent who would adopt a more balanced response at a calmer time. For some parents, how-ever, normal child behaviour is likely to be consistently negatively attributed what-ever the context. These parents are also more likely to be unresponsive or negatively responsive to their child's needs, unrealistic in their expectations of the child's behaviour, and may have difficulty in empathising with the child and showing the child warmth, love and affection (Frude 2003).

> Parenting is an active process of socialisation which involves the interpretation of children's behaviour. This interpretation is reflected back to children in ways which shape their behav-iour and which make a significant contribution to the schemas that children themselves develop.
>
> (McDonald 2001, p. 62)

The quality of the parent–child interaction is a significant factor in physical abuse:

> We would expect there to be more frequent and more hostile disciplinary encounters when the quality of the relationship between the parent and the child is relatively poor. These con-frontations may then escalate so that aggressive attacks become relatively common, and this will increase the probability that the child will one day be injured in an attack.
>
> (Frude 2003, p. 200)

Parents who physically abuse their children do not, on the whole, intend to injure them. Physical injuries are more commonly the result of a loss of control than a pre-meditated attempt to harm the child. As a strategy to control behaviour and enforce discipline, an action motivated by anger is likely to be ineffective, and parents who resort to harsh discipline methods for minor incidents are more likely to adopt ever more severe punishments to maintain a sense of control in the face of challenge.

Reder *et al.* (1993), in their study of 35 major inquiries into child deaths, also highlight the 'escalating' nature of abuse:

> The majority of the children ... had been beaten, bruised and sometimes tortured for a long time prior to their deaths. In some instances their injuries had already led to hospital admis-sions. Jasmine Beckford and her sister Louise were taken into care following admission to hospital with fractures but they were later returned to their family. (p. 45)

An assessment of likely physical harm to a child therefore has to incorporate an understanding of the nature of the relationship between parent and child, including the circumstances in which physical abuse is likely to be triggered. Frude (2003, p. 194) argues that this assessment has to include 'an appreciation of the interaction between the parent and the child in the hours, minutes and seconds before the assault'.

Jasmine Beckford was killed by her stepfather Morris Beckford on 5 July 1984. Little is recorded about the events which led to her death at the age of 4½ years but the consultant forensic pathologist recorded that Jasmine was thin and emaciated due to chronic undernourishment, there were multiple old scars consistent with the effects of a severe beating conducted within the period of a day or so leading up to her death, and the fatal injury had been caused by a blow to her head (London Borough of Brent 1985, p. cxxxvi).

During the 3 years of professional involvement with the family, however, there was no assessment of the relationship between Jasmine and her stepfather, although after her death the guardian *ad litem*'s report shed light on the nature of the relationship between Morris Beckford and his stepchildren. The guardian's report is based on interviews with Beverley Lorrington, Jasmine's mother:

> He was strict with the children, expecting that they instantly obeyed him. He wanted to teach them things that were too advanced for them (e.g. alphabet, numbers) and would become extremely angry if they could not learn. From the time that Jasmine and Louise came home on trial, they were both subject to physical abuse from their father ... Both Jasmine and Louise were frightened of him.
>
> (London Borough of Brent 1985, p. lxxii)

In the case of Sukina Hammond, the events leading to her death are clearly and harrowingly outlined in the Inquiry Report. They began with Sukina, then aged 5, and her sister being asked by her father to spell their names which they were unable or unwilling to do. When asked again they still did not respond. Sukina's father then hit Sukina on the hand with a ruler repeatedly asking her to spell her name. The attack escalated and resulted in her death (Bridge Child Care Consultancy Service 1991). The Inquiry Report identifies concerns from professionals about the relationship between Sukina and her father, with reports from the nursery that Sukina was very fearful of her father and was scared that he might 'beat up on me'.

For Morris Beckford and Sukina's father, the 'trigger' that led them to physically injure their children was based upon their children's ability to read. Little is known of Sukina's father's early upbringing, but it is known that Morris Beckford had an extremely violent childhood, that his parents were prosecuted on charges of ill-treatment and neglect and that he spent some time in care. Morris Beckford was also classified as 'educationally subnormal' and the report states that 'his subnormality was educational and not intellectual' (London Borough of Brent 1985, p. 42).

This indicates that Morris Beckford underachieved in school, and it is very likely that this influenced his desire to ensure that his children could read. There is no record of Sukina's father's schooling, but with the backdrop of the underachievement of many African–Caribbean boys in the education system (Commission for Racial Equality 2003) as a context, it is not hard to see why the ability to read should acquire such significance for both of these men.

For many black minority ethnic families, as for many white families, education can represent the chance to escape poverty and environmental disadvantage and, for these families, educational aspirations can strongly influence the way in which they discipline their children. Many families will achieve this through sanctions which have no harmful effect on the child, and many black families might not focus on education but have other priorities; however, for a very small minority of families, their desire to ensure that their children fare better than they did in the education system may lead them to misdirect their anger in the punishment of their children.

Inquiry Reports into the deaths of white children also contain examples of professional assessments that do not explore parent–child relationships, and it is not possible to establish whether practice would have been different had Jasmine or Sukina been white. What can be asserted, however, is that the impact of racism can distort the way in which professionals relate to black parents and interpret their behaviour, and it is within this context that race, culture and ethnicity become significant in influencing professional judgement:

Assumption based on race can be just as corrosive in its effect as blatant racism ... racism can affect the way people conduct themselves in other ways. Fear of being accused of racism can stop people acting when otherwise they would.

(Neil Graham QC, in the Laming Report 2003, p. 346)

There is evidence that professionals did not engage effectively with Morris Beckford or Sukina's father and were, as a result, unable to assess their capacity to parent. Both men were African–Caribbean and both had a history of in-family violence, although there is no evidence that they posed a threat to professionals who worked with them. In Sukina's case, the descriptions of her father made up a contradictory picture:

In meeting the professionals we were struck by the very wide range of descriptions given of Sukina's father, for example we heard him described as 'gentle, vicious, flamboyant, aggressive, deferential, caring, cold'.

(Bridge Child Care Consultancy Service 1991, p. 85)

In addition, the report states that various professionals said that they felt fearful of meeting Sukina's father before they met him.

African–Caribbean men are particularly vulnerable to negative racial stereotyping in which associations with violent crime, aggressive behaviour and irresponsible parenting are commonplace. Such generalisations obscure the specific characteristics of particular individuals and can create a sense of fear or avoidance based upon a perception rather than direct experience. In Tyra Henry's case, 'positive' racial and gender-based stereotyping was cited as having a likely effect on professional practice. In Sukina's case it is likely that negative gender-based stereotyping discouraged professionals from establishing a working relationship with Sukina's father to undertake an accurate assessment of the risk he posed to Sukina.

Whether or not this stereotyping was apparent to professionals, Sukina's father felt this to be the case:

Sukina's father felt that he experienced racism from various professionals and wrote a letter of complaint.

(Bridge Child Care Consultancy Service 1991, p. 84)

The report identifies that fear of being accused of racism can have an adverse impact on an assessment of the needs of an individual child. For Sukina, as for Jasmine Beckford, a lack of knowledge about the circumstances in which abuse was likely to occur, combined with an absence of information about the quality of the relationship between father and child, provided a poor foundation for an accurate assessment of risk to the children.

Culture is not an explanation for abuse, nor is fear of being accused of racism a reason for inaction. Black children deserve to be offered the same rights of protection as white children. It is not culture or race itself that makes black children vulnerable to abuse, it is the impact that these issues can have on professional practice which is at issue.

This is clearly evidenced by the views of various professionals in the Victoria Climbié case, and a number of examples are cited in the Laming Report:

On more than one occasion, medical practitioners who noticed marks on Victoria's body considered the possibility that children who have grown up in Africa might be expected to have more marks on their bodies than those that have been raised in Europe. This assumption, regardless of whether it is valid or not, may prevent a full assessment of those marks being made.

(Laming Report 2003, p. 345)

The response of Lisa Arthuworrey (Victoria's social worker in Haringay) to observations of Victoria's behaviour is also an example:

Lisa Arthuworrey said that when she heard of Victoria 'standing to attention' before Kouao and Manning she 'concluded that this type of relationship was one that could be seen in many Afro-Caribbean families because respect and obedience are very important features of the Afro-Caribbean family script'. Victoria's parents, however, made it clear that she was not required to stand in this formal way when she was at home with them.

(Laming Report 2003, p. 345)

Much has been made of the fact that Lisa Arthuworrey was a black social worker of Caribbean origin, and it is likely that such a statement from a black worker would be seen to carry weight in racial and cultural terms. There is a danger, however, in setting up 'cultural experts':

To use black workers to gain information on black cultures ... is misuse of black workers' time, as well as inappropriate professional practice. It is easy to see how this approach has proved attractive for many workers struggling to make their responses more appropriate to the needs of black communities. Many black workers have been seduced by the kudos that a cultural perspective can bring to their own professional status.

(Dutt & Phillips 1996, p. 179)

Evidence subsequently suggested that Victoria's behaviour was motivated by fear rather than respect, but the cultural explanation provided allowed the behaviour to be 'normalised', thus disconnecting it from the circumstances which gave it meaning. It is interesting to note that this statement was not challenged by other professionals, despite the fact that Victoria was from an African rather than a Caribbean background.

Just as cultural stereotyping of black minority ethnic parents will lead to inaccurate assessments, generalisations about children from these communities will also lead to erroneous judgements. All professionals need to ensure accuracy of information. Not to do so for black families, even where a black worker has given a culturally based explanation for behaviour, is to abdicate professional responsibility. An example of this is a statement from the Consultant Paediatrician, Mary Rossiter:

I was aware that as a white person I had to be sensitive to the feelings of people of all races and backgrounds, both clinically and with professionals. Maybe some social workers felt they knew more about black children than I did.

(Laming Report 2003, p. 346)

A consultant paediatrician needs to have the skills to diagnose non-accidental injury in children from all ethnic backgrounds. A misguided deference to the notion of cultural expertise belies the need to ensure that all children are safeguarded regardless of racial, cultural or ethnic origin. The identification of which families might pose a risk to their children has to be done by analysing the particular circumstances for the family, taking into account the individual, family and community dimensions of their lives rather than by generalising in relation to a type.

This approach to assessments is embodied in the *Framework for the Assessment of Children in Need and their Families* published in 2000 by the Department of Health, Department of Education and Employment and the Home Office in response to research and Inquiry Reports. Although published shortly after Victoria's death, the framework provided in this guidance would have assisted professionals greatly in their assessment of Victoria had it been available to them because it would have allowed information to be collated and understood in a much more comprehensive way. The Assessment Framework:

provides a systematic way of analysing, understanding and recording what is happening to children and young people within their families and wider context of the community in which they live.

(DoH *et al.* 2000, p. viii)

Any assessment under the Children Act 1989 has to use the 'assessment triangle' (see Fig. 13.1) to establish the extent to which parents have the capacity to meet the child's needs within their family and environmental context. Unlike previous national guidance, the Assessment Framework recognises that social, economic and environmental factors as well as family and community supports can affect the way in which parents are able to parent their children.

There is a direct link between the physical and mental well-being of children and their families and their economic and social circumstances. Living in poor housing, with a very low income and access to limited community resources would present a challenge for any parent, and those who do are often overwhelmed by their circumstances to the extent that parenting their children will be affected by the stresses of economic hardship.

The Children Act 1989 recognises that parents in these circumstances require further state support and s.17(3) and s.17(6) allow local authorities to provide a range of assistance to families where a child is in need. An assessment under the Assessment Framework will help professionals to target their intervention by identifying what is working well and the areas where the family requires additional support to meet the child's needs.

There is a difference between parents who experience difficulties in meeting children's needs as a result of social and economic circumstances and those who are unable to meet children's needs because they are unable or unwilling to provide an adequate standard of parenting, even with the appropriate level of professional assistance.

The definition of 'neglect' in *Working Together to Safeguard Children* (DoH *et al.* 1999) makes this distinction clear. Neglect is:

the persistent failure to meet a child's basic physical and/or psychological needs, likely to result in the serious impairment of the child's health or development. It may involve a parent or carer failing to provide adequate food, shelter or clothing, failing to protect a child from physical harm or danger or the failure to ensure access to appropriate medical care and treatment. It may also include neglect of, or unresponsiveness to a child's basic emotional needs.

(DoH *et al.* 1999, p. 6)

Although neglect can be exacerbated by material disadvantage, research (Stevenson 1998) shows that its cause is more multifaceted. Although many black minority families do experience disadvantage, this does not mean that more black minority ethnic children are neglected: 'there is no evidence – and one would not expect there to be – that serious neglect ... is more common amongst one group than another' (Stevenson 1998, p. 38). Many black families parent children very well, despite the environmental pressures. Their wider family, religious and cultural links can be strengths in the face of adversity and many have parenting skills that can help them to parent children effectively in difficult circumstances.

This does not mean that there are no individual, family or cultural differences in how parents approach the task of parenting. The Assessment Framework sets out the six 'dimensions' of parenting capacity, to be covered in any assessment under the Children Act 1989. These are: basic care, ensuring safety, emotional warmth, stimulation, guidance, and boundaries and stability. The challenge for professionals is to ensure that they account for difference whilst still maintaining a baseline standard in making judgements about the quality of parenting relative to the needs of the child.

In cases of suspected neglect, a distinction also has to be made between difference and deficit. For black minority ethnic families, cultural stereotyping can lead to negative assumptions about the care provided by black families, based on a notion of perceived inferiority of lifestyle or child care practices. Neglect is not about difference, it is about a persistent and severe deficit which results in significant impairment of the child's health and development. Cultural variations do not result in such detrimental outcomes for the child, and neglect cannot be explained by cultural factors.

Many children who are physically abused also experience emotional abuse or neglect, although physical abuse can occur alone. Jasmine Beckford, Sukina Hammond and Victoria Climbié were all neglected as well as being physically and emotionally abused. For Jasmine and Sukina, the scale of the neglect remained undetected by professionals until the Inquiries following their deaths.

In Victoria Climbié's case, the amount of evidence submitted to the Inquiry allows for a much more detailed insight into professional practice than was possible with either Jasmine or Sukina, and presents an opportunity to identify the impact that issues of race, culture and ethnicity had on the identification of and response to her abuse.

Professionals made observations about Victoria's appearance and behaviour which indicate that she was neglected by her aunt, Marie-Therese Kouao, from the outset, but in the process of seeking to establish Mrs Kouao's entitlement to services, an assessment of Victoria's needs was entirely overlooked.

The focus on 'entitlement' to resources for refugee and asylum-seeking children and young people results in children having to lie about their age, vulnerability and circumstances to gain access to resources and leads to exploitation by adults who may misuse children for their own profit.

Ealing Social Services supported Mrs Kouao until July 1999 when they established that she had made herself intentionally homeless. They offered to accommodate Victoria under s.20 of the Children Act 1989, which Mrs Kouao refused. It is probable that Mrs Kouao was reluctant to let Victoria out of her care for financial reasons, since to do so would have reduced her chances of accessing any services.

Throughout her involvement with Haringay Social Services, from August 1999 to her last contact with them in November 1999, Mrs Kouao continued to request rehousing. On 28 October 1999 Mrs Kouao was told that she was not entitled to rehousing and that only children who were at risk of serious harm would be accommodated. Four days later Mrs Kouao made an allegation that Carl Manning had sexually abused Victoria. Mrs Kouao withdrew the allegation the next day: this was the last day that any professionals saw Victoria alive – she died in February 2000.

In late 1999 the neglect and physical abuse of Victoria dramatically escalated. It appears that when Mrs Kouao realised that her chances of accessing housing and support were not enhanced by Victoria's presence she became more of a burden to her.

In *Beyond Blame*, Reder *et al.* (1993) explore the reasons why the children in the 35 Inquiry Reports they examined were fatally abused. They conclude that a significant feature leading to the vulnerability of some children as compared to others lies in 'the meaning of the child':

A child can mean different things to different parents. Traditionally a child is considered to carry the hope and aspirations of the parents, who are prepared to sacrifice some of their own personal gratifications to further the child's development. However, the vicissitudes of family life always colour the picture and many factors contribute to the meaning that parents attribute to children generally or to one child in particular.

(Reder *et al.* 1993, p. 52)

To establish the vulnerability of a child to continuing harm, we need to understand what a child represents to their parents and the factors that will increase or reduce that vulnerability. In Victoria's case, alongside the profit motive, there is also evidence that Mrs Kouao's links with the 'Mission Ensemble pour Christ' from August 1999 affected her behaviour with Victoria.

Pastor Orome at the Mission Ensemble Church formed the view that Victoria was possessed by an evil spirit, and that this was causing Victoria's strange behaviour (Mrs Kouao had said that Victoria was putting excrement in food) and her injuries. Pastor Orome said that he assumed Mrs Kouao was Victoria's mother and that she would love her daughter because she had given birth to her. He said that he prayed for her to be delivered from witchcraft, but denied that he had told Mrs Kouao to abuse or punish Victoria. Carl Manning, in his statement to the Inquiry, said that Mrs Kouao had on occasions referred to Victoria as 'Satan'.

This raises serious questions as to the role of religious beliefs as a contributory factor in child abuse. Along with Sita Kisanga, who was convicted of child cruelty in 2005 because she believed her 8-year-old victim to be 'possessed' by evil spirits, Marie-Therese Kouao also attended a fundamentalist black church. Religious beliefs and spirituality are significant for many black minority ethnic families who may find the support of religious organisations of great help in difficult circumstances. Religious beliefs do not make a parent injure or neglect a child, but for a small minority of parents they may contribute to abuse where the parent or carer is already predisposed to think negatively of the child.

Statutory agencies need to ensure that they take a balanced approach to the issue of religion, recognising the support provided by such organisations, but also being aware that religious institutions do not always prioritise the protection of children. There has been much concern over the responses from Christian churches, both Catholic and Protestant, to suspected child abuse. Lessons learned about the protection of children in these settings need to be extended to other religious settings, including temples, mosques and black churches.

Summary of the key issues

The research indicates that many black families experience social, environmental and economic disadvantage, but that the most disadvantaged minority ethnic groups do not generally access family support services. The introduction of the Children Act 2004 and the duty on local authorities to improve the well-being of children in relation to the government's five priority outcomes for children (physical and mental health and emotional well-being, protection from harm and neglect, education training and recreation, the contribution made by them to society, and social and economic well-being; s.10 Children Act 2004) may help to improve outcomes for children from these communities, but there is still much to be achieved in this area.

There is a great deal more to be understood about the role that ethnicity plays in the child protection system, although research indicates that ethnicity and culture do affect the referral, intervention and registration process. There is a need for more effective tracking of cases so that decision making can be more effectively monitored with regard to ethnicity and culture.

The introduction of IT-based recording systems such as the Integrated Children's System (which centralises the recording of information for all children who are assessed by social services, whether they are in the child protection system, children in need or children looked after) and the Common Assessment Framework (where any professional can initiate an assessment of a child they are worried is not meeting their potential in relation to the five priority outcomes in the 2004 Children Act) will provide the technology to achieve this, but whether this opportunity will be realised has yet to be seen.

Although information is available about physical abuse and neglect and black minority families, there is little known about emotional abuse and sexual abuse in these communities. Indications are that there is an under-reporting of these issues from children, families and professionals, but the reasons for this have not been explored to any satisfactory conclusion in research studies. Given the taboos surrounding sexual abuse and the challenges in evidencing emotional abuse, statutory agencies need the support of black communities to ensure that those children who are vulnerable to these forms of abuse can be protected. The low rates of referral indicate that there is a real lack of trust in professional intervention on the part of black communities.

An issue of continuing concern is the over-representation of black children in the care system, particularly the over-representation of children of dual heritage. As a significant proportion of these children have lone white mothers and are likely to have limited contacts with black communities, there is a real need to address the needs of these children and to identify what support provision is most effective for these children and families in preventing the children coming into the care system.

Conclusion

Ethnicity and culture are a part of every person's identity and, as such, they help to inform and to shape our attitudes, values, expectations and behaviour with our family, our friends, our communities and our children. Culture can help us to understand the context in which abuse takes place, but it does not explain why one parent from a specific cultural background harms a child while another from the same cultural background does not. Culture is important to white communities just as it is for black families, but it is never used as an explanation as to why abuse occurs in white English families.

Research helps us to understand the factors that contribute to children's vulnerability to abuse and statistics will inform us about demography of communities and patterns of professional response, but the protection of black and minority ethnic children requires more than knowledge; it requires attitudinal change.

Outcomes for children will not change until issues of ethnicity and culture are effectively integrated into assessment, planning, intervention and review for all children in need and in need of protection:

There is some evidence to suggest that one of the consequences of an exclusive focus on culture in work with black children and families is [that] it leaves black and minority ethnic children in potentially dangerous situations because the assessment has failed to address a child's fundamental care and protection needs.

(Ratna Dutt, in the Laming Report 2003, p. 345)

Key points and messages for practice

- Evidence suggests that black and minority ethnic families may be less likely to be referred to or access family support services. It is therefore important that professionals consider what community-based resources may be useful to families as this may help to alleviate problems at an early stage.

- There is a longstanding over-representation of children of dual heritage in the care system. Most of these children have white mothers and black fathers. There is a need for professionals to consider how these families can be better supported within the community.

- Child abuse occurs in all communities but myths about cultural patterns of abuse can influence professional judgement and the safeguarding of children. Professionals need to ensure that their judgements are based on sound evidence rather than cultural assumptions.

- The need to gatekeep resources and establish legal entitlement to services for children who are refugees or asylum seekers, or who are the children of refugees or asylum seekers, should not detract from the need to ensure that these children are safeguarded.

Annotated further reading

Barn R 1993 Black children in the public care system. Batsford, in association with British Agencies for Adoption and Fostering, London
    Outlines detailed research undertaken in a London authority on black children within the care system, and draws important conclusions in relation to the care paths of black children.

Bridge Child Care Consultancy Service 1991 Sukina – an evaluation report of the circumstances leading to her death. Bridge Child Care Consultancy Service, London
    Includes an analysis and recommendations as to the impact of race and culture on the decisions made in relation to Sukina.

Butt J, Box L 1998 Family centred: a study of the use of family centres by black families. REU, London
    A research study which identifies the extent to which family support is provided to black families, and identifies ways in which it could be provided more effectively.

Dutt R, Phillips M 1996 Race, culture and the prevention of child abuse. Report of the National Commission of Inquiry into the Prevention of Child Abuse, Vol. 2: Background papers. TSO, London
    Identifies the issues in relation to child protection and black families and presents a model for strategic intervention to address these issues.

Dutt R, Phillips M 2000 Assessing the needs of black children and their families. In: The framework for the assessment of children in need and their families practice guidance. TSO, London
    Provides guidance to professionals as to how to implement the Assessment Framework with black children and families.

Jones A, Butt J 1995 Taking the initiative: a report of a national study assessing service provision to black children and families. NSPCC, London
    This study looks at the extent to which services are meeting the needs of black children and their families. It includes the views of black children and young people, and provides a black perspective in child protection.

London Borough of Lambeth 1987 Whose child? The report of the Panel appointed to inquire into the death of Tyra Henry. London Borough of Lambeth, London
    One of the few inquiry reports on a black child that includes an analysis of the impact of race on the case.

Thoburn J, Chand A, Proctor J 2005 Child welfare services for ethnic minority families: the research reviewed. Jessica Kingsley, London
    A very helpful resource, collating all of the recent research in relation to black and minority ethnic families in relation to child welfare, with a very helpful opening chapter by Beverley Prevatt-Goldstein setting the current context in relation to race, culture, ethnicity and child care practice.

Useful websites

Commission for Racial Equality – Although funded by the Home Office, this organisation works independently of the government to promote good race relations and help eliminate unlawful discrimination. It undertakes research and provides guidance on how organisations can fulfil their legal obligations under Race Relations legislation: www.cre.gov.uk

Department for Education and Skills – Provides the latest child welfare legislation and guidance in downloadable form, including available statistics in relation to race and ethnicity and child care services: www.dfes.gov.uk

National Statistics Online – Provides a useful resource for governments statistics, including statistical research on ethnicity: www.statistics.gov.uk

REU – Formerly the Race Equality Unit, REU undertakes research and development projects in social care. It has a publications list and can be contacted at: www.reu.org.uk

9 Safeguarding children with disabilities

Deborah Kitson and Rachael Clawson

INTRODUCTION

The keynote presentation at a Barnardo's conference entitled 'Children with learning disabilities: how are their voices heard?' stressed the fact that children's voices are not heard clearly enough by people working, living or caring for them. Too often their voices are not heard until their abuse has become obvious and impossible to ignore. Discrimination of all kinds is an everyday reality for many disabled children, and it is therefore important that stereotyped assumptions of their lives, needs, communication and physical and emotional well-being are avoided by all professionals and agencies. For disabled children from black or ethnic minority families discrimination can be compounded by racism at institutional, cultural and personal levels.

Extensive evidence suggests that disabled children are more vulnerable to abuse than their non-disabled peers (Senn 1988, Cooke 2000, NSPCC 2003). Government guidance outlined in *Working Together to Safeguard Children** (DoH *et al.* 1999) and *The Framework for the Assessment of Children in Need and Their Families* (DoH *et al.* 2000) acknowledges that disabled children are particularly vulnerable to abuse and makes it clear that they are entitled to the same levels of protection and assessment of their needs as non-disabled children. The guidance also makes it clear that the same thresholds to safeguarding from harm apply to disabled as to non-disabled children (DoH *et al.* 1999).

To understand disabled children and the way that disability, and consequently they, are perceived, it is important to consider society's changing attitudes over the years, and the impact of research and the legislative framework on what has become generally recognised as good practice. Indeed, it is our attitudes over the years that have at times placed disabled people at increased risk. Later we will explore how present attitudes continue to impinge on the protection we offer and the work that we do with disabled children.

It is important to view how societal attitudes towards people with disability have evolved over time and the impact that these attitudes have had on them: how they are regarded, where they live and how they interact with the wider society. It is all too easy to assume that we have reached an era of equal opportunity, mutual respect and a recognition of our human rights as set down in the Human Rights Act 1998. Many people with disability would disagree.

This section challenges this assumption by looking at the history of disability and by discussing the myths that still exist today, their impact on the way that the community regards disability and more specifically how social care agencies work with disabled children.

Folklore referred to people with disability as 'changelings' and the work of elves and demons. In the sixteenth-century the Swiss physician, Paracelsus (Ryan &

---

* The most up-to-date version of this document was published by HM Government in 2006. For a full discussion of this, see Chapter 11.

Thomas 1987, Digby 1996) talked of fools, pure and uncorrupted, and later Lutheran Christianity questioned whether such people were truly human (Goodey 1996). In the eighteenth-century along with 'enlightenment' there were attempts to educate those referred to as 'idiots' and hence asylums emerged. Later in the nineteenth century the Industrial Revolution changed attitudes significantly (Fraser 1984): 'idiots' were regarded as economically unproductive and the workhouse was introduced, offering long-term institutional care and therapeutic intervention (Gladstone 1996). Later still came a scientific interest in eugenics which influenced many people's thoughts about disability (Ryan & Thomas 1987). Indeed, in 1945, post-war disillusionment with the eugenics movement contributed to the birth of the National Health Service in 1948 and the reclassification of asylums as mental handicap hospitals.

At this time legislation reflected changes in the way that disabled children were treated. Relevant policy and legislation will be outlined later in the chapter. The following section will consider available research which highlights the prevalence of the abuse of disabled children.

Research

There is a wealth of research which demonstrates that disabled children are more vulnerable to abuse and neglect than their non-disabled peers (Westcott 1991a, Kelly 1992, Miller 2003).

Awareness of the abuse of disabled children has grown since the 1960s, with most of the research coming from the USA; research in the UK has been fairly limited. Westcott (1991a) reviewed 22 studies published between 1968 and 1990 and found only three British studies. As there is little statistical information available on the abuse of disabled children in Britain, we do not know how many disabled children are abused, what happens to them or whether abusers are identified and/or prosecuted (Cooke 2000). There is also little research in relation to disabled children's experiences of the criminal justice system. This is significant as poor statistics will result in an underestimation of the experience of abuse among disabled children (Morris 1999).

In the past, research has been limited in terms of methodology. Westcott (1991a) found that there was a lack of a clear definition of disability and no guiding theory or hypothesis. She also points to the fact that there is a failure to involve disabled people in research (Westcott 1994). The actual extent of abuse is therefore unclear. Kelly (1992) reviewed available research evidence and estimated that the extent of abuse of disabled children ranged from 25 to 83%, thus highlighting the problems in methodology (see Creighton, Chapter 2, in this volume, for a full discussion of this issue).

Research undertaken in the 1990s and beyond has highlighted the previous methodology problems, and large scale research in the USA has demonstrated clearly the prevalence of abuse amongst disabled children as compared with non-disabled children. For example, Crosse *et al.* (1993) found disabled children were abused 1.7 times as often as non-disabled children (Cooke 2000) and, following analysis of computer records of more than 40 000 children in an American city, Sullivan and Knutson (2000) found disabled children were 3.4 times more likely to be abused or neglected (Miller 2003).

More recently, research undertaken by the Ann Craft Trust (Cooke 2000) highlighted the need for local authorities to collect and analyse data relating to disabled children subject to child protection procedures in their locality. Although the number of disabled children subject to procedures should provide an indication of the prevalence of abuse, Cooke's (2000) study revealed that many local authorities are unable to provide this information and there is often a lack of a common definition of disability. Morris (1998) also noted that social services departments fail to record statistics in relation to disabled children and there is little guidance on how disability is actually defined.

Many social workers inputting data onto computer systems have not been given clear guidance in the past as to how to record a child's disability and/or computer systems do not have information installed to enable the worker to record appropriate information. Our own experience is that this is now changing; some local authorities have developed clearer definitions of disability and use more sophisticated software which has been developed in discussion with social workers using it. However, the correct inputting of data still relies on abuse of disabled children being recognised as such.

Cooke points out that suggestions have been made that it is discriminatory to separately identify disabled children within a recording system as it highlights their 'victim' status. However, the Children Act 1989 identifies disabled children as requiring special care and the UN Human Rights Committee states 'the principle of equality may require affirmative action in order to diminish or eliminate conditions which cause discrimination' (Cooke 2000, p. 5).

Without collecting statistical information it is impossible for local authorities to have an overall picture of the number of disabled children who are abused and to therefore make any connections between disability and abuse. This information is vital if authorities are to have an informed view when putting together policies and provisions or services to offer the best chance of prevention or protection to disabled children. Without adequate research the authorities are in a weak position from which to develop policy and practice (Kelly 1992, Cooke 2000). Indeed the National Working Group on Child Protection and Disability made a recommendation in its report (NSPCC 2003) that the DfES should review the current child protection system in respect of disabled children and include the collection and analysis of data concerning disabled children and abuse.

Local authorities are currently in a prime position to reconsider the policies and protocols for safeguarding disabled children. The advent of new 'children's services' departments brought about by the 2004 Children Act and the change from Area Child Protection Committees to Local Safeguarding Children Boards is an opportunity for these issues to be revisited. One example of good practice in this area is a local authority setting up a disabled children's subgroup which feeds into the LSCB to ensure that the needs of disabled children are addressed.

It may be assumed that, given their heightened vulnerability to abuse, disabled children would be over-represented on the child protection register, yet research clearly demonstrates that this is not the case. One implication of this is that disabled children are not offered the same levels of protection as their non-disabled peers.

Further proof of this can be found in *Achieving Best Evidence in Criminal Proceedings* (Home Office *et al.* 2002) which addresses the needs of disabled children as witnesses within the criminal justice system. Clear guidelines for the interviewing of disabled children are given, including the use of specially trained individuals to aid the interview process in order to ensure that the account of what disabled children have witnessed can be to the standard needed by the criminal justice system. However, despite this and the introduction of Special Measures (outlined later in the chapter), research demonstrates that fewer disabled children are given the opportunity to be interviewed as part of a criminal investigation than their non-disabled peers and fewer cases get to court (Cooke 2000, Love *et al.* 2003).

In addition, there is very little research relating to disabled children's own experiences of the criminal justice system. The understanding and knowledge of those involved in investigating abuse of disabled children varies enormously and many assumptions are made, one commonly held assumption being that the disabled child will not be a credible witness or that it is not in the child's best interest to follow the investigation through to court. It is sometimes assumed that disabled children are not telling the truth, particularly if they have difficulty recalling specific facts about the incident. It appears that a high level of training and awareness raising are needed for all professionals involved in the criminal justice system if disabled children are to be given the same rights as non-disabled children.

The following section will consider legislation and government initiatives which impact on safeguarding disabled children from harm.

Legislation and government initiatives

The first Parliamentary Act that considered the protection of disabled people and a societal responsibility to regulate was passed in 1845. The Lunatics Act was concerned with the unlawful detention of people in private asylums. Soon after, the Education Act 1870 introduced compulsory education and this led to a growing awareness of an 'uneducable underclass'. The Mental Deficiency Act 1913 introduced compulsory detention for those certified 'mentally defective' and, as a result, increasing numbers were locked away in asylums with no support available to those living in the community.

The 1959 and 1960 Mental Health Acts provided the framework for mental health services which were, for the most part, taken up by people living in the community with their family carers. A number of public inquiries, including the Ely Hospital scandal in 1967, outraged the public and brought to their attention the conditions in which people in institutional care were living. This led to the 1971 White Paper *Better Services for the Mentally Handicapped* (DHSS 1971) in which targets were set to reduce the number living in institutions. A steady but diminishing number continued to be admitted to institutional care but the Jay Report (Jay 1979) advocated a faster pace of change and promoted the social model of disability. The Griffiths Report (Griffiths 1988), highlighting the difference between 'rhetoric and reality' in the provision of community-based services, was followed by the NHS and Community Care Act 1990 which was considered radical in its time, introducing as it did the assessment of need to access services in the community.

A number of recent policy and legislative initiatives designed to address the needs of all children have included disabled children specifically for the first time. The Children Act 1989 sets out the underlying principle that disabled children should be seen as children first, and although it has been criticised as being disablist and geared towards the needs of non-disabled children, it represented an important step forward in the recognition of the need for services specifically aimed at meeting the needs of disabled children (DoH 1991b). Standards are buttressed by guidance on the implementation of the Act (Volume 6): *Working Together to Safeguard Children* (DoH *et al.* 1999) and the *Framework for the Assessment of Children in Need and their Families* (DoH *et al.* 2000). The legislative and policy framework enables us to understand the context in which the safeguarding needs of disabled children are addressed. The Assessment Framework guidance states:

The cultural context in which assessments of disabled children take place is not a neutral one: disabled children and adults face major barriers to participating as equal members of our society. (p. 74)

Children Act 1989

Within the Children Act the local authority has two main responsibilities to all children:

1. Within s.17 of the Act it is the general duty of every local authority to safeguard and promote the welfare of children within their area who are 'in need' (s.17(1)). Disabled children are deemed 'children in need' by virtue of having a disability and are therefore entitled to an assessment of need. The Act also places a duty on local authorities to provide services to minimise the effect of disability and to provide the opportunity to lead lives which are as normal as possible (Schedule 2 (ix)).
2. Where a local authority is informed or has cause to suspect that a child is suffering harm or is likely to suffer significant harm, s.47 of the Act places a duty on the local authority to make any enquiries necessary to decide whether they should take action to safeguard or promote the child's welfare.

Volume 6 of the guidance is specifically aimed at working with disabled children and their families. This guidance notes that 'Children with disabilities are particularly vulnerable. They have the same rights as other children to be protected' (p. 46). Questions have been raised as to whether the principles laid down in legislation do in fact safeguard disabled children from harm. This question may partly be answered by considering whether local authorities and other agencies are equipped to work with disabled children in the child protection process.

Working Together to Safeguard Children 1999

Working Together provides specific although limited guidance in relation to the abuse of disabled children. It acknowledges that disabled children are more vulnerable to abuse and stresses the fact that standards and safeguards should be the same for them as for non-disabled children (the revised version of this document was published in April 2006; see Lyon, Chapter 11, in this volume).

Framework for the Assessment of Children in Need and their Families 2000

The Assessment Framework is designed to be inclusive of all children in need and to provide a framework for multi-agency assessment. In the past many standard assessment frameworks were developed with only non-disabled children in mind, with disabled children needing to 'fit in'. The Framework was developed as a multi-agency assessment tool, meaning that there should be one comprehensive assessment of a child which incorporates the views of all agencies working with the child. However, in practice, the extent to which the Framework is used to aid multi-agency assessment is not clear, and many disabled children continue to undergo a variety of assessments from different professionals and agencies in order to ensure that a holistic view of their needs is obtained. In terms of assessing a child's need to be safeguarded, possible indicators of abuse or significant harm may be difficult to separate out from the effects of a child's impairment, particularly if the child has multiple impairments (Westcott 1994) and a multidisciplinary approach to assessment, involving all professionals/carers who know the child best, including a consideration of the various settings the child is exposed to, is essential (DoH *et al.* 2000, Marchant & Jones 2000).

The Assessment Framework guidance for practitioners, issued as an aid to completing the assessment, contains a specific chapter on assessing the needs of disabled children and their families. It gives a clear foundation and practical advice for assessing potential abuse of disabled children and suggests that those undertaking assessments consider the following points:

- Are the key adults in the child's life aware of the increased vulnerability of disabled children to being abused?
- Are standards for safeguards within services in place and regularly monitored?
- Can the child access the safety channels that exist for all children (e.g. helplines, complaints procedures, advocacy services)?
- If not, what alternative safeguards can be put in place?
- Have any concerns about possible significant harm been carefully considered and been the subject of appropriate enquiries?

The guidance also gives examples of the necessity to consider the needs of disabled children carefully and to avoid assumptions to ensure that they are protected:

A seven year old boy's constant masturbation was 'explained' by his autism and his attempts to touch adults sexually were initially attributed to his confusion about boundaries. Several years later his father was convicted of sexual assault of all three children in the family.
Extensive bruising to the face, chest and arms of an eleven year old was said to result from falls during epileptic seizures. Medical advice was that the bruising was incompatible with falling and child protection procedures were initiated.

(DoH *et al.* 2000, p. 92)

Every Child Matters 2003/Children Act 2004

Every Child Matters sets out an agenda for proposed changes in reshaping services to all children and is given legal force in the Children Act 2004. The duties and functions of local authorities arising from the Children Act 1989 remain unchanged but the way services are delivered will change as they become integrated around the child and family. Listening to children and involving children are at the heart of the way services are to be delivered and the focus is very much on local change (DfES 2004b, 2004c). The challenge will be how disabled children are included in this process.

The Children Act 2004 also places a duty on local authorities to obtain the wishes and feelings of all children who may have an assessment or provision of services under s.17 of the 1989 Children Act or be subject to child protection enquiries under s.47 as far as is reasonably practicable and consistent with the child's welfare. It remains to be seen how far this will improve communication with disabled children. Social workers and other professionals involved need to be equipped to communicate with all children to ensure wishes and feelings are obtained. Issues of communication are referred to later in this chapter.

National Service Framework

The Children Act 2004 gives a clear focus for change but in itself is not enough to implement the changes needed at a local level. Published in September 2004, the *National Service Framework for Children Young People and Maternity Services* sets out standards for the planning, commissioning and delivery of children's services in England and Wales. The NSF is a 10-year programme which aims to ensure high quality and integrated health and social care; it will play a key role in helping children to achieve the five outcomes in *Every Child Matters*.

The NSF is in three parts and has 11 standards: Part one has five standards which apply to all children, Part two has five standards which apply specifically to children and young people with specific needs and Part three has one standard which addresses the needs of women and babies throughout pregnancy and the first 3 months of parenthood (DoH 2004). All standards apply equally to disabled children. The standards can be found in the *Change for Children – Every Child Matters* Executive Summary produced by the Department for Education and Skills and the Department of Health (2004a).

Standard 5 relates to safeguarding all children:

All agencies work to prevent children suffering harm and to promote their welfare, provide them with the services they require to address their identified needs and safeguard children who are being or who are likely to be harmed.

Arguably the NSF builds a framework from which disabled children can clearly benefit and in which there will be a framework for their views to be heard. The Department for Education and Skills and the Department of Health have published best practice guidance to aid this process in relation to Standard 8: *Disabled Children and Young People and those with Complex Health Needs* (DfES/DoH 2004b).

Standard 8 considers the need to safeguard disabled children from harm and is consistent with previous government guidance in outlining that disabled children are more likely to experience abuse than non-disabled children. The guidance stipulates that Area Child Protection Committees should have a system in place for safeguarding disabled children and that their specific needs are addressed in comprehensive, inter-agency safeguarding children protocols. It also stipulates that safeguarding protocols need to include agreement in relation to:

- consulting with disabled children and organisations advocating on their behalf about how best to safeguard them
- the development of emergency placement services for disabled children who are moved from abusive situations
- the systematic collection and analysis of data on children subject to child protection processes
- safeguarding guidance and procedures for professional staff working with disabled children
- training for all staff to enable them to respond appropriately to signs and symptoms of abuse or neglect in disabled children
- guidance on contributing to assessment, planning and intervention and child protection conferences and reviews
- disability equality training for managers and staff involved in safeguarding children work
- regular reviews and updating of all policies relating to disabled children.

Speaking Up For Justice 1998/Youth Justice and Criminal Evidence Act 1999

In 1998 an interdepartmental working group on the treatment of vulnerable or intimidated witnesses in the criminal justice system published a report entitled *Speaking Up For Justice* (Home Office 1998). The report recommended that there should be special measures to enable vulnerable or intimidated witnesses in a criminal trial to give their best evidence. This included measures for all children and vulnerable adults. The 1991 Criminal Justice Act permitted certain child witnesses in cases involving sexual abuse or violence to give their evidence-in-chief in the form of a video-recorded statement. This report extended this measure and included others; the Memorandum of Good Practice was revised accordingly and renamed

Achieving Best Evidence, covering guidance for vulnerable or intimidated witnesses, including children. It describes good practice in interviewing witnesses in order to enable them to give their best evidence in criminal proceedings. Section 2 refers exclusively to children.

All 78 recommendations in the *Speaking Up For Justice* report were accepted and those that required legislative changes were incorporated into the 1999 Youth Justice and Criminal Evidence Act. The special measures provided are:

- screening the witness from the accused
- evidence by live link
- evidence given in private
- removal of wigs and gowns
- video-recorded evidence-in-chief
- video-recorded cross-examination or re-examination
- examination of the witness through an intermediary
- aids to communication.

Witnesses eligible for special measures are:

- a witness who is under the age of 17 at the time of the hearing
- a witness who suffers from a mental disorder within the meaning of the Mental Health Act 1983, and who has a significant impairment of intelligence and social functioning, or who has a physical disability or disorder
- a witness whose evidence, in the opinion of the court, is likely to be diminished by reason of fear or distress about testifying.

In the case of a child witness, there are some special provisions. For example, there is a presumption that a child witness will give evidence-in-chief by way of video unless this would not improve the quality of the child's evidence. The use of Special Measures has a clear impact on the ability of the witness to give evidence and therefore on the likelihood of securing a conviction:

I didn't want to see him but wanted to make sure everyone in the court knew what he had done to me. He'd done it before to my friend and got away with it. I was worried people in court would be put off by the [BSL] interpreters or that they would think I'd made it up because that's what he told them. I was really happy that the interpreter told my side of the story just as I said it and that people in court believed me. I don't think I could have been that brave if I had to see him in court.

(12-year-old deaf girl known to the authors who was sexually abused by her stepfather – he was convicted on the basis of her evidence)

What is abuse?

The Children Act 1989 (Part IV, s.31) defines harm as 'ill-treatment or the impairment of health and development':

- development means physical, intellectual, emotional, social or behavioural development
- health refers to physical or mental health and ill-treatment including sexual abuse and forms of ill-treatment that are not physical
- harm means ill-treatment or the impairment of health or development; whether the harm suffered by a child is considered significant depends on the child's health or development as compared with what one could reasonably expect of a similar child.

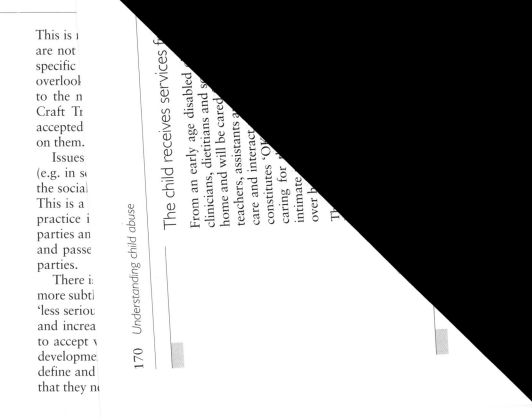

This is
are not
specific
overlool
to the n
Craft Ti
accepted
on them.

Issues
(e.g. in s
the socia
This is a
practice i
parties an
and passe
parties.

There i
more subtl
'less seriou
and increa
to accept
developmer
define and
that they n

Child protection and principles of good practice

There is a need for a 'rights-based' approach to services to ensure disabled children receive protection that is equal to that received by non-disabled children (Marchant & Page 2003). As demonstrated, research tells us that disabled children are more vulnerable to abuse than their non-disabled peers and our values and attitudes have an enormous influence over the way they are treated and the way they regard themselves – both crucial factors when considering their need for protection. If attitudes change, their vulnerability will reduce.

Vulnerability factors were summarised by Westcott and Cross (1996) as being 'negative social values: the general message that society gives to both disabled children and to potential abusers is that disabled children are worth less than non-disabled children'.

This reinforces the power imbalance between the child and the abuser and decreases further the likelihood that the child will try to disclose, or to be heard if they do so. To grow up from an early age to the realisation that you are worth less than the children next door will ensure low self-esteem and an acceptance when you are treated in an unfair and abusive way. Low self-esteem goes hand in hand with low expectations, low aspirations and feelings of low self-worth, all of which impact on the child's vulnerability to abuse.

When I was a teenager I was beaten by my mum and dad. I didn't know why. I was really confused. They took me away into a home. I couldn't talk to someone. I was too scared. The teachers wouldn't understand. They didn't have time for things like that. I hope they're different now. You need to talk to someone on your own. (Personal communication 2005)

...rom a number of different people

...children are seen by many professionals – therapists, ...cial workers. They may receive short breaks away from ...or by a number of carers. At school they have contact with ...nd volunteers. This gives them the message that any person can ...with them, and it may be difficult for them to understand what ...care' and 'not OK care' when there are so many different people ...hem in so many different ways. For example, if the child receives ...personal care from a number of people in various ways with no control ...ow care is delivered, they will not understand what is acceptable or abusive:

There's no way you can say 'no' to what a doctor does to you: they just damn well do it. When you're a kid you don't have any choice about it ... they lifted my nightdress, they poked here and they pushed there without asking me ... in front of a load of other people it was absolutely no different. I didn't say 'no' to any doctor, the porter actually was to me doing absolutely nothing different at all than any doctor or nurse had ever done.

(Westcott 1993, p. 17 – adult sexually abused by porter as a child)

The child becomes used to their body space being 'invaded' through disrespectful experience of health care and personal care

Many disabled children need the assistance of others with their personal care tasks – toileting, dressing, bathing, eating, etc. Although there is a possibility that they are at risk of harm from abusive carers, there is a bigger issue here. If intimate care is not offered in a sensitive way, taking regard of the child's individual needs and respecting privacy and dignity, then the child will become accustomed to being treated in a less than respectful way and will always tolerate this treatment without complaint. If a child is accepting of being treated poorly they are likely to be accepting of more serious abuse without complaint. It is crucial that from an early age the child understands their right to be treated in a way that they are happy about and their right to complain when this does not happen:

I had been bathed by so many people over the years I thought that what she was doing was just another way of being bathed and I had to put up with it. I did not realise that I could complain – nobody told me. (Personal communication 2003)

This teenage girl could have told somebody that the female carer in the home was masturbating her when she assisted her in the bathroom – she had good verbal communication. In fact her behaviour had changed – she became withdrawn and reluctant to join in activities but, though noted by staff, no-one had considered that she may have been being abused (see indicators section later in the chapter).

The child received little or no sex education

Many older people with learning disabilities have grown up without any sex or relationships education. Sex education equips people not only to develop positive and meaningful relationships but also to understand and protect themselves. Most of us learn in a variety of ways, including formal education, peer group learning, parent and sibling advice and experience. These channels are not available to many disabled people who do not have the same opportunities to learn from their peers, are protected in a way that inhibits their experiences and are often treated as children rather than future adults. Nowadays, children are more likely to receive sex education – many special schools acknowledge the importance of including it in their curriculum and mainstream schools offer sex education as part of Personal and Social Education (PSE). Concerns, however, are that this will not be suitable for children in special educational needs schools and consequently their parents may refuse permission for them to participate. In support of this, the NSPCC/Council for Disabled Children report *Safeguarding Disabled Children in Residential Special Schools* (2004) found few schools had clear plans for sex education for students:

I remember that time when your body changes. It was horrible. I had pains. They just said 'That's growing up'. It didn't really help. I can remember not having any pubic hair and no breasts. Was I developing correctly? It was a mixed class so I couldn't ask there. (Personal communication)

The child spends a lot of time away from home

A number of disabled children are in receipt of short breaks away from home: some may be in residential care or education and therefore are cared for by many people without consistency in their care or in the information and guidance that they receive.

The child spends time in segregated services

This engenders much debate. Integration is regarded as the way forward but sometimes without enough regard for the individual needs of the child. Integration (e.g. in schools) assumes that the child is able to look after themselves in that environment. Support to meet their needs is often a concern and an unsupported child will be vulnerable and at risk of being exploited by their peers.

The child is targeted by abusers because they appear unlikely to complain successfully to others

There is evidence to suggest that perpetrators target disabled people for a number of reasons which increase their vulnerability. The child may not be able to communicate clearly what has happened to them, either because they do not have verbal communication or because their carers do not understand their method of communication. Most children are able to communicate and it is vital that carers ensure that they 'listen' to them, whether by using words, signs, gestures, art, etc. Disabled children do not always understand that they can complain and do not know how to do so. Carers may not allow them the time required to raise their concerns, or believe them when they do. When the child complains too often, they are considered to be a nuisance. The cry for help is misunderstood as an inappropriate yearning for attention (see communication section later in the chapter).

I tried to tell my social worker what was going on at home but she was always in a rush – she said she would see me later but she never came back. So I changed my mind and put up with it. Anyway she was friends with my mum and dad so she would not have done anything. (Personal communication)

Family care and residential schools

Additional factors that can increase the child's vulnerability should be considered here. Many families experience isolation and little support in caring for their disabled child. They may be reluctant to ask for support as it can be misread as an inability to cope. Or the support may have been offered at a time when the family were still trying to come to terms with their situation, wanting privacy and not understanding the needs of their family. Families need the support when they are ready without feeling that professionals will consider that they are not managing.

Some disabled children have disabled parents who have additional difficulties accessing support (Cooke 2004). Those parents will often be even more reluctant to request help in case it is viewed as an inability to parent. They may find the information difficult to understand so do not receive the help to which they are entitled or they may have difficulties accessing community facilities. These factors place more stress on the home situation and leave the family, and subsequently the child, increasingly vulnerable.

Children living in residential homes or schools may also be particularly vulnerable to abuse and, as a result of their isolation, receive the least protection (Westcott 1993, DoH 1997, Williams & Morris 2003). Society deems it acceptable for disabled children to be cared for in residential environments from a young age due to their 'high level needs'; it is debatable as to whether the same thinking would be applied to non-disabled children. There are no comprehensive statistics available but all estimates indicate that the majority of disabled children who live away from home are in residential schools rather than substitute families. Disabled children in residential school may not have access to support or a safe person with whom to confide concerns or worries; many do not have access to an independent advocate. Children may not be aware of their right to complain or how to do this, they may be resident in schools a long way from home and have little contact with parents or other family members. Very little is known about their experiences from their own point of view (Williams & Morris 2003). Paul *et al.* (2004) highlighted the importance of facilitating regular face-to-face contact between parents and school staff in order that the child's needs be properly met:

I was sent to a school a long way away from home, I think it was because I was naughty at home and Mum and Dad didn't want me to live with them anymore but they said it wasn't because of that. I was sad and cried a lot but didn't have anyone to tell, I was worried that if I told [my key worker] she would be angry with me because I didn't like school.
(13-year-old girl with learning disability – personal communication)

Children can sometimes be placed in residential schools where placements are available rather than one that meets their needs. The needs of the child may not have been adequately or holistically assessed. In addition, many disabled children living in residential schools are not given the protection of 'Looked After' (s.20 Children Act 1989) status. This may mean that their care is not regularly reviewed by the local authority and their views not sought on a regular basis by social workers or the placing/funding agency (Williams & Morris 2003). It is often not clear which agency has overall responsibility for monitoring the placement, i.e. if the placement is funded solely by the local education authority, social services may not even be aware of the child.

The above issues will all impact on how well a child in residential school or home is safeguarded from harm. Paul *et al.* (2004) found a range of levels of child protection awareness in their research. They found that special residential schools often did not receive the degree of support and awareness of child protection and disability that they could expect from child protection services, either in their own locality or from the placing authority. Staff on the whole received little in the way of external child protection training. Schools also differed in the level of support they had received from the local authorities in drawing up child protection procedures.

Societal attitudes and the disabled child

In addition to the increased vulnerability of disabled children, the current child protection system often does not offer the necessary protection for a variety of reasons. Historically the focus of child protection services has been non-disabled children (Middleton 1992). However, over the past decade the level of awareness of the increased risk of abuse for disabled children has risen significantly and, as noted previously, principles of good practice are included in government guidance. However, applying the principles in practice, particularly if the child has a communication impairment, can be a challenge. The risk remains that the rights of disabled children are not protected and they continue to receive an unequal service (Marchant & Page 2003).

Any discussion relating to disabled children and child protection needs to be placed within the wider social context. The attitude of society towards disability can in itself create barriers to inclusion and so increase the vulnerability of disabled children. An understanding of the societal context in which disabled children are abused is essential to the development of antidiscriminatory services (Westcott 1994).

There are many reasons as to why disabled children are not safeguarded from harm to the same extent as non-disabled children. In working with disabled children, practitioners can easily collude in accepting standards of care that would not be accepted for non-disabled children. A really useful question to keep in mind when undertaking an assessment is: Would I consider that option if the child were not disabled?' (DoH *et al.* 2000, p. 80). Edwards and Richardson (2003) state that issues will only be raised where there is a recognition of child protection concerns but that there are many blocks to referrals being made, including:

- assumptions that a disabled child will not make a 'credible witness'
- concerns not always being recognised as child protection issues
- behaviour or physical symptoms sometimes being seen as the result of the child's impairment rather than an indicator of abuse
- use of medication – it can be misused but seen to be in the child's best interest
- a reluctance to challenge carers
- a reliance on carers to speak for the child or explain behaviour or symptoms and a ready acceptance of explanations by professionals involved
- the loss of the child's welfare if the prevalent view is that support is needed – the emphasis can be placed on support for the carers rather than the child's welfare.

Research has shown that many social workers believe that disabled children do not receive the same protection as non-disabled children for a number of reasons, including non-recognition of abuse, an unwillingness to recognise abuse and a lack of training (Cooke 2000). Morris points out that a wider interpretation of ill-treatment is required as many abusive experiences of disabled children are not recognised by the adults in their lives (Morris 1998, in Cooke 2000).

Even where a child protection concern is recognised and a referral is made, barriers continue to exist in disabled children accessing protection services through their needs being adequately assessed (Edwards & Richardson 2003):

- Assessments can be dominated by the child's impairment
- It can be difficult for the social worker to remain confident in their own expertise when challenged by a carer who knows the child well
- Existing timescales do not allow for additional time that may be needed
- The child's views are often not sought
- There is a prevalent view that carers are doing their best.

Indeed, Cooke (2000) argues:

There is always anxiety about possible subconscious collusion between social services and either the parents or foster carers who care for disabled children – feelings which encompass the idea that such caring people deserve support not criticism – so very careful assessment has to be carried out if the child is to be protected. (p. 28)

As noted previously, in most circumstances good practice would demand that assessments are multi-agency and include the views of all those who know the child best (e.g. teacher, teaching assistant, speech and language therapist, physiotherapist, occupational therapist, health visitor, school nurse, paediatrician, portage worker, family centre staff, carers in short break units, etc).

Where an assessment recommends that child protection enquires need to be made, there are barriers to adequately making those enquiries (Edwards & Richardson 2003):

- Not enough attention is paid to all sources of information
- Disproportionate weight may be given to medical evidence
- It might be difficult to identify a perpetrator as the child is in contact with many people
- The police are less likely to investigate abuse of a disabled child
- Social workers' attitudes and assumptions have an impact – they may doubt abuse has occurred or find it difficult to obtain evidence and so may be more willing to take the risk of not taking any action
- If initial child protection thresholds are not recognised, the case will not get to conference stage and key opportunities to protect the child are then lost.

In addition to the above, Edwards and Richardson (2003) point out that there are barriers to safeguarding disabled children in other parts of the system; for example, families with a disabled child are less likely to be referred to support services as services do not have the necessary 'expertise' and disabled children may be left in an abusive situation because of a lack of alternative appropriate foster or residential placements. Cooke found fewer disabled children had a change of residence than their non-disabled peers, and although this could be viewed as positive as support may be in place, it could also be seen as a result of no alternative placement being available. Research and our own practice experience also demonstrate that disabled children have fewer opportunities to access post-abuse therapeutic intervention, particularly if they have additional communication needs. However, social workers and other professionals can work creatively to address some issues for children and young people (see Case example 1).

Case example 1

Tom is 15 years old; he has epilepsy and a learning disability. He was removed from his birth parents aged 3 due to issues of neglect and placed with a number of foster families until he was adopted at age 6. His adoptive father died 2 years later. Tom was placed on the child protection register aged 14 due to issues of neglect and emotional abuse by his adoptive mother who then refused to allow him to continue living with her.

Tom had an extremely turbulent time in the following months; he experienced a number of foster placement breakdowns and exclusions from the special school he attended. His social worker recognised that he was not able to make sense of what was happening to him or to put his life experiences into context, so worked closely with a teacher from school who had known Tom since he was 3 to put together a 'social story'. This included photos of all foster placements and information about important life events, including where his adoptive father was buried. The social worker and teacher used this tool effectively once Tom had settled to help him gain some understanding of his life experience. Following a more settled period Tom was able to access support through the Child and Adolescent Mental Health Service.

Communication

Communication is a key issue in relation to safeguarding disabled children and the child protection process.

One of the most basic human rights is that of being communicated with and consulted about decisions affecting your life. This right is fully recognised in the UN Charter of Children's Rights, the Children Acts of 1989 and 2004, and most of the guidance produced alongside legislation and government initiatives. The test to local authorities and other agencies is the extent to which this is applied to children with communication impairments. Marchant and Page (2003) point out that the biggest barrier to communicating with disabled children continues to be the attitudes and behaviour of professionals and the failure to follow guidance.

Disabled children and young people communicate in a variety of ways. Some may have a reduced or lost ability to communicate or their ability is affected by the way they process language. For example, a child with autism may use verbal language but experience difficulties with processing language used. All children are able to give information regarding their feelings – for example, whether they are happy or sad, comfortable or uncomfortable, etc. Marchant and Page (2003) state:

Ascertaining how and what a child communicates is key to safeguarding them, whatever their level of impairment. We know that it is possible to recognise signs of contentment or distress in the youngest of infants and we need to ensure that our definitions of communication are inclusive and not discriminatory. (p. 62)

There are a wide range of communication systems used by children and young people. The list is not exhaustive but systems may include British Sign Language, Braille, Deaf Blind Manual Alphabet, Blisssymbolics, Makaton, PECS (picture exchange communication system), facial expressions, body language, sounds, finger pointing and eye pointing. There are also a number of pieces of equipment available, for example the Liberator or VOCA (voice output communication aid); this involves personalised words being placed into the equipment (e.g. names, lessons at school, food, etc.) that the child can choose by pressing a key. However, communication is still determined by those inputting the language:

I wanted to tell them at school that I didn't like the way one of my carers talked about me to other people but at the time I didn't have the right words.
(Adult with a learning disability – personal communication)

There is a need for all professionals to acknowledge and accept that communication occurs in a wide range of ways. Disabled children with communication impairments are discriminated against through a lack of understanding of their communication needs. Marchant and Page (2003) state:

We see it as vital that communication is understood as more than the use of speech and language and that all professionals' working definition of communication includes the wide range of ways children make their wishes and feelings known ... We regard it as the right of children that adults take responsibility for initiating communication, for maintaining it and for repairing it when it 'breaks down'. (p. 60)

Research undertaken by the Ann Craft Trust found that social workers did not think disabled children had a fair share of attention when it came to abuse investigations and this was related to time constraints, particularly if the child had a learning disability or communication impairment (Cooke 2000).

Communication is the absolute key to safeguarding disabled children from harm, both in terms of communicating with the child and communication between/within agencies involved. Communication needs should be an integral part of any assessment of disabled children, including assessments relating to child protection issues. The views that both professionals and carers hold in relation to the ability of a disabled child to communicate can be key in deciding whether abuse is actually reported and then the process that is followed.

All these issues have an impact on the child protection process and ultimately on whether a disabled child is adequately safeguarded from harm. For example, if the child does not have the choice of words, symbols or signs to tell what happened, does not feel they are being listened to or is not given access to a person to tell, the information will not be made available. One of the social workers interviewed in Cooke's research stated:

It is likely that a number of cases of abuse of disabled children do not come to light because people do not know what to look for and also because the children might not be able to speak out about the abuse.

(Cooke 2000, p. 31)

If professionals do not have the skills to communicate with disabled children the information which could be key to safeguarding them from harm will be lost. There is also a danger of relying on carers or parents to speak for or interpret for the child, particularly if that carer is implicated or suspected of being involved in an abusive situation. The social worker's role is to seek and represent the views of children; these views are not always the same as the view of the parent or carer. However, it is often easier for non-disabled social workers to relate to the non-disabled parents than the disabled child. Frequently we do not know what disabled children think because we do not ask them and we expect parents to answer for them (Middleton 1992).

It is all too frequent that disabled children's views are not included in assessments of need, including child protection enquiries. Our own experience has been that assessments sometimes state the child 'cannot give views due to disability' or is 'unable to communicate wishes and feelings' or the box which should contain this information is simply left blank. The reasons for this may vary: they could be related to timescales for completing assessments or to the assessor's level of skill and inclination. Social workers with the appropriate skills and understanding to ensure children's views are heard and represented unfortunately tend to be in the minority. It is crucial that work is done in conjunction with professionals who can communicate with the child to obtain their wishes and feelings and to gain a view of what it is like to live that child's life. Professionals involved need to make every effort they can to enable disabled children to communicate their views and make choices – if this is not the case, wrong decisions could be made.

Planning the investigation

It is vital that social workers and other professionals or carers working with disabled children are equipped with knowledge of safeguarding issues and have the appropriate skills to communicate with children. A lack of understanding from professionals may result in confusion or misinterpretation over what the child is saying.

Although in the past many communication systems have not included appropriate words, signs or symbols for intimate parts of the body, sexual activity or physically abusive actions, a growing awareness of the need for change has led to resource packs being published (e.g. Triangle and the NSPCC 'How it is' is a resource that will help professionals undertaking child protection investigations to better understand what disabled children want to tell them).

Any decision to investigate abuse of a disabled child must be planned and include prior discussion in relation to:

- the preferred communication methods of the child
- where the interview should take place
- who should interview the child
- whether any additional facilities or equipment is needed
- whether someone with a specialism in the child's communication should be included.

It may be useful to hold a strategy meeting involving all those who know the child best to identify the most appropriate way of proceeding. Any subsequent meeting (e.g. child protection conferences, core group meetings, review conferences, looked-after reviews) should always include professionals who know the child best and a person who can obtain the wishes and feelings of the child to act as an advocate if necessary.

The social worker needs to identify any barriers to communication that might impact upon an investigation or further work, and involve other professionals (e.g. speech and language therapists, teaching assistants, etc.) if necessary, especially if the child uses a method of communication which is personal to them. Professionals need to be aware, however, of the implications of using family members and/or carers to interpret for a child, particularly if they may be implicated in the abuse.

Our own experience has been that there is a need for more co-working and skill sharing amongst the teams in undertaking child protection work. The child protection skills of social workers working with disabled children can easily become rusty if not used frequently; confidence levels of workers can also be affected. Communication skills, confidence and understanding of issues relating to disabled children can be lacking in mainstream teams. Co-working can have positive results, both for the child and family and the social workers involved (see Case example 2).

Case example 2

This practice example concerned a mother of an 8-year-old girl with physical and learning disabilities. The mother was a single carer who had a level of learning disability herself. She also misused alcohol and neglected the needs of her child. The child's name was placed on the child protection register and legal advice was sought regarding removing the child from the mother's care.

Both social workers had specific areas of knowledge and skill and together devised a child protection plan and a way of enabling the mother to work with all agencies concerned and of communicating with the child to establish her views. The work had a positive outcome, with the child remaining with the mother with support and her name was removed from the child protection register. Both social workers felt they had learned a great deal from each other and would feel more confident in future in terms of their assessments and accessing appropriate support.

A 12-year-old boy with autism and a moderate learning disability alleged he had been hit by one of his carers. He was video-interviewed by the police but was unable to give any evidence. The police felt they could not pursue the matter. However, the social worker persuaded the police to reconsider and involve the child's speech and language therapist and another carer whom the child knew well and trusted. A second interview was planned with the boy's needs taken into account – at this interview he was able to say what had happened to him.

Even where other professionals may be reluctant to pursue child protection procedures, social workers can be instrumental in ensuring good practice is adhered to and in effecting change (see Case example 3).

Organisational issues in protecting disabled children

Very different cultures have existed between the field of social work with disabled children and child protection social work. In general terms, families with a disabled child are viewed as entering a voluntary relationship with Social Services, since many families would not be known to the service if their child was not disabled. Social workers enter relationships with a family that may last many years; relationship boundaries may become blurred, with the family viewing the social worker as a friend and the social worker accepting this role. Historically, the emphasis has been on supporting a family to care for their child with little weight given to obtaining the child's wishes and feelings or paying heed to them. Social workers may have excellent skills and knowledge in terms of disability issues and support services available, but may have received little child protection training or may not have had the opportunity to build skills in this area of practice. Some social workers may shy away from child protection issues or concerns as they find them too difficult on an emotional and practical level to deal with. All these factors have an impact on the recognition and investigation of child protection concerns and thus the protection of disabled children. Cooke (2000) found that social workers working in a specialist disability team may experience great difficulty in separating their 'supportive role' from their 'investigative role' in a family well known to them. In addition, parents who felt the social worker was a friend may feel betrayed. One social worker interviewed felt their team was 'cut off' from the mainstream team and they were considered of 'less importance' by mainstream social workers. There can be a lack of understanding and indeed interest in the complexity of the role of social workers working specifically with disabled children.

In contrast, 'child protection' work is viewed as the local authority carrying out its duty to safeguard children. Families may very well not be willing participants and are not necessarily viewed as voluntarily entering a relationship with their social worker. In child protection work, the parents' abilities often come into question – the child is not seen to be 'at fault'. In work with disabled children, however, the opposite can be true – parents' abilities are praised and the child's behaviour may be seen as being 'at fault' and the reason behind, or the explanation for, any concerns raised.

Disabled children require knowledgeable social workers if they are to be protected from abuse. This raises the question as to whether child protection work should be undertaken by 'specialist' social workers working with disabled children or social workers who work in mainstream teams who are 'specialists' in undertaking child protection investigations. Cooke's (2000) research demonstrated that there was a good case to be made for a specialist disability team to carry out child protection work as well as assessment and providing support. All social workers interviewed said they would welcome more training on disabled children and abuse issues.

Conclusion

The issue of disabled children and child protection has been receiving a higher profile over the past few years and is gaining a wider understanding. Recent government initiatives and legislation contain the grounding for improving protection structures and including disabled children in this process. In addition, some local authorities are changing the structures for working with disabled children and developing more comprehensive policies and procedures for safeguarding them from harm.

The Report of the National Working Group on Child Protection and Disability (NSPCC 2003) called for the DfES to develop a national strategy for safeguarding disabled children, including the improvement of current child protection systems and promoting good practice. The Report recommended a number of strategies to be put in place by Area Child Protection Committees (or future equivalent bodies), including the provision of mechanisms for consulting with disabled children, training to ensure that child protection workers have the necessary skills in working with disabled children, the development of emergency placements and therapeutic support, and clear policies and procedures for child protection concerns involving a disabled child. These strategies need to be put in place to ensure disabled children have equal access to systems designed to protect all children from harm.

Key points and messages for practice

- Research shows that disabled children are abused more often than non-disabled children.

- Disabled children are more vulnerable to abuse than non-disabled children.

- Disabled children have the right to the same protection as non-disabled children.

- Disabled children can communicate. Consider all methods of communication. The disabled child will be able to communicate even if they cannot do so verbally.

- Child Protection Teams and Disability Teams need to work together to ensure that the disabled child is offered the same protection as the non-disabled child and policies and procedures for the safeguarding of children should specifically address the needs of disabled children.

- Do not assume that a disabled child's injuries are associated with his/her disability.

- Disabled children need the same access to post-abuse support as non-disabled children.

Useful websites

Ann Craft Trust – www.anncrafttrust.org
Barnardo's – www.barnardos.org.uk
ChildLine – www.childline.org.uk
Department for Education and Skills – www.dfes.gov.uk
Kidscape – www.kidscape.org.uk
National Society for the Prevention of Cruelty to Children – www.nspcc.org.uk
Respond – www.respond.org.uk
Scope – www.scope.org.uk
Stop it Now! UK & Ireland – www.stopitnow.org.uk
Voice UK – www.voiceuk.org.uk

Abuse in institutional settings

Ian Butler

INTRODUCTION – SPECIAL PESSIMISM?

In 1836 the Clerk of the Bedford Union wrote to the Poor Law Commissioners seeking permission to have:

writing omitted as part of the schoolmaster's instruction in the workhouse, and that he teach reading only. The Board do not recommend this on the score of economy, but on that of principle, as they are desirous of avoiding a greater advantage to the inmates of the workhouse than to the poor child out of it, withdrawing thereby as much as possible any premium or inducement to the frequenting of the workhouse.

(Pinchbeck & Hewitt 1973, p. 503)

This historical anecdote can be made to illustrate several themes that find echo in this chapter. Firstly, it serves as a reminder that residential care in particular, but also other extrafamilial forms of care, have their origins in very specific forms of Poor Law provision for children that were characterised by insensitive, neglectful, deliberately stigmatising and punitive regimes that carried some degree of official sanction. Thus it makes the point also, that the abuse of children living away from home is not a new phenomenon.

Secondly, it demonstrates that the particular experiences of children living away from home have to be understood in the context of the general experiences of children of the time. Whilst one of the defining characteristics of public care might be the degree to which children and young people are removed from the wider community, institutional practices are embedded in the prevailing social construction of childhood and in the dominant professional cultures of the period.

Thirdly, it illustrates how individuals in positions of authority can devise schemes and strategies within the boundaries of particular institutions which, however misguided or malicious, nonetheless have a plausibility and even a logic to those with a motive to pursue them.

The main value of setting contemporary concerns over children living away from home in a broader historical perspective, however slight, is in order to contextualise and to limit the sense of crisis that often characterises debate in this area. This is not to argue for complacency but simply to suggest that taking a longer view may help to offset the 'special pessimism' (DHSS 1985b) that many social workers and parents share in relation to public care and which can seem to defy any hope of achieving positive and sustainable change. It has even been suggested that 'the 21st century is the time to break the umbilical cord of public care' (Ritchie 2005, p. 765) on the basis that there is 'no evidence that public care reduces risk of significant harm' (p. 764).

From its wider international perspective, a major UK voluntary childcare organisation goes even further and, in a document about residential care entitled *The Last Resort*, argues for 'a significant global reduction in the use of institutional care as a solution for children who are in need of care and protection' (Dunn *et al.* 2003, p. 3) on the basis that residential care is 'associated with *increased* risk to children' and that family forms of care 'can also prove unsatisfactory for the child and carers' (Dunn *et al.* 2003, p. 3, my emphasis; see also UNICEF 2005). These aspirations, however, have to be set against the 24% rise in the actual number of children looked after in England between 1994 and 2004 (to 61 100 at 31 March 2004 and 94 900 over the course of the whole year) and a 22% rise in the rate per 10 000 children in the general population over the same period (National Statistics 2005). It seems certain therefore that the needs and interests of children living away from home will require our attention for some time yet.

This chapter examines what is meant by 'institutional abuse' before considering the form and content of recent policy responses. Together, these considerations then form the basis for an exploration of some contemporary practice issues and how these might be addressed.

Review of the literature/research: a catalogue of abuse?

Despite the well-documented experiences of generations of children living away from home (Heywood 1969, Pinchbeck & Hewitt 1973, Hendrick 1994, DoH 1998a, Butler & Drakeford 2005a), the concept of 'institutional abuse' has only relatively recently entered the discourse of child protection. In 1992, Bloom reported just a handful of papers dealing with the subject in the American social work literature since 1980 (Bloom 1992) and, in 2003, Barter noted that 'UK research has yet to prioritise the area of institutional abuse' (Barter 2003, p. 2). Perhaps not surprisingly therefore, much of the literature in the field remains concerned with attempts to define the term and to describe the phenomena to which it refers. There is no universally accepted definition as yet and both elements of the phrase remain problematic.

In its everyday sense, the term 'institution' tends to conjure up the regimented, impersonal and large scale provision of residential care for children developed in the asylums, 'barrack schools' and workhouses of the eighteenth and nineteenth centuries. This sense of the term as referring to specific *sites* of abuse, despite the virtual disappearance of these particular forms of provision in the UK, is still reflected in the literature. With the exception of a relatively small number of studies describing the experiences of children attending boarding schools (Campbell-Smith 1983, ChildLine 1997), the phrase has been most commonly invoked to refer specifically to establishments for children in public care. It has been noted, however (Doran & Brannan 1996), that this reflects a past 'bias' in professional and political discourses towards institutions for working class and vulnerable children.

More recently, hospitals (Kendrick & Taylor 2000), churches (Commission to Inquire into Child Abuse 2005) and army bases (DfES 2005c, para. 10.5) have begun to be included as potential 'sites' of child abuse. After the accumulation of evidence for the existence of neglectful and brutalising regimes over many years (Liebling & Krarup 1994, Howard League 1995, 1996, Utting *et al.* 1997, Goldson 2002), even young offenders institutions, secure training centres and secure units are specifically identified by government in the latest (draft) version of *Working Together* (DfES 2005c) as housing children 'who may be particularly vulnerable' to abuse (DfES 2005c, para. 10.1). By identifying particular sites of abuse in this way, not only is a useful distinction made between familial and extrafamilial forms of abuse but awareness of the particular vulnerabilities of certain groups of children is substantially raised.

Gil, in still the most frequently cited account, defines institutional abuse as:

> any system, programme, policy, procedure or individual interaction with a child in placement that abuses, neglects or is detrimental to the child's health, safety or emotional and physical well-being, or in any way exploits or violates the child's basic rights.
>
> (Gil 1982, p. 9)

Gil goes on to define 'system abuse' as 'perpetrated not by any single person or programme but by the immense and complicated child care system, stretched beyond its limits and incapable of guaranteeing safety to all children in care' (p. 11) (see also Moss 1990, Stein 1993, Utting *et al.* 1997).

In relation to such system abuse, the literature on residential care in Britain, both academic and administrative, since the 1980s (DHSS 1985b, Milham *et al.* 1986, DoH 1991c, Parker *et al.* 1991, Berridge & Brodie 1998, Brown E *et al.* 1998, Sinclair & Gibbs 1998) provides too many illustrations of how, through 'drift', under-resourcing, inadequate planning and poor decision-making processes, the social, educational, health and life chances for children looked after away from home have been diminished. In foster care too, there is evidence (NSPCC 1995, Verity & Nixon 1995, Berridge 1996, Wilson *et al.* 2004) of how poor relationships with carers, a high number of unplanned moves from placement to placement (which interrupts schooling and weakens parental and community links), as well as poor patterns of communication and inadequate complaints procedures, have a detrimental effect on children whilst in care and afterwards. It is important to remember, however, noting the caution over 'special pessimism' made earlier, that despite such failures, overall outcomes for children in residential and foster care are generally favourable (DHSS 1985b, DoH 1991c, Bullock *et al.* 1993, Berridge & Brodie 1996).

Against a background of major structural inadequacies within the wider child care 'system', at the level of the individual institution, particular regimes or practices (an approximation of Gil's 'programme, policy or procedure') may also be constituted as abusive. Examples include the misuse of medication to manage challenging behaviour (Shaughnessy 1984) and the development of idiosyncratic and ill-founded 'therapeutic' regimes, such as the 'regression therapy' practised by the convicted paedophile Frank Beck in Leicestershire children's homes in the 1970s and 1980s (Kirkwood 1993). The practice of 'Pindown' operated in Staffordshire children's homes (Levy & Kahan 1991) is another example of the abuse of 'expert' knowledge used to justify harsh and abusive regimes, in this case imposing severe restrictions on children's liberty through subjecting them to humiliating and degrading forms of containment.

Kendrick and Taylor (2000) identify 'programme' abuse in the hospital care of children too, citing general practice in relation to pain control and the specific instance of the high death rate of babies undergoing heart surgery at Bristol Royal Infirmary (see Kennedy I 2001). They also cite evidence of 'system abuse' in similar terms to that found in relation to public care, noting in particular the presence of geographical disparities in health care provision for children across the UK.

Thomas (1990), however, has cautioned against understanding institutional abuse simply as a function of wider system or regime-specific abuse in that these are 'inert structures awaiting human operationalisation' (p. 10). In recognising the centrality of human agency in any abusive practice, the concept of institutional abuse begins to overlap with what is usually referred to as 'organised abuse', another elusive category.

Bibby (1996b, pp. 5–6), defines organised abuse as:

- the systematic abuse of children, normally by more than one male.
- It is characterised by the degree of planning in the purposeful, secret targeting, seduction, hooking and silencing of the subjects.
- Institutional and ritual abuse are but specialised forms of organised abuse.

By implication, Bibby associates organised abuse primarily with sexual abuse. His subsuming of institutional abuse into the broader category of organised abuse is arguable, but is consistent with the finding of some Inquiry Reports that the techniques used by single perpetrators are similar to those used by multiple perpetrators (see National Commission of Inquiry into the Prevention of Child Abuse 1996). By this reading, the systematic, covert and predatory abuse of children by Frank Beck in Leicestershire would constitute organised abuse and so be a form of institutional abuse, whereas the practice of 'Pindown' in so far as it was not characterised by 'purposeful, secret targeting, seduction' etc. would not. Accordingly, it would follow that it may be reasonable to consider organised abuse as an instance of institutional abuse rather than vice versa.

This may be no more than a matter of semantics. What is common to both positions are the enduring characteristics of any formal provision made for children looked after away from home, namely its relative 'invisibility' and the endemic inequality of power relations between children and adults, reflecting similar power relations in society more generally (see Wardhaugh and Wilding 1993). It is these factors in particular that permit abuse to take place and to remain undetected. Both residential and foster care in particular are essentially 'private' activities that tend not to command wider public attention or interest other than through the reports of 'scandals'. Children looked after are accordingly relatively isolated (Ayres 1989, Sobsey & Varnhagen 1988). Largely unobserved, such children are also uniquely vulnerable for other reasons in that they will already to some degree have had their self-esteem and support networks weakened by whatever experiences have brought them into institutional care (Solomons *et al.* 1981, Kelly 1992). In particular, children who have been subject to previous sexual or physical assaults prior to admission are more vulnerable to further abuse (Colton & Vanstone 1996, Macleod 1999).

Children with disabilities are also particularly vulnerable (Crosse *et al.* 1993, Jones 1994, Paul & Cawson 2002), as are those who are regarded as more difficult to work with for behavioural or other reasons (Blatt & Brown 1986). Such factors accentuate the powerful positions of adults in whose care children are placed. Such adults are routinely in a position to make life-changing decisions for the young people they are looking after. As Westcott (1991b) has observed, children in institutions are a 'voiceless population, having no control over decisions affecting their current and future placements, and no influence over the quality of care they receive' (pp. 12–13).

How far general or specific failures in the provision of out-of-home care can be said to constitute abuse is, of course, debatable. If one takes the view that 'abuse in institutions comprises any system which violates the rights of a child to a healthy physical and psychological development' (Doran & Brannan 1996, p. 156), then any failure to provide effective and compassionate care would constitute abuse. If one takes a position further along the spectrum of what might be regarded as abusive, by introducing the concept of 'significant harm' (Children Act 1989), for example, then a narrower range of activities and experiences would fall within the category of child abuse.

It is in this sense that both elements of the concept of 'institutional abuse' are problematic. In terms of the site of the abuse and the form it takes, and the manner in which it is pursued, any definition runs the risk of being either too wide or too narrow in its scope. On the other hand, if institutional abuse is regarded as a complex phenomenon, multicausal and appearing in a variety of forms, then Stein's (1993) conclusion, extended to include all forms of substitute care, is a useful starting point for further action. He argues that we should discard at the outset, any idea of finding a crude homogeneity in the abuse of children living away from home and discard an implicit standard or single response in addressing such abuse (see also Colton 2002).

Definitions of abuse that derive from the actions of the adults involved, rather than from the experiences of children, are perhaps inevitably inadequate and unsatisfying (Southall *et al.* 2003). Internationally, and indeed in some jurisdictions within the UK, an understanding of abuse that is founded on a recognition of the formal rights of the child, as defined in the UN Convention on the Rights of the Child, offers both a boundaried definition of abuse and specific directions for protective or remedial interventions. For some, at least, institutional care is a 'rights issue' (Dunn *et al.* 2003, p. 3). Articles 2 (principle of non-discrimination), 3 (best interests of child) and 6 (right to survival and development) of the UNCRC may be particularly relevant in the case of children living away from home (see Dunn *et al.* 2003, pp. 11 ff.). Notwithstanding the importance of a rights-based approach, however, La Fontaine (1994), in the context of organised abuse, has noted that 'even the best constructed definition is a poor substitute for acquiring systematic knowledge' (p. 230). Where such knowledge derives from the documented experiences of children (Butler & Williamson 1994, Butler 1996, Macleod 1999), consequent definitions may be of more conceptual and practical value.

A further difficulty remains, however. Without a more precise or at least consensual definition, calculations of both the type of abuse perpetrated upon children living away from home and the questions of its incidence and prevalence become almost impossible to address. There have, perhaps for this reason, been few systematic surveys of incidence or prevalence reported in the literature. American studies (Rindfleisch & Rabb 1984, Powers *et al.* 1990, Blatt 1992, New York State Commission 1992) and studies in the UK (Westcott & Clement 1992) would suggest that abuse in institutions is more common than for the child population more generally and that much goes undetected (see also Waterhouse 2000). For example, the NYS Commission calculated the rate of abuse in institutional settings as 87 per 1000 children as against 28 per 1000 children in the general population.

Rindfleisch and Rabb (1984), on the other hand, found a much lower substantiated incidence rate of 10 per 1000 children in institutional care in their study. However, any extrapolation, particularly from American studies, where forms of provision and constructions of abuse differ from those found in the professional and administrative literature in the UK, must be considered as tentative (Westcott 1991b, pp. 11–12). Evidence is stronger in relation to the gendering of certain forms of abuse, with boys featuring more strongly in relation to physical abuse and girls more strongly in relation to sexual abuse (Rosenthal *et al.* 1991, Westcott & Clement 1992).

In the absence of any more definitive accounts, perceptions of the incidence and prevalence of abuse in residential care in the UK have been mediated by the several reports of various 'scandals'. In summarising the findings of several inquiries, the

National Commission of Inquiry into the Prevention of Child Abuse (1996) concluded that:

The catalogue of abuse in residential institutions is appalling. It includes physical assault and sexual abuse; emotional abuse; unacceptable deprivation of rights and privileges; inhumane treatment; poor health care and education. (p. 19)

In relation to foster care, there is perhaps more cause for optimism but little more solid a foundation of systematic knowledge on which to base it. Thomas (1995), in his review of the largely North American literature, found that 'estimates of the incidence of abuse in foster care vary considerably, not least according to the measures and definitions used' (p. 35). The same observation is made in an earlier study by Benedict *et al.* (1994). In the UK, Gallagher (2000), in his small scale study using a very narrow definition of institutional abuse (close to Bibby's, cited earlier), reported a higher incidence of sexual abuse in foster homes than in residential settings (but both lower than in community settings – see also Lindsay 1997). An earlier study by Verity and Nixon (1995) reported that allegations of abuse were made in 4% of foster homes, of which 22% were deemed founded but which in a further 20% of cases it was not possible to decide either way.

From the fragmentary data available, it seems probable that child abuse is more frequent amongst children living away from home than amongst the population of children as a whole but the evidence is not strong. Whilst there remains a degree of uncertainty, or possibly even because there remains a degree of uncertainty, about how many children suffer at the hands of those whose job it is to care for them, the case for further research, continued vigilance and direct action remains a persuasive one.

Policy issues

The political and practice landscape of childcare in the UK has changed almost beyond recognition over recent years as several chapters in this book illustrate (e.g. Chapters 1 and 17). Devolution, the major reallocation of responsibilities for children between the Department of Health and the Department for Education and Skills, the emergence of new structures for the local delivery of services and a fundamental reorganisation of education and training in social care, predicating a reconceptualisation of the children's workforce, should all bear on the broader context in which services for children in public care and elsewhere are delivered. It is beyond the scope of this chapter to enumerate in detail all of the areas that have been subject to scrutiny as part of this extraordinary policy interest. Our focus is on institutional *abuse* rather than institutional *care*; however, taking the widest possible definition of the former, the distinction may be considered to be one without a difference (Stuart & Baines 2004, Butler & Drakeford 2005a).

Much of the impetus for change developed, ostensibly, out of the modernising agenda of New Labour. The *Government's Objectives for Children's Services* (DoH 1999a) specifically linked targets for improvement in areas relevant to the better care of children living away from home to broader policy initiatives to tackle poverty, educational disadvantage and health inequalities (paras 9–12). These targets, incorporating elements from the 'Quality Protects Programme' and from *Modernising Social Services* (DoH 1998a), carried the prospect of increased resourcing and strict accountability based on performance. They included, for example:

- reducing the number of changes of placement for children (para. 1.2)
- improving the educational achievements and health outcomes of looked-after children, especially those from ethnic minorities (paras 4.1, 4.2, 4.4)

- improving leaving care services (paras 5.1, 5.2)
- ensuring effective complaints mechanisms.

The early indications are that, in some areas, including educational attainment and health outcomes, looked-after children are faring better than previously although less well than their counterparts in the general population (DfES 2005d).

Less progress has been made in relation to employment at 16 and in relation to reducing criminal activity by looked-after children (DfES 2005d). Notwithstanding the low baseline from which these measures commenced, progress towards reducing the harmful effects of the broader child care 'system' on children looked after away from home is at least in the right direction. The programme of work arising from the Laming Inquiry into the death of Victoria Climbié (Laming Report 2003), the *Every Child Matters* agenda, should further assist in the general development of out-of-home care in that it envisages substantial improvements in the recruitment, training and reward of foster carers. Additionally, reviewing the provision for looked-after children and identifying priorities for improvement should form a key part of the local needs analysis process and the children and young people's plan (CYPP) which every authority was required to have in place by April 2006 as part of the *Every Child Matters* and Children Act 2004 reforms.

To ensure the delivery of its targets, the government introduced a new set of regulatory arrangements and inspection mechanisms via the Care Standards Act 2000. The Act, *inter alia*, established the National Care Standards Commission (replaced by the Commission for Social Care Inspection in April 2004) which sets national minimum standards (NMS) for children's homes, fostering services, boarding schools and residential special schools. Regulatory frameworks have also been developed for children in other settings, including National Service Frameworks for children in health care settings. Such managerialist devices are not without controversy (see Butler & Drakeford 2005b) but they seem to have found a secure place within the practice of social work in the UK.

A more discrete and focused set of initiatives more specifically directed at the level of the 'programme or individual' have also been developed as a consequence of the renewal of policy and professional interest in out-of-home care since the early 1990s. The first Utting report of residential care (Utting 1991), the 'Warner Report' (DoH 1992a) written following the report into the activities of Frank Beck in Leicester's children's homes, and the second Utting report (Utting *et al.* 1997), have supported the introduction of a new language of 'safeguards' into the care of children living away from home. In particular, attention has been focused on ensuring that unsuitable people are prevented from working with children. The Protection of Children Act was passed in 1999 and provided a statutory basis for lists of such individuals which had previously been compiled on an informal basis. In 2002, the Department of Health (DoH 2002a) were satisfied that all councils had developed policies and procedures to meet the requirements of the Warner Report but that implementation was inconsistent and variable.

Practice was not as well developed in relation to fieldwork staff (DoH 2002a), however, nor in relation to foster care (Social Services Inspectorate 2002). The Department of Health expressed 'serious concerns' (DoH 2002a) over arrangements to check health service staff with substantial access to children. While Criminal Records Bureau checks are now routinely carried out on prison staff, they have not been conducted on staff already in post. The findings of the Bichard Inquiry (2004) (which followed the Soham murders) are still being integrated into formal guidance but already the Inquiry has demonstrated the potential weaknesses of filtering and screening systems which rely too heavily on evidence of past conviction only and which do not take a more rounded view of the suitability of individuals to work with children.

As well as finding themselves in the care of 'unsuitable people', children may also find themselves in unsuitable homes, which seek to serve too many purposes and which try to accommodate too wide a range of needs. The infrastructure of residential care has been steadily eroding (DoH 1998a) as a consequence of the lack of any effective strategic planning. Utting's original report (Utting 1991) and the contemporaneous Welsh Office equivalent (Utting *et al.* 1997) made a strong case for retaining and developing a broad range of placement provision to ensure adequate choice. In his first report, Utting describes such choice as a 'fundamental safeguard' (Utting 1991, p. 2). It is only in the context of a range of provision, differentiated by purpose and function, that individual homes meet individual needs and thus become 'safe places for children' (Utting 1991, p. 2). As well as providing opportunities for raising the quality of care overall, the development of placement choice reduces the risk of mixing abusing and abused young people (Utting 1991, p. 35, DoH 1999a, pp. 85, 92) and allows for the targeted training of appropriate staff (see also Sinclair & Gibbs 1998 and O'Neill 2002 for a fuller discussion of peer abuse in institutional care).

As far as training is concerned, government, especially since the publication of the results of the Climbié Inquiry (Laming Report 2003), has indicated that it is intent on filling the gaps in existing training programmes to ensure that all workers have 'an appropriate level of training in safeguarding children' (DfES *et al.* 2003, s.87). In addition, the burgeoning interest in evidence-based forms of practice have seen the development of a wide range of web-based resources to support improved practice (see examples at the end of this chapter) but considerable scope remains for developing inter-professional understanding through common training approaches.

In their exhaustive review of progress on safeguards for children living away from home, Stuart and Baines (2004, p. 6) have concluded that:

Progress has been made, as part of the social inclusion agenda, in improving the life chances of looked after children and they are now less marginalised than previously.

Stuart and Baines reinforce the point that the issue is increasingly one of implementation and ensuring that the remaining and most marginalised groups – including children with disabilities (particularly those in residential special schools), children in hospital settings for long periods, children who are privately fostered, younger children and children within the prison and secure systems ('the most worrying area in relation to safeguarding children': 2004, p. 10) – receive continuing interest and attention. They also note the lack of any overall strategic approach to providing choice of placement for children and conclude that 'little progress appears to have been made and out of authority placements remain a problem. Policy seems to have been developed in a piecemeal fashion ...' (2004, p. 7).

Implications for practice

The current draft version of *Working Together* (DfES 2005c) may prove influential in setting out the practice agenda that follows both specifically from the latest policy initiatives and from the experience of the last 10 years. This core guidance, at least in its draft form, devotes a whole chapter to 'Safeguarding and Promoting the Welfare of Children who may be Particularly Vulnerable', including children living away from home (s.10.2 ff.). *Working Together* recognises the importance of locating the safety of such children in the wider context of other child protection measures and in terms of the overall quality of care provided (s.10.3 ff.). It also sets out 'essential safeguards' (s.10.5 ff.) against which any specific child protection measures might be set. These basic safeguards include several elements already familiar from the literature. For example, a safe placement is one where:

- children feel valued and respected and their self-esteem is promoted
- there is an openness on the part of the institution to the external world
- staff and carers are trained in all aspects of safeguarding children
- complaints procedures are clear, effective, user friendly and readily accessible and that staff recognise the importance of ascertaining the wishes and feelings of children
- recruitment and selection procedures are rigorous
- clear procedures and support systems are in place for dealing with expressions of concern by staff and carers about other staff or carers.

The specific vulnerabilities of children in private foster care placements (s.10.13 ff.) are given prominence, as are the needs of children with disabilities (s.10.32 ff.) and the issue of peer abuse (s.10.38 ff.).

Working Together is explicit that 'when children are in hospital, this should not in itself jeopardise the health of the child or young person further' (s.10.28) and draws attention to the National Service Framework for young people. The importance of primary care staff in child protection work, particularly GPs, midwives and school nurses, has long been understood (e.g. Hendry 1997, Long & Smyth 1998) and is clearly articulated in *Working Together* at s.2.74, s.2.82 and s.2.87. Moreover, it has been substantially reinforced by the Royal College of General Practitioners (RCGP) and others (Carter & Bannon 2002) who consider 'active participation in child protection procedures ... unequivocally to represent a key component' (p. 9) of the work of the staff of primary care health trusts (PCHTs).

Post-Children Act 2004 structures have the potential for producing closer working with other professions, improved lines of accountability and closer inspection, yet for PCHTs, the aspirations of the Royal Colleges and the requirements of *Working Together* represent a considerable challenge. For example, Bannon *et al.* have concluded that 'training for GP registrars is currently unsatisfactory in terms of focus and availability' (Bannon *et al.* 2001, p. 259), noting their particular concern that 'a significant minority had received no training in this area whatsoever' (p. 259). For doctors, according to the *BMJ* (Kmietowicz 2004), the 'threat of complaints and ruined reputations' is driving them away from fulfilling their role in child protection, leaving 30% of posts where paediatricians take a lead in child protection unfilled. (And this was a full year before the General Medical Council's decision to strike off Professor David Southall, one of Britain's best known paediatricians, for his role as an expert witness in several high profile cases of children whom it had been alleged had died at the hands of their parents.)

The RCGP recognizes this challenge and identifies several barriers to more effective engagement by primary care staff in child protection, including inadequate training, personal and professional anxiety and uncertainties over the limits to confidentiality (Carter & Bannon 2002, p. 13). It is, however, disappointing to note that while the Royal College recognises the need 'for safeguards to be put in place in order to prevent the abuse of children by PCHT staff', it has nothing to say about the particular needs of highly vulnerable groups including those looked after away from home.

Working Together also updates the protocols for managing the various strands of an investigation (child protection enquiries, any police investigation and the employer's disciplinary proceedings) into any allegation of abuse where the child is living away from home in the light of the revisions to local arrangements for safeguarding children introduced by the Children Act 2004. However, in order for any investigation to commence, the abuse has to be recognised or at least suspected and there are aspects of the dynamics of institutional care that can inhibit this.

Westcott (1991b) identifies four such barriers: the lack of procedures/policies for reporting and investigating a complaint of institutional abuse; a tendency to see institutional abuse as the failure of an individual member of staff, not the institution; the 'closed' nature of institutions and the belief system surrounding them which rests on the assumption that out-of-home care is, almost by definition, of a higher standard of care than children would otherwise receive in their parental homes. Such barriers to the discovery of institutional abuse still exert an influence and practitioners need to be mindful of them. To this list might be added the difficulties faced by staff who 'blow the whistle' (Durkin 1982, Hunt 1998); the studied deviousness of the paedophile (Wyre 1996); the insidious effects of institutional racism (Marrett 1991); and the demotivating effect of the kind of dysfunctional cultures that can develop in an institutional setting (Whitaker *et al.* 1998; see also Glisson & Hemmelgarn 1998 for an account of the positive advantages of well-functioning organisational cultures).

By way of a balance, however, one might also note the devastating consequences that can arise for staff who are wrongfully accused of being an abuser. These can be particularly acute for foster carers (Carbino 1991, 1992). One possible practice response to the inadequate support they usually receive from social workers in such circumstances might be for carers to establish their own network of personal support in anticipation of such an event (Nixon 1997).

The greatest challenge facing practice, however, is one that lies at the heart of the abusive process and which is so easily accentuated in the semi-closed world of out-of-home care. Central to the very concept of abuse is the relative powerlessness of children. It is their relative powerlessness that makes them vulnerable to abuse and which prevents them acting for themselves or engaging others to end it. This powerlessness is deeply embedded in prevailing contemporary constructions of childhood, which generally conceive of childhood in transitional or deficit terms (see James & Prout 1991, Archard 1993). Child protection practice is uniquely prone to regarding children and young people *only* as vulnerable. They are, but they are also capable of being effective authors of their own biographies. Any practice initiative that seeks to truly protect children must seek also to empower them. Any convention, declaration, policy, procedure or protocol that does not have both as its means as well as its ends, increasing the capacity of children and young people to speak and act for themselves, is unlikely to prove as effective as one that does (Cloke & Davies 1995).

Summary

The abuse of children living away from home is a complex phenomenon. It includes a wide range of behaviours that take place in a variety of settings. It is difficult to set clear conceptual boundaries between discrete forms of institutional abuse and wider deficiencies in the quality of care provided for children and young people. It has been held that the wider child care system, once extended beyond its capacity to deliver, can directly be abusive or create the circumstances in which abuse can take place. Certain regimes or practices can also be abusive and institutional abuse can sometimes involve the organised activities of multiple or individual abusers. Certain characteristics of institutional care, of whatever type, also make children particularly vulnerable to abuse, i.e. the children's relative isolation, invisibility and powerlessness.

Perhaps in part because of the difficulties in defining the phenomenon, there is no structured knowledge base in this field and current estimates of incidence and prevalence are unreliable. Nonetheless, sufficient evidence has been revealed through inquiries into identified abuse, particularly in relation to residential care, for the phenomenon to be recognised as significant and to have created a substantial policy interest over recent years. There is some evidence that a more proactive and integrated approach to policy formulation is now being pursued and that it is producing improvements in the standards of institutional care and the safety of children and young people, although areas of weakness both in terms of settings (particularly in custodial settings) and certain groups of young people (especially children with disabilities) remain.

Practice initiatives which challenge prevailing contemporary constructions of childhood as merely a transitional phase, or which counter professional ideologies that rest on deficit models of childhood, can help reduce the likelihood of abuse in the first instance and manage the consequences in the interests of the child when it occurs.

Conclusion

The Poor Law Commissioners did not allow the Bedford Union to proceed in the way in which they had planned. They recognised that providing the workhouse child with every means possible, including the ability to write, was the only way to enable them to grow up and play a full and productive part in the life of the community. In fact, the Poor Law Commissioners worked assiduously and with some considerable success to improve the conditions of the pauper child.

Indeed, the lasting lesson of history is that the best protection against institutional abuse is an unequivocal political, professional and personal commitment to provide the best care for children and young people who have to live away from home. At the heart of any healthy system, as much as at the heart of a neglectful or abusive system, are the actions and beliefs of individual practitioners. Institutional abuse begins and can only be ended there.

Key points and messages for practice

- The abuse of children living away from home is a complex phenomenon. It is multi-causal and appears in a variety of forms and settings. Practitioners must not assume a spurious homogeneity amongst such children and young people, nor should they allow their practice to be driven by simplistic accounts or models of practice.
- The 'invisibility' of children in public care, as well as their relatively weak social networks, particular characteristics and histories may make them especially vulnerable to abuse. Practitioners should therefore be mindful of the cumulative vulnerabilities of looked after children which may simultaneously be obscured and aggravated by the experience of living away from home and they should be prepared to advocate on their behalf.
- A proper, professional understanding of the rights and entitlements of children in public care may help in identifying both general and specific failures to safeguard and promote their welfare.
- The provision of an adequate range of services for children who cannot live at home, differentiated by purpose and staffed to a level of expertise sufficient to deal with children and young people with complex needs, is essential to the proper safeguarding of such children.

Annotated further reading

Butler I, Drakeford M 2005a Scandal, social policy and social welfare, 2nd edn. BASW/Policy Press, Bristol

This book provides an historical context for some of the recent policy responses to the deficiencies identified in the provision of out-of-home care. It also provides a detailed account of some recent child care 'scandals', especially the events reported by the 'Pindown Inquiry' in 1991, which illustrate how easily abusive practices can develop within residential settings.

Macleod M 1999 The abuse of children in institutional settings: children's perspectives. In: Stanley M, Manthorpe J, Penhale J (eds) Institutional abuse – perspectives across the lifecourse. Routledge, London

This chapter, along with several others in the book, provides a useful account of the experience of abuse from the point of view of those with the most detailed knowledge; in this case, children and young people themselves.

Ritchie C 2005 Looked after children: time for change? British Journal of Social Work 35:761–767

This article provides a radical challenge to the notion that existing forms of provision can ever adequately meet the needs of looked-after children.

Stuart M, Baines C 2004 Progress on safeguards for children living away from home. Joseph Rowntree Foundation, York

This paper is a very thorough and detailed account of progress made towards meeting the various goals, aims and objectives that government has established for the better protection of children living away from home. In describing the shortfalls, the paper also illuminates some of the key dynamics that inform the provision of such services.

Useful websites

www.everychildmatters.gov.uk/socialcare/lookedafterchildren is that part of the Every Child Matters website that addresses the needs of looked-after children. It contains a number of valuable links to other DfES sites dealing with related issues.

www.voicesfromcarecymru.org.uk/main.htm is the website of Voices From Care Cymru. VFCC exists 'to create opportunities for all young people who are or have been looked after in Wales, to have a say about the issues that matter to them'. Although based in Wales, the site is relevant to any young person who is or has been looked after.

www.crin.org – the website of Child Rights Information Network – contains references to hundreds of reports, recent news and upcoming events, as well as details of organisations working worldwide for children.

www.rhrn.thewhocarestrust.org.uk/wct/user/index.jsp is a direct link to a page from the Who Cares? Trust designed to tell young people all that they 'need to know about being in care'. The Who Cares? Trust promotes the interests of children and young people in public care and works with all those interested in their well-being in England, Scotland, Wales, Northern Ireland and around the world. Access to their home page is via www.thewhocarestrust.org.uk.

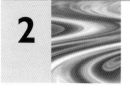
MANAGING THE PROCESS OF SAFEGUARDING CHILDREN

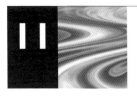

Child protection in the international and domestic civil legal context

Christina M. Lyon

INTRODUCTION

This chapter is not a mere updating of the chapter in the second edition but a substantial rewriting, as a great deal has happened in the field of child protection in the 5 years since the last edition appeared. A very serious word of warning must, however, be issued right at the beginning, which all readers are asked to bear in mind. Despite the fact that a large number of legislative reforms have taken place and a great many more cases have been heard before the courts, it has been necessary to reduce the length of this chapter substantially in order to embrace the other changes that have been included in this new edition. Such a reduction is not possible without reducing the utility and effectiveness of the chapter, and the details of many cases which would have helped the reader to understand the law have, therefore, had to be removed. The full version of this chapter appears on the website which accompanies the publication of this book (http://evolve.elsevier.com/wilson/child).

The focus in this chapter now has to be on the law in England and Wales as the same considerations mean that the comparable law in Scotland and Northern Ireland cannot be considered. It should be noted, however, that whilst the governing statute on the substantive law on child protection in Wales remains the Children Act 1989 as variously amended, the statutory provisions on the organisation of children's services in Wales are governed in the Children Act 2004 by separate provisions from those for England, and these will be noted at the relevant sections of the text. The title of this chapter has also changed because increasing recognition must now attach to the issue of whether the law in England and Wales complies with our international obligations under the various Conventions, Covenants and Charters, ratified by the UK government on behalf of its people. These include the European Convention on the Protection of Human Rights and Fundamental Freedoms 1950 (hereinafter ECHR), the most important of all these Conventions because it has been a part of our law since the implementation of the Human Rights Act 1998 on 2 October, 2000, and then, in date order: the International Covenant on Economic Social and Cultural Rights 1966 (hereinafter ICESCR); the United Nations Convention on the Rights of the Child 1989 (hereinafter the UNCRC); the Revised European Social Charter 1998 (hereinafter RESC) and the Charter of the Fundamental Rights of the European Union 2000 (hereinafter CFREU).

All of these Conventions, Covenants and Charters contain crucial provisions directing their signatories to abide by special duties to protect children and young people from abuse of any sort. Many of the readers of this text will only be familiar with the ECHR and the UNCRC, so it is important that it is understood by all who work in this area that these other Conventions are there to protect children and to be aware that bodies such as the European Committee of Ministers, supported by the European Network of Ombudspersons for Children, take them extremely seriously

(ENOC 2005) and are mounting campaigns against governments such as the UK seen not to be complying with the demands of such Conventions (Committee of Ministers 2005).

It is intended in this chapter to analyse the legal provisions in England and Wales, which are intended to provide the framework within which a range of State and voluntary agencies are expected to work together to prevent children suffering, or being at risk of suffering, significant harm at the hands of those looking after or caring for them (Fox Harding 1991, Parton *et al.* 1997). As far as England and Wales are concerned, these provisions are currently contained within at least three pieces of legislation: the Children Act 1989 (with its consequent Rules of Court, Regulations and Guidance as also amended by the Family Law Act 1996), the Adoption and Children Act 2002 and the Children Act 2004 (with its consequent Rules of Court, Regulations and Guidance). The Children Act 1989 (hereinafter CA 1989) was implemented in full in both England and Wales on 14 October 1991: the amending provisions relating to child protection issues to be found in Part IV Family Law Act 1996 (hereinafter FLA 1996), as well as those in the Adoption and Children Act 2002 (hereinafter ACA 2002) and the provisions restructuring the provision of services in the Children Act 2004 (hereinafter CA 2004), have all now been implemented.

This chapter will focus upon a critical analysis of the relevant statutory provisions as they apply in England and Wales, and on the judicial interpretation of these provisions in the courts in England and Wales.

Children's and parent's human rights as protected by the various international conventions, covenants and charters

The European Convention for the Protection of Fundamental Human Rights and Freedoms and the Human Rights Act 1998

When the Children Act 1989 was first introduced into the House of Lords by the then Lord Chancellor, Lord Mackay of Clashfern, it was described as 'the most comprehensive and far-reaching reform of child law, which has come before Parliament in living memory'. Such has certainly turned out to be the case. Nevertheless, if that was an apt description of that piece of legislation, it applies even more to the implications of the enactment of the ECHR in Schedule 1 of the Human Rights Act 1998 (hereinafter HRA 1998) and its consequent implementation across the whole of the UK from 2 October 2000 (Fenwick 2004). The potentially huge impact on the laws, practices and procedures relating to child protection in England and Wales effected by its incorporation in the HRA 1998 have already been felt, as can be seen in the number of cases in which children and parents have successfully complained to the courts of abuses of their human rights as protected by the ECHR. In the area of child protection, these cases have principally related to breaches by social services departments of children's rights under Articles 3, 6 and 8, to breaches of parent's or carer's rights under Articles 6 and 8 of the European Convention, and more generally to breaches by the state of Article 13 ECHR (see below).

Article 13 is not part of UK law as the government did not include it when it enacted the ECHR in Schedule 1 HRA 1998. The reason for not enacting Article 13 was that the government felt that the enactment of the HRA 1998 provided its citizens with access to the courts on any potential breach of the Convention. It overlooked the fact that if the courts had decided, as a matter of public policy, to exclude certain types of action from being brought in the courts on the grounds of public policy – for example, denying children the right to bring an action in negligence for the failure of social services to protect them – then this would deny the individuals effective access to a remedy before the courts as provided for in Article 13. The failure to enact Article 13 was thus found to be a breach of children's rights in cases such as *Z v UK* [2001] 2 FLR 612 and *E and Others v UK* [2003] 1 FLR 348 where the state's social services (in the Z case Bedfordshire, and in the E case Dumfries) were also found to have breached the children's Article 3 rights, and yet the decision of the House of Lords in the Z case, when it was originally *X v Bedfordshire CC* [1995] 2 FLR 276, and the decision of the courts in the E case meant that the children were denied access to an effective remedy before the courts as required by Article 13, and so this was breached as well.

The HRA 1998 extends to all UK citizens the right to take an action alleging breach of Convention rights (s.7(1)(a)) or to rely upon the ECHR in any proceedings which come before any British courts (s.7(1)(b)), and further requires various agencies including health authorities, social services departments and the police (which are all public authorities as defined in s.6(3)) to act in accordance with the rights conferred by that Convention. Space does not permit a lengthy explanation here but various Articles of the Convention will assume critical importance in child protection cases and procedures and will be referred to throughout the chapter as they arise. These will include:

- Article 2: 'Everyone's right to life shall be protected by law', which was alleged to have been breached by the police in *Osman v UK* [1999] 1 FLR 193, although the European Court found instead a breach of Article 6 (see below) and also arguably breached by the whole range of statutory agencies involved in the case of Victoria Climbié.
- Article 3: 'No-one shall be subjected to torture, or to inhuman or degrading treatment or punishment', found by the European Court of Human Rights to have been breached in the case of the child in *A v UK* [1998] 2 FLR 959 (who was beaten by his stepfather using a garden cane such that marks were left for several days and the child was taken by his natural father to a hospital, the decision in which has resulted in a change to the law on corporal punishment applicable in England and Wales), and in the case of the children in *Z v UK* [2001] 2 FLR 612 (the old *X v Bedfordshire CC* [1995] 2 FLR 276 case when heard in the English Courts) who were left in appallingly abusive and neglectful conditions for more than 3 years by social workers who were trying to work in partnership with parents under the principles of the CA 1989 but who forgot that the child should be the paramount focus of their concern (see Petrie, Chapter 21, in this volume).
- Article 5: 'Everyone has the right to liberty and security of person', an article which, so far, has not been imaginatively used by lawyers to protect children.
- Article 6: 'In the determination of his civil rights and obligations or of any criminal charge against him everyone has the right to a fair and public hearing within a reasonable time by an independent and impartial tribunal established by law', breached in *Osman* (see above) where the European Court of Human Rights stated that the Court of Appeal's decision in the domestic courts conferring a blanket immunity from being sued upon the police was a denial of the applicant's right of access to the court to sue for damages under Article 6 and in *Re L* [2002] 2 FLR 730 where the social services key worker failed

to communicate properly with the mother, who was further excluded from permanency planning meetings and from meetings with medical experts determining whether care proceedings should be commenced.

- Article 8: 'The right of every person to respect for his private and family life, his home and his correspondence, and further that there shall be no interference by a public authority with the exercise of this right except such as in accordance with the law and is necessary in a democratic society in the interests of national security, public safety or the economic well-being of the country for the prevention of disorder or crime, for the protection of health or morals, or for the protection of the rights and freedoms of others', breached in *F* v *Lambeth LBC* [2002] 1 FLR 217 where the boys were, to quote the judge, left to rot in children's homes without appropriate efforts being made to place them either back with their own family or in a substitute family.

- Article 9: 'The right to freedom of thought, conscience and religion; which includes the freedom to change one's religion or belief and freedom, either alone or in community with others and in public or private, to manifest one's religion or belief in worship, teaching, practice and observance, such right being subject to the same limitations as those governing the right to respect for private and family life'. In the case of *R on the application of Begum* v *Governors of West Denbigh High School* [2006] UKHL 15 (Times Law Report 23 March 2006), this right was judged by the House of Lords, upholding the decision of the High Court but overturning the judgement of the Court of Appeal, as not to include the child's right to wear a particular form of religious dress, in this case the jilbab, which covered the shape of the girl's arms and legs and her head, at school since this contravened the school's rules on uniform, which had, however, permitted her to wear the shalwar kameeze, consisting of a sleeveless tunic and trousers and headscarves. The provision allowing for the wearing of the shalwar kameeze in the school had been adopted following full consultation with parents, students and staff as well as with the three local Imams and, in the leading judgement in the House of Lords, Lord Bingham noted (at para. 33) that the school had taken immense pains to devise a uniform policy which respected Muslim beliefs in an inclusive, unthreatening and uncompetitive way and moreover that this satisfied the requirement of modest dress for Muslim girls (at para. 7).

- Article 10: 'Everyone has the right to freedom of expression which includes the right to receive and impart information', which would include the right to receive information with regard to reviews, on complaints procedures and information about children's rights to advocacy services under s.26A CA 1989.

- Article 14: 'The enjoyment of the rights and freedoms set forth in this Convention shall be secured without discrimination on any grounds such as sex, race, colour, language, religion, political or other opinion, national or social origin, association with a national minority, property, birth or other status', on the basis of which, since the European Court stated in *Botta* v *Italy* [1998] 26 EHRR 241 that Article 8 encompasses the right to physical integrity, it could be argued (although such an argument has not been made in the courts or in any academic articles on the subject) that s.58 CA 2004 is in breach of the child's right to be free from discrimination in the enjoyment of his Article 8 rights as it allows the defence of reasonable chastisement to be raised to a charge of common assault on a child, which cannot be raised in relation to anyone other than a child.

- Articles 1 and 2 of Protocol 1 of the ECHR, which in Article 1 provides that 'Every person is entitled to the peaceful enjoyment of his possessions' and Article 2 of which provides that 'No-one shall be denied the right to education, and that the state must respect the right of parents to ensure such education and teaching is in conformity with their own religious and philosophical convictions', unless these conflict with the state's obligations under state laws and policies to protect more vulnerable members of society, such as children, as confirmed in *Seven Individuals* v *Sweden* (Application No 8811/79 unreported 29 CDR 104) and confirmed in the UK courts by *R on application of Williamson* v *Secretary of State* [2005] 1 FLR 374 (see especially the judgement of Baroness Hale at pp. 395–401).

As can be seen from a very brief perusal of those Articles which may be deemed to be relevant to the issue of child protection, the implication of the guaranteeing of these rights by the implementation of the HRA 1998 on 2 October 2000 means that any agencies involved in the sphere of child protection must now ensure that their actions do not breach the fundamental rights secured to citizens – including, it must be emphasised, all children – under the Convention as implemented by HRA 1998. Those, therefore, who are working in the child protection arena would be well advised to access the *Core Guidance for Public Authorities: A New Era of Rights and Responsibilities* (Department for Constitutional Affairs (DCA) 1999), and they should be aware that all government departments have to review any proposed new legislation and procedures for which they are responsible in order to check their compliance with the relevant ECHR rights. The Minister concerned then has to certify at the beginning of the legislation that it is Human Rights Act compliant (HRA 1998, s.19).

The *Core Guidance* indicates that all staff need to be well trained in an awareness of the Convention Rights (DCA 1999, para. 81). Wherever possible, therefore, readers will be alerted to situations in which current law and procedures may conflict with the rights guaranteed under the Convention and where practitioners will have to be particularly alive to the issue of checking that their own individual practice complies with the demands of the Convention, and that they have received the relevant training on the subject.

The United Nations Convention on the Rights of the Child 1989

Whilst the ECHR is crucially part of our law as a result of the HRA 1998 and can give rise to actions being taken for and on behalf of children in the UK domestic courts, as well as still being able to take a case to the European Court of Human Rights if there is no effective remedy before the domestic courts, the UNCRC is not part of our law and no actions can be taken in the courts of England and Wales, or anywhere else, based upon alleged breaches of that Convention.

Nevertheless, since the UK ratified the UNCRC on 16 December 1991, and engages in the submission of regular reports to the UN Monitoring Committee as required by Article 44 of the Convention (see DoH 1994c, 1999c, UK Government's Written Replies 2002), it is clear that the government now takes it very seriously. All local authorities – including housing, social services and education, police authorities and health authorities – have signed up to it and are expected to comply with its requirements (DoH 2002a). This means that any profession engaged in work that relates in any way to children – all doctors and health professionals, education professionals, social work, social care work and all local authority and public authority personnel – will be bound by the demands of the UNCRC. The UNCRC can thus be said to be the aspirant gold standard by which our laws and the actions of various state bodies should be judged. This has been made apparent very recently by the important decision of the Court of Appeal in *Mabon* v *Mabon* [2005] 2 FLR 1125, where Rule 9(2A) Family Proceedings Rules 1991 (as amended) was interpreted by Thorpe L.J. as being capable of being interpreted so as to 'comply with the *UK's obligations to comply with both Article 12 UNCRC* and Article 8 ECHR to provide for the child's right to participate in decision making processes which fundamentally affect his family life'.

Increasingly, therefore, reference is made to the Articles of the UNCRC in the judgements of the UK courts, so whenever one is dealing with children and their families, one must also consider the relevant applicable articles of the UNCRC. In relation to child protection matters, the relevant articles include Article 3, Article 12, Articles 32–37(a) inclusive and, crucially, Article 19.

- Article 3, paraphrased, provides that: 'In all actions concerning children, whether undertaken by public or private social welfare institutions, courts of law, administrative authorities or legislative bodies, *the best interests of the child shall be a primary consideration* and that States must undertake to *ensure the child such protection and care as is necessary for his or her well-being*, and, to this end, shall take all appropriate legislative and administrative measures, and that States shall ensure that the institutions, services and facilities responsible for the care or protection of children *shall conform with the standards established by competent authorities, particularly in the areas of safety, health, in the number and suitability of their staff, as well as competent supervision*' (emphasis added).
- Article 12, as can be seen from the quote in *Mabon* v *Mabon* (above), crucially provides in 12(1) that 'children who are capable of forming their own views must be given the right to both express those views in all matters affecting him', which will include in all reviews, care planning meetings, and any other meetings discussing the child's life, which right is further reinforced in 12(2) where it states that 'the child must also be provided with the opportunity to be heard in judicial and administrative proceedings affecting the child either directly or through a representative', which ensures that children should be able to participate fully in complaints procedures themselves and in order to be able to express their views properly should have the right to an advocate provided pursuant to the new s.26A CA 1989 (see below), as well as being properly represented in all judicial proceedings and other administrative processes in which the child's life is being made the subject of a decision.

Articles 32–37(a) UNCRC seek to protect the child from all forms of abuse of whatever sort. Thus:

- Article 32 provides for the state's obligation to protect children from engaging in work that constitutes a threat to their health, education or development.
- Article 33 provides for the child's right to protection from the use of narcotic and psychotropic drugs and from being involved in their production or distribution.
- Article 34 provides for the child's right to protection from sexual exploitation and abuse, including prostitution and involvement in pornography.
- Article 35 provides for the protection of the child from involvement in their sale, trafficking and abduction.
- Article 36 provides for the child's right to protection from all other forms of exploitation not covered in Articles 32, 33, 34 and 35.
- Article 37(a) provides that no child shall be subjected to torture or other cruel, inhuman or degrading treatment or punishment (a mirror image of Article 3 ECHR).

■ Article 19 UNCRC interestingly provides that: 'States Parties shall take *all* appropriate legislative, administrative, social and educational measures to protect the child from *all forms of physical* or mental violence, injury or abuse, neglect or negligent treatment, maltreatment or exploitation, including sexual abuse, while in the care of parents, legal guardians or any other person who has the care of the child.' Article 19(2) goes on to provide that: 'Such protective measures should, as appropriate, include effective procedures for the establishment of social programmes to provide necessary support for the child and those who have the care of the child, as well as for other forms of prevention and for identification, reporting, referral, investigation, treatment and follow-up of instances of child maltreatment and as appropriate for judicial involvement.' In respect of both these provisions of Article 19, it must be admitted that both the law and the practice as thus far implemented (for example by s.58 CA 2004 in England and Wales) fails to accord the necessary State and institutional protection and support for children.

Arguably, UK legislation has everything the wrong way round in seriously failing to provide suitable educational measures designed to enable children to adopt preventative strategies but this may partly arise out of the difficult position adopted by the UK Government in relation to the issue of corporal punishment of children by their parents. Since the enactment of s.58 CA 2004 allows for parents in England and Wales to raise the defence of reasonable chastisement (but only in relation to a charge of 'common assault', so it should be noted that there is no such defence if the offence charged is 'assault occasioning actual bodily harm', 'wounding' or 'causing grievous bodily harm') and thus they retain the right to hit their children, then the provision of educational programmes enabling children to adopt appropriate preventative strategies when put into abusive positions could provoke physical problems to be faced by all concerned.

Nevertheless, it is interesting to note that *Working Together to Safeguard Children* (HM Government 2006a, para. 1.30, applicable to England, and see Welsh Assembly 2006) provides that physical abuse may involve 'hitting a child'. It seems inconceivable, therefore, that the Department of Health could have been responsible for issuing a Consultation Paper on the issue of '*modernising* the law relating to the physical punishment of children, so that it better protects children from harm' (DoH 2000a) and that its support for the continued legality of physical punishment should be set 'in the context of the Government's wider policy aims in support of families' (DoH 2000a, para. 1.7). They then went on to state a principle which is not only totally irreconcilable with Article 19 UNCRC, but also with the principles of Articles 8(1) and 8(2) ECHR, as implemented by the HRA 1998, in that it stated that it needed 'to achieve a balance between the right of parents to exercise their parental responsibilities and to bring up their children as they think best, without undue interference from Government, the responsibility of parents to bring their children up safely, *and the right of children to be protected from harm*' (DoH 2000a, para. 1.8).

The requirement to reform the law on the parental right to physically chastise children was brought to the fore by the ruling of the European Court in *A v UK* [1998] 2 FLR 218. In that case, an application had been made on behalf of Child A by his natural father to the European Court of Human Rights on the basis that the injuries sustained by his son at the hands of his stepfather reached such a level of severity as to be in breach of Article 3 ECHR, which provides that 'no-one shall be subjected to torture, or to inhuman or degrading punishment or treatment' (see above). The European Court concluded that there had been a breach of Article 3 and that domestic law in the UK did not give adequate protection to the child. It further ruled that the UK should immediately consider reform of its laws and that damages in the sum of £10 000 should be paid to Child A for breach of his human rights under the Convention. The Department of Health seemed to be totally oblivious of the mixed message that they are providing to its population at large as much as to the social work practitioners who have to work within the context of guidance issued by the government. It would seem totally incredible that a twenty-first century modern government could suggest on the one hand, in guidance to child protection workers, that hitting a child may amount to physical abuse (*Working Together*, HM Government 2006a, at para. 1.25) whilst on the other hand declaring that hitting children is a process which it not only endorses but thinks should be part of a government's wider policy aims in support of families! (For further details, see Lyon 2000, 2004.)

The government has, since the Consultation, reformed the statutory law on corporal punishment by enacting s.58 CA 2004, which has been in force since 15 January 2004. This provides that the defence of reasonable chastisement can now only be raised in relation to a charge of common assault (i.e. the most minor form of assault) under s.39 Criminal Justice Act 1988 (see above), but no longer as a defence to charges brought under s.18, s.20 or s.47 Offences Against the Person Act 1861 (OAPA 1861) or as a defence to a charge of cruelty to children under s.1 Children and Young Persons Act 1933 (CYPA 1933). Effectively, therefore, the parental power to discipline a child as set out in s.1(7) CYPA 1933 has been repealed (s.58(5)). To bring the civil law into line with this, s.58(3) provides that 'battery of a child causing actual bodily harm to the child cannot be justified in any civil proceedings on the ground that it constituted reasonable punishment', and subsection 4 provides that 'for the purposes of sub-section (3) actual bodily harm has the same meaning as it has for the purposes of section 47 OAPA 1861'. Effectively, therefore, to cause 'actual bodily harm' the injury must leave more than very short-lived, transitory marks and must not result in cuts or abrasions to the skin.

Debates on this provision in both the House of Commons and the House of Lords revealed just how bizarre may be the approach which the prosecuting authorities now have to take (Hansard 2004). In addition to the provision in s.58, practitioners should be aware that when the courts are trying to determine whether the defence is legitimately raised in relation to a charge of common assault they must follow the directions of the Court of Appeal in *R* v *H* [2001] 1 FLR 431. This decision effectively now requires that the court, in determining whether the punishment can be deemed to be reasonable so as to allow the use of the defence, should have regard to all the circumstances of the case such as the nature and context of the treatment, which is to be interpreted as including the defendant's behaviour and reasons for administering the punishment, as well as to the factors which were laid down by the European Court in *A* v *UK*, including the duration of the punishment, its physical and mental effects and, in some instances, the sex, age and state of health of the victim.

In reality, as the author has questioned elsewhere (Lyon 2004, 2006b), it is doubtful whether most social workers or parents in the population of England and Wales, and certainly not the children, have understood both the changes in the law and their potential significance for those children who daily experience more than the lightest of taps. It is undoubtedly the case that the new law offends against Article 19 and that the UNCRC Monitoring Committee, when it next reviews the law on child protection in England and Wales, will be aghast that such a provision remains on the statute book contravening recommendations which it made first in 1995, and then again in 2002 (UNCRC Monitoring Committee 1995, 2002).

Other important Covenant and Charter Articles for the protection of children

Articles 10(1) and 10(3) of the International Covenant on Economic Social and Cultural Rights 1966, ratified by the UK in 1966, provide that both 'the widest possible protection be given to families while responsible for the care of children' and that 'special measures of protection should be taken by states on behalf of all children and young persons'. The UN Committee on Economic, Social and Political Rights, which is responsible for monitoring a state's performance of its obligations under the Covenant, reported in 2002 (UNCESPR 2002) its view that the UK's Fourth Report to the Committee had demonstrated its continuing failure in its obligations under the Covenant to provide such 'special protection to children' by retaining the legal right of parents to corporally punish children.

In the context of Europe, Article 3 of the Charter of Fundamental Rights of the European Union provides that 'everyone has the right to respect for his or her physical and mental integrity', Article 24(1) provides that 'children shall have the right to such protection as is necessary for their well being' and, crucially, Article 17(1)(b) of the revised European Social Charter 1996 provides that: 'With a view to ensuring the effective exercise of the right of children to grow up in an environment which encourages the full development of their personality and mental capacities, the Parties undertake to take all appropriate and necessary measures designed to protect children and young persons against negligence, violence or exploitation.' The Council of Europe Committee of Ministers is deeply unhappy with the continued legality in some states of violence against children. The urgency with which it now views the need to outlaw corporal punishment of children throughout the member states is revealed in the adoption by the Committee of its response (Committee of Ministers 2005) to the call made by the Parliamentary Assembly of the Council of Europe for 'member states to ban all corporal punishment of children' (Parliamentary Assembly Debate 23 June 2004). Thus, the Committee of Ministers has declared that there is a need in all member states not complying with Article 17, of which the UK is one, to begin 'a coordinated and concerted campaign for the abolition of violence against children' (Committee of Ministers 2005).

Focus on the relevant legislative framework

The CA 1989 has, in almost 20 years, generated much mythology around its provisions and interpretation in law and in practice. Too many social workers, seniors and managers still rely on accounts of statutory provisions rather than themselves consulting the actual provisions of statutes, rules and regulations. This needs to change in order that children may be properly protected by practitioners. It is for this reason that the annotated reading set out at the end of this chapter provides the three essential texts which should be in the personal library of all those who work in child protection. As Lord Laming justly commented: 'The law is fundamentally sound; it is in the understanding of it and its implementation that workers across the field in child protection fail' (Laming Press Conference, 28 January 2003). The CA 1989, as amended by FLA 1996, ACA 2002 and CA 2004, deals with much, though by no means all, of the civil family law relating to children in England and Wales. Adoption law, although amended by small parts of the CA 1989 (see s.85 and Schedule 10), remains a separate civil code, formerly under the Adoption Act 1976 but now under ACA 2002. Nearly all the provisions of ACA 2002, creating a brand new adoption regime in England and Wales, were implemented on 30 December 2005. Children are subject to a vast plethora of other civil law statutory provisions and case law, such as education, child abduction and child support legislation, which impinge upon their lives in many different ways but which are, like adoption, beyond the scope of this chapter (but see Baginsky and Green, Chapter 17, dealing with education, and Williams, Chapter 20, dealing with criminal law provisions relating to child protection, in this volume).

This chapter therefore focuses entirely on the civil legal framework in England and Wales for protecting children. It would, however, be wrong to confine ourselves to thinking in this area solely of the civil justice system, since the legislation goes much further, at least in its underlying philosophy, than merely to define the terms upon which access to the courts may be sought (see DoH 1989a). Thus, as will be seen, there are provisions expressly designed to foster the development of preventative strategies and approaches, principally now by children's services authorities in England (s.17 CA 2004) and Wales (s.25 CA 2004), but also by other agencies (see s.17 and Schedule 2, Part I, para. 1, CA 1989). Note that *Working Together to Safeguard Children* (HM Government 2006a) has now adopted throughout the guidance the terminology of 'local authority children's social care department' as the term for the body responsible in the local authority for delivering services to children and for providing for their protection under the various statutory duties laid upon local authorities under the CA 1989 and under the administrative guidance laid down in *Working Together* and other associated documents. The term 'children's services authority' formed in many local authorities by the amalgamation of children's social services and education is, however, the body charged under the CA 2004 with the duty of promoting and safeguarding the welfare of children within their area. As *Working Together* has done, therefore, it is intended to use the term 'local authority children's social care departments', abbreviated to LACSCDs, to embrace the old terminology of local authority, and the term 'children's services authorities', abbreviated to CSAs, will be used only to indicate the duties owed by such bodies (usually the combined social services for children and education services) under the CA 2004. There are also very important provisions in Parts VI–XII of the CA 1989, governing the duty of LACSCDs to secure the welfare and protection of children in whatever environment they are being looked after away from their parents, whether this is in LACSCD children's homes, homes run by voluntary organisations or private bodies, day nurseries or child-minding facilities, private foster places, independent boarding schools, residential health facilities run by private individuals or in hospitals.

As well as considering the provisions of the legislation, one needs to note other directives that have been issued as a result of the failures of the different organisations that have responsibility for the welfare of children, as identified in the Laming Report (2003). Thus, for those working in the National Health Service, the *National Service Framework for Children and Young People* (DoH/DfES 2004) provides in *Standard 5* that 'All agencies must work to prevent children suffering from harm and to promote their welfare, provide them with the services they require to address their identified needs and safeguard children who are being, or who are likely to be harmed.' This, however, is a Standard and not a legal provision and so breach of it, in itself, cannot give rise to legal actions, although it could be cited in support of allegations that a particular part of the health service or a health service employee had failed in their duty of care to an individual and that this conduct was not in compliance with the standards expected in the Framework.

The legal framework provided by the CA 1989, as amended, is contained not only in the provisions of the statute but also in Rules of Court and in a large number of Regulations, often referred to by lawyers as 'secondary legislation'. Such Rules of Court and Regulations are as binding as the statutes themselves upon those to whom they relate and in respect of those whom they seek to protect (see, for example, the Family Proceedings Court (Children Act 1989) Rules 1991, as amended very many times, and the Children's Review Regulations 1991 as amended by The Children's Review (Amendment) Regulations 2004 for England and Wales). In addition, the legal framework provided by the Acts, the relevant Rules of Court and Regulations is further supplemented by guidance issued by the government departments most closely involved with issues of child protection, i.e. the Department for Education and Skills, the Department of Health and the Home Office, as well as, in the case of Wales, by the Welsh Assembly. Principal responsibility for issues relating to children in England, and thus for the issuing of such guidance, is now vested in the Department for Education and Skills (DfES) although *Working Together* (2006) itself has been issued in the name of HM Government.

Guidance on the CA 1989, much of it issued in 1991, runs to many volumes, including most crucially for those working in the field of child protection, *Working Together to Safeguard Children – A Guide to Inter-agency Working to Safeguard and Promote the Welfare of Children*, which is updated much more frequently. The latest version was published in April 2006 for England by Her Majesty's Government and for Wales by the Welsh Assembly. This critically important guidance was redrafted by the DfES for England (DfES 2005a) although ultimately published by HM Government (2006a) for England and for Wales by the Welsh Assembly (2006). *Working Together* must be part of the daily working tools of any professional working in the field of child protection in England and Wales.

Such guidance from government departments is issued pursuant to s.7 of the Local Authority Social Services Act 1970, which requires local authorities in their social services functions to act under the general guidance of the Secretary of State. As such, the guidance does not have the full force of legislation, but it *must* be complied with, unless local circumstances indicate exceptional reasons which would justify a variation. Practitioners should note that there has never been a case in which any local authority has successfully argued that they were justified in breaching such guidance because of exceptional circumstances: thus, for example, a shortage of staff or resources and arguments that a case had been referred to the housing department, which caused delay, have not been accepted as an excuse for failing to conduct a core assessment within the 35-day time period provided for in both *Working Together* and the *Framework for the Assessment of Children in Need and their Families* (DoH *et al.* 2000, National Assembly for Wales/Home Office 2001) (seen most recently in *R on the application of AB and SB v Nottingham City Council* [2001] 3 FCR 350).

It should also be noted at this stage that Circulars issued by government departments concerning the implementation of the provisions of statutes or regulations occupy a similar position; for example, Local Authority Circular 1999/29 *Care Plans and Care Proceedings under the Children Act 1989* (DoH 1999b) (see further below). Responding to a number of concerns about issues of child protection affecting those children who are looked after by children's services authorities, the government has issued a series of Circulars through the Department for Education and Skills associated with the implementation of the Children Act 2004 and the *Every Child Matters: Change for Children* programme (DfES 2004b, 2006).

The civil legal framework

Court structures and proceedings

A detailed discussion of these can be found in the full version of this chapter on the website and also in both Lyon (2003) and Priest and Wildblood (2005), referred to in Annotated further reading at the end of this chapter (see also Lane, Chapter 18, in this volume).

Prevention

LACSCDs and CSAs in both England and Wales (for the relevant provisions on CSA duties for England, see ss.10–24 CA 2004, and for Wales, see ss.25–34 CA 2004) are placed under very wide-ranging duties by s.17 CA 1989 (as amended by ACA 2002) to safeguard and promote the welfare of children within their area who are in need and, so far as is consistent with that duty, to promote the upbringing of such children by their families by providing a range and level of services appropriate to those children's needs. Pursuant to that, s.17(2) CA 1989 goes on to provide that, for the purpose of facilitating the discharge of their general duty under s.17, CSAs must have specific regard to their duties and powers set out in Schedule 2, Part I, CA 1989. Under the provisions of Schedule 2, para. 1, a duty is imposed upon LACSCDs to take reasonable steps to identify the extent to which there are children in need within their area. It is further provided that LACSCDs must publish information about services provided by them and by voluntary organisations, pursuant to their duty under Part III, CA 1989, and that they must take such steps as are reasonably practicable to ensure that those in England and Wales who might benefit from the services receive the information relevant to them.

The CA 2004 amended the CA 1989 to provide by s.17 CA 2004 that CSAs must, from time to time, prepare and publish a plan setting out the authority's strategy for discharging their functions in relation to children and relevant young persons (s.17(1)). The first of these plans were to be submitted to central government in April 2006 and are referred to as the Children and Young People's Services Plans (CYPSPs): they are intended to meet the five *Every Child Matters* (ECM) outcomes (for more on this subject, see Creighton, Chapter 2, in this volume). These CYPSPs consist of very detailed programmes which must demonstrate that CSAs are taking seriously the issues of providing services to all children in need and for children and young people generally, and for the greater protection of all children as well as for those children that they are required to look after or that they have formally looked after, referred to in the legislation as relevant children. CSAs throughout England and Wales will be publishing a series of information leaflets setting out details of their CYPSPs and the services which are provided in the locality for all children and young people.

The CA 1989 provides in s.17(10) and (11) a very wide definition of children in need. Thus, a child shall be taken to be 'in need' if:

- they are unlikely to achieve or maintain, or have the opportunity of achieving or maintaining, a reasonable standard of health or development without the provision of services for them by a LACSCD under the Act
- their health or development is likely to be significantly impaired, or further impaired, without the provisions to them of such services

- they are disabled, and for these purposes a child is disabled if they are blind, deaf or dumb, or suffers from a mental disorder of any kind, or is substantially and permanently handicapped by illness, injury or congenital deformity or such other disability as may be prescribed.

As was noted above, s.17(10) is indeed a very wide definition and many LACSCD information leaflets and CYPSPs seek to restrict the all-encompassing definition in order to 'gatekeep' limited resources available to departments for prevention. In many of the information leaflets, as well as in the CYPSPs, a high profile is given to the LACSCD's duty to safeguard children, and it has formerly been made clear that children in need of protection would be given a high priority in the provision of services (see variously Chapter 2 of successive copies of the *Children Act Report,* DoH 2003a). It remains to be seen whether this will continue to be the case under the new legislation.

Building on this 'preventative' approach, the CA 1989 goes on to provide in para. 5 of Schedule 2 that LACSCDs must take reasonable steps, through the provision of services under Part III, to prevent children in their areas suffering ill-treatment or neglect. As if to emphasise the point that children who abuse are, potentially, equally to be viewed as children in need as those children who are abused, the LACSCD is also required to take reasonable steps under the CA 1989 to reduce the need to bring criminal proceedings against children within its area and to take reasonable steps to encourage children in its area not to permit criminal offences (para. 7 Schedule 1, Part II, CA 1989). (For a thorough-going analysis of the concept of the 'child in need', see Bedingfield 1998.)

One of the underlying philosophies of the CA 1989 was its emphasis on partnership with families with children in need and further a reinforcement of the emphasis on preventative support through services to families. In the Department of Health's guidance it was clearly stated that 'it would not be acceptable for an authority to exclude any of the three categories describing children in need – for example, by confining services to children at risk of significant harm which attracts the duty to investigate under s.47' (DoH 1991d).

As has already been identified, the methods by which LACSCDs establish which children require safeguarding services will depend upon the measures for inter-agency collaboration in the identification process laid down by the Local Safeguarding Children Boards (LSCBs) as established under s.14 CA 2004. The LSCBs are further charged (s.14(1)(a)) with the duty of coordinating 'what is done by each person or body represented on the Board for the purposes of safeguarding and promoting the welfare of children in the area of the authority by which it is established'. How these Boards will work out in practice remains to be seen but their duties and functions are considered in the new Local Safeguarding Children Boards Regulations 2006 and in detail by Luckock in Chapter 14 (this volume).

A coherent prevention policy and plan is therefore necessary if CSAs are to take seriously their duty under s.10(2) and s.11(2) CA 2004 in England and s.25(2) and s.28 in Wales to safeguard the welfare of children within their area. (For a more detailed examination of this, see Lyon 2003, Chapter 4.2.) Sections 18 and 19 CA 2004 impose further duties on the new directors of CSAs (s.18), as well as on the lead member for children's services in the local authority council (s.19), to be accountable for the responsibilities of ensuring the promotion and safeguarding of children's welfare so that no-one can in future avoid personal responsibility for the failures by a particular CSA to safeguard a child, as happened in the Climbié Inquiry (Laming Report 2003).

Other preventative measures can also be identified within the provisions of the CA 1989, including the provisions in s.17(3) that any service provided by an authority in the exercise of its functions may be provided for the family of a particular child in need, or for *any member of their family*, if it is provided with a view to safeguarding or promoting the child's welfare. It is important to realise, therefore, that where an abused child is suffering at the hands of a family member – whether a parent, an older sibling or some other relative living in the family – it may be the case that the local authority will seek to provide services for those family members in order to attempt to safeguard the child who has suffered, or is at risk of suffering, significant harm.

Where it is felt desirable that an abusing member of the family should move out of the family home, Schedule 2, para. 5, CA 1989 could be used to encourage the perpetrator to move out of the premises and to provide accommodation for them. Use of this provision, of course, depends upon the cooperation of the perpetrator and, where one is considering the case of child perpetrators, who may well have been abused themselves, it may be more appropriate to consider the provision of accommodation under s.20 CA 1989, together with other necessary services such as psychiatric, psychological or social work assessment.

The use of both the service of accommodation under the legislation and other support services for such children will, of course, depend upon the level of cooperative partnership achieved between parents and workers. The necessity for LACSCDs to resort to s.20-type provision may be obviated in situations where the authority feels confident that the non-abusing parent will obtain relevant necessary protective measures in the form of domestic violence injunctions or orders, including exclusion orders or ouster orders, under the relevant provisions of the domestic violence legislation (see Part IV, FLA 1996 for England and Wales). The relevant ouster and anti-molestation orders obtainable under this legislation are available to partners of perpetrators of domestic violence where they, or their children, have experienced such violence. Both types of order can be obtained in an emergency and also provide for longer-term orders to be granted in a variety of different circumstances.

In recognition of the fact that children in such situations may need the benefit of protection provided by LACSCDs to support the parents in whose care they might otherwise remain, amendments to the CA 1989 were made by Schedule 6, FLA 1996. These amendments effected the insertion of new s.44(A) and 44(B) and s.38(A) and 38(B) into the Children Act. These provisions enabled the courts to include special exclusion requirements in both emergency protection orders (s.44(A)) (hereinafter EPOs) and interim care orders (s.38(A)) (hereinafter ICOs). The detail of these provisions can be found in the full version of this chapter on the website.

It has long been recognised, although it only seemed to be officially acknowledged for the first time in the Cleveland Report (Butler-Sloss 1988), that removal of the perpetrator is far better than seeking to remove the child, and thus every support should be given to the non-abusing parent if they are prepared either in the immediate or long term to seek remedial action using the domestic violence legislation or, alternatively, by using the provisions which can be attached to EPOs and ICOs set out above, in an effort to keep the child in the family setting. In those situations where police action has resulted in the removal of either an adult or child perpetrator, the necessity for the local authority to use any of the empowering provisions such as s.20 or Schedule 2, para. 5, or even the additional protective measures linked to EPOs and ICOs, will have been removed, either because the perpetrator has been remanded in custody or by the imposition of bail conditions in respect of an adult perpetrator, or in a remand to local authority accommodation in the case of a child perpetrator.

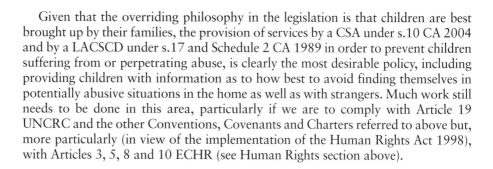

Given that the overriding philosophy in the legislation is that children are best brought up by their families, the provision of services by a CSA under s.10 CA 2004 and by a LACSCD under s.17 and Schedule 2 CA 1989 in order to prevent children suffering from or perpetrating abuse, is clearly the most desirable policy, including providing children with information as to how best to avoid finding themselves in potentially abusive situations in the home as well as with strangers. Much work still needs to be done in this area, particularly if we are to comply with Article 19 UNCRC and the other Conventions, Covenants and Charters referred to above but, more particularly (in view of the implementation of the Human Rights Act 1998), with Articles 3, 5, 8 and 10 ECHR (see Human Rights section above).

The process of identification and investigation

Suspicions about whether 'a child is suffering or is likely to suffer significant harm', which is the first of the threshold criteria that need to be satisfied in relation to a range of orders under the different pieces of legislation, may arise in a variety of different ways. It should be noted that where concern surfaces about whether a child is suffering or is likely to suffer significant harm in private family proceedings which are already before the court, such as a residence order or domestic violence application (s.8(4) CA 1989), the court has the power under s.37 of the CA 1989 to direct a local authority to investigate whether there is a need to bring care or supervision order proceedings in respect of such a child. While the LACSCD is conducting such an investigation, the court can consider whether it is necessary to make either an ICO or interim supervision order (hereinafter ISO) as was done in the case of *Re H* [1993] 2 FLR 541. The judge in that case also made a prohibited steps order under s.8 CA 1989, forbidding the natural parents from seeking to assume possession of, or be in contact with, the child without the court's further order (see also *Re CE* (s.37 direction) [1995] 1 FLR 26). Note that a s.37 direction must not be used as a means of appointing a children's guardian to represent the child where there is no real prospect of a CO or SO being made, and it should further be noted that a local authority must not be made a party to private law proceedings if it decides, following its investigations, not to seek a CO or SO (see further *F v Cambridgeshire County Council* [1995] 1 FLR 516). Another example of the use of s.37 where the judge gave excellent guidance about its use arose in *Re M* [2003] 2 FLR 636 (which is reproduced in full in the chapter on the website).

More often than not, in situations where it is suspected that a child is suffering or is likely to suffer significant harm, the child is a member of a family with whom social services are or have been already working (as was the case in *Re M* [2003] above) or concerns about the child have already become known to a number of different professionals, all of whom are working with the child and the family (see Farmer & Owen 1995). Dale *et al.* (1986a) reported that in well over 75% of cases that ultimately found their way into the courts, the family or the child was already known to the various helping agencies and was already the subject of considerable concern.

Pursuant to s.47 of the CA 1989, a LACSCD, in particular, is under a duty to investigate whenever it is provided with information that may suggest that a child living or found within its area is suffering or is likely to suffer significant harm, or where it is informed that such a child is already the subject of an EPO obtained by some other person, limited to the National Society for the Prevention of Cruelty to Children (NSPCC), or where the child is in police protection (see below). Where information is passed to the NSPCC, the LACSCD may also undertake appropriate enquiries and investigations – for example, s.44(1)(C) and s.31(1)(9). In order to undertake such investigations, the LACSCD is required to consult with a range of other agencies to enable it to decide what action it should take to safeguard or promote the child's welfare. The LACSCD may also request other agencies to assist them in such enquiries and investigations (see s.47(5)(9)(11) and (12). (These processes are described in much fuller detail in Lyon 2003, Chapters 4 and 5.)

The meaning of 'significant harm'

The basis for deciding to embark upon an investigation or to invoke any of the procedures to be described hereafter is that the child about whom one is concerned *is suffering or is likely to suffer 'significant harm'*. This concept is therefore the trigger for much of what may follow in the way of an investigation, and it is also the ground to which the various concerned agencies and the relevant courts must look when deciding whether to apply for orders, to exercise any special powers or, in the case of the courts, to make orders.

'Harm' is defined by s.31(9) CA 1989, as amended by ACA 2002, as meaning 'ill treatment or the impairment of health or development' and such impairment can arise from seeing or hearing the ill-treatment of another; development is defined as meaning 'physical, intellectual, emotional, social or behavioural development'; health is defined to include 'physical or mental health'; and, finally, ill-treatment is defined as including 'sexual abuse and forms of ill treatment which are not physi-cal'. When looking to satisfy the criterion of 'significant harm', it is the case that the court may be satisfied that the child is suffering from 'significant harm' if any one of the three types of harm envisaged in s.31(9) is present. This is indeed the guid-ance offered by the government in *Working Together* (HM Government 2006a), which states that each of these elements has been associated with more severe effects on the child, and/or relatively greater difficulty in helping the child to overcome the adverse impact of the maltreatment. It also points out that 'sometimes the process of suffering such harm is a continual process' but that 'sometimes, a single traumatic event may constitute significant harm, e.g. a violent assault, suffocation or poisoning' (HM Government 2006a, para. 1.25).

Neglect is, of course, included in harm and, as *Working Together* makes clear, it encompasses the persistent failure to meet a child's basic physical and/or psycho-logical needs likely to result in the serious impairment of the child's health and development (HM Government 2006a, para. 1.33). Thus, for example, the parents of the children in *Z* v *UK* were said to have been guilty of neglect since the psy-chiatrist giving evidence to the European Court in the case described the failure by both parents to meet the needs of the children in any way, including their emotional needs, as the worst example of the damaging effects of child neglect and abuse with which she had had to deal in over 20 years of practice (Stevenson 1998a, Iwaniec *et al.* 2004). Emotional neglect may obviously be just as damaging to a child's development as more obvious forms of injury or ill-treatment. The grounds for intervention can thus be seen to be very wide and, indeed, the Court of Appeal in *Newham London Borough Council* v *AG* ([1993] 1 FLR 281 at 289) empha-sised that the words of the CA 1989 must be considered but are not meant to be unduly restrictive when the evidence clearly indicates that a certain course of action should be taken to protect a child, a point reiterated by Thorpe J. in *Re A* [1993] 1 FCR 824.

The condition as to 'significant harm' is drawn with reference to the child con-cerned, so that those conducting the investigations, and the courts who may be called upon to make orders, must look at the position, characteristics and needs of each particular child. The criteria which may trigger off an investigation and the subsequent making of orders are intended to cover both situations, where the child has suffered, or is likely to suffer significant harm and the two may be linked together. Clearly, an investigation relating solely to past events is unlikely to proceed much further unless it is being linked in some way to the evidence that the harm is likely to continue (see *Re M* [1994] 2 FLR 577). It was stated very clearly in that case that a court could make a care order on the grounds that the child had been suffering significant harm at the point at which the local authority had initiated protective action in respect of the child. This case is, even now, still the leading authority on the interpretation of this aspect of the statutory threshold, and has been applied in later cases (see *Re K* [1995] 1 FLR 675). However, in *Re G* [2001] 2 FLR 111 it was stressed that this does not mean that the local authority may not rely on information obtained after the date of intervention (in this case expert assessments) nor on later events, which were capable of proving the situation that had existed at the point of the initiation of protective action.

As to looking at the likelihood of the future possibility of harm, as indicated by the words 'likely to suffer significant harm', the investigating agency, in consultation with other professionals concerned with the child, must seek to establish that there would be a greater risk to the child in leaving them in their current situation and by seeking to provide the services to ameliorate the situation or, in the worst case, by seeking the child's removal through an application for court orders. Were an application to be based on the issue of the future possibility of harm by reference to past events, then the House of Lords has determined (in *Re H and R* [1996] 1 FLR 80) that the standard of proof required of the likelihood of past events is proof on the balance of probabilities, except that where the allegation is an extremely serious one the evidence required to satisfy the court that there was a real possibility of harm to a child must be inherently more probable.

The harm suffered or apprehended must be 'significant' and, where this turns on the issue of health or development, the child's health or development will be compared with that which could reasonably be expected of a similar child (s.31(10) CA 1989). As far as the word 'significant' is concerned, *Working Together to Safeguard Children* (HM Government 2006a, para 1.25) states that:

There are no absolute criteria on which to rely when judging what constitutes significant harm. Consideration of the severity of ill-treatment may include the degree and the extent of physical harm, the duration and frequency of abuse and neglect, and the extent of premeditation, degree of threat and coercion, sadism, and bizarre or unusual elements in child sexual abuse. Each of these elements has been associated with more severe effects on the child, and/or relatively greater difficulty in helping the child overcome the adverse impact of the ill-treatment … More often, significant harm is a compilation of significant events, both acute and long-standing, which interrupt, change or damage the child's physical and psychological development. Some children live in family and social circumstances where their health and development are neglected. For them, it is the corrosiveness of long-term emotional, physical or sexual abuse that causes impairment to the extent constituting significant harm. In each case, it is necessary to consider any ill-treatment alongside the family's strength and support.

(For a fuller consideration of the concept of 'significant harm', see Adcock & White 1998 and Horwath, Chapter 13, in this volume.)

It is clear therefore that minor shortcomings in the health care provided, or minor deficits in physical, psychological or social development, should not give rise to compulsory intervention unless they are having or are likely to have serious and lasting effects upon the child. Prior to implementation of the CA 1989, the Lord Chancellor, Lord MacKay of Clashfern, also stated that: 'Unless there is evidence that a child is being, or is likely to be, positively harmed because of failure in the family, the State, whether in the guise of a local authority or a court, should not interfere' (MacKay 1990).

The comparison to be made with a similar child is not without problems, however, since one is required to compare this subjective child with that hypothetically similar child. There has been very little reported case law on the particular issue of 'the similar child' before the English courts. The issue did come up for early consideration by the court in the case of *Re O* [1992] 2 FLR 7, where Ewbank J. took a very robust view of what constituted a 'similar child'. In this particular case he was dealing with a young girl aged 15 who had been truanting from school and the issue was whether she had suffered harm compared with the hypothetically similar child. In Ewbank's view, a similar child in this case meant 'a child with equivalent intellectual and social development, who has gone to school, and not merely an average child who may or may not be at school' (p. 12). Clearly, if a child is disabled in some way, and this has affected their health and development, the investigating agency must ask itself what state of health or development could be expected of a child with a similar disability.

As to whether 'similar' involves any consideration being given to the child's background, the Lord Chancellor, at the time of debates on the Children Bill, stated that it could be suggested that background, as opposed to attributes, should be left out of account. He observed that 'the care that a parent gives to his child must be related to the circumstances attributable to that child in the sense of physical, mental and emotional characteristics' (Hansard 1989). The Department of Health, however, in its *Guidance and Regulations, Volume I – Court Orders* (DoH 1991e) states that 'account may need to be taken of environmental, social and cultural characteristics of the child' (para. 3.20). In terms of assessing whether consideration should be given to the child's cultural, religious or social background when comparing with the hypothetical similar child, there are, however, different views amongst the academic commentators. Thus, Freeman has argued that cultural pluralism ought to be relevant and that Muslim children, Rastafarian children and the children of Hasidic Jews may be different and have different needs from children brought up in the indigenous, white, nominally Christian culture (Freeman 1997, Brophy 2000, 2003, Brophy *et al.* 2003a).

On the other hand, Bainham (1993) has argued that allowances for cultural differences ought not to be made except at the welfare stage in the proceedings since, by definition, the threshold criteria set the minimally acceptable limits of behaviour towards children to be tolerated in English society and under our child protection laws. He further argues that, as such, English society has a right to expect everyone from whatever cultural background to comply and that, in any event, allowances for ethnic background take insufficient account of the widely divergent attitudes to child rearing held by the indigenous population (see also Korbin, Chapter 7, in this volume). The courts have failed to resolve this issue, although it could be argued that the decision of Wilson J. in *Re D* [1998] Fam Law 657 appears to lean more in Bainham's direction. The judge made a care order in this case in respect of a child of a Jamaican mother, who had been severely beaten with a belt suffering consequent cuts and bruises, held out of a window and threatened with eviction from the home when the mother was under stress. Wilson J. commented:

There are many real cultural differences even within ordinary white British society. Today in England and Wales we are not a collection of ghettoes but one society enjoying the benefit of the composition of very many racial and cultural groups and one society governed by one set of laws. It would concern me if the same event could give rise in one case to a finding of significant harm and in another to a finding to the contrary.

He did, however, acknowledge that 'if a child can say to himself or herself "my brothers, sisters, and friends are all treated in this way from time to time: it seems to be part of life" then that child may suffer less emotional harm than a child who perceived himself to be a unique victim'. It would therefore seem that further guidance on this issue in the context of a multicultural society is required from a more culturally mixed court.

While the child protection agencies, when investigating issues of significant harm, will obviously have to be sensitive to such racial, cultural and religious issues (see more on this in Lau 1997, and Korbin, Chapter 7, and Phillips, Chapter 8, in this volume), what the Lord Chancellor was clearly indicating himself in debates upon the Children Bill was that the agency should focus clearly on the needs of the particular child when contrasting their development with that of a similar child.

Processing the investigation further

The provisions in s.47 CA 1989 (s.47 investigations by LACSCDs are considered in detail in Bell, Chapter 15, in this volume) which go on to deal with provisions governing the investigation by LACSCDs, provide that enquiries must in particular be directed towards establishing whether an application should be made to the court or whether it should exercise any of its powers under CA 1989, which could include the provision of services pursuant to s.17 of the Act (see *Working Together* (HM Government 2006a, para. 5.44). Such alternative action may well be considered in the context of an initial child protection conference (see Bell, Chapter 15, in this volume). Section 47 provides for a range of measures to be taken to enable the LACSCD to pursue its investigation, including provisions to allow it to gain access to property in order to see the child (although it should be noted that such provisions do not authorise the local authority to gain access by force) or in terms of engaging the assistance of other agencies to help it process the investigation further.

Where the LACSCD's investigation under s.47 is impeded or frustrated in any way by the unreasonable refusal of access to the child, it should be noted that such refusal may constitute grounds for the CSA seeking an EPO (under s.44 CA 1989) or invoking the assistance of a police constable, either to exercise police powers of protection (s.46) or simply to exercise the police powers under s.17(1)(e) Police and Criminal Evidence Act 1984, which allows the police to enter any premises, if need be by force, in order to protect any person believed to be under threat to their life, limb or liberty.

It should be noted that by this stage of the investigation, as many details as possible relating to the child should have been gathered, including the child's name, address, names of parents, names of others in the household, name of the family's general practitioner (GP), details of any nursery or school that the child attends, and details of the family's or child's social worker, if there is one. The next step will be to check with both the efile and the child protection register. According to *Working Together* (HM Government 2006a, at p. xxv), child protection registers will remain in place until 2008 by which time it is hoped that local authorities will have in place the necessary IT systems to enable them to record child protection plans on all children at risk. The purpose of the efile, provided for by s.12 CA 2004, is to provide all professionals in due course with immediate electronic access to a file on any child for whom there is a unique identifying number and which will alert any of the professionals in contact with the family to any potential concerns which may be ongoing in relation to any child in the family. The purpose of the child protection conference is to record that the child is the subject of an inter-agency child protection plan and to ensure that the plans are formally reviewed every 6 months at least.

Wherever there is time, as well as checking the efile, and the child protection register where it continues, the agency involved may also check with the health visitor, school, education welfare department, the probation service, family GP, the police, the criminal records office (Bichard Inquiry Report 2004) and the NSPCC. All such checks provide essential information, but it might be that speed is of the essence and therefore action is required without being able to make all the desired enquiries.

The initial child protection conference (see paras 5.80–5.109, *Working Together to Safeguard Children*)

It may therefore be the case that while the next step in a non-urgent situation would be discussions within an initial child protection conference setting, such discussions may actually have to be postponed until after the taking of emergency action. In a non-emergency situation, where there is felt to be a risk of harm that has not yet materialised, there may well be ongoing work within the family which has identified a looming crisis. In such circumstances, it may be possible to convene an initial child protection conference with all the relevant personnel. An opportunity is thus provided for giving measured consideration to taking further legal steps, such as obtaining a child assessment order (s.43 CA 1989, hereinafter CAO) or the institution of proceedings for an ICO or ISO (see s.31 and s.38 CA 1989). (For a fuller discussion on the substance of child protection conferences, see *Working Together* (HM Government 2006a, paras 5.80–5.135) and see also Bell, Chapter 15, in this volume.)

Where more measured consideration is possible, the initial child protection conference may have recommended that it is more appropriate to engage in informal social work involvement with the family, together with the provision of additional services from a range of other agencies. The provision of such services is made possible by s.17 CA 1989; if services from other agencies are to be provided, this may require the invoking of s.27 CA 1989. Under s.27 and its comparable provisions, a LACSCD may request the help of one or more other agencies, including health and housing, in performing duties to provide services under the relevant provisions of the Act, and those agencies must comply with such a request unless they can prove that it is not compatible with their own statutory or other duties, or it unduly prejudices the discharge of any of their functions. The recommendation to provide services, and the monitoring of the provision of such services in terms of the effects on the family, does, of course, leave open the option of taking more formal legal action through the institution of proceedings for a care or supervision order if and when this might be required.

Making the child the subject of a written child protection plan

As will be seen in Chapters 12, 13 and 15, it should be noted that the initial child protection conference's decision-making power includes devising a child protection plan (HM Government 2006a, paras 5.102–5.109) and the allocation of a key worker (HM Government 2006a, para. 5.108). The key worker must be a worker from one of the child care agencies with statutory powers – either the LACSCD or, less usually, the NSPCC (para. 5.108) (see Horwath, Chapter 13, and Bell, Chapter 15, in this volume, where these matters are considered in detail). The plan must be in writing and is, of course, dependent upon the full core assessment of the child and the family having been undertaken in accordance with the *CAF* and the *Assessment Framework* described in detail in Chapter 13. *Working Together* states that the child protection plan should conform to the exemplar for the child protection plan (DoH 2002a), also examined in detail at Chapter 13. The plan can then be revisited at subsequent child protection review meetings or conferences.

It must be noted, however, in relation to all these types of meetings that parents, other carers and the child, where old enough, must be invited to attend and enabled to participate properly and thoroughly in such meetings by being given the appropriate information and evidence which may be discussed at such meetings. To do otherwise could amount to a breach of the parent's or child's rights under Articles 6 and 8 ECHR, as seen in the case of *Re L* [2002] 2 FLR 730. Munby J., in the English courts, examined the linkage between Articles 6 and 8 and in this case found breaches of both because a mother had not been invited by the local authority to be present at a whole series of crucial meetings, had not been given crucial documents and had not been communicated with properly by the authority's key worker in the case.

Nevertheless, despite all the best endeavours of those involved at the initial child protection conference where a child protection plan has been drawn up, or in those situations where the recommendation was merely more informal social work involvement and the provision of services, things can go wrong and emergencies may intervene. Thus consideration may have to be given to a more formal legal approach by invoking the provisions relating to ICO or ISO proceedings, applications for CAOs or, in more urgent situations, the invoking of the emergency powers relating to EPOs.

The invoking of formal legal proceedings in relation to the issue of child protection is not an easy issue for the relevant government department seeking to provide guidance. Whilst guidance in relation to the use of court orders has been issued, further consideration now needs to be given to the impact upon the relevant processes of the implementation of the ECHR brought about by the Human Rights Act 1998 (see above). Social work practitioners must therefore bear in mind not only the messages to be derived from the Department of Health's own publication, *Child Protection: Messages from Research* (DoH 1995a), and subsequent research, but also the overriding imperatives prescribed by the legislation and Article 8(2) of the Convention that one must act to protect and safeguard the child's health.

Emergency action

Applications for emergency protection orders

Where, therefore, there is reasonable cause to believe that a child is likely to suffer significant harm if either the child is not removed to accommodation provided by or on behalf of the applicant, or does not remain in a place in which they are then being accommodated, *any person* may make an application for what is termed under the CA 1989 s.44 an 'emergency protection order' (EPO). Such an application may be made by any person pursuant to s.44(1)(a) CA 1989, and may be made without notice and without the other parties being present to a single magistrate. Such without-notice applications for EPOs may also be made by any of the relevant child protection agencies using s.44(1)(a). (For interesting accounts of the use that is being made of EPOs by different authorities around the country, and that many more applications are made each year than the official statistics reveal, see the work of Masson & Winn Oakley (2004) and Masson (2005).)

Local authorities and the NSPCC in England are given additional rights to apply for orders under s.44 in case of emergencies. Thus, in the case of an application made by a local authority, s.44(1)(b) provides that where enquiries are being made with respect to the child in pursuance of an investigation, and those enquiries are being frustrated by access to the child unreasonably refused to a person authorised to seek access, and the applicant's social worker has reasonable cause to believe that access to the child is required as a matter of urgency, the court may make an EPO authorising the removal of the child to accommodation provided by social services, or the child's detention in the place in which they are being accommodated, such as, for example, a hospital. Almost identical provision is made with respect to officers employed by the NSPCC (see s.44(1)(c)).

Care must again be taken in relation to the use of emergency powers that there is justification for using such an approach and that in taking such steps the authority is not acting in breach of the parent's or child's rights to private and family life under Article 8 ECHR. In addition, the court must also ensure that it is not adding to such potential breaches by being overly assertive in pressing on with a case where the parent is asking for more time to instruct legal representation, thus itself acting in breach of Article 6 the right to a fair trial. Both these points are illustrated by the case of *Re P, C and S v UK* [2002] 2 FLR 631 (considered above in the section on Human Rights and where use of an EPO in the precise circumstances of that case was held to have been a breach of the parents' rights under Articles 6 and 8, although the court did concede that there would be circumstances where no notice would be appropriate where necessary to safeguard the child's health and her rights). Details regarding the duration of EPOs, conditions which may be attached to them, and provisions regarding applications to be made for discharge of the orders, are provided in s.44 and s.45 CA 1989.

It should be noted that the general principles governing the making of decisions by the courts concerning the upbringing or welfare of children also apply to the making of EPOs (see s.1(1) CA 1989). Thus, the courts' primary consideration has to be the welfare of the child, although the court is not required to have regard to the welfare checklist provided in s.1(3) CA 1989 as this is not applicable to EPOs (s.1(4) CA 1989). It should be pointed out, however, that no court should make an order under the Act unless it considers that doing so would be better for the child than making no order at all (s.1(5) CA 1989 – termed by the author the 'positive advantage' principle). It must be remembered that, in addition to obtaining an EPO and the additional powers concerning warrants obtainable under the Act, the legislation contains the power for the applicant to ask for exclusion requirements to be linked to EPOs, as described in more detail above.

As has been noted, EPOs may be made without notice. Although the previous *Working Together* guidance stated that whilst the court has power to direct a hearing where all the parties are present, 'the very fact that the situation is considered to be an emergency requiring immediate action will make this inappropriate or impracticable in most cases' (DoH 1999b, para. 4.46). No such guidance on the legal process is contained in the new version, however (see *Working Together*, HM Government 2006a). Generally, such applications will be made in the magistrates' family proceedings court and there is no provision for a hearing to take place in any of the higher courts. Since these orders are specifically to deal with emergencies, in many cases applications may have to be made to a single magistrate because such emergencies generally arise when the courts are not sitting, such as at night or over the weekend. The previous guidance stated that, 'in certain situations, giving parents notice of the application might be to place the child in great danger' (DoH 1999b, para. 4.36), although this advice is not repeated in the 2006 document. Where, as is generally the case, such applications are heard without notice, the rules demand that the applicant serve a notice of the application and a copy of the order within 48 hours on the parties to the proceedings (usually the parents), anyone else with the care of the child, and the local authority where it is not the applicant. The rules stress the critical requirement of informing parents of their rights and responsibilities under the order and clearly spell out such conditions as to medical, psychiatric or other assessment as may have been provided for in the directions accompanying the order. It should be noted that the various provisions providing for EPOs, and their duration without right of appeal for 72 hours, potentially breach Article 6 of the European Convention, which guarantees the right to a fair hearing by a court when it is determining anyone's civil rights and obligations (see *X Council v B and Others* [2004] EWHC 2015 Fam.). Since the granting of EPOs and their duration crucially affect the enjoyment of the parents' rights and exercise of their obligations towards their child(ren), it may be argued that these provisions breach the requirements of the Convention.

Practitioners should ensure, wherever possible, that they identify the child who is to be made the subject of an EPO but s.44(14) does provide that, where this is not possible, the applicant should nevertheless provide such identifying information as will enable the lawful execution of the order. Finally, it should be noted that there is no appeal to a High Court judge against the magistrates' refusal to grant an EPO. If the magistrates have not been satisfied as to the grounds required to the issuing of an EPO, there is no appeal against this decision, which was confirmed in the case of *Essex County Council v F* [1992] Family Law 569.

Police powers

In addition to the provisions for any person or LACSCD or the NSPCC in England being able to seek court orders authorising the removal or detention of a child from or in a specified place, the Act also provides the police with the ability to exercise police powers of protection without resort to the courts. These powers are exercisable by any police officer under the provisions of s.46 in England and Wales. In England, Wales and Northern Ireland, the police powers may be exercised for up to 72 hours – see s.46(6) CA 1989, Borkowski (1995) and work done by Masson and Winn Oakley (2004). These powers confer upon the police a very wide power to remove children from dangerous situations in which they might find them on being called out to cases involving domestic violence, disturbance or in response to any other information being laid before them. The police further have a role in assisting with the execution of EPOs, where the applicant feels that it is necessary to obtain a warrant to be able to enter the premises on which a child might be, if need be by force (see s.48(9) CA 1989).

Acting on suspicions that the child is suffering or is likely to suffer significant harm

Where there are merely concerns or suspicions that a child is suffering or is likely to suffer significant harm, the local authority in all the jurisdictions and the NSPCC in England may seek an order, usually from a Family Proceedings Court in England and Wales, for a CAO (see above). In the circumstances of *X Council v B and Others* (above) Munby J. considered that a CAO would have been more appropriate than the use of a without-notice EPO. Before granting a CAO, however, the court must be satisfied on the balance of probabilities that the applicant has reasonable cause to suspect that:

1. the child is suffering or is likely to suffer significant harm
2. an assessment of the child's state of health or development or the way in which they have been treated is required to enable the applicant to determine whether or not the child is suffering or is likely to suffer significant harm

3.   it is unlikely that such an assessment will be made, or be satisfactory, in the absence of a CAO.

Since an application for such an order is likely to be a planned response to concerns, the various court rules provide that the application must be made on notice and this underlines the fact that the order should not be made in emergencies (see the Family Proceedings Court (CA 1989) Rules 1991, r.4(1)). The CAO must specify the date by which the assessment is to begin and can nominate the person who is to do the assessment. Practitioners should be advised that this is really the best way of proceeding since it would be acutely problematic if the person so nominated subsequently refused: it is suggested therefore that prior consent from the person conducting the assessment is sought. Finally, the order can have effect for such period not exceeding 7 days beginning with the date specified in the order. It should be noted that the general principles governing the making of decisions by the court concerning the upbringing or welfare of children also apply to the making of child assessment orders (s.1(1) and (5) but not s.1(3) or (4) – see above).

Concerns about children in other situations

It should, of course, be pointed out that where suspicions of abuse arise in certain other situations, the LACSCD may have the power simply to remove the child rather than being required to go to court to obtain an order to do so. This would be the case where the child is being 'accommodated', pursuant to s.20 CA 1989 or pursuant to a CO made under s.31 CA 1989, and concerns about the child have developed as a result of the child's care in a particular children's home or other residential placement, or where the child is being cared for by foster parents (see also s.25 CA 1989).

Applications for care or supervision orders

Where concern over actual or potential significant harm to a child has not escalated suddenly, resulting in the need for an EPO, consideration should be given instead to initiating CO or SO proceedings by way of issuing an application for such an order in the family proceedings court. Such action may also be taken following on from an EPO, the exercise of police powers of protection, the result of a s.37 investigation, or the obtaining of evidence pursuant to an assessment done under the provisions of a CAO, and in each case where LACSCDs have then determined that these initial orders must be followed up by longer-term protective orders such as COs or SOs in England and Wales.

Preliminary hearings or other issues to be determined at the first interim care or supervision order hearing

Before the issuing of an interim order, or the hearing of such, the court may, pursuant to s.32 CA 1989 and the Protocol for Judicial Case Management (Step 3, para 3.4, and see crucially Lane, Chapter 18, in this volume), hold a preliminary hearing to determine the correct forum for the case (i.e. which court would be best to hear the case), who are to be made parties, and the appointment of a children's guardian (under s.41, and see Head, Chapter 19, in this volume). Legal Aid is automatically available for the child, who will be represented by their own solicitor as well as by a children's guardian (see Chapter 19), and for the child's parents or the person having the care of the child at the time of the initiation of the proceedings. Solicitors representing children are drawn from the Children's Panel, a specialist panel instituted by the Law Society comprising solicitors who are deemed to be properly qualified to represent children in care proceedings. This unique system for the dual representation of the child in care or supervision order proceedings (by a solicitor representing what the child wants, where the child is capable of giving such instructions, and of the children's guardian representing the child's best interests) was considerably strengthened by the provisions in the CA 1989 and the relevant rules of court made thereunder (see Munby 2004).

Practitioners should note that an application for a CO or SO will not result in the making of one or the other orders at the first time of application. It is most unlikely that a court at the first hearing would ever be able to be satisfied of the various threshold criteria laid down in s.31, and then of the demands in s.1(5) CA 1989, as to be able, immediately, to make a CO or SO. This is why, of course, s.38 CA 1989 in England and Wales provides for the making of ICOs or ISOs. It must be stressed, however, that where a LACSCD makes an application for an ICO or ISO as their first application in proceedings for COs and SOs, these will not be the only orders available to the court because s.38(3) CA 1989 also provides that the court may make a residence order, although if it does so it must also make an ISO with respect to the child unless satisfied that the child's welfare will be satisfactorily safeguarded without an interim order being made. As the old *Working Together* guidance stated (DoH 1991e, para. 3.35), 'the two main objectives of these powers are to enable the child to be suitably protected whilst proceedings are progressing where this is required, and to see that interim measures operate only for so long as necessary'.

It should also be noted that ICOs and ISOs may be made either following a s.37 direction by the court to a LACSCD to investigate the child's circumstances, or indeed at any stage where it is felt that further investigation or assessment of the child by the LACSCD is required and that more time is needed. It is provided in the Act that an interim order made on the date of first application for a CO or SO shall cease to have effect on the expiry of the period of 8 weeks beginning with the date on which the order is made. If second or subsequent interim orders have to be made, in order to allow for further investigation on behalf of any of the parties, such orders can only last for periods of up to 4 weeks at a time. At the expiry of each of the relevant dates, a further application for a new ICO or ISO has to be made and the courts again have to continue to be satisfied of the threshold criteria laid down in s.31(2) CA 1989. The threshold criteria that have to be satisfied before the court can make ICOs or ISOs are the same as those required for the making of a full CO or SO under the provisions of s.31(1); the only difference is that where the court is looking to make an ICO or ISO it cannot do so 'unless it is satisfied that there are *reasonable grounds* for believing that the circumstances with respect to the child are as mentioned in s.31(2)'. In addition, it should be remembered that the requirements of both s.1(3) and s.1(5) CA 1989 must be observed. The fact that both these requirements have to be observed, in addition to the welfare paramountcy principle in s.1(1) CA 1989, is laid down in s.1(4), as the making of an ICO or ISO is an order under Part IV of the Children Act 1989 and is thus incorporated as being 'the circumstances' mentioned in subsection (4) in the opening words of s.1(3) CA 1989.

ICOs and ISOs are therefore similar to full COs or SOs in that the welfare checklist *does* apply to such orders whereas, as was noted earlier, the welfare checklist does not apply to any applications being made to the court for EPOs or other protection orders such as CAOs.

The 'threshold criteria'

It must be remembered that before the court can make an ICO or ISO, it has to be satisfied that there are reasonable grounds for believing that the circumstances with respect to the child are as mentioned in s.31(2). In addition, of course, a court can only make a CO or SO under the provisions of s.31(1) CA 1989 if it is satisfied of the so-called 'threshold criteria'. Providing practitioners keep in mind that, under the requirements for ICOs and ISOs, one simply has to establish that there are 'reasonable grounds for believing that the circumstances with respect to the child are as mentioned in s.31(2)', then there should be no difficulty in obtaining an interim order if one so satisfies the court. To establish what exactly is required it is necessary to look at the terms of s.31(2) CA 1989 which provides that 'a court may only make a CO or SO if it is satisfied:

(a) that the child concerned is suffering, or is likely to suffer significant harm; and

(b) that the harm, or the likelihood of harm is attributable to:

   (i) the care given to the child, or likely to be given to him if the order were not made, not being what it would be reasonable to expect a parent to give to him; or

   (ii) the child's being beyond parental control'.

There are therefore a number of different constituent elements contained within the so-called 'threshold criteria'. The first element of this (as already discussed) is that the child at the centre of the proceedings 'is suffering or is likely to suffer significant harm'. The issue of the standard of proof required, since care proceedings are civil proceedings, is therefore proof on the balance of probabilities, with stronger evidence being required in respect of more serious allegations as required by the case of *Re H and R* [1996] 1 FLR 80 and the approach of Lord Nicholls in that case has since been confirmed as the correct one by the Court of Appeal in *Re U* [2004] 2 FLR 263 as a result of cases coming before the courts following the decision in *R v Cannings* [2004] 1 FCR 193 (see above, and the website in relation to the debate on *Re H and R*). It has to be remembered, of course, that in applications for ICOs or ISOs, all that has to be proved at this stage, as contrasted with that which must be proved at the final hearing of the application for the CO or SO, is that the person making the application for the interim orders has 'reasonable grounds' for believing that the circumstances with respect to the child are as mentioned in s.31(2) and s.38(2) CA 1989.

Having therefore established that the applicant has reasonable grounds for believing that the child is suffering or is likely to suffer significant harm, then one must go on to establish that the harm or likelihood of harm is attributable to the care given to the child or likely to be given to the child if the order were not made, not being what it would be reasonable to expect a parent to give to the child, or that the child is beyond parental control. In looking at the issue of the care being given to the child, many academics have argued that this first alternative of the second limb has always posited a standard of care rather than that it was the care in every case to be given to the child by a parent. In other words, one was talking about an objective standard of parental-type care which one would expect a parent to ensure that the child received, rather than that the limb was focusing on care which could only be given by a parent or parents. Others, however, had argued that this first alternative in the second limb of the threshold criteria was focusing exclusively on the fact that the care given to the child was not that which would be reasonably expected to be given by the child's parents themselves.

This issue came up for consideration ultimately by the House of Lords in *Lancashire County Council* v *B* [2000] 1 FLR 583, where it was determined that the phrase 'care given to the child' referred primarily to the care given by a parent or parents, or other primary care givers, but where, as in this case, care was shared, the phrase could be taken to include the care given by any of the caregivers. Their Lordships found that this interpretation was necessary to allow the court to intervene to protect a child who was clearly at risk, even though it was not possible to identify the source of the risk. Their Lordships emphasised that it by no means followed that because the threshold conditions had been satisfied, the court would go on to make a CO, and when considering cases of this type, judges should keep firmly in mind, in the exercise of their discretionary powers, that the parents had not been shown to be responsible for the child's injuries. The steps taken in this case had been those reasonably necessary to pursue the legitimate aim of protecting the child from further injury, which was an exception to the guarantee for respect for family life contained within Article 8(1) of the European Convention, as provided for in Article 8(2). Nevertheless, the court upheld the making of the CO in respect of the child as being the only way to guarantee the protection of the child. Similarly, in the cases of *Re O and N and Re B* [2003] 1 FLR 1169, the House of Lords held that where a child suffered significant harm but the court was unable to identify which parent had been the perpetrator, or indeed whether both had been, then the court should proceed at the welfare stage on the footing that each of the parents was a possible perpetrator and then, in the light of that, determine whether a CO was better for the child than making no order at all.

The second alternative to the second limb of the threshold criteria is that the harm or risk to the child is attributable to 'the child's being beyond parental control' (see s.31(2)(b)(ii)). Again, there have been remarkably few reported cases on this particular alternative. Nevertheless, in *M* v *Birmingham City Council* [1994] 2 FLR 141, a 'wayward, uncontrollable, disturbed and periodically violent' teenager, who had originally been accommodated by the local authority under s.20, was made the subject of a care order by the court, despite her mother's evidence that she could in reality control the child. On the evidence of the teenager's own behaviour, the court was unable to agree with the mother and found that the child was beyond the parents' control and therefore not likely to receive the requisite degree of care necessary to prevent her having suffered, continuing to suffer and being likely to suffer significant harm. Stuart-White J. indicated that s.31(2)(b)(ii) might apply to a state of affairs which may be in the past, present or future. In *M* the teenager concerned was in local authority accommodation but the courts nevertheless held that the child was beyond the parental control of both mother and partner and thus it has been argued that the reference to 'parental' control is wide enough to include non-parents caring for a child, at least where they have parental responsibility.

It should also be said that it is possible, although certainly not necessary, for both the alternatives of the second limb to be satisfied at the same time. In the case of *Re O* [1992] 2 FLR 7 (and see above), Ewbank J. indicated that the situation of the child not attending school in the circumstances of that case established *either* a lack of reasonable parental care *or* the child being beyond parental control, as required for each of the alternative limbs to be satisfied.

In addition to satisfying the court that there are reasonable grounds to believe that the threshold criteria laid down in s.31(2) of CA 1989 are satisfied, the applicant for an ICO or ISO is further required to satisfy the court that making an order is better for the child than making no order at all – the 'positive advantage' principle provided by s.1(5) – and that the court has had regard to the welfare checklist laid down in s.1(3). Moreover, as well as satisfying all the requirements of s.31(2) and s.38(1)(2)(3), social workers applying for ISOs would be well advised to read the further conditions laid down in the remaining provisions of s.38. It has already been stated that the first ICO or ISO can last for a period of anything up to 8 weeks but that second or subsequent orders can only last for a period of 4 weeks at a time. Where the court makes an ICO or ISO, it is also able to give such directions (if any) as it considers appropriate with regard to the medical or psychiatric examination or other assessment of the child; however, the legislation further provides that if the child is of sufficient understanding to make an informed decision, they may refuse to submit to the examination or other assessment (s.38(6)).

In the first case on this point under the section where an interim care order had been made, and a 15-year-old girl had refused to comply with the direction as to psychiatric assessment made upon her, and indeed refused to emerge from the bedroom in which she had barricaded herself for several months, the local authority instead resorted to the inherent jurisdiction of the High Court under s.100 CA 1989. Douglas Brown J. in *South Glamorgan County Council v W and B* [1993] 1 FLR 574 ruled that the High Court, under its inherent jurisdiction, had the power to override the child's right to object granted by Parliament in the statute and contained in the provisions of s.38(6). This is, of course, the point at which children's rights to their own autonomy collide with children's interests in being protected (see Lyon 1994). From the point of view of the social work practitioner, therefore, if such a direction has been obtained, either in an EPO (see s.44(6) and (7)) or in a CAO (see s.43(7) and (8) or in s.38(6)), then if the practitioner believes that the child's greater protection demands their wishes being overruled, resort will have to be made to the High Court under the provisions of s.100 CA 1989 in order to enable the Court's inherent jurisdiction to be invoked and the child's wishes overruled.

It should also be noted that, in relation to ICOs and ISOs, the court can also include a direction that there is to be no medical or psychiatric examination or assessment, or that there should be no such examination or assessment unless the court directs otherwise. These provisions are clearly intended to enable the court to retain control of the situation and to ensure that no unauthorised medical examinations or assessments are performed on a child without the protection conferred by the provisions of s.38.

It would appear to be the case that the courts have been fairly insistent that interim orders, instead of final care orders, should always be used if important evidence remains outstanding or unresolved; for example, where assessments of the child are still being made under the provisions of s.38(6) and their outcome is awaited, and most especially where such assessment will assist the court in reaching its final decision as in the case of *Re C* [1997] AC 489. The House of Lords' ruling in this case confirmed that where the court deems that any assessment, whether medical, psychiatric or otherwise, is necessary to enable it to reach a final decision, then the local authority will have to comply with the orders and directions issued by the court, regardless of the costs that may be incurred. In the critically important case of *Re G* [2006] 2 FLR 67, the House of Lords has re-emphasised the point made in *Re C* above that such assessment must solely be for the purpose of obtaining information to enable the court to reach a conclusion on the case. Thus, they stated that what is directed under s.38(6) must clearly be an examination or assessment of the child, including where appropriate the child's relationship with her parents, the risk her parents may pose to her and the ways in which those risks may be avoided or managed, all with a view to enabling the court to make the decisions which it has to make under the Act with a minimum of delay. The House of Lords in *Re G* went on to stress that any services which are provided for the child and his family must be ancillary to that end and must not be an end in themselves and thus the provisions of s.38(6) cannot be used to ensure the provision of services either to the child or his family. Whilst Kennedy R (2001) has put forward the view that maintaining a distinction between two necessary aspects of clinical intervention – namely information gathering, which as a matter of law can be funded, and treatment, which as a matter of law cannot be funded – is bizarre, the House of Lords in *Re G* has categorically determined that s.38(6) cannot be used to provide services which the clinician identifies as being crucial to effect a change in the family.

The hearing for a final care or supervision order

It had been hoped that with the passing of the CA 1989 in England and Wales, delay in civil child protection proceedings would be a thing of the past. As the years went on, however, delay became an ever more serious problem, with public law cases on average taking at least as long as they used to pre-implementation of the Children Act and in some cases longer. In both *Avoiding Delay in Children Act Cases* (Booth 1996) and, very importantly, in the Lord Chancellor's Department's *Scoping Study* in 2002 (LCD 2002), the causes for delay were identified and it was recognised that most cases were taking at least a year. Consequently, the *Protocol for Judicial Management in Public Law Children Act Cases* was drawn up and issued in 2003 ([2003] 2 FLR 719). This provides that care cases must generally take no longer than 40 weeks to reach a conclusion and lays down strict timetables to be observed by all litigants in such cases (for more detail, see Chapter 19).

Once all the investigations and the medical, psychiatric or other assessments have been completed, the local authority has filed its care plan and the children's guardian has completed their report in respect of the child, the court will be ready to proceed to the final hearing of the application for a CO or SO. The standard of proof required at the final hearing goes beyond that which has been required thus far for the issuing of CAOs, EPOs, ICO or ISOs. By s.31(2), the court may only make a CO or SO if it is satisfied *on the balance of probabilities* that the child concerned is suffering or is likely to suffer significant harm, and that the harm, or likelihood of harm, is attributable to:

(i)   the care given to the child, or likely to be given to him if the order were not made, not being what it would be reasonable to expect a parent to give to him; or

(ii) the child being beyond parental control.

The requisite standard of proof has already been discussed in relation to the various limbs of s.31(2), as has the issue of the comparison of a child's health or development with that which can reasonably be expected of a similar child (see above). Once the court is satisfied that the relevant limbs of s.31(2) have been established, the court must then go on to consider which order, if any, it should make. Thus, once the threshold criteria have been established, there is yet another stage for the court, sometimes described as 'the welfare stage', which requires the court to determine which order it should make based on what is in the best interests of the child. Thus, it is only where the constituent elements of s.31(2) have been proved that the court will be able to consider whether or not a CO or SO is the most appropriate course of action or whether indeed it should support the making of other private law orders such as a residence order.

Consideration must be given to the possibility of other orders since, pursuant to the Human Rights legislation, the courts have determined in *Re B* [2003] 2 FLR 813 that there is a vital judicial task to be performed between finding the threshold criteria crossed and endorsing the making of a care order. Thus, the Court of Appeal stated in that case that where the application was for a care order empowering the local authority to remove a child from the family, the judge could not make such an order without considering the rights of the adult members of the family and of the children of the family under Article 8 ECHR. Thus the court could not sanction such an interference with family life unless it was satisfied that it was both necessary and proportionate and that no less radical form of order would achieve the essential end of promoting the welfare of the children.

In order to assist the court in determining whether and which order to make, various parts of s.1 CA 1989 are held to be relevant to the court's determinations, thus:

- s.1(1) CA 1989 provides that when a court determines any question with respect to the upbringing of a child, then the child's welfare shall be the court's paramount consideration
- s.1(4) provides that where the court is considering whether to make care or supervision orders, it must apply the provisions of s.1(3), the welfare checklist
- where the court is considering whether or not to make one or more orders under the Act with respect to a child, then s.1(5) applies, which provides that the court shall not make the order, or any of the orders, unless it considers that doing so would be better for the child than making no order at all (the 'positive advantage' principle).

As well as being bound by these various principles of s.1 CA 1989, the court will also have before it the report of the children's guardian reviewing the history of the child's case and making recommendations to the court based on the investigation and interviews with all the parties concerned including the child, where the child is old enough to put forward any views. Consideration of the guardian's report will enable the court to make a better informed choice as to which order, if any, it should consider making. In addition, however, it should also have before it the LACSCD's care plan. The submission of this to the court is now required under the provisions of s.31A CA 1989 (as inserted by ACA 2002). (With regard to the required date of submission, see paragraphs 51–53 of the *Protocol for Judicial Case Management in Public Law Children Act Cases* ([2003] 2 FLR 719) considered in detail in Chapter 19.) As to the format of the plan, regard must be paid to the guidance now contained in LAC (99)29 entitled *Care Plans and Care Proceedings under the Children Act 1989* applicable to England (DoH 1999b; on the issue of concurrent planning, careful consideration should be given to Wall 1999), and in NAFWC 1/ 2000 for Wales. Appendix F of the *Protocol* makes it clear that both interim and full care plans must be provided to the court in compliance with the demands of these documents (see Chapter 19).

In its Final Report in 1997, the Children Act Advisory Committee (Children Act Advisory Committee 1997) drew attention to the problems faced by some local authorities in drawing up care plans where the satisfaction of the threshold criteria depended on proof of specific facts, such as 'had a child been sexually abused or non-accidentally injured and, if so, by whom?' As has been pointed out, there might have been no prior history of inadequate parenting or social services involvement; however, until those questions could be answered, a care plan could not sensibly be made and that might lead to unacceptable delays in the proceedings. The solutions suggested by the Committee, approved by Bracewell J. in *Re S* [1996] 2 FLR 773 and adopted in the *Protocol,* is that there should effectively be a 'split hearing': the first hearing – now referred to in the *Protocol* as the Preliminary Hearing or a 'substantial fact finding hearing' (para. 6.1 *Protocol* and see above) – should be held to determine whether the threshold criteria are met by proof of the relevant facts; and then, once the criteria had been proved, the Final Hearing – which must be by the same judge who has heard the preliminary hearing – should be held to consider the care plan and the relevant various reports and to decide what order, if any, should be made. In the case of *Re CD and MD* [1998] 1 FLR 825, the court criticised the local authority for its delay in seeking a CO and for not applying at a much earlier stage for a split hearing in relation to the issues.

At this second 'welfare stage', therefore, once the court has had an opportunity to read the guardian's report and any other expert report which might be before it, it must then determine whether or not the making of an order is better for the child than making no order at all (the so-called 'positive advantage' principle). (For a detailed consideration of the two-stage process, including the issue as to the benefits to the child of the making of an order, see the judgement of Booth J. in *Humberside County Council* v B [1993] 1 FLR 257.) The court may be of the opinion, perhaps as a result of the guardian's report or consideration of the care plan, that the making of a CO or even a SO would actually be the wrong order to make: the provision of s.1(4) CA 1989 enables the court to decide whether to make one of a range of orders which are available under the CA 1989, including the making, where relevant, of any of the s.8 orders which could be made in conjunction with a SO. (The orders available under s.8 CA 1989 include a residence order, a contact order, a specific issues order and a prohibited steps order; the provisions of s.8 should be consulted for the precise scope of these orders.)

Any of the s.8 orders can be made, however, in conjunction with a SO. Thus, for example, the LACSCD may have applied for a CO in respect of a child but the guardian's report may recommend the making of a residence order in favour of grandparents or other relatives, and the making of other s.8 orders in respect of the parents, such as a contact order in favour of the mother and a prohibited steps order in respect of the father. Where the LACSCD or the court considers that contact should be supervised in any way, potentially this can be achieved by the making of a s.16 family assistance order (see the comments of Booth J. in *Leeds City Council* v C [1993] 1 FLR 269). In order to determine that any order which the court makes is in the paramount interests of the child (see s.1(1) CA 1989), the court is required to consider the terms of the welfare checklist set out in s.1(3) CA 1989. These provisions set out for the court a very extensive checklist relating both to the background and the circumstances of the individual child, as well as to the capability of any persons who might be seeking orders in respect of the child or in relation to whom the court is considering making any one of the orders available under the Acts. Where the court is proposing to make a care order, the LACSCD should, under the provisions of s.34(11) CA 1989, further submit to the court the arrangements which are being proposed for the child to have contact with members of their family. Where the court is proposing that there should be no contact, or the family or child do not agree with the arrangements being proposed, an application will have to be made to the court to determine issues of contact under the provision of s.34 CA 1989 (for further information, see Lyon 2003, Chapter 10). Section 34(1) CA 1989 broke new ground by creating, for the first time, a presumption of reasonable contact with a child in care, which was emphasised in the cases of *Re B* [1993] Fam. 301 at 311, *Re E* [1994] 1 FLR 146, *Berkshire County Council* v B [1997] 1 FLR 171 and *Re T* [1997] 1 All ER 65. It should also be noted that the effects of the decisions of the European Court of Human Rights in *K and T* v *Finland* [2000] 2 FLR 79 and *S and G* v *Italy* [2000] 2 FLR 771 make it more difficult for the local authority to provide justification for decisions which would limit or terminate contact between the child and his parents than would justify the initial decision to remove the child from his parents' care.

Where, in a final hearing for a CO or SO, the court has determined that one or the other order should be made, despite the availability of other orders under s.8, then the provisions of ss.31–33, s.35 and Schedule 3 would have to be consulted in detail. These provide respectively for the effects of the making of a care order or a supervision order and, in the provisions of Schedule 3, the additional conditions which may be attached to a supervision order.

Additional protection available through the courts

Whereas in most situations the making of a CO or SO will be sufficient to guarantee the long-term protection of the child who has suffered, or is at risk of suffering, significant harm, there may be situations in which the LACSCD will need additional protection for the child, or specific guidance in relation to some aspects of the care of the child. Where this is necessary, and where it is not possible by any other means (including the use of the provisions of CA 1989) to acquire such protection, the LACSCD may have to seek to invoke the inherent jurisdiction of the High Court to obtain the relevant orders (see s.100 CA 1989).

A LACSCD, which has a child in its care pursuant to a CO under s.31, is unable to use or benefit from the provisions of s.8 providing for the issuing of a prohibited steps order or a specific issues order (see s.9(1) CA 1989). Instead, the LACSCD would have to apply to the High Court to be given leave to make an application for an order providing relevant protection under s.100 CA 1989. The High Court in each jurisdiction may only grant leave where it is satisfied that the result the LACSCD wishes to achieve could not be achieved through the making of any other order under the provisions of the CA 1989 and there is reasonable cause to believe that if the court's inherent jurisdiction is not exercised with respect to the child, the child is likely to suffer significant harm (s.100(4) CA 1989). The situations in which the High Court's inherent jurisdiction may be invoked by the LACSCD include those situations where an injunction is required to prevent an abusing parent or child from going near or having contact with the child who has been made the subject of a CO and is in need of protection, as was the case in *Re S* [1994] 1 FLR 623. It may also be invoked where a medical procedure is required in respect of the child, the child's parents are refusing to give consent, and the relevant health authority or trust is concerned about accepting the consent provided by the local authority holding the CO, even though they are legitimately able to give it by virtue of the fact that making the CO has conferred parental responsibility on them under s.33(3) CA 1989 (for further detail on this, see Lyon 2003).

Appeals

Appeals in care and contact order proceedings are dealt with in full in the Chapter on the website.

Protecting children in care

In order to cater for a large number of difficult situations with regard to the standard of care exercised in respect of children being looked after by a LACSCD, whether pursuant to a CO or to s.20, the CA 1989 provides for a system of review of cases to enable the child's voice to be heard (see s.26(1)(2) CA 1989 as amended by ACA 2002). In order further to protect the child, as a result of the amendments made by ACA 2002, the CA 1989 now provides that:

- the child's care plan must be considered at every review
- there should be such a plan for all looked-after children
- an independent reviewing officer should chair the review
- where they consider it necessary, the child's case can be referred to a children's guardian to determine whether or not the case should be referred to the courts (see s.26(2)(e)(f) and (k); for further details, see Lyon 2005).

Where a child is complaining about harm occurring in a residential home provided by the LACSCD, a home provided by a voluntary organisation or a foster home, then *Working Together to Safeguard Children* (HM Government 2006a, paras 9.3, 11.5 and 11.25) advises that LACSCDs must take such complaints seriously and investigate in the same way that they would complaints about abuse occurring within the family setting (see Butler, Chapter 10, in this volume). *Working Together to Safeguard Children* (HM Government 2006a) states that 'experiences show that children can be subjected to abuse by those who work with them in any and every setting'. It goes on to point out that 'all allegations of abuse of children by a professional, staff member, foster carer or volunteer (from LSCB member agencies) should therefore be taken seriously and treated in accordance with local child protection procedures ... It is essential that all allegations are examined objectively by staff who are independent of the service, organisation or institution concerned' (HM Government 2006a, para. 11.5).

Both the system of reviews and the representations procedure (established by LACSCDs under s.26(3) CA 1989 and the new Children Act 1989 Representations Procedure Regulations 2006) are intended to ensure that children's complaints could properly be brought to the surface, particularly in the wake of residential child care scandals such as Leicestershire, Ty Mawr, Castle Hill, St Charles, Melanie Klein and Kincora. Although those scandals had surfaced prior to the implementation of the Children Act 1989 in England and Wales in October 1991, unfortunately, further residential child care scandals have emerged even since the implementation of the supposed protective procedures (see also Butler, Chapter 10, in this volume). The Utting Report (Utting *et al.* 1997) and the Waterhouse Report entitled *Lost in Care* (Waterhouse 2000) revealed that, even where children attempted to complain and to use relevant procedures, their complaints were not listened to and this was supported by the findings of the Joint Inspectors in 2002 (DoH 2002a) and again in 2005 (Commission for Social Care Inspection 2005a, HM Government 2006b). Although the government put a great deal of money into the *Quality Protects* programme, making money available for LACSCDs to spend in achieving greater access for children to complaints procedures and other sources of support such as Children's Rights Officers, it was decided that further reforms were necessary. Thus, s.26A CA 1989 was inserted by ACA 2002, providing for children to have access to advocacy services in order to be assisted in making complaints and representations, and new guidance, *Get It Sorted*, was issued (DfES 2004d) together with, in 2006, the issuing of new Representations Procedure Regulations (see above) designed to ensure that children will find it much easier to make a complaint; for example, representations can now be made orally under Regulation 6.

It remains to be seen, however, whether enough has been done to ensure that children feel confident when making complaints about the system (Lyon 2006a). Paradoxically, the Care Standards Act 2000 (s.72) provided for a Children's Commissioner for Wales to be an independent officer to whom children could refer their complaints, and the Commissioner's powers were extended by the Children's

Commissioner for Wales Act 2001. Part I of the Children Act 2004 now makes provision for a Children's Commissioner for England but the legislation does not provide the office with similar powers of investigation as that possessed by his counterpart in Wales: indeed, he is prevented from conducting such investigations into individual cases (s.2(7) CA 2004). There is also no duty on England's Commissioner to promote children's rights but rather only to promote their views and interests with regard to the ECM five outcomes (s.2(2)(a)–(e) CA 2004). Many commentators have therefore queried whether or not England's Children's Commissioner will turn out to be a toothless tiger (Lyon 2006b).

It has to be remembered that a child living within the system, be it in residential or in foster care, is not easily able to access relevant information about the complaints or representations procedure, and much more has to be done pursuant to the guidance issued in *Get It Sorted* to guarantee such access and to provide children with information as to the availability of advocacy. Once a child is possessed of the relevant information with regard to the complaints procedure, there is then a two-stage process to be engaged in by the LACSCD, which should involve independent members. The reason why greater consideration is being paid to the issue of children having access to an advocate to represent them is as a direct result of the report *Getting the Best from Complaints – The Children's View* (Office of the Children's Rights Director for England 2005), which found that it is such a formal and difficult process for children: there is such an imbalance of power between the child seeking to make representations and the panel sitting to hear such representations that it is at least questionable whether such procedures really do guarantee the further safety and protection of children or, indeed, comply with the provisions of Article 6 on fair trial under the European Convention (Lyon 2005, 2006a). To suggest, as some politicians have done, that more children should be placed in foster homes or that they should be more quickly adopted is potentially to jump from the frying pan into the fire: foster care or adoption are not necessarily the safest or even the best solution for some children and finding the right foster or adoptive home may not be easy (Prime Minister's Review of Adoption 2000).

Conclusion

What has been provided here is a brief analysis of the legal provisions available to protect children under Parts IV and V of the Children Act 1989, as amended, and of the new framework for children's services provided in the CA 2004, examined in the context of the ECHR and the UNCRC and the other relevant Conventions and Charters. As was indicated in the Introduction, the provisions in Parts VI–XII of the CA 1989 also seek to extend protection to children in whatever environments they are being looked after, but in many situations, if there are concerns about the child suffering significant harm, resort will have to be made to the relevant orders contained in Parts IV and V of the CA 1989.

To many working with children and families, resort to the courts will be seen as a failure of all the agencies and systems designed to prevent children suffering harm. Whilst to a certain extent this may be true, it must also be acknowledged that there are situations in which resources, however plentiful, will simply make no difference or where serious and sudden outbursts of violence towards children can be neither predicted nor, in many cases, prevented.

Much does, however, remain to be done in the field of educating children so that they might develop their own preventative strategies and little effort has been put into this area, either by central or local government and particularly not in schools, despite the rhetoric of *Every Child Matters* and the clear message that children and young people want to be safe (DfES 2003a). Slogans such as 'information is power' and 'forewarned is forearmed' spring readily to mind when considering the plight of many youngsters who have to act in ignorance of what could be achieved, if only they had been taught appropriate strategies in compliance with the demands of Articles 8 and 10 ECHR. Of course, this raises the concern that discussing strategies and raising the profile of the issue of child abuse may encourage a proliferation of unfounded allegations, but the evidence provided by research into the incidence of child abuse and the testimony of adult survivors must make it all the more certain that we should work towards the notion that prevention is always, but always, better than cure – see *Childhood Matters* (National Commission of Inquiry into the Prevention of Child Abuse 1996).

It remains bizarre that the government should have enacted s.58 CA 2004, providing that parents can continue to hit children, when this measure was opposed by over 360 professional organisations and voluntary organisations working with children, including the Royal College of Paediatricians. The government, yet again, will be censured by the UN Monitoring Committee in 2007 when it considers the UK's next report but it has also now become a target for censure from the European Council of Ministers (see above). Less than 40 years ago, society accepted that men should not be allowed to hit their female partners or wives and legislation was enacted in the Domestic Violence and Matrimonial Proceedings Act 1976 to ensure that women would be adequately protected, not only through the appropriate enforcement of the criminal law but also by giving them appropriate and effective civil remedies, now reinforced by the Domestic Violence Crime and Victims Act 2004, passed in the same year as s.58 CA 2004. Yet women today are amongst the supporters of the retention of the parental right to hit children. Children are now the only members of society who can be legitimately subjected to assault by bigger, more powerful people and the question must be asked as to why they should continue to be subject to this special age-related discrimination under the law. Children should have an equal right to physical integrity under Articles 5 and 8 of the ECHR, such rights to private and family life having been determined by the European Court of Human Rights to encompass the right to physical integrity in *Botta* v *Italy* [1998] 26 EHRR 241, and an equal right to the protection of these rights under the law, as guaranteed by reading Article 14 in conjunction with Article 8.

As Kofi Annan, the Secretary General of the UN, has put it in answer to the question 'Why make a special case for children?', 'Much of the next millennium can be seen in how we care for our children today. Tomorrow's world may be influenced by science and technology, but more than anything it is already taking shape in the bodies and minds of our children.' So how much do we care for our children in England and Wales today?

- Be thoroughly familiar with the relevant legal provisions relating in any way to child protection in the Children Act 1989, as variously amended, and the Children Act 2004. Never, ever rely on secondary sources for information on the law. Always have your own copies of the relevant legislation, regulations and rules as updated. Remember that, as Lord Laming stated: 'There is nothing fundamentally wrong with the law relating to child protection, the problem lies with those who fail to implement it properly because of a lack of knowledge.'

- All practitioners operating in the field of child protection must, in compliance with the *Code of Practice for Social Care Workers* (General Social Care Council 2002), ensure that they are fully aware of all the relevant law relating to their areas of practice and ensure that they obtain the relevant training in those areas. Once they have made known their training needs to their employers it is then the responsibility of the employers to provide the relevant training.

■ Remember to be honest with children in indicating that the law and legal proceedings are not a cure. They are literally a measure of last resort when all other appropriate measures to safeguard and protect the child have failed. The law is a very blunt instrument for dealing with the problems and difficulties of such children but the court's and your concern is to try to do what is in the paramount interests of each child.

■ Be thoroughly familiar with the demands of the Human Rights Act 1998 and, in particular, with the requirements of the ECHR contained in Schedule 1 HRA 1998. This is now part of UK law and can thus give rise to actions in the courts. Also be thoroughly familiar with the provisions of the UNCRC 1989 and other relevant Conventions, Covenants and Charters, but be careful not to mislead children as these are not part of English or Welsh law. If your practice is truly in line with the requirements of both the ECHR and the UNCRC, as well as all other Conventions, Covenants and Charters protecting children and young people, you will not go far wrong.

Annotated further reading

Her Majesty's Government 2006 Working together to safeguard children – a guide to inter-agency working to safeguard and promote the welfare of children. TSO, London. Online. Available: www.everychildmatters.gov.uk/workingtogether

This document states that it must be read together with several other pieces of guidance published earlier by various government departments. These include Working Together to Safeguard Children involved in Prostitution *(DoH 2000);* Working Together to Safeguard Children in whom Illness is Fabricated or Induced *(DoH 2002);* Complex Child Abuse Investigations – Inter-agency Issues *(Home Office, DoH 2002);* Female Circumcision Act (1985), Female Genital Mutilation Act 2003, Home Office Circular 10/2004; Young People and Vulnerable Adults Facing Forced Marriage – Practice Guidance for Social Workers *(Association of Directors of Social Services Departments, DfES, DoH, Home Office, Foreign and Commonwealth Office 2004) and* Guidance on Allegations of Abuse made against a Person who works with Children in Appendix 4 of Working Together *(HM Government 2006).*

Lyon C M 2003 Child abuse, 3rd edn. Family Law, Bristol

Prest C, Wildblood S 2005 Children law: an interdisciplinary handbook. Family Law, Bristol

This contains very little by way of narrative or explanation but does contain most of the relevant statutes, with some annotations, statutory instruments, Practice Notes and Directions, which professionals will need in order to understand the much more detailed narrative account to be found in Child Abuse *(Lyon 2003, above).*

All three of these taken together (including all the related volumes of Working Together*) form a comprehensive account of the legal process.* Child Abuse *by C M Lyon is a very detailed narrative and does not reproduce vast tracts of the legislation as these can be accessed in* Children Law. Child Abuse *includes all the changes made by the Adoption and Children Act 2002 and anticipates many of the changes in the Children Act 2004, and begins with a recommendation from the President of the Family Division that it should be required further reading for all those practising in the field of child protection, including judges. It is written from a practitioner's perspective in clear and comprehensible language.*

Child Abuse *covers all aspects of the child protection process from prevention using Part III CA 1989, through core assessments, strategy meetings, child protection conferences and reviews, and all stages in care proceedings including the submission of care plans and the judicial case management protocol for use in care proceedings through to appeals in such cases. It also includes separate chapters dealing with: evidence in care proceedings; criminal proceedings arising out of the allegations of child abuse, whether taken against adults or against children; contact issues; representations procedures and judicial review, which are used when it is alleged that a CSA employee has made a wrong decision; the national and international legal and social policy context; forms of child abuse; issues in child abuse; and, given the emphasis on it in the Children Act 2004, inter-agency cooperation. The book concludes with an analysis of: the impacts of the Victoria Climbié Inquiry report; the pressures with which those working in child protection have to deal; the* Safeguarding Children *report; and a consideration of the approaches which may be taken by the UN Monitoring Committee when it next considers a UK report in 2007.*

Useful websites

www.alc.org.uk – Association of Lawyers for Children. Access information on lawyers belonging to the Association of Lawyers for Children, all of whom are usually on the Law Society Child Care Panel and thus have experience of acting for children in care and supervision order cases.

www.bichardinquiry.org.uk – Bichard Inquiry report on the deaths of Holly Chapman and Jessica Wells.

www.cafcass.gov.uk – The Children and Family Court Advisory and Support Service (CAFCASS) website has parts devoted to both children and practitioners but if you are going to direct children to the children's part of this website make sure you think they will understand the material as much of what is on the site for children is written with adults in mind – see, for example, the section for children on the European Convention on Human Rights which is part of UK law.

www.carelaw.org.uk – A Guide for Young People in Care. A much better website for children in care than the CAFCASS website and has a good section on Human Rights.

www.childabuselawyers.com – Association of Child Abuse Lawyers. Access information on lawyers belonging to the Association of Child Abuse Lawyers, who might therefore be expected to be familiar with the issues in care and supervision order proceedings, especially where abuse or neglect of any sort is at issue.

www.nagalro.com – A useful website for those doing guardian work for children in care and supervision order proceedings.

www.there4me.org – A website from the NSPCC for 12–16 year olds with advice on a whole range of matters.

The Commissioner for Children websites in England and Wales

For England the Commissioner's website is: www.childrenscommissioner.org

For Wales the Commissioner's website is: www.childcom.org.uk

The English Children's Rights Director, Roger Morgan, also has a separate website: www.rights4me.org.uk

The Victoria Climbié Inquiry Report, previously available on the Department of Health website, is now available at www.everychildmatters.gov.uk/ _files/ 6728E64BAB0ED84EABA7B374C36758DA.pdf

A more detailed list of useful addresses and websites is provided on the website.

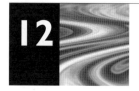

12 Making enquiries under Section 47 of the Children Act 1989

Corinne May-Chahal and Claire Mason

INTRODUCTION

In some cases it doesn't really make any difference whether it's cultural or not, the matters covered by the lilac book will only be as good or in depth or as relevant as the person using it. … Some [assessments] are excellent and some are very very poor, because there's a tick box, some rely too heavily on the tick boxes. What they do is they answer the questions but they don't pull it together at the end. So it isn't really an assessment, it's a collection of information.

(Brophy *et al.* 2005, p. 66)

The process of making enquiries is authorised through Section 47 (s.47) of the Children Act 1989 and directed by local procedures, all of which cover the requirements stated in *Working Together to Safeguard Children** (HM Government 2005a). Such procedures can only offer a broad outline; they cannot convey every aspect of the enquiry. Much rests on the ability of professionals to identify and obtain the right information and, crucially, to *analyse* the significance of that information as evidence of actual or likely significant harm. The death of Victoria Climbié and the resulting inquiry led by Lord Laming pointed to shortfalls in the child protection system (Laming Report 2003). Sadly, as the government admits, no service can ever protect every child (DoH *et al.* 2003) but the latest policy agenda *Every Child Matters: Change for Children* (DfES 2003a) aims to place the protection of children from harm within a framework of universal services. As a consequence, the making of enquiries under s.47 and the analysis of information obtained through them must be reviewed within this inter-agency and partnership context. This chapter reviews key changes in the making of enquiries stemming from the government's response to the Laming Inquiry (Laming Report 2003) and the Joint Chief Inspectors Report *Safeguarding Children* (DoH 2002a), embodied by *Every Child Matters: Change for Children* (DfES 2003a) and the Children Act 2004.

From *Messages from Research* to *Every Child Matters*

During the early 1990s, a number of studies were carried out in the UK, the USA and Australia, which showed that child welfare agencies had been dealing with very dramatic increases in allegations of 'child abuse' and neglect (Thorpe 1994, DoH

---

* The most up-to-date version of this document was published by HM Government in 2006. For a full discussion of this, see Chapter 11.

1995a, Parton *et al.* 1997). However, at the same time as political and professional demands for investigating these allegations increased, the results of investigatory activities did not lead to a commensurate increase in the number of children who were found to have been significantly harmed or injured. The suspicion that many of these child protection referrals may actually have been expressions of concern about children in need more generally were confirmed by the UK government report which summarised a number of studies into English and Welsh child protection services. The publication of *Messages from Research* (DoH 1995a) summarised 20 studies and demonstrated that despite the intentions of the Children Act 1989 there had been little progress in moving towards a more needs-led approach to safeguarding children.

By implication, these and other findings indicated that there was a widespread mistaken categorisation of child care referrals as 'child protection' rather than 'children in need' and that local authority social services departments should have been paying closer attention to the way in which referrals were handled before making the decision to make enquiries under s.47.

The causes of this problem were and continue to be both varied and complex. One obvious factor has been the public criticism of social workers and their managers which has occurred after each inquiry into child deaths, the most recent of which (Laming Report 2003) suggests that much closer and detailed attention needs to be paid to referral-taking activities at the 'front door' of agencies as well as ensuring assessment activity is not just about 'risk' (Mason *et al.* 2004).

The 'front door': making the decision to enquire under s.47

Following outcome research into careers of children entering the child protection system, Thorpe (1994) found that many children who were subject to s.47 enquiries could be more appropriately classified as child concern or children in need without significant harm. A classification system was developed that enabled local authorities to provide more specific services, reduce the number of s.47 enquiries, initial case conferences and children becoming looked after. The criteria for making this decision (Thorpe & Bilson 1998) were as follows:

Section 47 – Child protection

1. Information has been offered that clearly indicates a child has been harmed or injured, or an adult has behaved in a way that would normally cause harm or injury, and an investigation is needed to clarify this information.
2. It is necessary to clarify whether the alleged actions were deliberately intended to cause harm or injury or were the consequence of an accident or excessive discipline.
3. Allegations have been received from a number of different sources.
4. Reports are required from other professionals in health, education and criminal justice who have first hand evidence of the alleged harm or injury.

Section 17 – Child concern

1. Parents are having difficulties and support is required to help look after children.

2. An assessment is needed to clarify the type of support required and which agency is most appropriate to deliver this support.
3. The moral character of parents is given as a reason for concern over care of the children.
4. General concerns are expressed about care of the children but no direct allegation of harm is made.

There are many reasons why a child may be classified as being 'in need' that are not linked to maltreatment, including disability. However, Thorpe and Bilson (1998) are attempting to distinguish between reasons that might previously have led to a child protection enquiry by providing a third category – child concern – which will include some false positives and negatives and some children in need. Such cases can sound quite serious child protection reports when they are referred but when the information is questioned, allegations often turn out to be concerns rather than actual or likely significant harm (May-Chahal & Coleman 2003).

A further opportunity to divert families away from unnecessary s.47 enquiries is provided by the new Common Assessment Framework introduced in *Every Child Matters* (DfES 2003b):

Some frontline services, such as the police, schools and health, may refer children to social services without a preliminary assessment of the child's needs. As a result, social services may be overwhelmed with inappropriate cases, and children and families may undergo initial assessments unnecessarily. Frontline professionals such as pastoral staff in schools, who may already have trusting relationships with the child or parent, may be in a better position to discuss initial concerns with a child or parent, and work with them over time, than a social worker with whom the family has had no previous contact.

(DfES 2003b, p. 57)

The importance of multi-agency working is, of course, not new but the emphasis on the role of the other statutory agencies is changing. They should no longer act simply as 'reporters or detectors' of problems and concerns but actually become the main players in enabling families to find resolutions. The Common Assessment Framework (CAF) forms one part of the wider *Every Child Matters: Change for Children* programme. The CAF shares the domains as set out in the *Framework for the Assessment of Children in Need and their Families* (DoH *et al.* 2000). This should help to address problems relating to the number of inappropriate referrals for s.47 enquiries to social services and the number of 'children in need' being referred with child protection concerns because of differing interpretations of language and thresholds (DoH 1995a, DoH *et al.* 2003). Further, by reducing the number of inappropriate enquiries, resources may be released to provide more responsive services to a wider range of vulnerable children in need. Implementation of the CAF will enable agencies to meet their obligations to cooperate to improve well-being and to make arrangements to safeguard and promote the welfare of children as set out in Children Act 2004 s.10 and s.11 (DfES 2005e).

Initial research suggests that the CAF could potentially halve the number of referrals to local authority (LA) social care (Mason *et al.* 2004), thus providing a further opportunity to redirect resources to support those children most in need of services. Mason *et al.* (2004) sampled referrals entering LA social care and analysed them according to a classification system of s.47, s.17 and CAF. In addition to the finding that cases originally responded to as s.47 could have been categorised as s.17 using the already established diversion criteria (Thorpe & Bilson 1998), it was found that 49% of cases could have been categorised as CAF. In the LA where the research was conducted this could have potentially reduced the need for s.47 enquiries thus offering a more collaborative and less intrusive intervention between parents and professionals. Cases classified as CAF in this research (Mason *et al.* 2004) were those where:

- the child was referred by another accountable professional
- more information was required with regard to the problem in a multi-agency context
- there were other accountable professionals already involved with the family who, in light of this previous involvement, were in a better position to undertake a common assessment as a tool for working with the family.

Assessing significant harm

As part of the wider 'refocusing' agenda, the government introduced the *Framework for the Assessment of Children in Need and their Families* (DoH *et al.* 2000) which aims to encourage a comprehensive assessment of a child regardless of whether they have been referred as 'in need' or suffering significant harm, characterising the move away from incident-driven, investigative 'risk' assessments so heavily criticised throughout the 1990s (Audit Commission 1994, DoH 1995a, Gibbons *et al.* 1995b). However, research suggests that the degree to which local authorities have achieved this aim is varied. The problems encountered (Horwath 2002, p. 199) have included:

- practitioners not paying equal attention to all domains of the child's context
- lack of attention to anti-oppressive practice
- assessments being dominated by a social services agenda
- assessments being driven by timescales
- organisations failing to recognise the impact of an incident-driven culture on implementation.

A national evaluation carried out by Cleaver and Walker (2004) found that implementation of the Framework was most effective in councils where there was strong leadership, a clear implementation plan involving managers and practitioners, and adequate and flexible training. The findings also support Jack and Owen's claims (2003) that the three domains were not assessed equally, with environmental factors, including the effects of poverty and housing, not being given adequate attention.

In addition to improving the assessment of need, there had been some optimism that 'refocusing' would herald a move away from a 'risk' orientation in child protection enquiries towards a more inclusive, supportive approach (e.g. Houston 2001). However, Parton *et al.* (1997) predicted more pessimistically that, although the technology may change as in the form of the CAF, practices are likely to remain investigative and risk based because of the underpinning ideology and dominant understanding of 'child abuse'. 'Child abuse', from its (re)discovery in the 1960s (Pfohl 1977), was understood as something deliberate, physically done (or not done when it should have been) to a child, by a parent or family member, which had psychological causes (Corby 2000). It has also come to be constructed as something that has definable and detectable risk factors, even though these may be contested (Cleaver *et al.* 1998). This dominant understanding, however, has been found to gloss over a range of parenting practices and childhood contexts that do not fit well within it.

In both England and Europe, the majority of referrals for 'physical abuse' concern excessive corporal punishment where parents are under stress but following normative disciplinary practices to excess (May-Chahal & CAPCAE 2006). Most child sexual assault cases also fall outside the traditional stereotype of incest or intrafamilial relations, with the majority of cases concerning peers and those outside the family in the UK (May-Chahal & Cawson 2005) and in the US (Bolen 2001). Despite this, research suggests that these traditional understandings of 'child abuse' continue to frame and filter services (Aldgate & Statham 2001, Bolen 2001) at the level of referral (Spratt 2000) and assessment (Mason *et al.* 2004).

The success of the Framework and the 'refocusing' agenda in the making of enquiries depends, therefore, upon individual and agency culture. Where an agency appears to be 'in denial' about the need to refocus and the emphasis is prescriptive and narrow, the Framework is reduced to a mere information-gathering tool within the enquiry process, the focus continuing to be incident driven (Horwath 2002). Conversely, at the integrated end of the spectrum where 're-focusing has been addressed at both strategic and operational levels and at an inter-agency level' (Morrison 2000, p. 367), then the Framework is likely to have supported a change in practice that is in keeping with the spirit of the Children Act 1989, is 'needs led' and incorporates families' strengths.

Working in partnership

A great deal has been written about working in partnership with both parents and children and this is a key principle underpinning the making of enquiries under s.47, with the importance of working cooperatively with parents emphasised in *Working Together* (HM Government 2005a). Research has suggested that working in partnership with families leads to better outcomes for children (Cleaver 2000) and the views from children and families show that their expectations of the enquiry process are high. Practitioners must obtain trust through demonstration of their competence (PAIN *et al.* 1997). In addition, those about whom enquiries are made valued honesty and respect, demonstrated in terms of recognising rights and individual needs and including these in decision making. Practical applications would be keeping to plans, scheduling meetings to take account of need, respecting wishes in allocating workers (particularly in relation to ethnicity and gender) and ensuring that everyone feels they have been listened to. Fairness was also important and is demonstrated through enquiries being conducted in a just and open manner. Information is central: children and families require clear, comprehensive information, at a level which reflects their knowledge and understanding. Shemmings and Shemmings (1996) identify four key conditions for building partnership which summarise these principles:

- openness and honesty
- answerability
- even-handedness (avoiding rigidity combined with fairness)
- sensitivity.

Each of these principles is relevant to the making of enquiries, as they are to all child welfare practices. From research on the implementation of the Framework for Assessment, Cleaver and Walker (2004) also found that parents valued a shared perspective, between parents and social workers, on the difficulties that families were facing.

The term 'partnership' is in itself often assumed to be commensurate with empowering and liberating practice; however, as Holland and Scourfield (2004) point out,

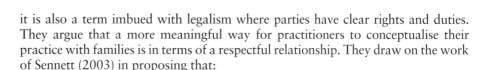

it is also a term imbued with legalism where parties have clear rights and duties. They argue that a more meaningful way for practitioners to conceptualise their practice with families is in terms of a respectful relationship. They draw on the work of Sennett (2003) in proposing that:

> Reluctant clients of child protection teams may not be able to control the fact of being 'seen' (made visible) by the authorities but they should indeed be able to control the *conditions* of their visibility [original emphasis]. They need not be objectified and demeaned by inhumane bureaucratic responses.

(Holland & Scourfield 2004, p. 32)

Analysis of policy issues

Information sharing

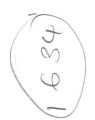

The Laming Inquiry clearly exposed shortfalls in the sharing of information across agencies relevant to s.47 enquiries. Workers expressed confusion regarding what information to share and with whom (DoH *et al*. 2003). The publication of *What to do if You're Worried a Child is Being Abused* (DoH 2003b) included an Information Sharing Appendix in an attempt to begin to tackle this confusion. However, recognising that more fundamental issues needed addressing, the government set out a radical agenda for overhauling the processes for information sharing. *Every Child Matters: Next Steps* (DfES 2004a) and the statutory guidance on the Children Act 2004 (s.10, Duty to cooperate) clearly set out how local areas are expected to improve their information sharing. The Children Act 2004 makes provision under s.12 for the implementation of information sharing indices or databases in each local authority, which will allow agencies to share basic information about a child. The initial evaluation into the Trailblazer sites (Cleaver *et al*. 2004a) indicates that there are varying practices with regard to the level of information placed on these shared indices, particularly in relation to concerns regarding a child.

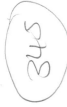

   Information sharing is crucial in the making of enquiries under s.47. However, it is one thing to share information and another to make sense of it. For example, in a report by the Thomas Coram Research Unit (2003) into use of child protection registers, three-quarters of child protection register custodians reported concerns about the effectiveness of inter-agency information sharing. The report points to the fact that in nearly a third of cases the custodian of the register believed that people gained false reassurance from the fact that a child was on the register, whereas in another third of cases they believed that because the child was not on the register this indicated that there were no safeguarding concerns.

   Communication between professionals has long been recognised as a key issue in child protection and surfaces with alarming frequency in child death inquiries (Sinclair & Bullock 2002). The general laws that are of relevance to information sharing are as follows:

- The Common Duty Law of Confidence
- The Data Protection Act 1998
- The Human Rights Act 1998.

The government is currently consulting on its guidance for information sharing through the publication of *Cross Government Guidance on Sharing Information on Children and Young People* (DfES 2005f). The following key principles on information sharing are set out (DfES 2005f, p. 5, s.2.1) to guide what is a complex and contentious area:

- The safety and welfare of a child or young person must be the first consideration
- There must be a legal basis for sharing information
- The information shared should be relevant to the purpose for which it is being shared
- Practitioners should be open and honest with children, young people and their families
- Consent to share information should be obtained
- Information should be accurate, held securely and kept for no longer than necessary
- Good practice dictates that the consent of the child, young person or parent to share information should be sought and a clear explanation given as to why the action is necessary. However, if seeking consent is judged to place a child in danger of significant harm then consent should not be sought before sharing information.

Far less guidance has been given on how to analyse information, on the way in which sense is made of it and how to identify what is important to attend to and what might be misleading.

Making a referral to local authority social care

The Laming Inquiry (Laming Report 2003) and the Joint Chief Inspectors Report (DoH 2002a) highlighted how workers were frequently confused by the various volumes of guidance relating to the Children Act 1989 and were unclear about what to do when they had concerns about a child. In response to these criticisms the government set about clarifying guidelines for safeguarding children. If there is clear evidence that a child has been significantly harmed or injured, or if there is a likelihood of significant harm or injury, then a referral should be made directly to LA social care as outlined in *What to do if You're Worried a Child is Being Abused* (DoH 2003b) and *Working Together* (HM Government 2005a). Both documents set out the expectation that full information about the child is recorded at *first point of contact* (as recommended by the Laming Inquiry). Workers are thus expected to record information with regard to the child's name, address, date of birth and names of persons with parental responsibility.

Working Together (HM Government 2005a) clearly sets out the procedure for making a referral to LA social care and explicitly states that the nature of the concern and the needs of the child and family should be clarified. It should also be established whether the referrer believes the child to have been maltreated, what the basis for these concerns might be and whether urgent action is needed to keep the child safe. Measures have been introduced following the Laming Inquiry that seek to make the process of making a referral more accountable. All referrals by telephone should be confirmed in writing within 48 hours and a written referral should be acknowledged by LA social care within a day of receiving it. If a referrer has not received an acknowledgement within 3 working days they should recontact LA social care. LA social care then has 24 hours in which to decide its next steps. If the decision made is to take no further action then the referrer should be informed.

The initial assessment

Once a referral concerning significant harm is made to LA social care, enquiries should be guided by the Framework for Assessment (see Horwath, Chapter 13, in this volume). In the first instance this will invoke an initial assessment that should:

- be completed within a maximum of 7 working days of the date of referral
- be carried out using the framework set out in the *Framework for the Assessment of Children in Need and their Families*
- address the questions:
  - What are the needs of the child?
  - Are the parents able to respond to the child's needs?
  - Is the child being adequately safeguarded from significant harm, and are the parents able to promote the child's health and development?
  - Is action required to safeguard and promote the child's welfare?
- involve seeing and speaking to the child (according to age and understanding and within a timescale appropriate to nature of the concern) and family members as appropriate
- draw together and analyse available information from a range of sources (including existing records)
- obtain relevant information from professionals and others in contact with the child and family (this includes seeking information from relevant services overseas if the child has spent time abroad).

LA social care are required to ascertain the children's wishes and feelings about services and this should be given consideration prior to a service being implemented. They should:

- seek parents' permission before discussing a referral about them with other agencies, unless such a delay or discussion may place a child at risk of significant harm
- ask is this a child in need? (s.17 of the Children Act 1989)
- ask is there reasonable cause to suspect that this child is suffering, or is likely to suffer, significant harm? (s.47 of the Children Act 1989).

These questions are underpinned by the principle of meeting the needs of all children brought to the attention of services, and recognise that even where significant harm has not been substantiated the child and their family may still have needs that should be addressed. They also prioritise participation and a respectful relationship between professionals, parents and children. Any action plan developed from the initial assessment should be discussed with the family unless this may place the child in danger of significant harm.

Most cases do not go to court but an eye to the statutory dimension of enquiries remains. The court has powers to concern itself with assessment at emergency or interim stages and with the child's contact with parents. There are ranges of orders that can be brought into the s.47 enquiry process to enforce social work intervention. In relation to this, three orders were created by the Children Act 1989: an emergency protection order (EPO), a child assessment order (CAO), and a recovery order (*Working Together* provides details of these). In addition, the police have powers to take children in immediate danger into police protection, and to obtain warrants to search premises. If the case goes to court, before it is heard there can be an initial hearing called a directions appointment. This will give directions to everyone concerned about how the case should proceed and can include:

- agreement on a timetable for the case
- appointment of a children's guardian
- decisions about whether the case should be transferred
- consideration of attendance of the child
- other directions as appropriate, e.g. contact or assessment.

Joint working

There is a very clear mandate that the police and social services should work together wherever there is a case which may constitute a crime against a child and every Local Safeguarding Children Board is required to develop clear policies and procedures with regard to joint enquiries (HM Government 2005a). *Working Together* (HM Government 2005a) is currently consulting on amendments to the requirements to re-emphasise guidance so that the police 'are notified as soon as possible where a criminal offence has been committed against, or is suspected of having been committed against, a child – unless there are exceptional reasons not to do so' (HM Government 2005a, p. 73, s.4.18).

Strategy discussions decide how joint working should be undertaken and will be held in all cases where there is the suspicion that a crime has been committed. *Working Together* (HM Government 2005a) sets out the purpose of a strategy discussion as being to share information, agree the conduct and timing of any criminal investigation, and plan how the s.47 enquiry should proceed. If it is considered that the child is likely to suffer immediate harm, then an agency with statutory powers should act quickly to secure the immediate safety of the child, which may necessitate the bypassing of the initial assessment process. Such emergency action should be quickly followed by s.47 enquiries structured by the domains of the Framework for Assessment.

The Youth Justice and Criminal Evidence ACT 1999 and the Memorandum of Good Practice

Given the salience of the consideration of criminal proceedings in the making of s.47 enquiries it is important to understand the implications for the child as a victim of crime and thus as a potential witness. In practice, very few cases result in criminal prosecution, but this possibility influences the way in which children must be interviewed where it is suspected a crime has been committed. The Youth Justice and Criminal Evidence (YJCE) Act 1999 builds on the reforms originally introduced by the 1988 and 1991 Criminal Justice Acts, reflecting a concerted policy shift towards making the process of giving evidence easier for children and young people. Changes to the way in which children are allowed to give evidence have proceeded incrementally. The Criminal Justice Act 1991 abolished the competency requirement, allowed for committal proceedings to be bypassed under certain circumstances, and permitted video-recorded evidence to be admitted, but only for evidence-in-chief. The YJCE Act 1999 introduced special measures that effectively provide for implementation of the 1987 Pigot recommendations if these measures are applied for and agreed. Thus children may be heard in private and may be aided by the use of interpreters. These changes, combined with an increase in awareness of child sexual abuse cases and the desire to prosecute them, have served to intensify the focus on the child victim as a potential witness. This is because evidence gained at the early stages of enquiries, including interviews with the child, could be relevant later on and will be gathered with prospective use in mind.

The offences that apply to the making of video-recorded interviews cover physical assault, cruelty, neglect and sexual assault. The interview should equate with a witness statement of the first detailed account given to the police and should be conducted as soon as is practicable. There are three reasons for this:

1. There has been much controversy over the possible contamination of evidence by practitioners and parents prior to the initial interview.
2. In the light of research on memory and recall it is considered better to get as recent an account as possible from the child.
3. A recent complaint has more validity in law. As a consequence, video interviews have now become an important consideration early on in the enquiry process.

The interview structures the child's early contact with professionals and will be phased, as follows:

- *Rapport* – This stage helps the child to relax and supplements the 'base line' knowledge obtained in planning. Crucially, it allows the interviewer to explain the ground rules for discussion, such as the acceptability of saying 'I don't know' or 'I don't understand'.
- *Free narrative* – The child is asked to recall everything they can remember about the alleged offence in their own words. Prompts can be made about information mentioned by the child, for example: 'Did anything else happen?'
- *Questioning* – This stage begins with open-ended questions and progresses to specific, non-leading questions, closed questions and, as a last resort, leading questions. The aim is to ask as few questions as possible, to elicit as much free narrative as possible, and to avoid leading questions which are likely to be edited out and invalidate the interview.
- *Closure* – It is essential to make sure that the child is not in distress at the end of the interview. Neutral topics can be returned to, the child should be asked if they have any questions, and a contact name and telephone number given.

Children who have been the victim of serious offences may be distressed and in need of immediate help. The *Memorandum* emphasises that these are not therapeutic interviews, and that once they have been completed, it should be possible for 'appropriate counselling and therapy' to take place. The Crown Prosecution Service should be informed about this. An advantage, and this was the intention, is that this way of interacting does not pre-judge an allegation and assume that something has happened. It encourages all to keep an open mind. As such, practitioners involved with the child are advised to abide by the basic rules of evidence, including avoidance of questions which assume disputed facts or suggest an answer (leading questions), steering away from talk about previous statements or what others have said (hearsay) and avoiding reference to the character of the accused.

UN Convention on children's rights

The British Government ratified this Convention in 1991. It is relevant to the making of enquiries in at least two ways. First, it sets out basic rights that pertain to all children. These are broadly covered by the Children Act 1989 and include:

- all actions concerning the child should take full account of their best interests
- the rights and responsibilities of parents are respected
- the child's right to express an opinion and to have that opinion taken into account in any matter or procedure affecting the child
- the right to obtain and make known information and express views unless they violate the rights of others
- the right to protection from interference with privacy, family, home and correspondence, and from libel/slander;
- the State's obligation to protect children from all forms of violence perpetrated by parents or others responsible for their care.

Secondly, a number of investigations may concern the assessment of behaviours that are alleged to be bad for the child. In this context the following rights apply:

- the child's right to freedom of thought, conscience and religion, subject to appropriate parental guidance and national law
- the child's right to meet with others and to join or set up associations, unless the fact of doing so violates the rights of others.

Practice implications of research and policy

Expanding the surveillance of childhood and parenting

Despite its intention, there is potential that the opening up of assessment practices through the new processes of CAF and information sharing could lead to the expansion of the purview of 'child abuse' and 'risk of abuse' rather than a reduction. This could lead to a parallel increase in enquiries being made under s.47. To avoid such an undesirable outcome it is important to understand parenting practices in their situated context, and to enquire into and to work with all domains of the CAF to reduce the likelihood of significant harm. The DoH (2000e) clearly states that assessment (making enquiries) and intervention should go together – it is not a case of assessing and then providing services. The process is iterative and dynamic and assessment is not, in itself, a service for children.

Competing interests and selective concerns

There are competing interests in the enquiry process, to do with rights, responsibilities, need, protection, prosecution and justice. All of these must be balanced with optimum outcomes for children in mind. Individual workers will have to come to judgements in each particular case and within different working arrangements. Much hinges on the relationship in the field between social workers, the police and other professionals when trying to balance protection, prosecution and welfare. In addition, a great deal depends on the moral and cultural framework within which individual practitioners operate, particularly in relation to their understanding of the causes and characteristics of parental violence to children, children's rights, parental competence and participation. The implications for practice are twofold. Firstly, decision making should be guided by the needs of the child and not the balance of power in social and working relationships. Opportunities to raise questions about this should be built into the enquiry process. Secondly, practitioners need opportunities to review and be more objective about their decision-making criteria, and to learn how these might affect enquiries and their outcome.

Research on the referral process shows that it is selective in ways that may have been inappropriate, with an overemphasis on specific children and their carers:

1. Research clearly indicates that children in all social groups can experience physical, emotional and sexual violence and neglect and that a large amount of significant harm to children is not reported (May-Chahal & Cawson 2005). Thus, many children and their carers either find their own solutions outside the safeguarding system or they remain in harmful situations. Most children referred for LA social care come from socio-economically disadvantaged groups; it is therefore likely that there is a social class bias operating in the s.47 enquiry process.
2. In the context of this bias, families referred for child protection reasons may not contain children in need of safeguarding but rather they may be referred by mistake (false positives). In such circumstances it is unlikely that the enquiry process will lead to the uptake of family support services unless there is a clear non-judgemental and inclusive approach.
3. There is an indication that children of black and ethnic minority families remain marginalised and whilst guidance and policy must take account of ethnicity and need, in practice black and minority ethnic children continue to be over-represented in the looked-after system.
4. Research suggests that disabled children may be more vulnerable to interpersonal violence yet there is considerably more that needs to be done to ensure that their access to equitable initial assessments becomes a reality (Westcott 1999; see also Kitson and Clawson, Chapter 9, in this volume).
5. There is a gender bias in child protection which is not directly and overtly addressed in policy and practice (Otway 1996, Scourfield & Campling 2002), despite clear gender issues being identified in various research studies: the high proportion of men who appear to be child sexual offenders, the higher proportion of girls who appear to be their victims (Finkelhor & Dzuiba-Leatherman 1994b), the high proportion of single female parents referred for child protection concerns (Thorpe 1994) and the focus on mothers and mothering in the enquiry and assessment process (Farmer & Owen 1995, Parton *et al.* 1997) (see Featherstone, Chapter 6, in this volume, for a further discussion of gender issues in child protection).

All of these selective concerns are legitimated by the need to protect or otherwise support children in need. The implications for practitioners engaged with parents and children in s.47 enquiries, simply stated but still difficult to put into practice, amount to the need for application of clear antidiscriminatory practice principles (Thompson 1997).

A shift from treating children's accounts forensically

Since the admissibility of video-recorded evidence was introduced, there has been an increasing emphasis on obtaining evidence for both criminal and care proceedings, and the impetus in such cases has been to establish the validity of an allegation and identify who was responsible, particularly in child sexual abuse cases. This has meant that children's contributions to the enquiry process have been either as victims who may be potential witnesses, or more generally as objects of evidence. The shift in policy contained in *Every Child Matters* and *Youth Matters* heralds a change towards more participatory, information-sharing approaches with children and young people. The enquiry process must actively involve children and seek information not for validity, but to engage with them in the process of assessing need. This means developing more participatory approaches to the making of s.47 enquiries.

A key issue in developing a participatory approach is that of confidentiality and we consider that the government guidelines outlined above in relation to information sharing provide a clear framework on which to build. The main area of difficulty will be agreement (between children and professionals or between parents and professionals) on what constitutes significant harm that ultimately should be reached in consultation with all those involved wherever possible and appropriate to the age of the child concerned. Failure to obtain the child's agreement and consent may well result in the child retracting the allegation or otherwise undermining the assessment.

Recording

Records must be accurate and clear, reflect all the work that is being done and all information known regarding the family. Records are accountable. The court may use them, children, families and other professionals can access them and they may be scrutinised under case review procedures. Distinctions must therefore be made between fact, opinion and hearsay, and confidentiality of source information should be respected.

The medical examination

Medical evidence is important for three reasons: to reassure the child and family that there is nothing physically wrong, to ensure that the child receives appropriate treatment wherever necessary, and to obtain forensic evidence for use in court proceedings.

Once again the general principle of obtaining the informed consent of the child and family applies. This means that the medical examination should be carefully explained to the child, in an age-appropriate way. Where the parents do not consent, but the child does, the 'Fraser*' ruling applies. Gender of examiner is important and children should be given a choice. There has been some concern that the medical examination can contribute to a feeling of 'secondary abuse' for the child, however sensitively the practitioner may handle it, particularly in cases of sexual assault. When consent is refused, an EPO or CAO can be applied for. However, grounds for carrying out a medical examination need to be very clear in such cases.

The Laming Inquiry (Laming Report 2003) makes some important recommendations in relation to the medical examination. Firstly, it outlines that if the examining doctor believes that taking a detailed history directly from the child is in the child's best interest then this should be done even without the consent of the carer. Secondly, if there is dissent amongst medical professionals regarding a diagnosis of

---

* Following the Gillick case and a ruling by the House of Lords, people under 16 who can understand what is proposed, and the implications, are competent to consent to medical treatment regardless of age. A set of guidelines known as Fraser Guidelines set out the criteria that should be met before considering a child 'competent'.

deliberate harm then there should be a full, detailed and documented discussion regarding these differences and, if necessary, further opinion should be sought (DoH *et al.* 2003).

Conclusion

This chapter has presented a review of research, policy and practice in relation to making enquiries under s.47 of the Children Act 1989. The enquiry process is essentially an information gathering and an information sharing exercise. It requires the skills of judgement and engagement in order to assess and balance the immediate and long-term interests of the child, the need for prosecution and justice, the need for appropriate intervention and respect for individual privacy and freedom. Key components of the process are the ability to justify actions in these terms and to carefully record all information. The initial contact with the child and family set the tone for the rest of the process. It is therefore vitally important that the practitioner is able to engage with the child and their carers in a way that reduces the strong feelings of anger, denial and fear that the process can generate.

Key points and messages for practice

- Take a critical approach to information and consider firstly whether the application of Common Assessment Framework arrangements is more appropriate than a referral to local authority social care.

- Critically analyse information and make a judgement about whether a referral would be more effectively dealt with for the child and family through s.17 procedures.

- Work in a way that is respectful of children, young people, their carers and their situations.

- Carefully reflect on what information is shared, for what purpose, whether the legal framework is contravened and how it is intended to analyse and use the information.

Further reading

Department of Health, Department for Education and Employment, Home Office 2000 Framework for the assessment of children in need and their families. TSO, London

Department for Education and Skills 2005 Working together to safeguard children and Local Safeguarding Children Board regulations.
This consultation document is downloadable from www.dfes.gov.uk/consultations/conResults.cfm?consultationId=1365

Department of Health 2003 What to do if you're worried a child is being abused. DoH, London. Online. Available: www.safeguardingchildren.co.uk/managed/files/dfes-what-to-do.pdf

Useful websites

For all the latest developments relating to the *Every Child Matters* agenda, visit the DfES website at www.everychildmatters.co.uk. CAF and ISA initiatives can be obtained by following the relevant links.
The Joint Chief Inspectors website gives information regarding their inspections and provides access to their latest reports – www.safeguardingchildren.org.uk
Publications from the DfES are accessible through their website at www.dfes.gov.uk/publications. It also has a link to HMSO.

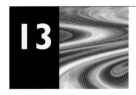

13

Safeguarding children: the assessment challenges

Jan Horwath

INTRODUCTION

Assessment is a routine aspect of child welfare work. Any practitioner who comes into contact with a child and their family is likely to be involved in assessments. These assessments may be specific and specialised; for example, an assessment of the needs of a child with regard to a hearing impairment. Alternatively, they may be multifaceted, requiring the involvement of a diverse range of professionals. This is likely to be the case when assessing the needs of maltreated children – the subject of this chapter.

Effective assessments, in cases of child maltreatment, are crucial if the assessments are to inform meaningful planning and interventions likely to promote better outcomes for children and their families. Sound assessment practice is dependent on professional knowledge and skills and the ability of professionals to work together with each other, the child and the family to identify the child and family's needs (for further detail, see DoH 2000c). It should be borne in mind, however, that child protection assessments are likely to be influenced by a range of factors such as perceptions of abuse, values and beliefs, which may affect the approach and can result in a loss of child focus (Reder *et al.* 1993, Munro 1999, Buckley 2003, Horwath 2005a). It is all too easy to provide a theoretical overview about assessment without considering the challenges encountered by professionals when applying the theory to practice. However, if practitioners are to complete child-centred assessments it is important that they are not only aware of the assessment task and process, but they also need to be aware of the factors that can distort the assessment and in addition have the ability to prevent or rectify any distortion. It is with this in mind that the aims of this chapter are both to explore the key components of effective assessment practice in cases of possible child maltreatment and to consider the range of factors that influence individual assessment practice.

The first part of the chapter centres on the assessment task and the second part on the assessment process in relation to safeguarding and promoting the welfare of children. Throughout the chapter the challenges encountered by front-line staff when assessing children where there are concerns about maltreatment will be considered.

Assessing children: a changing task?

Child protection is referred to in *Working Together to Safeguard Children** (HM Government 2005a, p. 19, para. 1.19) as 'the activity which is undertaken to protect

---

* The most up-to-date version of this document was published by HM Government in 2006. For a full discussion of this, see Chapter 11.

specific children who are suffering or at risk of suffering significant harm'. Based on this definition, the purpose of assessment in child protection work can be described as 'identifying the needs of children who are suffering or at risk of suffering significant harm in order to intervene in their lives to safeguard and promote their welfare'.

This definition immediately raises the question: 'What are the needs of a child who is suffering or at risk of suffering significant harm?' The way in which this question is answered will influence the way in which the assessment task is interpreted and the types of intervention considered to meet the needs of the child. Unfortunately, there is no definitive answer to the question. Interpretation of significant harm is influenced by perceptions of maltreatment, government policy, research and practice developments. This can be understood by considering the changing interpretation of the assessment task in child protection work that has occurred in England over the last 30 years.

The 1970s and 1980s

During the 1970s and 1980s, government placed considerable emphasis on developing child protection systems to both standardise practice and promote a forensic approach towards child maltreatment (DoH 1995a, Parton *et al.* 1997, Stevenson 1998b, Horwath 2001). However, an emphasis on gathering forensic evidence led to an assessment focus on specific incidents of possible maltreatment (DHSS 1982, DoH 1991a, Gibbons *et al.* 1995b). This approach lent itself far more readily to the identification of physical abuse and to a lesser extent sexual abuse (Parton 1995). As cases of neglect and emotional abuse were not as readily identified through specific incidents, they were more likely to be filtered out of the system (Gibbons *et al.* 1995b). However, Gibbons *et al.* (1995a) found that a single abusive incident does not necessarily cause long-term difficulties for children. In the long term, a negative environment, most notably one of low warmth and high criticism, is more likely to have a detrimental effect on the health and well-being of a child.

The Orange Book

The late 1980s witnessed the introduction of government assessment guidance designed to assist long-term planning for children considered to be suffering or likely to suffer from significant harm. This guidance was called *Protecting Children: a Guide for Social Workers Completing Comprehensive Assessments* (DoH 1988a) – generally known as 'The Orange Book'. It was underpinned by a developmental approach towards the assessment of a child and should have had a positive impact in shifting the focus of assessment of significant harm from specific incidents to the developmental needs of children. However, the Orange Book was not used widely or imaginatively, and its application was limited to its specific purpose, i.e. comprehensive assessments and planning for children on the child protection register* (Katz 1997, Stevenson 1998b). Despite the limited way in which the Orange Book was used in practice it was and indeed remains very useful for the assessment of cases of possible maltreatment as it explores issues over and above the incident of abuse.

---

* An English system for recording all children who are believed to be suffering or likely to suffer significant harm and are subject to multi-agency child protection plans.

The Children Act 1989

The Children Act 1989 was set to change practice interpretation of the assessment task. The Act places an emphasis on working with a wide range of children – children in need. This included children unlikely to achieve a reasonable standard of health and development (s.17(a)) and children where concerns exist about the significant or likely significant impairment to health and development (s.17(b)). Despite the wider assessment remit, a report entitled *Child Protection: Messages from Research* (DoH 1995a), which summarised the main findings of 20 research studies on child protection practice completed before or in the early stages of implementation of the Children Act 1989, showed that the assessment task continued to focus on obtaining forensic evidence (Parton 1995). Samra-Tibbetts and Raynes (1999) concluded that the narrow interpretation of the assessment task meant many children in need received only a minimal assessment whilst those considered to be suffering or likely to suffer significant harm were often over-assessed.

Despite this emphasis on assessing children suffering or likely to suffer significant harm, the assessment and subsequent plan focused on the identification and elimination of risk and danger at the expense of the identification of children's developmental needs and the prevention and therapeutic responses that were likely to meet these needs (Audit Commission 1994, Cleaver & Freeman 1995, DoH 1995a, Cleaver *et al.* 1999, Ayre 2001). Wider issues that could affect the health and development of a child such as poverty and racial harassment were rarely identified and tackled (Parton 1995, Lymbery 2003).

The publication of *Messages of Research* in 1995 by the Department of Health led to an increased awareness amongst professionals that they should be focusing on identifying and planning to meet the *needs* of children who were suffering or likely to suffer significant harm. However, practitioners found themselves in a position where limited resources meant work with children was service led rather than needs led (NCH Action for Children 1996). In this situation, the focus became accessing the available resources and completing assessments with thresholds and eligibility criteria for services in mind. Emphasis remained on short-term interventions – the quick fix. In addition, practitioners were confused as to *how* to assess the needs of children. The result was that assessment practice varied and assessments were often unfocused (Social Services Inspectorate 1997a, 1997b). In order to clarify the assessment task practitioners required more explicit assessment guidance than was currently available.

A framework for assessing children in need and their families

Clarification came with the *Framework for the Assessment of Children in Need and their Families* (DoH *et al.* 2000) introduced by government in 2000. The Framework, which continues to underpin assessment practice in England, takes an ecological approach towards assessment. This means 'an understanding of a child must be located within the context of the child's family (parents or caregivers and the wider family) and of the community and culture in which he or she is growing up' (DoH *et al.* 2000, p. 11, s.1.39). This approach is based on the principle that, in order to safeguard children and promote their welfare, the assessment task for practitioners involves identifying the developmental needs of the child, considering parental capacity to meet these needs and the impact of wider family and environmental factors on the child and family. The assessment task can therefore be broken down into three *domains*. The guidance goes further and identifies *dimensions* that need to be explored in relation to each of the domains (see Fig. 3.4, p. 62). The Framework and the accompanying practice guidance outline what practitioners should consider when assessing the various domains and dimensions of what is commonly referred to as the 'assessment triangle'.

For the first time practitioners in England have been given a clear answer to the question: 'What are the needs of a child who is suffering or at risk of suffering significant harm?' In addition, the guidance makes explicit the principles underpinning the Framework and the way in which these should inform the interpretation of the assessment task.

These include (DoH 2000c, DoH *et al.* 2000, Rose 2001, Ward 2001):

- A child-centred focus: When completing the assessment, consideration should be given to the impact of maltreatment, parenting and the community context on the particular child in question.
- Rooted in child development: This means recognising the importance of each aspect of development for the particular child as well as considering the significance over time in the child's life (Rose 2001).
- An ecological approach: The practitioner should consider the child in the context of their world. That includes immediate and extended family, school and community.
- Working with the child and family: The child and family are the ones experiencing life together. Unless their perceptions of the situation are obtained, practitioners will not have a full picture (this is discussed in detail later in the chapter).
- Building on strengths as well as identifying difficulties: The dimensions of the assessment triangle are deliberately neutral in terminology. The aim is to encourage practitioners to approach each dimension by considering both strengths and difficulties. This approach should inform planning by building on strengths and addressing weaknesses.
- Multidisciplinary practice: The assessment task in cases of possible maltreatment is multifaceted. It can only be completed effectively if those with the particular knowledge and skills to assess each of the dimensions work together (this is discussed in detail later in the chapter).
- Based on equality of opportunity: The dimensions of the assessment triangle are not culturally specific and can be used to assess the needs of children irrespective of culture and complexity of need.

Further principles are considered in the next section.

A criticism that has been made of the Assessment Framework is that the focus on the 'needs' of children marginalises concerns about risk (Corby 2000, Calder 2003a). Indeed the term 'risk' is not used in the Framework or accompanying guidance. Calder (2003a) argues that a failure to use words like 'risk', 'dangerousness' and 'child abuse' can lead to a distortion of purpose when completing assessments, minimising the potential risk of significant harm posed by perpetrators of abuse. Assessing risk of significant harm by taking into account the abusive behaviour of particular parents/carers is integral to the application of the Assessment Framework. Risk assessment is about making a prediction regarding possible outcomes for children, i.e. 'making judgements under conditions of uncertainty' (Munro 2000, p. 44). The predictions and judgements, in cases of maltreatment, usually centre on the dangerousness posed by carers, i.e. 'the risk of a serious negative outcome' for the child (Hagell 1998, p. 83). Based on these definitions, the only way in which practitioners are able to assess risk of dangerousness is to consider ways in which parenting capacity impacts on the developmental needs of the child in both the short and longer term. Thus the assessment task, when assessing risk of significant harm, remains gathering and making sense of information with regard to the three domains of the Assessment Framework, more specifically assessing:

■ perspectives on the nature of the harm or abuse
■ the short- and possible long-term impact on the child's developmental needs
■ individual parent/carer issues
■ parent/carer relationships with each other, the child and extended family
■ parent/carer's ability and motivation to meet the needs of the child
■ family, social and community influences and resources
■ interactions between the family and professionals

(adapted from Dale *et al.* 2005, p. 155).

The assessment process

Adcock (2001, p. 76) describes assessment 'as the collection and evaluation of information relevant to the identified purpose'. The 'identified purpose' in cases of child maltreatment has been discussed above. The *way* in which the information is collected and evaluated – the assessment process – is explored in this section.

However, before beginning to explore the assessment process in detail it is necessary to give consideration to three further principles underpinning the Assessment Framework (DoH *et al.* 2000) as these will influence the interpretation of the assessment process. These principles are as follows:

■ Assessment should run in parallel with actions and interventions: In other words, as the needs of the child and family are identified, these needs should be met and reviewed.
■ Assessment is an ongoing process, not a single, one-off event: This means that practitioners should not only assess the immediate needs of the child in relation to safeguarding their welfare but also the longer-term needs of the child and their family. In addition, the effectiveness of actions and interventions designed to meet these needs should be revisited to ensure the changing needs of the child and family are met.
■ Assessment should be grounded in evidence-based practice: The assessment should draw on theory, research, policy and practice 'in which confidence can be placed to assist in the gathering of information, its analysis and the choice of intervention' when planning to meet the needs of the child (DoH *et al.* 2000, p. 1, s.1.1).

The author, together with Buckley and Whelan (Buckley *et al.* 2005), devised a five-stage model outlining the process practitioners should follow if they are to effectively assess the needs of vulnerable children and their families. This model was developed in the Republic of Ireland in collaboration with senior managers, trainers and front-line staff from three health boards (now known as the Health Service Executive). It is of particular value because it not only draws on the literature on assessment but is also informed by the views and experiences of professionals from a diverse range of disciplines who participated in the study. Another advantage is that the process model is not country specific and is therefore of relevance to practitioners working in various settings in different jurisdictions. The five stages are:

■ Responding
■ Protecting
■ Devising

- Gathering and reflecting
- Sharing, analysing and planning.

Each of these stages will be considered in the context of the English Assessment Framework, focusing on the assessment process following referral to local authority (LA) children's social care. The five stages outlined above begin once a referral has been received by social work services. There is, however, an assessment stage that occurs before this: the decision to make a referral. This is considered below before the model is explored in detail.

Making a referral

Research into referral practice indicates both a lack of consistency amongst professionals as to when and how to refer a case to social work services and confusion as to the criteria for defining a child in need (Birchall & Hallett 1995, Gibbons *et al.* 1995b, Horwath 2005a). The Common Assessment Framework (CAF) (DfES 2004e), which is being introduced in England, may go some way towards improving the quality and consistency of referrals between agencies. The CAF uses the same domains as the Assessment Framework and provides a national standardised approach to conducting an assessment of the needs of a child or young person and deciding how those needs should be met. It is designed for early identification of children's needs. Whilst child protection concerns would warrant an immediate referral to LA child social care, the police or the NSPCC, the fact that all those working with children and their families will be using the CAF should embed a common language amongst professionals for discussing needs and should encourage the use of an evidence-based approach when identifying concerns. In addition, where the CAF indicates that the child has urgent needs that result from concern about significant harm, information gathered will feed into the specialist assessment process.

Yet, no matter how detailed the guidance on referral task and process, a range of factors seem to influence referral practice. Zellman (1990) studied these factors in relation to doctors' decisions to refer to cases of child abuse. He summarised these as 'bad for me', 'I can do better than the system' and 'not reportable'. The author, who completed a study in the Republic of Ireland of referral practice in cases of child neglect, found these factors appeared to influence the way in which other professionals in addition to doctors approached referrals. I noted an additional factor: 'be sure – report everything'.

- 'Bad for me' appears to be associated with fear of litigation or violence from parents or anxiety about the community's negative response towards those referring cases.
- 'I can do better than the system' was associated in the Irish study with professionals' lack of confidence in the ability of social work services to meet the needs of the child and family.
- 'Not reportable' was connected to professionals operating high thresholds with regard to maltreatment or anxieties about making inappropriate referrals.
- 'Be sure – report everything' appeared to be motivated by a fear of making a mistake by not referring possible abuse cases.

These findings are supported by Dalgleish (2003, p. 97) who concludes that 'referral thresholds are influenced not by case information but by the values placed on the consequences by the decision-maker'.

Responding to referrals

Returning to the five assessment stages described above, the first stage of the assessment process follows a referral to social services with concerns that a child may be suffering significant harm. At this stage the social worker is required to gather basic information about the child and family. However, it is also necessary to clarify (HM Government 2005a, p. 73, para. 4.17):

- the nature of the concerns
- how and why they have arisen
- what appears to be the needs of the child and the family.

Based on this information, the social worker should identify whether there are concerns about maltreatment, the evidence for these concerns and whether to consider urgent action to ensure the child is safe from harm. In effect, the social worker, in consultation with other professionals, makes what Hollows refers to as a 'holding judgement' (2003, p. 68), This is designed to ensure safety and create stability for the child whilst attempting to keep options open for longer-term planning (Munro 1997, cited in Hollows 2003). Assessment at this stage is crucial in terms of identifying both the *urgency* of the referral and also the *intensity* of the level of inquiry (Munro 2000). The LA should decide and record the next steps of action within 1 working day from the point of referral. Responses may include no further action, referral to other services or the initiation of an initial assessment.

The initial assessment

This is a brief assessment of the child and family and should be completed within 7 working days from the point of referral (DoH *et al.* 2000). Cleaver and Walker (2004) found only 38.5% (*n* = 866) of referrals proceeded to initial assessments, with child protection concerns being the most frequent reason for an initial assessment. Of the cases that went on to have initial assessments, only 10% were carried out on young people over 15 years of age. In 27% of the cases there were concerns about parenting issues and 61 of the cases were rated by the research team as having multiple problems.

Protecting the child(ren) from immediate harm

In cases where there are concerns that a child is suffering or is likely to suffer significant harm, the social worker has to consider whether the evidence indicates that there is an immediate threat to the safety of the child. Practitioners should consider whether the child has been seen recently and what signs and indicators of abuse were noted. In addition, information should be obtained about the alleged perpetrator and the contact the child continues to have with this person. As part of this assessment it is important to identify whether there is a carer available who can offer both immediate and also long-term protection to the child and other children in the household whilst the assessment is being completed. When gathering this information the practitioner may become aware that a criminal offence against a child may have taken place. In these situations they should inform the police as soon as is possible and work in partnership with the police to ensure the needs of the child and family are identified and met alongside criminal investigations. When assessing immediate harm and the need for protection, it is all too easy to focus on a specific incident without placing this in a context. In a number of situations this can result in no further action when in fact, as for example was the case for Victoria Climbié, daily life was intolerable for the child (Laming Report 2003).

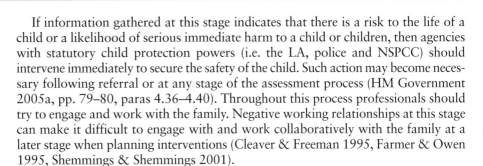

If information gathered at this stage indicates that there is a risk to the life of a child or a likelihood of serious immediate harm to a child or children, then agencies with statutory child protection powers (i.e. the LA, police and NSPCC) should intervene immediately to secure the safety of the child. Such action may become necessary following referral or at any stage of the assessment process (HM Government 2005a, pp. 79–80, paras 4.36–4.40). Throughout this process professionals should try to engage and work with the family. Negative working relationships at this stage can make it difficult to engage with and work collaboratively with the family at a later stage when planning interventions (Cleaver & Freeman 1995, Farmer & Owen 1995, Shemmings & Shemmings 2001).

Devising the assessment

The strategy discussion

Any assessment requires careful planning (Milner & O'Byrne 2002, Parker & Bradley 2003, Holland 2004). In cases of suspected maltreatment this planning is likely to occur at a 'strategy discussion'. This should ideally take place at a meeting but may happen over the telephone. The discussion is likely to involve LA children's social care, the police and other appropriate professionals such as teachers and health personnel. The professionals involved should be of sufficient seniority within their organisations to contribute to the discussion and make decisions. The purpose of the discussion is to share information and decide whether to proceed with a s.47 enquiry designed to establish whether a child is suffering or is likely to suffer significant harm. If it is agreed that the child is suffering or is likely to suffer significant harm, the following should be considered (HM Government 2005a, p. 81, paras 4.42 and 4.43):

- Planning the conduct and timing of any criminal investigation
- Agreeing on immediate action required to safeguard and promote the welfare of the child
- Determining whether legal action is necessary
- Agreeing a plan for completing a core assessment under s.47 of the Children Act 1989.

At this stage little information may have been gathered as part of the initial assessment. Although there may be physical evidence of injuries or sexual abuse it is not always present and evidence of emotional abuse or neglect may only become apparent after a more in-depth and longer-term assessment.

Planning the core assessment

The core assessment is 'an in-depth assessment which addresses the central and most important aspects of the needs of a child and the capacity of his or her parents or caregivers to respond appropriately to these needs within the wider family and community context' (DoH *et al.* 2000, p. 32, para. 3.11). A core assessment should be completed in 35 working days. The core assessment is the means by which a s.47 enquiry is carried out (HM Government 2005a, p. 82, para. 4.47). When planning the core assessment the following must be considered:

- Ways in which the core assessment will be completed: This should include identifying the information required, taking account of the domains and dimensions of the Assessment Framework, about the child and their family. In addition, consideration should be given to possible sources of this information and ways in which the information will be obtained and recorded.

- Who should be interviewed and for what purpose? Interviews should be held with:
  - the child
  - in most cases the parents/carers
  - individuals personally and professionally connected with the child.
  In addition to interviews, plans should be made for observations of the inter-actions between the child and carers, specific assessments and examinations (e.g. psychiatric, psychological, community-based family-centre assessments or independent social work assessments). Consideration should also be given as to who is best placed to complete these interviews, observations and assess-ments, and when.
- A multidisciplinary approach: A qualified and experienced social worker from LA children's social care should have lead responsibility for the assessment. However, health, education and other services have a statutory duty under Part III of the Children Act 1989 to help the LA carry out s.47 enquiries.
- Ways of engaging the child to ascertain their wishes and feelings: Particular attention should also be given to the way in which this is managed if the child is to be interviewed as a victim of a criminal offence in line with *Achieving Best Evidence in Criminal Proceedings: Guidance for Vulnerable or Intimidated Witnesses, including Children* (Home Office *et al.* 2002).
- Particular requirements, taking account of race, ethnicity and learning or physical disability.
- The needs of siblings and other children who may have been in contact with the abuser.
- Engaging the family.

(Adapted from HM Government 2005a, p. 82, para. 4.43.)

Engaging children and young people

Cleaver and Walker (2004) found that professionals were not very effective at engaging children and young people in the assessment process. They conducted eight interviews with children who had been the subject of an assessment and found that they did not think their social workers had always spoken to those they consid-ered important and who could make a valuable contribution to the assessment. The children found it difficult talking to social workers about personal and family issues and also felt that their views were frequently discounted or disbelieved. In terms of the assessment process they did not understand the process and over half did not think social workers had shared possible actions and plans with them. Holland (2004, p. 85) provides the following suggestions for involving and representing chil-dren in assessments. Children should:

- have access to clear information
- be consulted about assessment methods
- decide how to express themselves (e.g. verbally, in writing) and whether to have views represented on their behalf
- have opportunities to build up relationships with social workers who are honest, reliable and provide assurances regarding confidentiality and its limits
- be confident that a holistic portrayal of their life will be conveyed.

Lord Laming (Laming Report 2003) is clear that a key aim of communication with children, or about children, is to gain a comprehensive understanding of a day in the life of the child. There are a number of ways in which practitioners can do this. For example, by using a clock and asking the child what they would be doing at different times. What is crucial is that practitioners get the minute detail that really provides

Box 13.1
Detail of a day in the life of a child

What happens about getting dressed and washed in the morning?	
	■ Are clothes readily available, clean and in a good state of repair?
	■ Are they appropriate for the weather and context (e.g. going to school)?
	■ Does the child have to find their clothes?
	■ Do they have their own clothing?
	■ What happens about washing body, hair, etc?
	■ Where is the child expected to do this?
	■ Is this supervised appropriately, bearing in mind the child's age and ability?
	■ Does the child wash and brush their teeth in the morning?
	■ Is this appropriately supervised?
	■ Are there facilities available (e.g. tooth brush, hairbrush)?
	■ Does the child have any special needs (e.g. are they incontinent)? How is this managed?

From Horwath (2007).

a clear picture of daily life for the child. Box 13.1 describes the kind of detail that is required about just one aspect of their daily routine in the case of a child where there are concerns about physical and supervisory neglect.

Engaging families

As identified above, engaging families in the assessment process is crucial if the assessment is to identify strengths as well as weaknesses (Saleeby 1992). This should be done sensitively and with respect. Workers should recognise the importance of building up positive working relationships with parents as, in the majority of cases, the outcome of s.47 enquiries is that children remain or are returned to their carers (DoH 1995a). Dale *et al.* (2005) evaluated the findings of 20 studies that sort the views of over 1000 parents and carers in the British Isles, USA and Australia who had experienced child protection enquiries. They noted some common themes and complaints, including families feeling that the child protection system is 'arbitrary and opaque' (Dale *et al.* 2005, p. 90), that they were treated unfairly and that they believed the interactions with practitioners were negative. The Assessment Framework has had a positive influence in terms of addressing the concerns of parents and carers. Cleaver and Walker (2004) found most parents reported that they felt consulted and involved in the assessment and planning process and that social workers had listened to them, gained and recorded their views.

Gathering and reflecting

Whilst gathering information about the child and family occurs throughout the assessment process, at this stage professionals, ideally with family members, work together to gather and collate information about the three domains. A variety of methods can be used to gather this information, including case records and consultation with other professionals and the child and family. Increasingly, assessment tools are being developed to assist practitioners gather information from the child and family. Table 13.1 provides a summary of some of the key tools which can be used not only to gather information but also to provide a framework for reflecting on and analysing information with regard to specific needs of children. Many of the tools draw on information identified in the literature or agreed by experts as indicating possible risk to children – hence they are described as 'consensual tools' (English 1999, Gambrill & Shlonsky 2000).

A note of caution is necessary when using tools and scales. Tools are designed to assist with the assessment and should not be used in isolation (DoH 2001b). In

Type of tool	Purpose
HOME (Home Observation for Measurement of the Environment) Inventory (Cox & Walker 2002)	A set of tools for assessing a child's home environment Comprises groups of scales for different age ranges that are scored as present or absent Scoring is completed using a mixture of observation of the home and carer–child interaction as well as parental report Covers aspects of parenting required to meet the developmental needs of the child and is useful in drawing the professional's attention to neglected areas
Family Assessment (Bentovim & Bingley Miller 2001, p. 6)	A range of methods and instruments designed to aid the assessment of family competence, strengths and difficulties Includes interview schedules designed to explore family organisation, character and history and a range of family tasks to assist families to talk or do things together Can also help to identify strengths in the family upon which it may be possible to build a planned intervention
Home Conditions Scale	Focuses on the physical home environment
Family Activity Scale	Designed to explore with carers the environment they provide for their children Gives practitioners some insight into the daily life of a child in this family
Parental Daily Hassles Scale	Assesses the frequency and intensity of 20 potential daily 'hassles' that carers experience when caring for children
Recent Life Events Questionnaire	Designed to assist the compilation of a social history Assists in assessing the impact of past events in the carer's life on current parenting
Adult Well-being Scale	Explores the feelings of the carer in terms of depression, anxiety and irritability, which can be useful in assessing the carer's ability and motivation to meet the needs of their child
Alcohol Scale	Seeks to establish how alcohol consumption impacts on the individual and to identify those with hazardous drinking habits which may influence their parenting capacity
Strengths and Difficulties Questionnaire	Focuses on the child's emotional and behavioural strengths as well as their difficulties
Adolescent Well-being Scale (Cox & Bentovim 2000)	Designed to gain some understanding as to how an adolescent feels about their life
Graded Care Profile Scale (Srivastava *et al.* 2003, 2005)	Designed to assist professionals assess different aspects or 'areas' of care (physical care, safety, love and esteem) against predetermined criteria; these areas are broken down into 'subareas' and specific 'items' To complete the assessment the practitioner grades each item on a five-point scale; each point on the scale has a description enabling the practitioner to rate what they have observed Scoring enables practitioners to identify areas of strength and weakness The GCP can be used alongside the Assessment Framework
Genograms	Family trees providing a visual representation of family relationships, including separations, divorce, deaths and transitory and long-term relationships
Ecomaps	A visual representation of the child and family within their wider family and community network Enables family members to identify strong, tenuous, positive and negative links

(Continued)

Table 13.1
(Continued)

Type of tool	Purpose
Culturagrams (Parker & Bradley 2003)	Information is gathered about immigration, community, contact with cultural institutions, values, beliefs, language, holidays and special events to determine the meaning and impact of culture on the daily life of children and their families
Life maps	Different analogies can be used such as a car journey, a road map, a game of snakes and ladders, strip cartoons, allowing individuals to identify positive, negative and significant experiences and events in their lives

addition, questions linked to the tools are dependent on making a judgement regarding acceptable standards, strengths and deficits. It is therefore important that practitioners give examples so that other professionals, and indeed the family, can be clear on what evidence judgements have been made. Further, a number of these tools are dependent on self-report. Practitioners should reconcile what the family tell them with what they actually observe and have learned from other sources. There is also a danger that carers and children may be over-optimistic in their responses when answering questions from professionals (Murphy-Berman 1994, Gershater-Molko *et al.* 2003, Stone 2003).

Another issue regarding the tools and scales concerns cultural sensitivity. Practitioners need to ensure that the tools used are relevant for all cultural groups and that possible risk factors are seen in the context of the cultural setting. This can be done by checking out with the family rather than presuming relevance (Murphy-Berman 1994, Munro 2000). Professionals also need to be aware that their own cultural values may influence the way they interpret and grade the information received.

Observation

An effective tool for gathering information which is often forgotten by practitioners is that of observation (Ellis *et al.* 1998, Tanner & Le Riche 2000, Caldwell & Bradley 2001, Holland 2004). In a recent study of child neglect the author found that in 15 out of 21 home visits, made by social workers following a referral, there was no evidence on the file that the child had been seen let alone observed within the context of their home environment (Horwath 2005b). Howe *et al.* (1999, p. 178) argue that the information required to not only make sense of the care-giving environment the child is experiencing but also the quality of relationships within the family can only be gained by observation. They go on to identify how observation can contribute to an assessment. This includes providing information about:

- the physical environment
- non-verbal behaviour between family members
- verbal communication
- parental consistency
- parental sensitivity and availability to the child and other children in the family
- the behaviour of children in different settings.

Five key questions

Professionals can feel overwhelmed by the amount of information that is collected as part of a core assessment. Buckley *et al.* (2005) have devised the following questions to assist practitioners reflect on the significance of the information obtained in order to inform planning to meet the needs of the child.

1. *What facts, observations and opinions do you have to support the information gathered?* By answering this question practitioners can begin to assess the quality of the information gathered.
2. *What does this mean in relation to the child's safety, welfare and development?* As indicated above, safeguarding and promoting the welfare of the child should be a primary consideration throughout the assessment. This question ensures that assessments remain child focused.
3. *How do practice experience, research findings and literature inform this part of your assessment?* Answering this question enables practitioners to begin to make sense of the information gathered. For example, by drawing on the literature in relation to the impact of drug misuse on parenting capacity, practitioners can begin to establish whether the particular parent's behaviour in relation to drug use is likely to impact on their ability to meet the needs of their child.
4. *Should an intervention be made now? If so, what?* As outlined above, one of the key principles underpinning the Assessment Framework is first recognising that needs are likely to become apparent at various stages of the assessment and second that practitioners have a responsibility to meet these needs as they are identified.
5. *Has the parent/carer engaged with the change process?* Professionals should consider the carer/carers' attitude towards change. For example, do they recognise the need to change their behaviour? Are they committed to making changes? How do they demonstrate this commitment?

Sharing, analysing and planning

Having gathered and reflected on information obtained as part of the assessment, concerns that a child is at continuing risk of significant harm may be substantiated. In this case an initial child protection conference should be held. However, collating and reflecting on information may indicate other courses of action are more appropriate ways for completing this phase of the process as shown in Figure 13.1.

In this chapter the focus for exploring the next phase of the assessment process will be the initial child protection conference. However, as shown in Figure 13.1, if the case is not considered at a child protection conference, plans for interventions may still be drawn up to meet identified needs. If this is the case, sharing, analysing and planning should take place at a case planning meeting following a similar process to that outlined in this section.

Sharing, analysing and planning occurs when the professionals who have been involved in the assessment and other relevant agencies' representatives come together, where appropriate with the child and family, to make sense of the information gathered and consider what, in light of research, practice experience and developmental theories, this means in terms of the needs of the child that are and are not being met. The purpose of this phase of the process is to use evidence-based practice to inform decisions and formulate a plan that will safeguard and promote the welfare of the child.

A number of dilemmas face practitioners at this stage of the process:

1. The initial child protection conference should take place within 15 days of the strategy discussion. Whilst this prevents delay in making decisions about the child and family, it means that the core assessment, which is expected to take

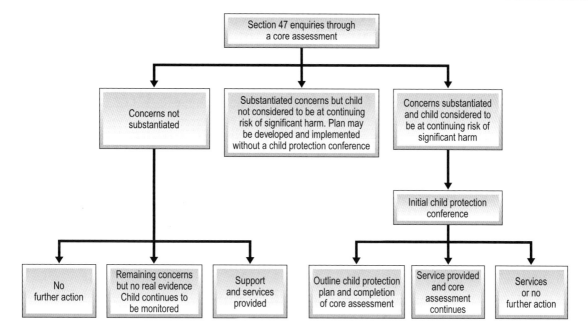

Figure 13.1
Different outcomes from gathering and making sense of information as part of s.47 enquiries.

35 days, is incomplete. Yet, the social worker from LA children's social care is expected to provide a written report to the conference that provides a summary and analysis of the information obtained to date as part of the core assessment. Holland (2004) found that problems such as staff sickness were often encountered when completing assessments which affected the information that could be gathered within the timescales. With this in mind, it is important that social workers emphasise the evidence base for concerns, bearing in mind the gaps in the information collected.

2. In cases of child protection, these assessments may take place in a hostile and stressful context which – as Corby (2000) notes – is not conducive to careful analysis.

3. The social worker has had a limited time in which to establish a working relationship with the child and family. For example, if the social worker has only met the child on one or two occasions they will have had little opportunity to build the trusting relationship in which a child is likely to talk openly and honestly about their wishes and feelings. It is not only social workers who face these dilemmas, other professionals are also required to ideally prepare a report or bring to the conference details of their involvement with the child and family.

Buckley *et al.* (2005) have identified four tasks that should be completed at the initial child protection conference. By completing these tasks it is anticipated that the members of the conference will go beyond just sharing information to reflect on the significance of the information in order to identify risk of significant harm, the developmental needs of the child and ways in which they can be met. These tasks are:

■ Sharing and analysing
■ Making sense of the information

- Making judgements about motivation and change
- Deciding what needs to happen next.

Sharing and analysing

This activity describes the review of information gathered to date in light of the concerns that led to the assessment and any concerns that arose during the assessment about the safety and welfare of the child. Practitioners often struggle with analysing information, providing a summary of information gathered rather than an analysis (Social Services Inspectorate 1997b, Cleaver & Walker 2004, Holland 2004). Cleaver and Walker (2004) found that social workers considered they were ill-prepared and poorly equipped for this task. As part of this activity, conference members should pay attention to both family and community strengths and vulnerabilities in terms of meeting the developmental needs of the child in both the short and longer term. The child's protective environment, the resilience of the child and their vulnerability to further maltreatment should also be considered.

Making sense of the information

Based on the analysis, members of the conference can attempt to answer the question: 'Is this child at continuing risk of significant harm?' If the answer is affirmative, the chair of the conference should determine which category of maltreatment the child has suffered. This will indicate to any professional consulting the child's social care record the primary presenting concerns when the child was subject to the conference (HM Government 2005a, p. 90, para. 4.83). When answering this question, consideration should be given to the information gathered and analysed. Conference members should consider the evidence that either the child *has* suffered significant harm or impairment of health or development as a result of maltreatment and this is likely to continue or the child *is* likely to suffer significant harm or impairment of health or development as a result of maltreatment. The crucial decision that needs to be made is whether the child is at continuing risk of significant harm and hence in need of a child protection plan. Hollows (2003, p. 69) refers to this as an *issues* judgement.

The following questions are designed to assist professionals make issue judgements in cases of maltreatment in order to inform plans to meet the needs of the child:

- What are the pre-existing and current factors that indicate the child is suffering maltreatment?
- What type of behaviour on the part of the carer/carers is of concern?
- Are these behaviours impacting on the health and well-being of the child? If so, how?
- What evidence is there to support this?
- What are the pre-existing and current strengths that protect the child from abuse and promote their welfare?
- What is there about the current situation that increases or decreases the likelihood that the health and development of the child will be affected through maltreatment?
- How does the current situation fit with past patterns of carer/carers' abusive behaviour?

Making judgements

It is complex enough making sense of information to decide whether a child is at continuing risk of significant harm but what is even more complex is making decisions about safeguarding the child from future harm and promoting their welfare. Hollows (2003, p. 70) refers to these decisions as *strategic* judgements. These involve professionals deciding how to respond to the identified needs of the child and family and developing plans that safeguard and promote the well-being of the child. Crucial to the way in which these judgements are made are the beliefs, knowledge, skills and practice wisdom that inform the way in which we make decisions.

Factors influencing judgement making

Taylor and White (2001) note two types of activity take place in relation to social work: practical–moral and technical–rational. These activities are equally applicable to multidisciplinary child protection practice. Technical–rational activity centres on evidence-based practice that draws primarily on procedures, research and theories to inform decision making. Practical–moral activity recognises that both workers and service users are individuals. In other words, we all have our own values, beliefs, anxieties and fears which are likely to influence our approach to child protection work. For example, we may have strong beliefs about the cases that should or should not receive services. This can distort our approach to assessments and inform judgement making, resulting in a loss of focus on the child: This may take a number of forms (DoH 1991a, Reder *et al.* 1993, Munro 1999, Laming Report 2003, Reder & Duncan 2004a), including:

- treating information discretely, being selective about the information gathered and recorded to raise or lower thresholds to meet the needs of the worker or parent rather than those of the child
- having fixed ideas about a situation and failing to change these views in light of additional information
- being over-optimistic or over-pessimistic about a child and their family's situation by focusing predominantly on strengths or weaknesses
- minimising concerns
- failing to focus on the child through over-identification with the carers or focusing on incidents of abuse rather than the effects.

Ability and motivation to change

Central to this judgement is determining whether the parent or carer has both the ability and the motivation to meet the needs of the child. In addition, if there are concerns about ability and/or motivation, are these issues that can be addressed through interventions and how will change be measured? The following questions should assist in making the judgement:

- What are the child's views on their situation? What do they want to change?
- What insight does the carer(s) have in relation to the impact of their behaviour on the child?
- What would need to change if the carer(s) were to meet the needs of the child?
- What are the indicators that carer(s) have the ability and motivation to make the changes required to promote the welfare of the child?

Making judgements about motivation is complex. Practitioners need to be clear as to whether within the assessment phase they are looking for actual change or potential for change (Holland 2004). Dale *et al.* (2005, p. 97) note that the negative responses of parents during assessment, such as frustration and irritation, can be inappropriately interpreted as evidence that they will not cooperate or are not motivated. They found that professionals can be 'almost paranoid' and 'think dirty', believing parents will 'fake good'. They stress the importance of keeping an open mind. Corden and Somerton (2004) recognise that some carers may appear demotivated but through actual engagement in intervention plans find motivation. For example, they may attend parenting classes because they are directed to do so with no intention of changing. However, they find that they actually do learn from this experience and consequently change their behaviours towards their children. Whilst some practitioners may be over-suspicious and negative towards parents, others can be over-optimistic and live in hope, believing in carers who agree to make changes when in fact there is no evidence that the carer has actively engaged in or sustained the required level of change. Moreover, the types of behaviour and attitude that need to change are likely to be deeply embedded, meaning that change will be a very slow process. This is a real problem for practitioners who need to assess whether sufficient change will occur at a pace that will meet the needs of the children in the family. In addition, the opportunities for change through the input of services within the current child welfare system are not geared up for slow change but rather for quick throughput and immediate results. Finally, practitioners need to be realistic about the type of change that can be achieved, particularly with chronic neglectful families. Patterns of chronic neglect can be so embedded within the family's style of functioning – carers having learned these behaviours from their own parents – that practitioners' expectations of what can change and at what pace are often unrealistic (Horwath 2007).

Planning and review

Having decided how to safeguard and promote the welfare of the child, the final stage of the assessment process involves making decisions about ways in which the 'how' will be translated into a workable child protection plan and contingency plan. Decisions also need to be made about the professionals who will be working with the family and child to meet their needs, the roles and responsibilities of all involved, timescales and systems for monitoring and reviewing progress.

Effective planning is likely to occur if practitioners and the family have clear, desired outcomes. Outcomes are specific statements of what the family and professionals are looking to achieve through the child protection plan. They are the final goal or end result. The outcomes should be developed in light of concerns about the significant harm the child is or is likely to be suffering and any identified unmet needs. The more specific the outcomes, the more likely that all those involved will share a common understanding of the aims and objectives of the child protection plan. Vague outcome statements such as 'protect the child from future harm' give little indication as to the specific needs of the child and the services and actions required to meet those needs. In order to achieve the desired outcomes for a child and their family, strategies or a coherent plan of action is required – this is the purpose of the child protection plan. The outcomes can be broken down further into objectives, with consideration given to how the objectives will be achieved, the resources required, the targets and the monitoring arrangements. In addition, the family and professionals need to develop short- and long-term indicators that provide evidence-based measures of the progress that is being made towards the final goal (Hogan & Murphy 2002). These measures provide the framework for evaluating the effectiveness of interventions. This should be done on a regular basis by the core group of professionals who will be working with the child and family to implement the plan and at child protection review conferences. Reviewing effectiveness is a crucial assessment task. The professionals, together with the child and family members, should be assessing whether the plan is achieving the agreed outcomes and adequately safeguarding and promoting the welfare of the child.

Recording

Assessment records provide the official account of the assessment task and process. They become the case history, acting as a point of reference for professionals and informing subsequent assessments. Hence, it is important that they are accurate and provide a detailed account of information gathered, the analysis of that information and how this informed planning. This means that recorded information should be jargon free. Moreover, there should be no room for ambiguity. For example, does the instruction from a supervisor on a file 'complete assessment', mean write it up, based on the information gathered to date, or carry on gathering information? This was a dilemma for a social worker highlighted by the Victoria Climbié Inquiry (Laming Report 2003, Raynes 2005).

Assessment recording in England centres on a series of forms designed to assist practitioners gather and make sense of the obtained information. Cleaver and Walker (2004) found that practitioners using these forms routinely failed to record the child's religion and the identity of relations not living in the household. Both of these are crucial. For example, in the 2001 Census, 77% of people in the UK stated that they had a religion and in the 1999 British Social Attitudes survey, 19% of those who stated they belonged to or were brought up in a religion attended a religious service at least once a month. By ignoring religion, practitioners may fail to identify a key influence and possible source of support for the family. Likewise, by failing to consider relatives living outside the family home practitioners may disregard individuals who are significant to the child.

Holland (2004) identifies an issue which is often forgotten by practitioners and others reading files: records cannot be neutral documents. The style in which they are written and the actual content of the report will be influenced by the author and their agenda. For example, if a practitioner is unhappy about a decision to leave a child at home, the recording is likely to be defensive, justifying the decision made – almost anticipating a possible inquiry if the case goes wrong.

The working context

Assessment practice will inevitably be influenced by the context in which it takes place. Staff vacancies, uncertainty about role, high staff turnover, absenteeism and inexperience will all influence the ability of front-line staff to complete assessments (Reder & Duncan 1999, Jordan & Jordan 2000, Jones 2001, Laming Report 2003). Moreover, organisational performance targets may place pressure on staff to prioritise the needs of the organisation rather than those of the child and family. One of the greatest challenges in terms of the working context is for professionals from different disciplines to work together effectively.

Although Inquiry Reports following child deaths consistently highlight poor outcomes for children when professionals fail to work together, little is known as to how effective multidisciplinary working can promote better outcomes for children. Yet, as described above, a multifaceted assessment is crucial if professionals are to take a holistic approach to assessing the needs of children and their families. Cleaver *et al.* (2004b) found that the Assessment Framework was an effective vehicle for engaging professionals from a diverse range of disciplines in the assessment and also clarified criteria used to define a child in need and professionals roles. However, these professionals also noted that poor social work practice, notably a failure to communicate outcomes of referrals and assessments, lack of agreement over the definitions and lack of resources identified as part of the assessment process hampered collaboration.

Reder and Duncan (2003) highlight the importance of understanding the ways in which professionals communicate with each other when working together in child maltreatment cases. They conclude that a range of interpersonal factors influence the meaning given by each worker and indeed each family member, when communicating with each other. They argue that communications, i.e. messages given and received throughout the assessment process, will be influenced by the preconceptions that individuals have of other agencies, their working context and the individual's feelings, values and beliefs. The individual will attribute meaning to messages based on what they perceive, see or hear which will be influenced by the above. In the following text, consideration is given to the way in which these influences affect referral and decision making.

Summary

The first few years of the twenty-first-century have been dominated by a desire on the part of policy makers and professionals to improve the quality of assessment practice in cases of children in need, including children in need of protection from significant harm. Improvements to the quality of assessments are likely to occur only if policy makers and professionals recognise the key points and messages for practice outlined below.

Key points and messages for practice

- The assessment task does not remain static; it changes depending on our developing knowledge and understanding of the needs of children and factors that are likely to influence outcomes for these children. Professionals must therefore have an up-to-date knowledge of both developmental theories and research about factors that are likely to influence child development.

- Assessment is an ongoing process of gathering information, making sense of this information, planning to meet the needs of the child and reviewing these plans. For this to take place, professionals working together to assess the needs of a child should ensure that they have a shared understanding of the assessment task and process.

- Crucial to effective assessment is recognising that practitioners are not automatons. Every professional brings with them their own values and beliefs, professional perspective, past experiences and personal issues that will influence their interpretation of child maltreatment and the way they interact with the child, family and other professionals. To this end, professionals should pay as much attention to the personal and professional factors that are informing their decisions as they do to the developmental needs of the child, parenting capacity and family and environmental factors.

- Agency context and inter-agency relationships will influence perceptions of what can be done and by whom. Professionals and their managers should therefore be aware of the way in which organisational goals and culture, resources and inter-agency relationships influence approaches to and engagement with the assessment process.

Further reading

Calder M C, Hackett S (eds) 2003 Assessment in child care. Russell House, Lyme Regis

Cleaver H, Walker S, Meadows P 2004 Assessing children's needs and circumstances. The impact of the assessment framework. Jessica Kingsley, London

Horwath J (ed) 2001 The child's world. Assessing children in need. Jessica Kingsley, London

Holland S 2004 Child and family assessment in social work practice. Sage, London

14

Safeguarding children and integrated children's services

Barry Luckock

INTRODUCTION

At the front of his Inquiry Report, Lord Laming (Laming Report 2003) has had reproduced a colour photograph of Victoria Climbié. It is a striking snapshot. Presumably taken a year or more before her murder, it presents Victoria brightly dressed in a yellow, red and black outfit and posh new trainers. Below the photograph is a quote from Antoine de Saint-Exupery's *The Little Prince* and a statement of dedication to Victoria. The quote had been selected to convey Lord Laming's sentiments in presenting his Report, 'I have suffered too much grief in setting down these heartrending memories', it says. 'If I try to describe him, it is to make sure that I shall not forget him.'

The intention is apparent. By placing Victoria within our direct gaze, readers are required to hold her in mind rather more effectively than had those professionals and managers who were supposed to support and protect her. This reinforces a central finding of the Inquiry. For although she 'was not hidden away' (Laming Report 2003, p. 3) during the 10 months she spent in England before her death, Victoria had still been 'abandoned, unheard and unnoticed' (p. 2) by the people responsible for her support and protection. In this period no fewer than three housing authorities, four social service departments, two police child protection teams, the NSPCC and two NHS hospitals had contact with Victoria. In each case, as Health Secretary Alan Milburn told the House of Commons on the day the Laming Report was published, 'the authorities and the agencies empowered by Parliament to protect children … did nothing to help her' (Hansard 28 January 2003, column 738).

The photographic strategy only partially succeeds. The dramatic presentation of Victoria at the outset is followed by a Report that proceeds, in meticulous detail, to record the events that led to Victoria's death. The Laming Report forces us to face the consequences of the 'gross failure of the system' (p. 3) designed to support and protect her. We learn exactly *when*, *where* and *how* individual responsibility was avoided and inter-agency working was confused and ineffective. In contrast we are not helped to make much sense of *why* children like Victoria can get lost from sight so easily, why individual professionals and their agencies were apparently so ready to avoid their responsibilities to intervene and to communicate their concerns and coordinate their efforts effectively. Instead, the Report, having brought her back into view, ends by losing her experience from sight once again in a list of organisational and procedural recommendations for enforcing agency and professional responsibility.

These recommendations are significant because of their influence on the major reforms to children's services that followed Victoria's death. Whilst earlier government attempts to reduce failures in child protection had focused on improved *cooperation between agencies,* the response to the Climbié case was to propose the *integration of their work*. This shift in approach was made clear by Alan Milburn, then Secretary of State for Health, in his response to the Laming Report:

Finally, Mr Deputy Speaker, Victoria needed services that worked together. Instead the report says there was confusion and conflict. Down the years inquiry after inquiry has called for better communication and better co-ordination. Neither exhortation or [sic] legislation has proven adequate. The only sure-fire way to break down the barriers between these services is to remove the barriers altogether.

(Hansard 28 January 2003, column 740)

This chapter describes the shift in child protection policy and practice that emerged out of the New Labour government programme of reform between 2003 and 2005, following the publication of the Laming Report and the *Every Child Matters* Green Paper (DfES 2003b). It outlines the organisational changes to children's services at both strategic and practice levels. In particular it explains how the policy of integration was intended to reconnect specific arrangements for protecting children from harm with broader policies to improve child well-being as a whole and to ensure that child safety and well-being became a 'shared responsibility' (DfES 2003, p. 64).

A second aim is to consider the likely effectiveness of the new approach. By embedding routine procedures to protect a small number of children at risk of harm within an integrated system of services for all children, the New Labour reforms aimed to build in communication and coordination both earlier and later in the process of safeguarding child welfare. Integrated practice was demanded for reasons of *prevention of harm*, enabling the effective identification of a wide range of 'additional needs' in children and the provision of appropriate support. It was also required for the *promotion of well-being*, once children had been made safe through the formal child protection process. Would this organisational and procedural response to failures of joint working resolve the avoidant agency and professional dynamics spotted but not explained by Lord Laming, and thereby enhance safe and supportive engagements with children?

Working together for child protection: research evidence and practice experience

The use of organisational means to coordinate potentially divergent social and professional objectives and practices in child welfare has for some time been a feature of social policy in England. Hallett and Birchall (1992) have distinguished this 'mandated coordination' (p. 33) from the voluntary arrangements discussed in the standard literature on 'interorganisational linkages'. Coordination itself is generally understood to occupy a position on a 'continuum of collaboration' (Thistletwaite 2004), somewhere between agency and professional autonomy at one end and full service integration at the other. In social policy the question has been how to facilitate sufficient coordination to ensure the achievement of common public goals whilst preserving the skills and resources of different agencies and professions. In the case of child protection in England and Wales, mandated coordination has produced a dual approach to what has formally become known as *Working Together* (DHSS/Welsh Office 1988). Central government (and wider public and media) concerns about the problem of child abuse going back over several decades (Home Office 1950, DHSS 1974a) have been translated into both *strategies for planning and cooperation* in local inter-agency networks and *procedures for joint working* in individual cases. This meant that the New Labour government, in considering the shift to integrated working, was able to draw on a body of research evidence and practice experience demonstrating the effectiveness or not of inter-agency and inter-professional working at both strategic and operational levels.

Three main sources of research evidence and practice experience were available. First, there were numerous Inquiry Reports, of which the Climbié Report was the latest. These enabled lessons to be learnt on the basis of worst case scenarios (e.g. DoH 1991a). The failures of communication and coordination exposed by Lord Laming, interpersonal and interorganisational alike, were shown to be perennial. Second, there were a number of research reviews and studies that enabled a more balanced picture of the effectiveness of 'working together' in child protection to emerge. In particular, the research reviews by Hallett and Birchall (1992) and the Department of Health (1995a) demonstrated that communication and coordination were able to provide an adequate measure of initial safety and support where cases could be readily fitted into routinised child protection procedures (Hallett 1995). Problems tended to arise at the *threshold* to these procedures and the services they triggered, especially where the nature of concerns and the responsibility for responding to them could not always be agreed (Gibbons *et al.* 1995b). They also emerged in *later case management and intervention* where, once decisions had been taken and protection plans agreed, it was often the social worker more or less alone who was left with the responsibility for promoting as well as safeguarding child welfare (Farmer & Owen 1995).

As we will see, the post-Climbié reform of children's services specifically addressed both these issues. Also influential in policy terms have been research findings on the nature of the policy process. Child death inquiries remind us of the gap that can emerge between agreed principles of intervention laid down in law and policy on the one hand and these day-to-day practices on the other. The nature of this gap, between the demands of 'the policy community' at the centre and the response of the local, front-line 'delivery networks', has been extensively debated in the public policy literature (Marsh & Rhodes 1992, Marsh 1998, Hill & Hupe 2002). This policy analysis has been productively employed in one major study of the effectiveness and reform of organisational arrangements for inter-agency coordination between the NHS and social services in child protection (Lupton *et al.* 2001). We will see later how the need for this gap to be managed effectively has been central to the children's service reform programme.

A third body of literature appears to have had less influence on government thinking on shifting the focus of 'working together'. This includes a diversity of studies and accounts in which the nature of the interpersonal and interorganisational *dynamics* played out in child protection are considered, in order that the failures and limitations of the *structures and procedures* of joint working might be better understood. Certain authors have developed *socio-political and cultural analyses* to account for the often confused and conflicted nature of professional communication and service coordination. The focus here is the uncertain and contested nature of child abuse and child protection and the negotiated nature of the political and professional response in a diverse, complex and democratic society. For example, Ferguson (2004) and Parton (2006) have shown how, in the shift from 'simple' or 'organised' to 'late' or 'reflexive modernity', these negotiations are increasingly visible and contested in nature, as hitherto private family relationships become seen as matters of public concern. Parton (2004) and Simmonds (2004) further remind us that which children and family lives become visible and eligible for inclusion in these processes has itself become a contested matter. For example, it was only after her death that the real identity of Victoria Climbié was finally established. Only then did the political and professional community in England actually come to accept responsibility for the experience of this transient black African girl, who had been in the country for some time but never part of the community.

From this socio-political perspective the coordination of the differing professional roles of social workers, health practitioners and the police cannot and should not be seen simply as a procedural matter. It is argued that there is no settled social agreement about what kind of problem child abuse and neglect represents or which kind of professional response best guarantees child safety (Parton 1985). Social work, on behalf of the local authority, was given full lead responsibility for child protection between 1971 and 1988 in order to provide a focal point of accountability. The *Working Together* procedures (DoH/Welsh Office 1988) confirmed the social worker as the key worker in case management for children on the child protection register. However, the earlier vision of the 'battered child' (Kempe *et al.* 1962) as the object of proper medical and health care concern has still been periodically revived, as the Climbié case attests, and health professionals have continued to exercise their authority in judgements and prescriptions where children are harmed. This medicalisation of child abuse, and the re-politicisation of child protection as a social issue generally, is best represented in recent times by the angry public debates about the accuracy and legitimacy of the diagnosis of 'Munchausen syndrome by proxy' (BBC News 2004). In the meantime, there has been a reassertion of criminal justice responses to child abuse, which is now seen as a matter of public protection as well as safe family life (Utting *et al.* 1997, Bichard Inquiry Report 2004, Kemshall & McIver 2004, Parton 2006).

In lieu of any settled agreement about child abuse, child protection strategic and day-to-day practice negotiations are not always readily or appropriately contained by formal procedures. Indeed, when the attempt is made to manage the intrinsically complex and contested nature of child protection by making the response bureaucratic (Howe 1992) and legalistic (King & Trowell 1992), this puts at risk the authenticity of engagements between children, parents and professionals (Ferguson 2004). The civil liberties of citizens may also be compromised where those bureaucratic procedures become developed into coherent systems of social surveillance (Parton, Chapter 1, in this volume).

Comparative research has provided a rather different perspective on the nature of effective and legitimate negotiations in child protection. The work of Cooper and colleagues (Cooper *et al.* 1995, Hetherington *et al.* 1997) is important here. In comparing a number of European child protection systems, they concluded that it was different *cultural* assumptions about the relationship between children, families and the state and contrasting *legal traditions* that were the most significant determinants of interpersonal relationships in practice. Defensive yet unsafe procedural responses might be a local problem. For example, conflict and confusion in inter-professional responses to child care concerns appeared to be reduced in France because the paternalist authority of the children's judge (*juge des enfants*) could be evoked by children, parents and professionals alike and this provided legitimate authority and case coordination in one unified role. Effective joint working followed from this. In the Flemish community in Belgium it was a combination of the 'confidential doctor' and a formal 'mediation committee' who had the measures of delegated authority and corresponding space and time necessary to negotiate agreements about abuse and protection before adversarial and bureaucratic legal and managerial arrangements took over. Drawing on this research Cooper *et al.* (2003) suggest that 'spaces' for negotiations based in trust and professional authority found in other child protection systems should be (re-)introduced in England. However, their argument – that these conditions must prevail if the personal, professional and agency avoidance of responsibility and engagement, exposed in the Climbié case, is to be overcome – has not had a noticeable impact on government policy.

Equally neglected in policy has been the *psychosocial* research literature on the dynamics of intervention and decision making in child protection. Here the case is made that the interpersonal relationships through which negotiations are conducted are influenced by the *psychology* as well as the politics and culture of child protection. Effective communication has been identified as the foundation of effective negotiations. Professionals must be able to communicate with both children and parents and with each other if concerns are to be identified and a coordinated response provided. Communication failures in each case have almost always been at the heart of inadequate practice, as a succession of child death inquiries has demonstrated (DoH 1991a, Reder *et al.* 1993, Reder & Duncan 1999, 2004). Reder *et al.* (1993) explain how the 'multiple relationship contexts' (p. 65) of inter-professional communication are affected by personal as well as organisational factors, such as professional role and identity and agency structure and demands. They use systems and social cognition theories to discuss the 'psychology of communication' (Reder & Duncan 2004) and argue that professionals need to develop a 'communication mindset' (p. 96). By this they mean a framework for making sense of the meaning of information and messages exchanged within the interpersonal relationships created when child care concerns arise. There are two key assumptions made here:

- information exchange is of no consequence unless a shared meaning can be attributed to it
- the interpersonal context in which communication takes place is a critical influence in the process.

Different commentators emphasise different aspects of this interpersonal context. Nonetheless, at heart there is the recognition that a 'communication mindset' is inhibited by a combination of key factors. In essence these concern the capacity of the practitioner, the agency and the inter-agency network to contain the uncertainty, anxiety and conflict created when a responsible professional comes face to face with likely abuse and neglect. Personal emotions, such as fear and anger, can get played out in professional conflicts over roles and responsibilities, values and priorities, and decisions and resources. For example, from a psychodynamic perspective, Rustin (2005) highlights the role of anxiety in the Climbié case. Identifying a 'defensive evasion' (p. 11) at the heart of inter-professional and inter-agency practice, she points to the intolerable emotional experience of practitioners in such cases. Workers with responsibility to act can get trapped between the disturbing reality of abuse on the one hand and a sense of impotence about their capacity to resolve it on the other. In this situation they are likely to avoid rather than grasp any opportunity to hold the experience of an abused child in mind in order to think carefully about what best to do. This 'avoidance of thought' (p. 17), especially in circumstances of insufficient resources, can be pervasive. Not thinking clearly leads to not writing things down and not putting minds together and sharing thoughts with others. According to this view, the fragmented and dislocated nature of the abused child's experience gets mirrored in the discontinuities and gaps in the professional response. Cooper (2005a) and Cooper and Lousada (2005) use the Climbié case as an example of what they term 'borderline welfare'. Here professional relationships remain false and shallow as painful realities get projected away from, rather than contained by and incorporated in, an effective emotional engagement.

White and Featherstone (2005) point to the moral and linguistic as well as the emotional aspect of communication, showing how professional narratives about what counts as the right thing to do become ritualised in practice and undermine the capacity for understanding the contrasting perspectives of other professionals. Munro (1999, 2002) also concentrates on the thinking processes of individual practitioners. From a cognitive perspective she demonstrates how information gathering and decision making in child protection is impeded as much by the intrinsic difficulties of reasoning in the face of limited knowledge, time pressures and conflicting values as by the emotional impact of the process or the ethical commitment of a particular professional identity.

It was in the face of research evidence and practice experience that pointed to the inherently ambivalent, contested and fragmented political, cultural, professional and psychological responses to child abuse and neglect that the New Labour government embarked on its programme of reform of child protection and children's services. Much less available was evidence or experience on the likely impact of reforms designed to move services further towards integration. Whilst government policy can claim to be based on evidence (albeit selective) of the negative effects of services that are poorly integrated, it cannot be said to draw on any substantial body of research that demonstrates the positive benefits of integration itself. There is much evidence about the factors (if not mechanisms) that facilitate or inhibit integrated working processes in children's services but hardly any on the impact of these processes on child well-being (Sloper 2004), not least in child protection itself. We return to the question of evidence later when we review the initial impact of the reform programme. Before this, however, the focus of the programme itself is discussed.

Working together: from a coordinated child protection system towards integrated children's services

Hallett (1995) suggests that the 1974 DHSS circular which provided the foundation of the child protection system 'constituted an administrative mandate to cooperate' (p. 4). She refers to the key policy assumption during this period that provides the context for this approach. This was the concern to maintain a structural separation between health and personal social services, in the belief that 'services should be organised according to the main skills required to provide them, rather than by any categorisation of primary user' (p. 5). This emphasis on distinctive professional skill rather than common 'service user' needs set the scene for the approach to 'working together' that was put in place after 1974. However, the administrative focus of this approach was further reinforced by the wider social influences already discussed. The longstanding cultural commitment to using the courts as a last resort to decide on but not manage cases of child abuse was accentuated by successive Conservative governments (1979–1997) which emphasised non-intervention in family life by the state and made limited resources available for voluntary support. In these circumstances local inter-agency strategies and procedures were effectively given the main responsibility for managing child protection yet little of the authority and few of the resources necessary to do so effectively.

When New Labour came to power in 1997 these core assumptions were more or less reversed. Instead of retaining a separation of services in order to preserve a diversity of professional skills, the aim now was to clearly identify the primary 'service users' and their needs and wishes so that those skills and services could be integrated around the task of meeting them. Children in their own right became the focus of concern and the improvement of their well-being the outcome to be achieved. In the place of a presumption of non-intervention in family life there was a belief in early intervention and new legal duties and powers (authority) and money (resources) to ensure effective implementation. Coordination became legally mandated and the administrative system previously established for the purpose of child protection was extended and refocused on the active 'prevention' of harm and 'promotion' as well as any reactive 'safeguarding' of child welfare. Rather than simply revising child protection processes and procedures, the aim was to implement a 'radical change in the whole system of children's services' (DfES 2004b, p. 4). Meanwhile, outside of children's services themselves, a parallel set of multi-agency public protection arrangements (Home Office 2003a) were put in place to manage risk to the public in general. However, this latter aspect of joint working is not our main concern here.

It is important to recognise that the refocusing of the child protection system within children's services has left intact most of the established processes and mechanisms for managing specific concerns about child safety. Within children's services themselves the dual process of 'working together' developed between 1974 and 1988 has been retained. Neither ideas from mainland European systems, intended to enhance space for negotiation (Cooper *et al.* 2003), nor proposals to separate investigative and supportive approaches (Parton 1997) to dealing with abuse and neglect have been adopted. Judicial protection (through the use of courts and orders) is still reserved for cases that cannot be safely managed within the administrative protection process. Indeed, both strategic inter-agency planning and day-to-day procedures for joint working in individual cases have been retained and strengthened. As we will see, social work continues to exercise the investigative, assessment and key work roles once concerns are referred to the children's services authority, and the Children Act 1989 duties still apply.

Whole system reform as a context for child protection

Every Child Matters (DfES 2003b) proposed a radical change to the statutory and organisational context in which child protection was to be practised rather than to the key processes and mechanisms for 'working together' in individual cases. The Green Paper ushered in what was known as a 'whole-system reform' (DfES 2004b, p. 2) of children's services. The intention was to embed the inter-agency child protection system, designed to safeguard the welfare of a relatively small number of abused and neglected children, within a new set of arrangements for providing integrated services for all children. The 'whole systems' approach altered the existing inter-agency child protection process in two main ways:

- by *extending* strategic and frontline joint working responsibilities and arrangements from specialist and targeted services, such as child protection planning, back into universal services and practice settings, including schools and primary health care – the aim here was to improve *early identification*
- by *refocusing* joint working at all levels of service (universal, specialist and targeted) around the support of individual children with 'additional needs' of whatever kind, and their parents – the aim here was the *prevention* of harm and the *active promotion* of well-being.

Whole systems approaches to the reform of public services had already been used in adult social care (Pratt *et al.* 1999, Audit Commission 2002). They were seen as the next stage in the shift along the line from separatism, competition and partnership approaches to service provision (Hudson 2004). The key components (Audit Commission 2002) were:

- a *shared vision* informed by 'service user' views
- a *comprehensive range of services* provided by multiprofessional teams
- *mechanisms* to enable 'service users' to navigate their way through the service system so they received the service they wanted when they needed it.

In the case of children's services, these three aspects were implemented by a combination of legal and managerial changes. The Children Act 2004 provided the 'legislative spine' (DfES 2004b, p. 5) of the reforms. It gave statutory force to the new, shared vision of a child-centred, outcomes-led approach to child welfare services. It sought to ensure arrangements for comprehensive and integrated services by consolidating and strengthening the lead role of the local authority (known now as the children's services authority) for service planning and coordination, whilst requiring a range of partner agencies and professionals to cooperate in communication and service provision. A change management programme, known as *Change for Children* (DfES 2004b), provided a framework for the development of effective local arrangements, to be developed under the auspices of 'children's trusts' (HM Government 2005b). At the heart of these was the extension of the key worker or 'lead professional' role, already widely used in specialist (e.g. disabled children) and targeted (e.g. child protection) services, to a wider group of children with 'additional needs'.

A shared vision: integrated services for improved well-being

The new vision of child protection is integrative and comprehensive. As *Every Child Matters* confirmed, the intention is to ensure 'we properly protect children at risk of neglect and harm within a framework of universal services which aims to prevent negative outcomes and support every child to develop their full potential' (DfES 2003b, p. 13). This resolved a longstanding debate within social work about the focus of services for children. During the 1990s it had been argued that 'child protection' had come to dominate practice at the expense of 'family support' and the case was made for a 'rebalancing' or 'refocusing' of social work (DoH 1995a). The separation of safeguarding/child protection from promoting/family support was proposed, for example by giving the police lead responsibility for investigation and protection (Parton 1997) or by creating a self-standing child protection agency (Kendall & Harker 2002).

Every Child Matters transformed the debate. Rather than concern itself simply with the focus of social work practice with children 'in need' or 'at risk', it concentrated instead on the nature of the outcomes expected for all children, whatever services they received. Instead of seeking to separate 'safeguarding' and 'promoting', and attach professional roles to each of them, the Green Paper proposed the greater integration of both to ensure these outcomes were achieved. The revised *Working Together* guidance (DfES 2005a) set out a cumulative definition of the objectives of child protection and linked this to the five well-being outcomes specified in the Children Act 2004. This served to retain the traditional commitment to minimising risk and harm to children 'in need', whilst embedding it in the contemporary policy of maximising opportunity for all children. Safeguarding and promoting welfare now involved:

- protecting children from maltreatment
- preventing impairment of children's health or development *and*

- ensuring that children are growing up in circumstances consistent with the provision of safe and effective care *and*
- undertaking that role so as to enable those children to have optimum life chances and to enter adulthood successfully.

Whilst the Children Act 2004 itself made no reference to the duty of agencies to promote equality of opportunity and eliminate discrimination, statutory guidance in relation to 'children's trusts' added this perspective (HM Government 2005b).

Strategic arrangements for integrated services

The Children Act 2004 confirmed the lead role of the local authority in planning and coordinating integrated services for children and extended requirements on partner and other agencies to cooperate with these plans and provide their own services in ways that would safeguard and promote child welfare. A new duty requiring the local children's services authority to set up Local Safeguarding Children Boards put local arrangements for coordinating the work of key agencies in relation to child protection onto a statutory footing. Taken together, these duties and powers provided a legislative context within which arrangements to cooperate could be used to facilitate integrated planning, commissioning and delivery of services. The Children Act 2004 itself did not require local authorities and partner agencies to pool budgets or merge their staff and functions, still less to recreate themselves as new agencies. Following consultation on the Green Paper, *Every Child Matters*, the government stepped back from setting out in legislation any new organisational structure for service integration (DfES 2004e).

Instead, the initial approach to integration was through the *Change for Children* programme and the local establishment of 'children's trusts' in each of the 150 children's services authority areas. Whilst a framework for the 'model of whole-system change' (DfES 2004b, p. 6) was designed centrally, its implementation was down to local management. In this way the *Change for Children* programme provided a management model for dealing with the concerns identified in the public policy literature about the gap between central government policy and legislation and local interpretation and action. 'Children's trusts' were intended to facilitate integrated front-line practice, where possible within multi-agency teams, by establishing mechanisms of *inter-agency governance and integrated strategy*. Government guidance emphasised the essential importance of 'robust inter-agency governance arrangements ... to drive the change processes and to create the framework for a new way of working' (HM Government 2005b). Trust Boards were advised, to enable senior managers of partner agencies to support the lead role of the Director of Children's Services. The Children Act 2004 requirement to produce the Children and Young People's Plan provided a focus for an integrated strategy and pooled budgets to enable joint commissioning.

Integrated front-line delivery

Specific mechanisms to ensure *integrated practice* itself, by coordinating intervention around the needs of children, are at the heart of 'children's trust' arrangements and 'whole systems' working. In the same way as the Children Act 2004 consolidated the lead role of the local authority in strategic service integration, the revised *Working Together* guidance (DfES 2005a) confirmed social work in the lead, or key work, role for children referred into the formal child protection process. Also retained was the *Framework for the Assessment of Children in Need and their Families* (DoH *et al.* 2000), now established as the standard tool for identifying need and informing decisions about services and support. Consistent with the core aims of extending front-line joint working responsibilities and arrangements from specialist and targeted services into universal services and practice settings, and refocusing joint working at all levels of service around the support of individual children and their parents, these two mechanisms of key working and standardised assessment were rolled out across children's services.

The *lead professional* role was created to ensure that service integration at the strategic level could be translated into joint working at the level of the individual child. Building on the experience of the key work role in child protection (Hallett 1995) and with disabled children (Townsley *et al.* 2004), the lead professional would provide a single point of contact for a child and family. The task was to support children and parents 'in making choices and in navigating their way through the system' (DfES 2005g, p. 8) as well as playing a more traditional case management and review role. This dual emphasis was in line with the idea, increasingly central in New Labour policy, that children (and their parents) were 'service users' with interests to express and choices to make as well as people with vulnerabilities who had need of direct support or care.

A *Common Assessment Framework* (CAF) (DfES 2004e) was developed with the aim of recording concerns at an earlier stage and have children with 'additional needs' for support referred to the appropriate specialist or targeted service. The success of this new practice tool depended on effective information exchange. A national network of indices of information about all children in the country was to be implemented by 2008 by which time the CAF would be fully in use. Indices would include basic information on each child, details of practitioners working with the child and a means of logging concerns. Common assessment and information sharing, in turn, were to be underpinned by a common core of skills and knowledge, applicable to all practitioners working with children and young people (HM Government 2005d). The intention was to embed a common practice language within children's services through the use of these roles, tools and processes and thereby help break down barriers to integrated working with children maintained by contrasting professional assumptions and practices. It was anticipated not only that children and families would benefit from a single assessment process but also that the reduction of repeat and overlapping procedures would save time and money.

A further assumption was that *new forms of multi-agency working* would emerge whereby different professionals would have their practice integrated not only by the use of common tools and processes but also by physically working more closely together. The co-located team was the preferred model of integrated working and a number of examples were available as the reforms were being introduced. Youth Offending Teams, Sure Start programmes and Behaviour and Support Teams were all offered as possible approaches. A multi-agency 'full service' hub with an integrated management structure and funded by pooled budgets was suggested (DfES 2005h). This full service approach to integration could be based in a local office or centre or in a school. In the latter case the policy of creating 'extended schools', that pre-dated the children's trust, was itself extended to ensure that there was at least one full service school in each local authority (DfES 2005i, Cummings *et al.* 2005).

The implementation of the three elements of the 'whole system' approach we have reviewed here – a joint vision, strategic coordination and integrated practice – puts the process of 'working together' in child protection into a radically new practice context. The narrow and defensive approach criticised in the Laming Report has been replaced by a broad and expansive redefinition of safeguarding and promoting welfare, in which positive outcomes for children are specified. The key duties and powers of the Children Act 1989 have been retained and the lead role of the local authority has been reinforced in relation to the safeguarding and promoting tasks. However, in extending the collaborative duty on agencies and requiring them to exercise it actively to improve the well-being of all children, the Children Act 2004 refocused State intervention. Non-intervention is to be replaced by early, preventive intervention. The *Change for Children* framework provided a model of organisational reform through 'children's trust' arrangements to ensure that children and families get an integrated response when 'additional needs' are identified. In all cases those children and families are now expected to play an active role, not only in negotiations about services and support in their own case but also in the process of service design as a whole.

How will this shift in focus, from a coordinated child protection system towards integrated children's services, affect the experience of practitioners, children and parents brought together by concerns about child safety? What evidence is there that the new approach will be more effective in managing the political, professional and personal tensions inherent in responses to child abuse and neglect?

Working together in integrated children's services: opportunities and risks for child safety and protection

The New Labour reforms consolidate and extend the dual approach to service coordination long established for 'working together' in child protection. New *strategies* for planning and cooperation in local inter-agency networks and new *practices* of joint working in individual cases are being put in place across the 'whole system' of children's services. In this respect two contrasting views about the likely success of the reforms might be expected. First, it might be predicted that the inherent and unsettling personal, professional and political dynamics stirred up by the task of safeguarding children will be further managed out of the system by the intensification of routinised procedures and their dispersal across a wider service terrain. This is similar to the conclusion reached by Parton (Chapter 1, in this volume) and others (Penna 2005) who fear the civil liberties as well as the bureaucratic implications. Alternatively, it might be anticipated that the intrinsic dynamics and conflicts will persistently break through these 'surface' (Cooper 2005a) responses and disrupt the apparent coherence of government plans at both strategic and practice levels. Early experience provides evidence on both sides.

At the *strategic level*, competing political commitments were already emerging within months of the initial implementation of *Change for Children*. On re-election in May 2005 the government embarked on further 'radical' reforms, in which market mechanisms of competitive services and (parental) choice rather than bureaucratic 'whole systems' approaches were placed centre-stage (PricewaterhouseCoopers 2004, HM Government 2005e). Evaluation findings on the early experience of 35 'pathfinder children's trusts' had in any case pointed to the 'sheer scale and complexity of the task' they had set themselves (University of East Anglia 2005, p. 1). With so many potential partners involved, the cost and effort required to develop an effective 'children's trust' called for high-level leadership and formal agreements, especially where there was no strong local tradition of joint working. However, intended partners such as GPs, schools and private sector service providers were already often absent from the process. Even if the resources necessary for the proposed expansion of integrated children's centres (replacing Sure Start programmes), extended schools and local service hubs are forthcoming, it is entirely certain that the political commitment to reassert choice over health and education in the individual case can easily be reconciled with the goal of preventative surveillance and support for children in general. The tension between the two aims reminds us that policy itself continues to embody contested values that might be expected to be played out in local practice.

At the level of *day-to-day practice* it is helpful to consider the early evidence of the impact of the children's services reforms at each stage of the 'working together' process.

Identification, early intervention and referral

The child protection system developed in England and Wales between 1974 and 1997 was criticised for its poor targeting of children. The main summary of government-sponsored research of the period concluded that too many children and families were unnecessarily 'caught up in the child protection process' (DoH 1995a, p. 25). However, a closer reading of individual studies also indicated that many children who were demonstrably being harmed were not effectively identified, supported and protected (Gibbons *et al.* 1995b). Thresholds to social work services and the formal child protection process remained unacceptably high (DfES *et al.* 2003). Victoria Climbié's death was a stark reminder of this. These contrasting findings indicate how important it is that those responsible for identifying children who do need to be made safe (as well as to be supported) have a clear understanding of how to recognise these children and what to do next. The integrated approach attempts to support effective identification not only to improve the referral process into the formal child protection system but also to provide early support to prevent 'additional needs' escalating into 'risk of significant harm'.

With regard to the introduction of a CAF, early research evidence might be seen as encouraging. It suggests that practitioners themselves working in universal services with the estimated three million children with 'additional needs' were keen in principle to switch to a common, holistic approach to the recognition and assessment of concerns (Peel & Ward 2000, Cleaver *et al.* 2004a, 2004c, Cleaver & Nicholson 2005). The introduction of joint training in relation to the 'common core' of skills and knowledge (HM Government 2005d) for all children's services workers might reinforce this shared commitment: just as social work learned to reconfigure the assessment and decision-making process for children 'in need' and 'at risk of harm' around standard frameworks and forms, so too might other children's practitioners.

However, even if practitioners are prepared to import routinised risk management systems into early intervention, practical and ethical issues may not easily be overcome. The *practical constraints* are familiar. There are significant technical challenges involved in the effective embedding of new work processes, especially where integrated ICT systems are concerned. More significant still are the cost implications of integrated early intervention. Even if the identification and referral of concerns is improved by common processes employed within integrated team-working in schools, centres and service hubs, the capacity of agencies and professionals to provide the additional services and support required remains in question. Whilst additional resources have been invested in workforce development, the extent of the ambition of children's services reform means that continued investment in additional and improved preventative services is expected increasingly to come from savings made elsewhere. This is on the assumption that integrated working will reduce costs by minimising overlaps in practice (e.g. by replacing multiple by single assessment). Early preventative intervention will save the cost of expensive remedial interventions later down the line.

It is often said this policy is evidence based and it is certainly the case that integrated early intervention programmes can have long-term cost–benefit effects, as the Headstart programme in the US has demonstrated (Schweinhart *et al.* 2004). There is also accumulating evidence about the elements of effective interventions in individual cases at all stages of childhood (Moran *et al.* 2004). The *Every Child Matters* early intervention and integrated services approach is consistent with these findings in general terms. However, careful study of the evidence reminds us that programmes and interventions are successful for children living in conditions of adversity only when service quality and professional skills are high (Melhuish 2004) and intervention is focused and consistent (Moran *et al.* 2004). As we have said, there is as yet no sound evidence that integrated working itself, led by a key worker or lead professional, actually results in improved child welfare outcomes (Sloper 2004). In these circumstances, where aspirations and responsibilities for improved child well-being are increased but resources are constrained, it might be anticipated that practitioners and managers will continue to act defensively.

The *ethical uncertainties* of active early intervention have also impeded initial progress towards integrated practice. Much of the research on early intervention assumes additional services will be welcomed by children and parents, whilst conceding that some of them will be 'hard to reach'. However, where those interventions are designed to identify risks to child safety, their capacity to reassure children and parents and to generate confidence and trust are of crucial importance. In this respect information-sharing arrangements have become the focus of particular concern. Leaving aside the sheer practicalities of establishing the kind of ICT capacity necessary to provide an index of all children that does actually provide the means of logging and communicating concerns, contrasting professional traditions of information gathering and exchange can be expected to continue to influence practice on a case-by-case basis.

As an example, during the period when the new *Working Together* guidance (DfES 2005a) was being drawn up, concerns about the risk to children of predatory sex offenders were heightened. This followed the Soham murders and the publication of the Bichard Report (Bichard Inquiry Report 2004), in which the failure of a police authority to properly record and share information about the known risks posed by Ian Huntley, the murderer of the two girls, was highlighted. This shifted the balance of the child protection response generally away from the principle of confidentiality to protect individual rights to privacy towards that of automatic information exchange to prevent risk and enhance child protection. As a result, local agencies began to draw up protocols that required practitioners to report to the police information they had from children and others about underage sexual activity (Munro 2005a). This raised questions once again about whose information this was and to what purpose it could legitimately be put by professionals. It also emphasised how conflicting social and political objectives (rights to privacy/rights to protection) changed the nature of the relationship between a child or young person and a professional responsible for managing concerns raised about them. Unsurprisingly, the shift towards a criminal justice response to protection angered health professionals, who traditionally prioritise the right to confidentiality of patients, including children (Ward 2005).

The *status* of information in relation to concerns about a child will remain a significant issue for day-to-day practice. The studies by Cleaver *et al.* (2004a, 2004c, 2005) of the initial trialing of the new information sharing and assessment (ISA) system showed how practitioners wanted access to simple and unequivocal guidance, especially legal advice, on what information people should share in which circumstances. However, it is not at all clear either that simple rules will be agreed in the face of competing political and professional principles or that rules will, or ought to, diminish disputes in individual cases.

The *meaning* of information is as equally contested as its status and ownership when concerns about children emerge. As we have seen, the research on the nature of professional judgement in circumstances where information is partial, uncertain and ambiguous shows how decisions about risk and response can get skewed. It is not unusual for common errors of reasoning to be exacerbated by the emotionally and ethically stressful nature of the child protection task (Munro 2002, Cooper 2005a, Rustin 2005). Research on the use of standardised practice tools, such as the *Framework for Assessment*, shows that structured approaches to identifying and assessing concerns do not in themselves solve the problem of making an informed judgement (Cleaver *et al.* 2004b, Cleaver & Nicholson 2005). As well as gathering and recording information, practitioners must be able to analyse it. Early identification in the case of Victoria Climbié failed not only because facts were not recorded and shared accurately but also because conflicting and avoidant interpretations of those facts were made by different professionals with contrasting roles and responsibilities. It may be that improved training (Reder & Duncan 2004) will enhance the analytical skills of front-line practitioners, especially where training is based on a common core of skills and knowledge. Professional skill and authority can create the conditions of trust needed for children and parents to share information too. Nonetheless, the evidence is that contrasting interpretations about the meaning to be attached to the facts gathered are pervasive (White & Featherstone 2005). This will be likely to affect how concerns, particularly about child safety, are identified and communicated, especially where decisions are made under pressure.

Assessment and protection

Where concerns are referred for a social work initial assessment and a decision about immediate protection, the long-established 'working together' procedures remain in place. Prior to the move towards an integrated approach, research and experience had shown that the initial social work assessment was likely to put considerations of service eligibility before those of child need. For example, the Laming Report criticised social services departments for spending 'a lot of time and energy devising ways of limiting access to services, and adopting mechanisms designed to reduce service demand' (Laming Report 1993, para. 1.52). Two joint inspection reports (Commission for Social Care Inspection 2005a, DoH 2002a) showed that social workers were maintaining very high thresholds to initial assessment and protection, only responding to cases indicating very high risk of harm. Specific groups of children, such as disabled children, older children and those living away from home, were given a low priority. The primary reason for high thresholds appeared to be a lack of social work staff and this put pressure on children, families and referring professionals alike to manage difficult situations without formal social work support.

In itself, integrated working will not solve this problem. Arguably the intended improvements to early identification of concerns might increase rather than decrease the pressure of referrals on the formal protection process and the social work service. The initial evidence from Sure Start suggests that this is not a foregone conclusion (Carpenter *et al.* 2005) and there will be a counterpressure to hold concerns within universal services, managed by the new lead professional role.

Nonetheless, until effective preventative interventions are developed at this level (or definitions of risk and harm to children relaxed) it is difficult to see why education, health and other front-line practitioners will want to take on greater responsibility for child protection when the existing 'working together' procedures must be used (DfES 2005g) and the lead role passed on to the social worker.

Planning

No substantive changes to the formal arrangements for the negotiation of protection plans have been made as a result of the children's services reforms. The system of child protection conferences and plans has remained in place despite suggestions that more participative means of negotiation, decision making and planning about protection and support could have been introduced (Cooper *et al.* 2003). Only the child protection registration process has altered, with the proposed social care record for all children replacing the specific child protection register for a few. Research findings continue to show that children and parents find participation difficult to achieve in the formal child protection process (Cleaver & Freeman 1995, Commission for Social Care Inspection 2005b). Children and parents must now be advised that they can attend case conferences and bring an advocate, friend or supporter but the legalistic and managerial focus of the decision-making and planning process persists.

Intervention and review

Once a protection plan has been agreed for a child, the conference must make recommendations about how agencies, professionals and family members should continue to work together. The social worker remains the key worker, and hence becomes the lead professional, and the core group is still the means by which the inter-agency protection plan and core assessment that underpins it is implemented. The formal review process follows.

Previous research demonstrated the extent to which inter-agency working, significant and effective at the early stages in routine cases, dissipated once the child's name was registered, the protection plan agreed and the social services department had taken on the key work role (Farmer & Owen 1995). It remains to be seen whether the new statutory framework will lead to the prioritising of joint working and targeting of additional resources required if the social work service is to be adequately supported in its lead professional role in protective intervention. First, there is clearly tension between the simultaneous demands for additional resources of early intervention services and specialist and targeted protective interventions. The hope of government, that increased investment in services such as Sure Start would lead to reduced demand for 'more intensive support' (DfES 2003b), has yet to be borne out in practice (Carpenter *et al.* 2005).

Next, there is also a good deal of research evidence to suggest that the development of more seamless models of teamworking is not a straightforward process. For example, the co-location of multi-agency professionals is only likely to succeed in achieving continuous and effective joint working if certain conditions are achieved. Separate professional, as well as shared inter-professional, roles and responsibilities need to be respected and supported, clear leadership has to be provided and adequate and reliable funding secured (Cameron & Lart 2003, Sloper 2004). Even so, it is important to remember that the integration of children's services may turn out to be at the expense of the fragmentation of other cross-agency relationships. The risk to effective joint working between adult services for parents with mental health problems and children's services has already been identified in research (Stanley *et al.* 2003, Stevenson 2005a).

Finally, there is evidence that the lead professional, or key work, role itself can impede rather than enhance effective joint intervention with children and families. In particular, research in the US has demonstrated that centralising service decisions about a child in a single case manager role can lead other professionals to reduce their own personal responsibility for involvement (Glisson & Hemmelgarn 1998). This tendency has already been detected in the English and Welsh system, where routinised working together may be effective in maintaining local inter-agency social networks but at the expense of any real shared responsibility (Hallett 1995, Glennie 2003). In these circumstances, if the key worker role is concerned mainly with coordination rather than with the development and maintenance of a personal helping relationship with the child and family, joint working can actually reduce the effectiveness of subsequent intervention. Similar findings for integrated working with disabled children have been reported, where the need of children and families for relationship-based support as well as practical service coordination is emphasised (Townsley *et al.* 2004).

These latter findings get to the heart of the problem with the *Change for Children* reform programme because they remind us of the extent to which the unruly emotional and demanding relational aspects of service reform have been displaced by the relentless concern with formal roles and procedures. This leads Cooper (2005a, p. 9) to call for:

a new kind of policy making ... one that is informed from start to finish by a concern to sustain connections between the fine grain of the transactions we ask staff and their managers to engage in, and the management and development of systems and structures.

Conclusion

We know that, despite the development of a sophisticated inter-agency child protection system in England and Wales over a 30-year period, significant numbers of children continue to be abused and neglected inside and outside their family home (May-Chahal & Cawson 2005). The New Labour reforms of children's services seek to safeguard and promote the welfare of these children by integrating professional responses where there are concerns about child well-being. Existing inter-agency responsibilities for 'working together' within the formal child protection system have been strengthened. This system, in turn, is more firmly embedded within a new set of statutory arrangements for joint working for early intervention and prevention. The objectives of the reforms are hugely ambitious, directly linking interventions to ensure child safety in cases such as Victoria Climbié with a programme of social investment designed to socially include all children and prepare them as active future citizens.

We have reviewed the likely opportunities for improving child safety and the possible risks associated with the reforms. One risk is that integrated services will extend professional communication and coordination at the expense of civil liberties. An alternative argument is that the very recognition of this risk, combined with the inflated social ambition yet narrow managerial focus of the reforms, will mean that emotional and ethical, and political and professional conflicts will continue to characterise child welfare practice, however much organisations defend against these dynamics. Resources will fail to match ambitions and disputes over both the status and meaning of information and the responsibility for managing the concerns conveyed will persist. In either case, on the evidence of traditional 'working together' practices, the increasingly pervasive and intensive routinisation of procedures may more or less contain and control concerns about children but at the expense of creating those conditions necessary for the development of the authentic and effective personal and professional engagements that were so absent in the case of Victoria Climbié. It is difficult to see how current children's services reform as it stands will provide the means by which children and parents might feel able to confide in the professionals about what is really going on in their lives and the professionals feel personally able to hear and respond to those concerns. Unfortunately, like the Laming Report recommendations that preceded the reform programme, it is this crucial consideration that has, once again, tended to be lost from sight in policy.

Key points and messages for practice

- Do not take government policy rhetoric at face value. Governments have to manage competing political demands and the 'whole systems' integrated services agenda may well be compromised by the marketisation of individual choice in health and education. In any case, adequate resources for change are not secure.

- Remember that structural and procedural responses to systems failures are double-edged. They can provide a measure of appropriate routine and response in inter-professional and inter-agency practice but they can also consolidate defensive and avoidant relationships.

- Effective communication and coordination are founded in relationships characterised by emotional attunement and a reflective 'mindset'. Policy for integrated services is largely silent on these matters.

- Conflict is intrinsic to child protection. Make sure you have arrangements in place to explore how it is affecting your practice with children, parents and other professionals.

Annotated further reading

Cooper A, Lousada J 2005 Borderline welfare. Feeling and fear of feeling in modern welfare. The Tavistock Clinic Series. Karnac, London
   This book presents a psychoanalytical account of avoidant professional practice in child welfare. It develops the trenchant exploration of the Victoria Climbié Report in Cooper (2005a); see also Rustin (2005).

Hallett C, Birchall E 1992 Coordination and child protection: a review of the literature. HMSO, Edinburgh
   This is a comprehensive review that provides a foundation for understanding why and how 'mandated coordination' developed as the means of 'working together' in child protection in England and Wales.

Reder P, Duncan S, Gray M 1993 Beyond blame: child abuse tragedies revisited. Routledge, London
   Together with their subsequent book, Lost Innocents: a Follow-up Study of Fatal Child Abuse *(Routledge, London, 1999), this book provides a powerful insight into the ways in which professionals failed to develop the 'communicative mindset' needed for safe practice in serious cases.*

Thistlethwaite P 2004 Integrated working: a guide. Online. Available: www.integratedcarenetwork.gov.uk
   This guide, along with others produced by the Integrated Care Network, provides a good source of information from a policy perspective on the managerial aspirations and challenges of the shift towards service integration.

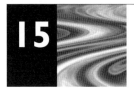

Safeguarding children and case conferences

Margaret Bell

INTRODUCTION

Case conferences are crucial tools in the management of children in need of protection. Indeed, despite criticisms of their unhelpful focus on risk assessment and the policy shifts toward a more overtly welfare-based child protection service, guidance under the Children Act 1989 (DoH 2000d) and more recently the Children Act 2004 (DfES 2005c), has confirmed the pivotal role of the initial child protection conference within the system. It remains an inter-agency meeting, held after Section 47 enquiries leading to the completion of the Outcome of s.47 enquiries Record (DoH 2002a) have established that a child may suffer, or be at risk of suffering, significant harm, where:

> those family members, the child where appropriate, and those professionals most involved with the child and the family, meet to ... analyze in a multi-disciplinary setting ... all relevant information, to make judgements about the likelihood of a child suffering significant harm in future and to ... plan how to safeguard the child and promote his or her welfare.
>
> (DoH 1999c, p. 69)

At the same time, in cases where children's safety can be assured, the guidance (DfES 2005c) recommends greater use of meetings 'of involved professionals and family members' (para. 4.62) where action plans are established and services provided. Such developments are to be welcomed as part of the broader based framework for meeting children's welfare needs. However, many of the complex issues in the management of conferences and other meetings in child protection remain. This chapter will, therefore, describe the background to the current situation and explore some of the main areas of continuing debate in relation to the purpose and scope of these conferences – including pre- and post-registration practice, assessments of risk and need, professional roles and responsibilities and the experiences of the participants. It will draw, in particular, upon the research of Farmer and Owen (1995), Thoburn *et al.* (1995), a research study undertaken by Bell of 83 initial child protection conferences in a northern city (Bell 1999), and another reporting 27 children's experiences of child protection investigations (Bell 2000b).

Background

Case conferences to register children at risk of abuse were set up following the publication of the Maria Colwell Inquiry Report in 1974. However, their central role within the child protection system, the status of the child protection register and its purposes remained ambiguous until 1988 when *Working Together** (DoH *et al.*

---

* The most up-to-date version of this document was published by HM Government in 2006. For a full discussion of this, see Chapter 11.

1991) made it clear that the primary function of the initial child protection conference was to provide 'a forum for the exchange of information between professionals'. Following the Children Act 1989, *Working Together* (DoH *et al.* 1991) confirmed that the initial conference was an essential component in protecting children. Inviting parents and children to take part in the meeting was advocated, and more detailed guidance on how to involve families was provided to Area Child Protection Committees by the *Challenge of Partnership* (DoH 1995b). Also in 1995 a number of research studies on the workings of the child protection system were published (DoH 1995a) and these have profoundly influenced the development of policy and practice.

On the positive side, the research studies confirmed the successful role of the initial conference in protecting from further harm children who were registered. In examining 120 conferences in two authorities, Farmer and Owen (1995) found that, 20 months after registration, 70% of the children were considered to be protected and in 68% of cases the child's welfare needs were met. At the same time, however, the research raised grave concerns at the shortcomings of the system. The work of Gibbons *et al.* (1995b) demonstrated that large numbers of children were filtered out of the child protection process at different stages without their needs being addressed. They concluded that since only one-quarter of abuse enquiries reached conference and, of those, approximately one-third were not registered, more flexible responses to child abuse referrals should be developed so that appropriate help could be provided. Other research studies clearly demonstrated that, as far as the families were concerned, the experience of the investigation overall and of being present in the meeting was often traumatic. Cleaver and Freeman (1995), Thoburn *et al.* (1995) and Bell (1999) concluded that more constructive ways of involving families in the conference needed to be established and that, wherever possible, other means of protecting children and of meeting their wider welfare needs should be found. Added to concerns raised by the research, Social Service Inspectors found variable practice, poor management of family involvement, poor quality of assessments and unclear child protection plans (Social Services Inspectorate 1997a). *Working Together to Safeguard Children** (DoH 2000d) endeavoured to respond to the strengths and shortcomings of the existing system by confirming the centrality of the initial conference while also defining the situations in which other routes for meeting children's needs might be used both prior to and after the initial conference. The death of Victoria Climbié in 2002, however, reactivated concerns about the assessment and management of children at risk of abuse. While the ensuing Laming Report (2003) determined that the difficulties related to the interpretation of the law, rather than the law itself, the need to promote more effective preventative services informed the recommendations in the subsequent Green Paper *Every Child Matters* (DfES 2003b) and the Children Act 2004. A key recommendation was the replacement of the child protection register with a more effective system: 'the focus should be on establishing an agreed plan' (p. 13) and, from 2007, registration on the child protection register will be replaced by the child becoming the subject of a child protection plan.

The present situation

Where there are child protection concerns and s.47 enquiries suggest that there is reasonable cause to suspect that a child is suffering, or is likely to suffer, significant

---

* The most up-to-date version of this document was published by HM Government in 2006. For a full discussion of this, see Chapter 11.

harm, a case conference may be held. Recent guidance (DfES 2005c) supports the earlier guidance in recommending that the professionals and the family members involved should first have 'a strategy discussion' to decide on the need for emergency action, further enquiries and the provision of interim services and support. In cases where the child's safety can be assured – for example, where the perpetrator has left the household – interventions other than proceeding to an initial child protection conference are encouraged. Family group conferences (paras 9.11–14) or other meetings are seen as providing possible alternatives.

However, where concerns are substantiated, an initial child protection conference should be held within 15 working days of the strategy discussion. Under the Children Act 2004, s.14(1), Local Safeguarding Children Boards replace Area Child Protection Committees, and are required to provide protocols specifying a required quorum for attendance, a list of who should attend and to lay out the method of decision making. An Initial Child Protection Conference Report (DoH 2002a) should be provided by the local authority social worker on each child under consideration, and other professionals should also contribute information, preferably in writing. (Note that *Working Together to Safeguard Children* (HM Government 2006a) has now adopted throughout the guidance the terminology of 'local authority children's social care department' (LACSCD) as the term for the body responsible in the local authority for delivering services to children and for providing for their protection under the various statutory duties laid upon local authorities under the CA 1989 and under the administrative guidance laid down in *Working Together* and other associated documents.)

The purpose of the initial conference is twofold: to consider whether the child is at continuing risk of significant harm and, if so, whether safeguarding the child requires inter-agency help and intervention delivered through a formal, detailed child protection plan. If both of these criteria are satisfied, the chair should determine which category(ies) of abuse or neglect the child has suffered. Currently a child protection register is held in each area and, where a decision is made to register a child, the category of abuse and details are recorded. In 2004, the number of children registered was 27 800, the largest category being neglect (41%) and the lowest sexual abuse (9%). However, following the concerns raised by Lord Laming that registration provides a false sense of security, and taking into account evidence that professionals do not reliably make checks (Greenfields & Statham 2004), from 2007 registers in England will be disbanded. Instead, the child(ren) will be made the subject of a child protection plan which should identify the risk factors, establish short- and long-term aims and objectives, and identify which professionals are responsible for what, and within specified timescales (DfES 2005c).

Each LACSCD is required to set up a social care IT system which will have an electronic care record for every known child. When the child is the subject of a child protection plan this will be recorded, so that all 'legitimate' agencies and professionals can obtain the relevant information. This information system will be supported by the Integrated Children's System which is currently being piloted in eight LACSCDs in England and Wales, and which is intended to support integrated assessments and information sharing across agencies by its electronic database. The child protection plan made at the conference should nominate an experienced social worker and, 10 days later, a 'core group' meeting should take place where a more detailed plan is operationalised, written agreements made and timescales appropriate to the child(ren) established. Within 35 working days a comprehensive assessment consistent with guidance in the *Framework for the Assessment of Children in Need and their Families* (DoH 2000e) should be undertaken. Within 3 months, and every 6 months thereafter, a review conference should be held to consider the child's developmental progress, against the intended outcomes, and de-registration is encouraged as soon as the child protection issues are resolved. The Integrated Children's System provides a number of electronic records (exemplars) for each stage of the process where all this information will be recorded.

This framework for child protection decision making thus represents a clear response to the concerns identified in *Messages from Research* (DoH 1995a) and in the Laming Report (2003), that the sharp focus on risk assessment which the conferences have traditionally assumed should be balanced with attention to the welfare needs of all family members. Whether the framework of the proposed system, including the abandonment of the register and the use of the Integrated Children's System, supports this shift in focus is a matter for debate. As Armstrong (1997) suggested, the requirement to merge child protection into the wider canvas of services for children has, at local level, produced confusion and a blurring of boundaries. In responding to a mass of other government initiatives – not all of which run in tandem – some authorities have neither the commitment nor the funding to resource the development of pre- and post-registration services alongside the development of universal, preventative, community-based services. The worry is that children diverted from the conference may remain unprotected, a concern reinforced by recent research on Sure Start which concluded 'the utilization of services by those with greater human capital left others with less access to services than would have been the case had they not lived in Sure Start areas' (Melhuish *et al.* 2005). At the same time it is unclear at this stage how the identification of children at risk, or increased service provision to them, will be enhanced by the move from registration to a child protection plan. The hope is that plans will be more detailed, owned by all the professionals involved and result in better resourced service provision.

To explore some of these issues in more detail I shall address the following core dimensions of the initial conference, and the related issues for other conferences in child protection:

- purpose – collecting and analysing information and making judgements of significant harm
- the social work role
- the experiences of parents and children
- the child protection plan and subsequent core group meetings and family group conferences.

Purpose

The objectives of conferences in child protection are to share and analyse the information presented, to make judgements about the likelihood of a child suffering significant harm and to decide, with the parents, family members and the child, the most appropriate future action. The initial conference has the additional task of deciding whether or not to place the child's name on the child protection register or, from 2007, to put in place a child protection plan. Each of these objectives is intrinsically problematic – in particular for the initial conference. Some arise from difficulties external to the conferences themselves, others from the complexity of the group process. First, I will discuss issues concerning the collection of information before the conference, and then explore some factors affecting the presentation and analysis of information within the conference.

Information collecting

It hardly needs saying that the quality of the decisions made by the conference is determined by the quality of the information made available to it. As reported above, there are concerns about the level of skill and expertise of the social workers undertaking assessments and the quality of information presented (Social Services Inspectorate 1997a). The Department of Health addressed this by the more detailed guidance in the Assessment Framework (DoH 2000e), by the introduction of the post-qualifying child care award in 2000 and by the guidance following the Children Act 2004 – *Working Together to Safeguard Children* (DfES 2005c). While early research on the use of the Assessment Framework (Cleaver *et al.* 2004b) suggests that initial and core assessments are improving, and that the Assessment Framework improves inter-agency collaboration and parental involvement, Horwath and Morrison (2000) are more sceptical, reporting that practitioners do not pay equal attention to all three domains of the triangle: 'parenting capacity and social context are marginalised'. It remains to be seen whether the new Integrated Children's System – comprising exemplars held on a database – provides the means for better and more analytical recording by social workers or can promote better inter-agency information sharing. At the end of the day it is likely to be the capacity of the authorities to manage and fund the technology, as well as the skills of the professionals, that will determine the use of the Integrated Children's System.

Whatever the system, the fact remains that the task of collecting and processing information for an assessment is immensely difficult. One of the difficulties in collecting information is in accessing family members. Bell (1999) interviewed 22 social workers about their initial assessments and found only three believed they had seen most of the child's primary attachment figures and only six had seen the child alone before the conference. Farmer and Owen (1995) reported a similar pattern. The social workers explained that this was because some of the adults were violent, some had mental health problems, some were not cooperative and sometimes language was a barrier. Other difficulties more recently identified surround the differences in approach and culture between adult mental health and child protection practitioners involved with the family (Tye & Precey 1999). Calder and Horwath (1999) suggest that collecting information can be particularly difficult from families from ethnic minorities, who construct barriers of secrecy because of their fear of racially motivated interventions. This is worrying since children from ethnic minorities are disproportionately represented in child protection registrations (Chand 2000). As Farmer and Owen (1995) suggest, in practice social work staff do not have sufficient understanding of cultural diversity, the effects of which – graphically illustrated in the case of Victoria Climbié – include poor engagements, poor assessments and delays in decision making (Ward *et al.* 2003).

There is increasing awareness that the emotional impact of the work (e.g. fear of violence) affects who is seen and what information is processed (Bell 2000a). Gibbons *et al.* (1995b) reported the presence of domestic violence in 27% of their sample of approximately 2000 child protection referrals. Farmer and Owen (1995) report higher rates. Milner (1996) found that social workers often failed to record the existence of violence in case notes or to report it to conferences, concluding that professional responses could be driven by the fear of intimidation and harassment, sometimes of a sexual nature. Edleson (1999) records a 30–60% co-occurrence of domestic violence and physical abuse in his review of studies. A more recent Australian investigation (Briggs *et al.* 2004) revealed that workers across a range of professions working with children were subjected to a variety of stressful and damaging behaviours that led to physical and psychological illness and 'burn out'. In analysing Inquiry Reports, Munro (1998) found that social workers 'lost' key bits of information and failed to make connections between the abuse of mothers and risk to children.

In so far as the children are concerned, workers may also avoid talking to them. The case of Victoria Climbié is a classic example, where, despite being known to a number of agencies over several months, no professional engaged her in any meaningful conversation. Laming identified a number of reasons for this, including the need for an interpreter and concerns about compromising future investigations (Laming Report 2003, p. 244). The social worker said she did not feel adequately trained – and there is evidence that practitioners lack the skill, confidence or knowledge to communicate with children, in particular children with communication difficulties such as disability or language.

It seems likely that avoidance and denial are among the strategies for managing the anxiety provoked by these transactions. The emotional response of the worker should, of course, be addressed in supervision so that its significance in the overall assessment can be considered. However, reports suggest that lack of managerial support is common and that the quality and quantity of supervision is often inadequate (Social Services Inspectorate 1997a). Concerns about staff recruitment and retention and inadequate resource provision are clearly relevant, and are being addressed by the workforce reforms laid out in *Every Child Matters* (DfES 2004a) and the establishment of a Children's Workforce Unit. The difficulties extend beyond social work to the other key professions; currently about one-third of posts for doctors designated for safeguarding children are vacant.

There is also evidence that social workers lack confidence in selecting information which is key to the conference. The research commonly describes how the focus of enquiry was on the incident of abuse, with less attention paid to family background or environmental factors which could provide explanations. In cases where families were already known to social services – 41% in Bell's (1999) study, two-thirds in that of Thoburn *et al.* (1995) – the social workers relied on information on file. However, Thoburn *et al.* (1995) found that social work files were unreliable sources of information on family circumstances in the year prior to referral – for example, a serious loss by death or divorce was not recorded. Munro's (1999) study of child abuse enquiry reports between 1973 and 1994 also noted professional failure to take a longer-term perspective and that past history was not used to assess current functioning. Farmer (1999) provides further evidence that constructions of risk made during the initial investigation were carried into the conference, fed into decisions about registration, influenced intervention strategies and were rarely questioned, even in reviews.

A number of factors, therefore, affect what information is collected, as well as the ways in which it is recorded, prioritised and presented. Other professionals, equally, may miss important bits of information, neglect to present them to the conference or fail to attend. The sparse attendance of general practitioners (GPs) at conferences has long been a source of concern. Polnay (2000) reports that nearly 50% of the GPs in her postal survey accorded child protection conferences low priority and could not spare the time to attend. Professional perspectives also influence expressions of concern and the ways in which these are prioritised (Cleaver & Freeman 1995). For example, in constructing a diagnosis of neglect, professionals from different agencies may apply different indicators of vulnerability. In such cases, health visitors are more likely to prioritise hygiene, whereas doctors look at bruises, teachers at learning difficulties and social workers at parenting skills.

Sharing information

Problems about quality coexist with matters of process and interpretation, some of which arise from the difficulties of inter-agency communication, some from poor training and support and some from the presence of family members in the conference. There now exists a substantial body of literature exploring the ways in which inter-professional communications are affected by issues of status and power. Hallett (1995) described how professionals, such as teachers who may only attend one conference in their career, do not feel part of the 'inner core' and hence believe their contribution is unimportant, or feel inhibited in speaking. This creates confusion because while these attenders feel they lack the knowledge and experience necessary, their contribution is perceived by others – particularly the children – to be very important. Other professionals, such as health visitors and school nurses who play a key part in the safety of younger children, struggle to be assertive in the conference which they experience as being dominated by social services. In the Victoria Climbié Inquiry, Laming also identified that 'status inequality' meant nurses felt their views were less important than those of other professionals (Laming Report 2003). Baginsky's work on teachers (2000a, 2003a; see also Baginsky and Green, Chapter 17, in this volume) also highlights the confusion and lack of information teachers have about child protection procedures, despite the fact that over half of them had been involved in at least one child protection conference. In some cases criminal proceedings are being pursued and this also alters the dynamics of the conference. Cooper *et al.* (2003) suggest that inter-professional trust is built up by positive personal experience which may be difficult to promote in a meeting where people do not know one another. Differing views on confidentiality compound the difficulties. In an attempt to decrease the dominance of social services, authorities employ chairpersons who are independent of line management. In any event, a skilled chairperson who commands authority and has good leadership skills is essential to the effective functioning of the conference.

It is generally accepted (see Thoburn *et al.* 1995, Bell 1999) that the presence of family members in the conference improves the quality of information available. Family members add to it and clarify key details, while the professionals are more rigorous and accurate in what they say. However, these benefits have to be balanced against some of the difficulties which have been identified. Some of the professionals in Bell's (1999) study found it difficult to express negative views about the family in front of them, fearing this might alienate parents and endanger their capacity to protect the child. From a health visitor:

I feel other information may have been presented and considered regarding the child's home situation, especially mother's lack of protective skills, if she had not been there. (p. 120)

At the same time, parents objected to information about their family background being shared in the conference, as well as to the professional interpretation of some events or behaviours as abusive. This was also inhibiting. *Every Child Matters* (DfES 2004a) suggests that, since the implementation of the Data Protection Act 1998 and the Human Rights Act 1998, professionals have even greater concerns about sharing information in front of the parents. Additionally, in some conferences, the family's presence was found to be distracting when they became upset, and there were logistic problems in managing conferences where, for example, the parents were separated and had secrets from one another or in situations of domestic violence. The role of the chairperson in managing these situations is key, but, again, they are dependent upon the quality of information made available before the conference to judge how these situations might best be managed, including whether anyone should be excluded. The guidance recommends that family members should only be excluded if there is risk of violence or intimidation. However, this information is not always known to the professionals before the conference.

Analysing information

Through experience and training professionals can become more experienced and skilled in presenting information which the family may not like to hear. However, there is evidence that they lack confidence in interpreting and analysing it. Howe (1999) has pointed out that collecting pieces of the puzzle is not enough: 'pieces have to be in place for pictures and patterns to be seen … and then move on to the analysis' (p. 195). There is continuing concern about the poor analysis of information and the absence of theoretical application. As described above, the focus is on describing incidents of abuse or neglect, with concerns accumulating, but with little evidence that the dynamics of the family situation or the social context have been analysed in relation either to causation or to the making of a protection plan. In considering why social workers are more interested in what has happened than why, Stevenson's (1995) conjecture that social workers deny the significance of socio-economic forces is supported by the research. Farmer and Owen (1995) and Gibbons *et al.* (1995b) found little reference to material factors relevant to the family situation. In the conferences in Bell's (1999) study, observation suggested that the social workers became uncomfortable when families described appalling social conditions which they could do nothing about. At the same time, Stevenson suggests, social workers who may be more willing to explore the dynamics of family functioning have lost confidence in, or understanding of, theories which might facilitate this. The move toward case management may increase uncertainty in this area because it requires less involvement in assessment of and direct work with families. Stevenson concludes that situations in which neither material circumstances nor family dynamics are adequately explored 'is the worst of both worlds and that the conference is operating with little or no explicit content and with little discussion of causation, of whatever kind' (p. 230).

Inter-agency processes also contribute to the lack of debate in the conference about aetiology. I have already identified some of the ways in which disagreements in the conference were suppressed. The professionals said they thought it important to present a united front to the parents and in some cases suppressed disagreement or diluted the negatives. The investigating social workers reported that decisions about registration were made beforehand and only rarely changed as a result of information heard in the conference. Hallett (1995) also noted an absence of dissent and conflict between the different professionals, concluding that there was a tacit agreement to avoid deeper differences in the way situations were perceived. Corby *et al.* (1996) provide evidence that parents are also inhibited from disagreeing with the professionals. The imbalance of power makes it difficult for them to speak and they fear making a bad impression. They conclude that the process of removing conflict from the conference, added to the parents' belief that the decision had already been made, is more likely to alienate parents and make them apathetic than to empower them. In the 110 conferences studied, the chairperson had a key role in encouraging and supporting the expression of different views and in managing conflict constructively, but was not always successful in achieving this.

All this suggests that the conference's primary function – to share and analyse information – is secondary to its instrumental function of managing professional anxiety in this highly charged area of risk. The idea of the conference offering mutual support in anxiety-provoking situations is not new. In 1980, Hallett and Stevenson accepted this as a valid part of the process. Farmer and Owen (1995) also suggest that the formality of the conference and the routinisation of the procedures serve to distance the participants from the emotional impact of the distressing information that had emerged during the investigation. However, while managing anxiety may provide an important function, the push to consensus makes it more likely that the chairperson supports the already determined registration recommendation from the social worker. While many chairpersons are highly experienced and skilled operators, a possible consequence is that the conference decision may not be owned by other professionals in the conference group. This will have implications for post-registration commitment. It will also influence the way in which the family – who are present but do not contribute to the registration decision – perceive the roles and responsibilities of the different professionals in subsequent meetings.

Judgements of significant harm

Clearly, a number of interconnected and complex factors affect the collection, sharing and analysis of information that is presented to the conference. However, chairpersons report that, even where information is shared openly, many of the professionals present in the conference shrink from giving an opinion on registration. The guidance detailing the process and content of 'Information for the Conference' emphasises the need to 'take care to distinguish between fact, observation, allegation and opinion'. However, it does not suggest how this can be done. Some of the problems here are philosophical – how are 'facts' defined, and how can moral judgements be justified? Much has been written about the moral nature of the discourse in child protection work (Wattam 1992; see also Parton, Chapter 1, in this volume).

The overview in *Messages from Research* (DoH 1995a) describes very clearly the ways in which thresholds for determining abuse differ historically and culturally and, as we have seen, they may also differ between practitioners in the conference. The rates of children on and added to registers, and the categories used, vary regionally (Gibbons *et al.* 1995b) and over time. For example, in 1997 the number of children registered under the category of neglect and emotional abuse is significantly higher than in 1993, whereas there was a reduction in the categories of physical and sexual abuse. However, there is little evidence of change in the way the threshold criteria are being applied. Since 1997, the number of children registered annually has remained fairly steady, at around 30 000. It is to be hoped that a positive outcome of the demise of the register in 2007 will be that the child protection plan is owned by all the key professionals in a way that registration is not.

There are real problems in distinguishing between fact, observation, allegation and opinion as well as in determining when the threshold of significant harm has been reached – or, indeed, how 'significant' is to be defined. Ayre (1998) reports that health professionals receive little guidance in judging what constitutes significant harm. Judgements of significant harm also require that culpability and intent are addressed. In cases of physical abuse and sexual abuse the medical evidence may be unequivocal in so far as the injuries and incident and the identity of the abuser are concerned. By contrast, in situations of marital breakdown or domestic violence, the children may suffer emotional abuse which is not identified because it remains hidden and is not the result of a specific act directed at the children (Bell 2003).

In cases of neglect there are unique difficulties in agreeing on the benchmark and in determining cause and effect. It is difficult to substantiate – it happens over time, although the conference agenda is built around a snapshot of the present – and proving intentionality or culpability may be implausible in the context of the environmental disadvantage in which many of these families exist. The following quote from one of the mothers in Bell's (1999) study well illustrates the gap between what parents and professionals consider to be abusive:

> I do smack my children, and I believe in smacking them. But I love them. I try to keep them clean, but it's impossible where we live. And how would you manage as a single parent with three boys under 5, no money and a stinking damp house? (p. 164)

Dingwall *et al.* (1983) suggested that intention should be one of the three types of evidence used to confirm child abuse – the others being the child's clinical condition and the nature of their social environment. The research has demonstrated, however, some of the ways in which information is presented as evidence and then used to construe responsibility or culpability for the abuse. Again, this raises issues about fitness for purpose. I have already suggested that the conference has an instrumental function which gets in the way of its primary purpose. Here I am suggesting that the conference is fulfilling a quasi-judicial function which is potentially unjust. The family members can hear what is said and contribute but – unlike the LACSCD – they do not have legal representation and are not well positioned to dispute 'the facts' or question professional opinion. Additionally, my interviews revealed that they are unclear about the basis of the registration decision and that the nature of their subsequent cooperation is 'voluntary'. All this raises questions about justice as well as process and effectiveness, especially where working in partnership is one of the imperatives.

The social work role

I have already mentioned some of the sources of personal and professional stress for social workers and suggested that contradictory demands are made on them in the conference. First, the social work role in relation to the family is complex. This role requires them, at different times, to act in different roles – as advocates, reporters, supporters, negotiators. Not all of these roles sit comfortably together. Lupton *et al.* (2001) point out that such ethical conflicts are also experienced by health visitors. Additionally, there are conflicts of role in acting for different family members whose interests may diverge. Separated parents, for example, may hold entirely different views on good enough parenting; or the child's right to be protected may conflict with what the child wants, or what the parents want. The interests and rights of wider family members may differ, but also need to be addressed and presented to the conference. Further conflicts of interest may be created by the need to act as an advocate for the family in the conference while at the same time gatekeeping and case managing the LACSCD's scarce resources. Arguably, the imperative to work in partnership renders the task even more difficult – especially when the LACSCD cannot provide the service the social worker believes the family needs.

Second, in pursuing s.47 enquiries, social workers walk a tightrope between the care and control functions of their work. In offering practitioners choices at each stage of the enquiry regarding which model of care planning best suits the family situation, *Working Together* (DoH 2000d, DfES 2005c) clearly emphasises the care dimension of their role. Where parents can be relied upon to protect their children – including in cases where serious concerns have been substantiated – they should be supported in doing so without resort to the initial conference, or without registration.

However, the critical decision as to how, when and by whom the threshold of entry into the child protection system is determined remains, and remains with the social worker. Deciding not to hold an initial conference may well place additional high risk demands on practitioners already under stress and over-burdened. Alternatively, in pursuing registration, social workers may be perceived by parents to be taking up adversarial positions in which they are accorded control, while not having access to the resources the families want to meet their care needs (Bairstow & Hetherington 1998). Again, hopefully the shift away from the more formal registration to a child protection plan will reinforce for families and workers the more positive aspects of their monitoring and intervention.

Family participation

The participation of families in the conference has, for some time, been regarded as a key component of partnership practice. Even before the Children Act 1989, some authorities had been including parents. Following the unequivocal guidance in *Working Together* (DoH *et al.* 1991), all authorities introduced family participation. Some favoured partial exclusion, believing the consideration of risk and registration decision could be compromised by the parents' presence; others (Farmer & Owen 1995, Thoburn *et al.* 1995) thought this the worst of both worlds from the parents' point of view. Early concerns about the impact of parents' presence on the decisions made, generally, have been allayed. In Bell's (1999) study, conferences with parents present were not less frequent, less well attended and did not lead to different registration outcomes. Professionals believed that most conferences were better with parents attending than without; the quality of information was better, and the parental perspective better appreciated. Parents who attended were, in general, glad that they were able to be present and believed that it was right that they should be present. However, one-third of the conferences in this study were rated as having particular difficulties linked to the presence of parents, such as those where the parents were denying the abuse (Bell 1999). Parents are now routinely invited to the conference, and there are attempts also to include the wider family. In 1996, 75% of parents attended conferences (Social Services Inspectorate 1997a). Of course not all parents want to attend and much depends upon the way in which they are prepared (Longstaff 1998). A particular concern raised by the research is that the mother is the target of much of the work pre-, during and post-conference. In Bell's (1999) study, 94% of the mothers were invited to the conference, as opposed to 44% of the fathers; 70% of the mothers attended and 24% of the fathers. Farmer and Owen (1995) found, further, that children were more likely to be registered if the mother was seen as responsible for the abuse or neglect. Such practices are potentially oppressive to men, women and children: while men are excluded, women are seen as carrying responsibility for protection of the child, and feel guilty when they fail. Equally, the child's key attachment may be to another adult altogether. While who gets invited to the conference should be a focus for the initial assessment, the evidence suggests that the net is not cast sufficiently wide and the spotlight is on the mother.

There are other thorny and important issues. All the research undertaken on parental participation has shown that, although many parents were glad to have attended, the conference was often experienced as intensely painful and humiliating. From one of the parents in Bell's (1999) study:

I don't think parents should go because it's too upsetting ... loads of people going through the same problem. If they'd understood how awful it was they'd have supported us. It felt like a trial with the police there. (p. 151)

Many of these parents questioned the relevance of the information presented which related to their family background or lifestyle, rather than the incident. They found the meetings too big and disliked the presence of police and of other professionals not directly involved. While three-quarters felt they had been listened to and fairly treated, most felt they had not influenced the decision of the conference.

There is still little research specifically on the experiences of black families. In tracking 120 conferences, Owen and Farmer (1996) found it difficult to locate cases where black children had been registered. Families were wary about participating, and women were discouraged by their male partners. Like their white counterparts, the black families reported distress and a sense of intrusion at being referred. None had asked for help and they had no understanding of what registration meant. Nevertheless, in 70% of these cases the family was engaged, and successful outcomes were enhanced when social workers were matched on the dimensions of race, gender and culture. Humphreys *et al.*'s (1999) study of Asian families who had attended conferences shows that, in spite of the good intentions of many individual workers, Asian families experienced a discriminatory service, such as lack of attention to the parents' health. In Bell's (1999) study more cases from ethnic minorities were described as difficult. It seemed, as happened also in the case of Victoria Climbié, that the professionals lacked confidence in making judgements about child care practice, while the families lacked confidence in or refused to engage with the system. As Korbin (1981) suggested, cross-cultural differences can produce, on the one hand, an unhelpful cultural relativism and, on the other, cultural blindness or superiority.

Language also presented difficulty; some words necessary, for example, to describe sexual abuse do not exist in other languages. Working with interpreters brought additional difficulty, especially when they – as they often did – belonged to the same community as the family. There were particular problems in some families where the women did not speak English, or were not expected by their male partner to take part in discussions. In others, the values of the parents and the child diverged – as in where they held differing opinions about acceptable sexual and marital partners, or family rites of passage.

The extent to which parents actively participate in the conference is thus questionable. Farmer and Owen (1995) estimated that parents contributed to the conference discussion in 44 of the 71 conferences they attended; in 15 cases their contribution was extremely limited and in only 11 cases did they participate in an exploration of the relevant issues. Thoburn *et al.* (1995) found that only 8% of the parents attending could be described as participating in the assessment of risk, and only 2% about registration. Farmer and Owen argue for greater use of parent advocacy but, as Stevenson (1995) points out, this carries the dangers (notably when the advocate is a lawyer) that the conference becomes an adversarial encounter which makes establishing partnership difficult. The focus on risk assessment, implying a disregard of wider welfare needs, also makes it less likely that the conference will be experienced as positive by parents.

Corby *et al.* (1996) suggest that the process of removing conflict from the conference, added to the parents' belief that the decision had already been made, is more likely to alienate parents and make them apathetic than to empower them. Perhaps it makes more sense, on the basis of the research evidence above, to talk about enablement rather than empowerment. For the parents in Bell's (1999) study who had participated, the strong sense of having been fairly treated seemed to lessen feelings of anger, to encourage a more rational response and to allow for a more positive social work relationship to develop. Their involvement in the process did seem to lay a firmer base from which to proceed in cases where they were not in denial. However, the extent to which such relationships can be described as partnerships is debatable.

Children's participation

Every Child Matters (DfES 2004a) has furthered the requirement that children participate in decisions about their care, and the guidance (DfES 2005c) is now very clear that 'enquiries should always involve separate interviews with the child' (para. 4.49) and that children have a right to participate. However, there is now general consensus that children's presence in the conference is rarely appropriate and that participation, which covers a range of processes, levels and activities, can take various forms and should be embedded in the longer term work. Attendance at the conference may be traumatising for some children. Others may be silenced or confused about what they feel. Mars (1989) found that black female children were less likely to disclose for fear of a racist response. The impact of the child protection system itself will create fear and uncertainty. In interviews with children about their experience of child protection investigations, one of the mothers in Bell's (2000b) study vividly described the impact on the family:

When they heard my child had an injury it was madness with police and social workers turning up and all the neighbours watching. It was so embarrassing. I felt all that was unnecessary. (p. 37)

As suggested above, social workers may find it difficult to engage with traumatised children. In Bell's (1999) study, only 27% of the social workers interviewed saw the child before the conference and the level of immediate post-conference activity – including talking to the child – was low. Although the child was more frequently seen in Thoburn *et al.*'s (1995) study this was not always with the parents' agreement, in which case it had a negative impact on future relationships.

Children are rarely present at the initial conference. Some authorities occasionally include adolescent children, and there have been projects (see Scutt 1998) using child advocates. The more recent research on children's views on being involved in child protection investigations has built on earlier work which concentrated on interviews with children looked after outside the home (Stein & Carey 1986). Barford (1993) talked to 11 children from four different families. He found that the social workers' initial contact was often surrounded in uncertainty, with some children wanting to speak but unable to, and others finding themselves expected to talk but unsure what to say. Shepherd (1994) found that younger children had very little understanding of the process. Shemmings (2000) interviewed 34 children about their experiences of attending an initial conference and reported a range of views, with children saying they needed preparation and independent representation, and that their view had not generally been sought. Bell's (2002) more recent study of 27 children aged 8–16 suggests that they are given information, but their understanding of what is happening is poor and their desire to engage, including attending the conference, was variable. A few who had not been invited wished to have been there; others were happy for their views to be presented by their social worker; yet others were uninterested or feared going. From a 16-year-old girl:

They asked me if I wanted to go … I didn't want to – nothing would have persuaded me – I didn't know what to say – I used to get all confused. My Mam used to go and talk about school – I just didn't want to hear it – couldn't be doing with it – it got me mad because I'd done nothing wrong – it was the family's fault. (p. 11)

The research is therefore common in finding variation. Clearly, different children want different things with regard to participation, and age is not the main criterion in determining attitude. Many of the children interviewed by Bell were troubled about confiding in a public meeting what was happening at home, fearing that adults would react in ways they did not want and that they would lose control of their lives. What mattered to them was that there was someone there for them who listened and took seriously what they said, and who they could trust.

It seems that children, like their parents, need a lot of help to enable them to exercise choice in relation to how they participate in the decision-making process. Essential prerequisites are a relationship of trust within which the trauma of the process can be contained, skills in communicating with children, and time and space within which information about what has happened and what will happen can be shared and digested. Real choices about the different ways in which the child's view can be heard need to be offered, including the use of an advocate, written messages, drawings and audio-tapes. Clearly the conference agenda must specify at which point the child's voice will be heard and the ensuing core group should always consider the child's wishes and feelings, and the ongoing need for children to be kept informed and seen alone. As with their parents, attention needs to be given to the gender and race of the social worker, and whether a change of worker after the initial conference would be appropriate. This should all be recorded in the minutes and written into the protection plan.

The child protection plan

The difficulties the initial conference faces in constructing a detailed child protection plan after dealing with the registration issues have been well documented. Farmer and Owen (1995) and Bell (1999) found that risk assessment had so dominated the majority of conferences that there was little time left to consider the second crucial element, the child protection plan. In Farmer and Owen's study, on average, only 9 minutes were devoted to the protection plan. Bell noted that the presence of parents increased the length of the meeting by 20 minutes, with the result that some professionals had to leave before important discussions on registration and planning took place. Further, as *Messages from Inspections* (Social Services Inspectorate 1997a) confirms, there is great variation in the quality of the plans made at the conference. Farmer and Owen (1995) noted variation from broad general statements to detailed specifications, and in over a third of the cases studied, important aspects were overlooked. As reported above, the recent guidance on the need to construct a detailed and specific child protection plan in place of registration should ensure that the plan receives greater attention in the conference, as well as at the core group meeting 10 days hence. The operationalisation of this will require a massive injection of additional resources, including investment in post-registration practice and service provision.

Poor post-registration practice has been identified in a number of studies. In exploring the practice of 22 social workers after the conference, Bell (1999) found that only six had visited the family in the week following the conference and inter-agency work was negligible. Hallett (1995) also described inter-agency collaboration as being 'much more highly developed up to and including the initial conference than it was thereafter' (p. 275). Calder and Horwath (1999) found that key workers felt overburdened by their responsibilities and that other agencies were reluctant to share the tasks. *Working Together* (DoH 2000d) and the recent guidance (DfES 2005c) reaffirm that the agencies involved should work together to cooperate in the post-registration work and lays out in much greater detail the management of core groups, written agreements and family group conferences, as well as the relationship between their responsibilities and those of the initial conference.

Although *Working Together* (DoH *et al.* 1991) had identified core group meetings as being the appropriate place where planning could be progressed and operationalised, there was no guidelines on who should chair them, whether parents should be present and whether they were making decisions which were properly the responsibility of the initial conference. The commitment of all members of the core group was not always high and procedures were not always adhered to. Calder and Horwath (1999) identified other issues for both practitioners and families in the core group, such as that family participation was reactive rather than proactive and that recording and written plans were poor.

In an attempt to address the lack of clarity and status of the core group as the focus for the post-registration work, *Working Together* (DoH 2000d, DfES 2005c) clarifies the respective roles of the conference and the core group in relation to the child protection plan. The conference should produce an outline child protection plan identifying risks, short- and long-term objectives and who should do what, and when; the core group has responsibility for developing and operationalising the plan 'as a working tool'. Membership comprises all professionals who have direct contact with the family and key family members, including the child, if appropriate. It should meet within 10 working days of the conference, and record agreed action. However, while the inter-agency component of the core group is reinforced, the role of the key worker remains complex and extensive:

> To lead the core group, to maintain responsibility for managing the multi-agency plan, complete the core assessment of the child and family, to co-ordinate the contribution of family members and other agencies, to put the child protection plan into effect and review progress.
> (DoH *et al.* 1999, p. 76)

A child protection plan exemplar (DoH 2002a) is included in the Integrated Children's System for this purpose.

While this clarification of responsibility is long overdue – and the Framework and Integrated Children's System exemplars provide the tools for conducting comprehensive assessments within a child-centred and ecological framework – the tasks are complex and burdensome. The role of key workers as managers is emphasised, but the question of whether they (or others) should carry out the work with the family remains unclear. Also unclear is the question of who should chair the core group. Some authorities have, for some time, used conference chairpersons to chair this meeting in acknowledgement that social workers lack the necessary status, experience and skills. What is essential is that other professionals are kept on board, and that the families' responsibility for their children's care is actively maintained.

Family group conferences

One of the mechanisms for establishing the responsibility of the family – as opposed to that of the professionals – is the family group conference (FGC). Originating in New Zealand (Wilcox 1991), FGCs are meetings where all members of the wider family, including the child, meet together, and propose to the professionals the best ways for them of safeguarding and meeting the child's needs. Initially there was speculation that FGCs might replace child protection conferences. However, in evaluating attempts in six authorities to introduce family group conferences, Marsh and Crow (1998) found that social workers experienced some difficulty in relinquishing the policing aspect of their role in child protection cases. By 2001, only 38% of local authorities in the UK had established FGCs, and these most commonly in youth justice and accommodation (Brown 2003). So, while the useful function of FGCs in care planning is confirmed by research (see Bell & Wilson 2006) the difficulties encountered in using them suggest that their use is more limited than was originally hoped. *Working Together* (DoH 2000d) concluded: 'Family Group Conferences do not replace, or remove the need for child protection conferences – but may be valuable for children in need where a plan is required for the child's welfare' (p. 78). However, the recent guidance (DfES 2005c) does include the suggestion that FGCs might be held also at the investigative stage (para. 9.11). Since the essence of FGCs is that the families discuss their problems and needs in the absence of the professionals, it will be interesting to see if social workers do feel confident to use them at this stage.

Conclusion

In the first edition of this *Handbook* (1995), Stevenson reviewed the knowledge base and research findings in relation to initial child protection conferences with reference to content and purpose, process, inter-professional cooperation and parent/child participation. This chapter looks again at those issues, re-examining some of the problems identified which still remain, while also exploring the ways in which progress has been made. The problems that still remain concern the ambiguous nature of the tasks and functions of the conference, the way in which the conference process can militate against quality inter-agency assessments of risk and need, and the adversarial nature of the encounter which can distress parents and make children's participation extremely difficult. Arguably, the difficulties identified in these areas are embedded in the system. Other models do exist which may be less adversarial. In comparing the experiences of English and French parents, Bairstow and Hetherington (1998) found that, while parents in both countries experienced similar problems, the English parents were more upset and less satisfied than their French counterparts. In France, as in Scotland, parents have direct access to the judge – or the panel – and experience the law as accessible and responsive to their needs. Most importantly, they felt the professionals were on their side. Although it seems ironic to propose that the ideology of rights which underpins our system mitigates against partnership, some of the evidence presented here in relation to the conference function and process leads to that conclusion.

However, despite the difficulties identified, there is evidence that our existing child protection system does succeed in protecting children from future harm and that, as Laming suggested, the structures laid out in the Children Act 1989 for safeguarding children are basically sound. It is their interpretation and implementation and the need for a greater injection of resources that will lead to its being more effective. Inter-agency collaboration is difficult, and the issues identified here cannot be wished away. Brandon *et al.* (2005) recommend that Local Safeguarding Children Boards establish a pool of experts to advise professionals about the group dynamics and the factors that cause professional tensions and cloud decision making, as well as about the individual children. Working together should be facilitated by the establishment of children's trusts and shared budgets, particularly with regard to closer working relationships with education and health.

We do not yet know whether the Assessment Framework will facilitate better assessments for every child conferenced or whether using the exemplars contained within the Integrated Children's System (which every LACSCD is required to do from 2006) will address some of the difficulties in information sharing that exist in conferences, reviews and related meetings. However, the structure that is provided for more thorough and detailed assessments of every child in the family, and the common assessment framework that is proposed, ought to encourage all professionals to talk the same language and to construct action plans that are timely and appropriate. The effects of disbanding the child protection register in 2007 will be important to track, and it is to be hoped that more effective child protection plans will result and be effected in its place.

As Morrison (2000) suggests, the effectiveness of the new systems seems to depend upon local factors, such as funding, leadership and technology, as well as the skills and ability of the workforce. Hopefully the proposed workforce reforms will improve career structures and encourage retention, while at the same time better working conditions will provide front-line practitioners with the support, supervision and resources they need to engage in the essential direct work and carry out the complex child protection tasks.

Finally, the development of frameworks for pre- and post-registration practice is encouraging if they reduce the need for more intrusive State intervention at all stages of the process. Services that are welfare based are more likely to promote opportunities for preventative and therapeutic work, both before and after conference, and research suggests that they are experienced as supportive by the families that attend (Platt 2001). Such developments need to be adequately resourced and delivered at community level, preferably by multidisciplinary teams (see Bell 2005). However, preventative initiatives should not lead to complacency. There is concern that, even where family support services exist, children who are at risk of harm may not be adequately protected without recourse to the initial conference. It must also be recognised that shifting the focus of work with children and families away from the heavy end of child protection to family support – an area traditionally staffed by unqualified workers – has left many social workers feeling confused and de-skilled and has contributed to the retention and recruitment difficulties identified above. As Laming said, doing the basic job properly is the best route to safeguarding and curbing harm to children and it is when workers are supported, well supervised and have access to training that they are most likely to operate effectively in the difficult domain of child protection conferences.

Key points and messages for practice

- An ICPC is an inter-agency meeting held after s.47 enquiries have established that a child may suffer, or be at risk of suffering, significant harm. The most recent government guidance (*Working Together*, DfES 2005c) has confirmed their central role within the child protection system, although the child protection register will be disbanded from 2007. In its place, a child protection plan will be put in place for each child where abuse is established and the Integrated Children's System will enable each LACSCD to hold information on electronic records.

- The child protection plan, nominating a key worker, should be developed at the core group meeting and should ensure that all professionals have a role in addressing the welfare needs of all family members within timescales that are appropriate to the needs of the child(ren).

- The tasks of collecting and processing information essential to the conference purpose are complex and difficult, and a chairperson skilled at managing group dynamics, inter-agency communication and the involvement of family members is essential to its effective functioning and good decision making.

- Within the context of expanding community-based child welfare services, and in cases where the child's safety can be assured, other inter-agency meetings should be held both before and after the initial child protection conference where action plans are established and a range of services provided.

- The effective safeguarding of children depends upon the skills and expertise of child protection social workers and their professional colleagues, and it is essential that resources are provided to fund the recruitment and retention of practitioners in statutory teams, and their ongoing professional development and training.

- Both pre- and post-registration work need to be developed on an inter-agency basis to ensure that the needs of children and of their parents, in particular in relation to mental health and substance misuse, are met. Adult and children's services could develop more effective systems for working more closely together and sharing information.

- Working together across social services, health and education should be facilitated by the establishment of children's trusts and shared budgets, and Local Safeguarding Children Boards should ensure that inter-agency training is developed and resourced and that expert consultation is available to practitioners.

- Involving parents and children in the decisions made at the conference is likely to lead to greater cooperation and understanding of what needs to change, what it is necessary to achieve and how. This requires early involvement with and preparation of the child's significant attachment figures and each child, that information and procedures are shared and, where possible, real choices are offered. Communication with families may require special skills and help with language differences, as well as a range of methods of presenting the views of the child(ren) and vulnerable adults to the conference.

16 Health practitioners and safeguarding children

Julie Taylor and Jo Corlett

INTRODUCTION

Health practitioners are not a homogeneous group. Even within the different professions there are identity and boundary issues. For example, midwives tend to dislike being referred to as nurses and it has become common practice to use the somewhat cumbersome phrase of 'nurses, midwives and health visitors' to reinforce the distinctions. Doctors, as everyone knows, are superior to nurses, but even within that group there are distinctions. Primary care is lower in status than front-line clinical practice and of course surgeons may be nearer to God than anyone else.

Although the above is a highly facetious start to a chapter that attempts to bring together some messages for 'health practitioners', it is important to point out that in a hierarchical NHS, professional pride, training and experience can still create divisions that are not always recognised outwith the health service, nor always acknowledged within. Increasingly, the Allied Health Professions (AHPs) can be added to this group, but currently there are 13 named AHPs and it would be wrong to assume that such alliances are always comfortable: physiotherapists may identify more with respiratory physicians than they do with podiatrists; mental health nurses may have more in common with some social workers than they do with accident and emergency consultants or speech and language therapists. Nonetheless, this disparate group is collectively referred to as 'health practitioners' and as such our chapter attempts to tackle some of the major child protection issues that are likely to confront this group, and to provide some guidance in terms of how these might be addressed. Whilst collaborative practice is a clear imperative for all, that we have not achieved it yet *within* health is an important consideration when we try to promote it *across* different agency groups.

This chapter takes as its starting point some of the messages for health practitioners that have come out of serious case reviews. It then deals specifically with some of the identifiable groups that have a particular or more frequent input into child protection, whilst acknowledging that this will never be a complete listing. The role of AHPs in child protection is not addressed, although there are overriding messages that cut across all health professional groups. Child protection is everyone's business and all health practitioners need to be alert to the possibilities that the patients and clients with whom they work may be victims of or, by omission or commission, perpetrators of, child abuse and neglect. The chapter then moves on to some of the broader initiatives, often multiprofessional, that have been introduced to try to give children the best possible start in life. We will take a particular look at health practitioners' roles in *Sure Start* and in assessing and supporting parenting. We will then round off the chapter with some of the general issues that need to be focused on more clearly.

Lessons for health from serious case reviews

The death of Victoria Climbié in 2000 shocked the nation, not only because of the extreme brutalisation to which she had been subjected over a sustained period of time, but because the array of service providers with whom she had been in contact failed to recognise that such abuse was taking place or to save her life. Within his summary, Lord Laming, Chairman of the Inquiry Committee commissioned to report on the circumstances surrounding Victoria's death, noted that there was a gross failure of the system to protect Victoria. In addition to contact with the local Housing Department's Homeless Person's Unit:

> Victoria was known to no less than two further housing authorities, four social services departments, two child protection teams of the Metropolitan Police Service (MPS), a specialist centre managed by the NSPCC, and she was admitted to two different hospitals because of suspected deliberate harm.
>
> (Laming Report 2003, p. 3)

Bad practice, lack of managerial accountability, limited cross-agency working and poor information sharing and recording are some of the issues highlighted within the report, which makes a total of 108 recommendations aimed at ensuring that this type of case never occurs again. Twenty-seven recommendations relate specifically to health care. Many are concerned with the need for detailed and accurate record keeping by both medical and nursing staff, including documentation of face-to-face discussions and recording of any suspicions raised by staff concerning deliberate harm. The recommendations also stress the need to ensure rigorous procedural systems are in place, aimed at safeguarding children about whom staff are worried. For example, a child should not be discharged from hospital without the permission of a senior member of medical staff, or without a documented plan for future care, or without an identified GP. These seem straightforward and indicative of routine good practice, but in the case of Victoria Climbié, such policies and procedures were not in place.

The need for training in the recognition of deliberate harm and child protection procedures for general practice staff (including GPs) and those working in liaison roles at the hospital/community service interface are also recommended in the report. Traditionally, it has been seen as the role of the health visitor to take the lead in child protection within community service provision. With the recent changes in legislation and the organisation of child protection, however, there is a need for health professionals other than health visitors to become more involved. All nurses working with children should receive training in child protection, as well as nurses who may be caring for parents whose children are vulnerable; for example, mental health nurses working with parents who have substance misuse problems (Crisp & Lister 2004).

Children and their families also need to be paid more attention. Brandon *et al.* (2005) suggest health and social care professionals generally are not good at listening to families and their concerns, particularly siblings who are often aware that abuse is occurring within the family. They recommend more use could be made of this 'expertise'. As such, any group working with families needs to be aware of, and receive training in, how to identify and deal with situations where child abuse is suspected. There also seems to be a need in general for health staff to improve their communication skills with children and their families. Research has suggested that nurses and other health workers do not communicate effectively (Hallstrom *et al.* 2002).

Most complaints to the NHS are related to issues of communication (Pincock 2004). There is therefore a need to equip health workers with the necessary knowledge and skills to communicate effectively with children and parents (Corlett & Twycross 2006), particularly in sensitive situations where deliberate harm is suspected. Observational skills are also crucial in practitioners being able to identify vulnerable children and high risk environments, but again, these skills are dependent upon training and continual updating.

The overriding message in the Laming Report is the need for workers to be more proactive in gathering and sharing information and to engage in multiprofessional approaches to safeguarding children. Information is often not collected, or is collected but not available to colleagues working in other professions, or is available but not actively shared. There is a need for more open and coordinated communication between the various agencies who might be involved with one particular child or family.

Similar concerns were highlighted in the Bichard Inquiry (2004), set up by the Home Secretary to investigate child protection procedures, particularly practices relating to the vetting of those who work with children, following the murders of Jessica Chapman and Holly Wells. Ian Huntley, subsequently convicted of their murders, had a previous police record of sexual offences not revealed by screening procedures, enabling him to be appointed as caretaker at the school attended by Jessica and Holly. During the case, it was suggested that information sharing was difficult because of data protection legislation. This assertion is rejected within the report, but the following comment is made:

Better guidance is needed on the collection, retention, deletion, use and sharing of information, so that ... professionals can feel more confident in using information properly.

(Bichard Inquiry Report 2004, p. 4)

Again, the need to collect better quality information and disseminate this to others is reiterated.

These and other highly publicised cases have resulted in a great deal of policy development aimed at safeguarding children now and in the future. In spite of this, the second joint Chief Inspectors' report published in July 2005 (Commission for Social Care Inspection 2005a) strikes a cautionary note, stating that whilst the need to safeguard children is now given greater priority across agencies, this is not always translated into practice. There are particular concerns regarding the safety of children who are disabled, living away from home or in health or secure settings (see Butler, Chapter 10, in this volume).

Nurses and midwives and health visitors

In this section we examine in more detail some of the different professional roles within nursing and midwifery. Whilst there is much overlap between different roles (e.g. health visitor versus lead nurse child protection), the distinct professional focus of each role has a particular bearing on child care and protection. Disentangling this is not always easy, however, because there remains a lack of consensus in the professions about the extent of health care professionals' involvement in child protection. Moreover, involvement in the identification or detection of child protection issues is still not easily accepted by many nurses (Crisp & Lister 2004). At the time of writing, there is ongoing dialogue between the Royal College of Nursing and the Department of Health, trying to map national core competences that can be linked to designated child protection doctors. Designated and lead nurses' competences are also being mapped against the Department of Health Assessment Framework (safeguarding children). The reality, however, is that there are significant variations in the way this crucial role is played, not only between each country in the UK but also between localities within each country. There is as yet no uniform model for lead and designated child protection nurses and it will be interesting to watch this crucial role develop.

Health visitors

Recent changes in role and title and a new registration point on the professional register have meant the established statutory health visitor role is undergoing considerable change. The specialist community public health nurse part of the register was established on 1 August 2004, with practice standards applied from August 2006. These changes have not yet been fully implemented, and while it used to be the case in the UK that all children under the age of five were assigned a health visitor who undertook regular checks on their development, practice across the UK is now more variable. Given their statutory and, until recently, universal role with all families, health visitors are in a unique position to recognise situations that are or could be abusive or neglectful.

Appleton's (1994) overview of the role of the health visitor in relation to child protection looked at three areas:

- health visitors' and clients' perceptions of the health visitor's role in working with vulnerable families in relation to child protection
- the identification of vulnerable families by health visitors and non-health visitors
- a review of their preventative work.

Drawing on such work in the previous edition of this Handbook, Rouse (2002) comprehensively outlined the history, development and political context of health visiting and we shall not therefore repeat that here. Whilst policy and training documentation emphasises and endorses the crucial role of health visitors in child protection, the truth is that this is a relatively small part of their overall public health and health-promoting role (Rouse 2002). Rouse suggested the health visitor role could be summarised as having three distinct emphases in child protection: primary, secondary and tertiary prevention. These categorisations are helpful and worth exploring in more detail.

Primary prevention

Primary prevention focuses on preventing the development of situations in which child abuse or neglect might occur, mainly through teaching or information giving. Rouse suggests that this is perhaps the most important role of health visitors in child protection. Given their universal contact with all families with young children, the health-promoting and educative role is crucial.

Rouse provided a useful list of practices that health visitors (and indeed other health practitioners) can employ in their primary prevention role; for example, the promotion of positive parenting practices. It is important to note, however, that it is not always so clear cut, since health visitors can have their own parenting beliefs that may or may not be transmitted to a family (Taylor & Redman 2004).

The literature has demonstrated repeatedly that stress is a crucial ingredient in child protection issues – see, for example, earlier work by Belsky (1980) and more recently by Sidebotham *et al.* (2001). Lending a 'listening ear' could certainly be productive in providing an outlet for stress and health visitors are in a very strong position to deal with some of the stresses caused by poverty and by the cultural, social and economic contexts of child abuse and neglect. Yet nurses and health visitors largely remain silent at a wider political level. There is an old saying which suggests that if you give a family a parcel of food you will feed them for a week. Give them a goat and you will feed them for life. A 'listening ear' is important, but collective attention to some of the wider stressors may be far more effective in the longer term.

The primary prevention role concentrates on parents. However, in practice, health visitors deal mainly with mothers and using the term 'parents' conceals a lack of attention to fathers. 'It is a major methodological flaw in child abuse intervention research to use the word "parenting" when in reality it is mothers who are studied' (Daniel & Taylor 2001, p. 48). Clarke and Popay's (1998) study revealed that many women (and indeed many fathers themselves) do not trust men to be good enough at a parenting role. In Chalmer's (1992) small study, health visitors tended to not engage with men, despite opportunities, nor did they have any real conceptualisation of the role they might have in parenting. Daniel and Taylor (2001, 2005) argued that fathers and father figures require more attention than is often afforded them by practitioners, both in assessing the potential risk they may pose to a child, but also assessing them as a potential asset. To use the term 'parent' may be ambiguous and if in practice this really means only mothering, then this should be explicit (see also Featherstone, Chapter 6, in this volume).

Secondary prevention

Secondary prevention is concerned with prevention of the development of stress and tensions leading to child abuse, mainly through surveillance, referral for support, identification of family stressors and other predisposers to child harm in the antenatal period, and giving meticulous attention to detail in collating indicators (if not evidence) of abuse and neglect (Rouse 2002).

This is very helpful for exploring some of the secondary prevention aspects of the role of the health visitor in child protection. It is, however, worth a little more unpacking. Rouse added a cautionary note concerning the identification of 'risk factors' in families, an aspect of practice that is relevant to all health practitioners but which is sometimes taken lightly. We shall therefore discuss it in more detail later in the chapter. Referring families for parenting support is also a useful suggestion and again, such programmes will be discussed later in the chapter.

Rouse's list of secondary prevention actions included discussing with families any causes for concern. In reality, however, this is never easy: if abuse is occurring, then a vigorous denial is likely and there is potential for great upset, suspicion and anger amongst family members. If abuse is not occurring, then stigmatisation and, increasingly, litigation are also possible outcomes.

It has been shown that health visitors see poverty, poor parenting, mental health problems and failure to thrive (FTT) as the four most frequent problems they face (McIntyre & Collinson 1997), all of which may be interrelated. This demonstrates some of the difficulties health visitors face in practice. Wright's (2005) discussion of weight faltering points out that whilst FTT is strongly associated with child neglect in professional understanding, in most cases FTT is primarily a behavioural or dietary problem. Nonetheless, although a minority, children who are abused or neglected are more likely to fail to thrive than other children, presenting a major challenge to health care professionals (Wright 2005).

Children are routinely weighed at regular visits and suspicions of FTT could stem from these. However, research has revealed that health visitors are not very good at detecting FTT (Batchelor & Kerslake 1990). Better results were found in Newcastle, where training and research have resulted in 80% of cases being identified by the health visitor (Wright & Waterston 1994). The situation is exacerbated by inaccurate and unreliable weighing equipment and poor record keeping (Batchelor & Kerslake 1990). The increased surveillance accorded to low-income families also cannot be ignored. Taylor and Daniel (1999) argued that some children with FTT could be falling into a gap between health and social care, where FTT could not be taken as a child protection issue by health care practitioners, but referral to a social worker, who could not diagnose a medical condition, was also problematic. Perhaps if weight faltering had been picked up more consistently in the case of Victoria Climbié, there may have been a different outcome.

The diagnostic criteria themselves, i.e. weight falling below the 3rd centile, have also been shown to be restrictive. Batchelor and Kerslake (1990) interviewed health visitors in this regard and revealed that children whose weight was below the 10th centile but above the 3rd were often a cause for concern. Because they could not be referred to a paediatrician until this happened, health visitors were almost willing the children's weight to fall so that action could be taken. Such a sustained drop is rare and it was findings such as these that led Wright and colleagues to develop a weight monitoring chart that diagnosed weight faltering more accurately, enough at least to trigger health visitor assessment and subsequent referral to a paediatrician (Wright 2005). FTT, therefore, provides a good example of situations in which concerns about communication and role boundaries can be important in day-to-day work.

Tertiary prevention

Tertiary prevention concerns prevention of deterioration, mainly through monitoring and support, where child harm seems to have occurred (Rouse 2002). Rouse (2002) usefully pointed to areas of child protection where the health visitor can have a significant role. Perhaps the central aspect of this tertiary supportive role, however, is one in which the health visitor may feel most comfortable, i.e. that of monitoring the child's health and development.

There is clear evidence, mostly stemming from the randomised controlled trials by Olds *et al.* (1995, 1997) in the United States, that nurse home visiting is effective at improving parenting skills, reducing child behavioural problems, reducing unintentional injury and enhancing support to mothers. Home visiting is not a universal service in the US, however, and not all studies have used trained home visitors. However, research has found that mothers visited by para-professionals, compared with controls, displayed greater sensitivity to their children and provided a more supportive home environment (Olds *et al.* 2005). Chaffin (2004) is critical of this work, however, demonstrating that the three home visiting programmes introduced by the Olds team are the only ones where there appear to have been consistently positive results. The evidence has been mixed, but recent systematic reviews have begun cautiously to suggest home visiting can have a beneficial effect. A large review by Kendrick *et al.* (2000) showed some evidence that home visiting could improve parenting and the home environment and recently, from their review, Hahn *et al.* (2005) concluded that home visiting programmes can be effective in reducing child maltreatment. Health visiting services are, however, a costly element of community health services in the UK (Bryans 2004).

Whilst nurses, and particularly health visitors may often be the first to suspect abuse or neglect, there remains some lack of clarity about their role (Crisp & Lister 2004). The welcome and increasing role of specialist and consultant nurses in child protection has the potential to coordinate and systematise health visitor practice effectively and it will be interesting to follow developments as these roles are shaped and evaluated. On the other hand, the recent emphasis on a public health role has the potential to clash with the traditional yet narrower role of supporting families (Crisp & Lister 2004). The next few years will be interesting as the new specialist community public health nurse role becomes established.

Midwives

There is growing acceptance that midwives have a pivotal role to play in child protection. Bennet *et al.* (2001) confirmed that over half the midwives they surveyed stated they had a role in child protection and that midwives required specific child protection training. As with health visitors, some midwifery services and policies are exerting pressure on midwives for them to be able to recognise adult behaviours and attitudes that might be predictive of risk of future abuse or neglect. As Chapman (2002) argued, however, a lack of objective prediction tools makes this an almost impossible task.

Domestic violence: a role for health visitors and midwives?

There is increasing acknowledgement of the risk to children caused by living in a household where intimate partner violence is occurring. Edleson *et al.* (2003) conducted telephone interviews with 114 battered women, where a quarter of them reported their children had been physically involved in the events. In another study, 52% of children who had been sexually abused reported spousal violence at home (Kellogg & Menard 2003). Research confirms that there is a substantial overlap between domestic violence and child maltreatment (Hartley 2002) and is therefore an issue that must be taken seriously. Children and young people are witness to violent and abusive behaviour in many ways. Rodwell (2005) summarises such research well. They may:

- be in the same room when the incident is taking place
- hear events as they unfold from another room
- witness physical damage to an adult or property following an incident
- become involved in the abuse accidentally while trying to intervene
- be used as a pawn to bargain or threaten with, particularly post-separation
- become the direct subject of abuse, which may be physical, sexual, emotional or a combination of these.

Health visitors and midwives are uniquely placed to identify families where there is intimate partner violence, yet perhaps this is not always effectively managed. Peckover's (2003) analysis of women's help-seeking from health visitors in the context of domestic violence found that women felt they would have appreciated a little more help. Rodwell's (2005) research with public health practitioners about their perceptions of their role in families where there was domestic violence found a lack of consensus amongst practitioners.

This was confirmed by Marchant *et al.* (2001), who conducted a postal survey of all NHS Trusts in England and Wales providing maternity services. Only 12% of units had a written policy for identifying women experiencing domestic violence, although 30% had some form of agreed practice. Very few had audited their practices, however, and only about half displayed material for women experiencing domestic violence. Less than half routinely offered women an appointment without their partner.

Increasingly, policy suggests that midwives and health visitors should routinely be engaging with the issue of domestic violence. Whilst there remain barriers to effective and complete participation in the screening and support of women (and by proxy, children), this is an area which is likely to have benefits in safeguarding children and is to be welcomed.

Other nursing roles in child protection

School nurses hold a pivotal, and sometimes unacknowledged, role in child protection. For many though, the ethical problems they experience in this regard and how these are managed has at times been viewed as 'setting them up to fail'. In one small study of their experience of ethical conflict, interviews with school nurses showed child protection issues emerged as a strong theme (Solum & Schaffer 2003). However, their isolation often made it difficult for them to share and resolve such dilemmas.

Paediatric nurses, with specialist training geared particularly to children and a different registration point from general nurses, are likewise in a unique position with regard to child protection. However, a combined Medline/Cinahl search using the key words 'paediatric nurse' and 'child protection' brings up not a single hit. So whilst the NMC and DoH state that safeguarding children should be integral to the curriculum, details of how this is interpreted are left to specific training providers. Children's nursing students may get up to 15 or 20 hours of teaching (over a 3-year course), whereas adult nursing students in some areas may get hardly any input on child protection (Thain J 2005, personal communication).

Children who have been abused are more likely to present to the Accident and Emergency (A&E) department than any other within the hospital setting. A&E nurses therefore have an important part to play in the detection of such abuse (Fagan 1998). Fagan's study of the role of A&E nurses dealing with cases of suspected child abuse found that all respondents could identify factors alerting them to the possibility of child abuse having occurred. Intuitive or 'gut' feelings were also important. However, most of the nurses within the study did not feel skilled in detecting and dealing with suspected child abuse. Those that did feel skilled saw this as being as a result of their experience and the informal knowledge they had gained whilst working within A&E.

Fagan makes the point that if these nurses saw themselves as skilled and knowledgeable as a result of their intuition and experience, rather than as the result of any education or training, bad practice could simply be perpetuated. The nurses in the study saw their role as being one of detection, rather than prevention, which Fagan suggests is somewhat restrictive since valuable opportunities may be missed for them to use their skills to prevent abuse occurring in the first place. Fagan does not expand on this preventative role. However, if nurses can identify children who may be at risk and bring their concerns to the attention of appropriate members of the multidisciplinary team, support strategies can be implemented which may prevent a family situation deteriorating to the extent that abuse is occurring.

Children who are being abused or neglected may attend A&E for reasons other than those related to the abuse, such as accidental injury or some health problem, whilst a disabled child may present because of a health problem related to their disability. A&E nurses caring for the victims of domestic violence should also be trying to ascertain whether any children have been victims of or witness to the violence. They are in a prime position to be able to help such children by alerting others to their concerns so that mechanisms of support can be implemented. However, these nurses need to be able to see beyond the presenting problem and to use their interpersonal and communication skills to probe a little deeper in determining families at risk.

Powell (1997) provides a detailed list of indicators of abuse that A&E staff should be aware of: bruising, burns, multiple fractures, adult bite marks, failure to thrive, frozen watchfulness, excessive sadness, self-mutilation, childhood overdose, indiscriminate attachment, precocious sexual activity, venereal disease, genital or rectal bleeding. Powell suggests the neglected child may also present as dirty, underweight and hungry. Differing explanations as to the child's injuries and delay in seeking treatment are also warning signs. Frequency of attendance is also important: children are often abused over a long period, with multiple injuries inflicted over time. A problem already discussed earlier in this chapter has been that of poor practice in relation to information recording and sharing, which in the past has made it more difficult to detect patterns of abuse and A&E attendance. The proposed *Children's and Maternity Services Information Strategy* (DoH/DfES 2005) should in future enhance the sharing of information between A&E departments, with all A&E and hospital admissions being recorded and available to staff at a new point of contact.

Because of the setting in which they work, A&E nurses may be in the position of being the first to detect or suspect child abuse. This is a highly emotive area and one in which any health professional, not just those working within A&E, may be reluctant to become involved if they are not confident in their knowledge, skills or expertise.

In a survey of 979 nurses, doctors and dentists in Northern Ireland working in primary care, Russell *et al.* (2004) found great variation in the ability and willingness of the three professions to report physical abuse. They found nurses and health visitors were more willing to come forward, even though doctors had seen more cases and were better able to recognise symptoms of physical abuse. Dentists in this study were the least able. Four themes arose from this survey:

- professional fear of misdiagnosis and its consequences
- professional uncertainty when reporting physical abuse (lack of clear guidelines)
- professional challenges to reporting (workload, red tape, lengthy reporting procedures, lack of sensitivity and support from social services and from colleagues)
- the need for multidisciplinary training.

Only education, training and supervision by experienced and skilled staff will give less experienced health professionals the confidence to be able to work proactively in situations where abuse is suspected.

There may also be fears that the therapeutic relationship with the child and/or the child's carers may be damaged. Confidentiality is highly valued in all the health professions and is not broken easily or without thought to the consequences of so doing. In cases where injuries are clearly the result of non-accidental harm, these obviously should be reported. However, many cases are not so clear cut and the nurse may only have suspicions to go on, particularly if the child is experiencing emotional abuse or neglect, rather than physical harm. Reid and Long (2002) warn of the way in which suspicions can get out of hand and irreparably damage the therapeutic relationship. Nurses, however, have both a professional and an ethical duty to report their concerns to named professionals with a responsibility and expertise for child protection and to remain objective in caring for the child and family.

Medicine

It seems somewhat contrived to separate medicine from nursing, midwifery and health visiting, as many of the issues already discussed are equally applicable. Nonetheless, there are some specific points that arise separately for doctors. Not least is that health-related suspicions may be referred to them in the first instance and the weight of responsibility is arguably therefore more burdensome.

Paediatricians

Paediatricians are probably at the forefront of health practice in relation to child protection. Referrals come to them; they are used to diagnose, investigate, confirm and refer suspicious and confirmed cases; and child protection issues, for many, make up a large percentage of their caseload. In an analysis of how community paediatrics has developed, Blair *et al.* (2000) performed a retrospective analysis of data collected routinely for contracting purposes in order to describe the current clinical workload of the modern community paediatrician. They concluded that the transfer of child health surveillance to the primary health care team has resulted in an increasingly specialised role for community paediatricians. In particular, this was centred on child development, disability and social and behavioural paediatrics.

Given recent media and legal attention, it is hardly surprising that there is a growing reluctance to enter paediatrics as a career. The striking off the register of Professor Sir Roy Meadow following his expert witness testimony in cases of sudden infant death syndrome, despite support from both the media and the medical community, sent out discouraging messages to paediatricians taking a lead on child protection. The Royal College of Paediatrics and Health has stated that paediatricians are increasingly being frightened away from child protection work due to fears of complaints from parents (Dyer 2005): a poll of College members suggested about one in six had been the subject of a serious complaint (Dyer 2005).

Taking a rights-based approach to their work with children also seems to be an important development for paediatricians. Marking the 15th anniversary of the UN Convention of the Rights of the Child (UNCRC), Waterston and Mann (2005) requested written pieces from a range of professionals in paediatrics, including a surgeon and a nurse, to offer their personal perspective on the meaning of children's rights. Some of the answers made reassuring reading: that those involved in paediatric medicine are aware of the rights of the child and are making sincere attempts to uphold these. Waterston (2005) suggests that the UNCRC is an essential framework for individual as well as public health practice in paediatric medicine.

GPs

Virtually all children are registered with a general practitioner (GP), although few have had formal training in paediatrics, an issue currently under review by the Royal College of Paediatrics and Child Health and the Royal College of General Practitioners (Craft 2005). Their traditional role has been one of assessing and treating sick children, although studies show that GPs recognise their need for training in child protection matters (Bannon *et al.* 1999a). In fact, it seems from a number of studies that GPs' participation in child protection issues causes them great anxiety and tends to be delegated to the health visitor (Bannon *et al.* 1999b, Simpson *et al.* 1994).

Waterston (2005) suggests that paediatricians and GPs also have a role in relation to bullying, given that this is a reasonably frequent concern arising in consultations. He suggests a graded response, from a general advisory/supportive role to one where input is provided to the local education authority on training on anti-bullying policies.

Assessment of parenting is also seen as a key issue for GPs in relation to a wide range of health-related issues, such as substance abuse, attention deficit hyperactivity disorder, teenage mothers, post-partum depression, learning disabilities, infant temperament, colic, diabetes, homelessness, child obesity, emotional support, child injuries, fruit and vegetable consumption, and conduct disorders.

Assessing parenting is a difficult and contentious area of practice. What emerges from the literature describing the quality of parenting is a clear picture of 'poor' parenting but much less detailed descriptions of 'good' parenting and little guidance about the threshold of what might constitute 'good enough' parenting. Thus, there remains a tendency to target 'bad' parents or families rather than seek solutions of greater complexity at a broader level (Taylor *et al.* 2000). (For a fuller discussion on this subject, see Daniel and Rioche, Chapter 24, in this volume.)

Increasingly it has been suggested that health visitors, school nurses and midwives should be trained to assess risk factors in parents in order to prevent child abuse and neglect. Although risk factors are important, so many have now been identified that it is difficult to know how they would be measured or analysed in a valid or reliable way. As Sidebotham (2003) highlighted, there is not as yet a strong evidence base regarding the effectiveness of risk assessment tools. Even so, there is an increasing emphasis on assessing parenting and screening for risk factors (Reder & Lucey 1995) and work continues to develop an empirically tested, accurate and consistent risk assessment tool (Warner 2003, Ryan *et al.* 2005). This is yet another child care and protection debate that is likely to rage, but according to Kaufman and Zigler (1992), it is statistically unfeasible to predict child abuse accurately. For health practitioners who are familiar with checklist approaches, awareness of the debate and judicious use of such instruments is advised.

Parenting programmes and family centres

Having urged some caution about parental assessment and the prediction of abuse and neglect, there has nevertheless been a recent proliferation in programmes designed to support parents. Parenting programmes have increased in popularity with groups such as health visitors, but there is a need for more extensive research into their effectiveness (Spencer 2003). Such programmes have a range of names and aims, and although the components of each can differ slightly between and even within programmes, there are increasing reports of success.

For example, programmes using the principles of family therapy as a way of dealing with children's behavioural and emotional difficulties can be useful (Johnson *et al.* 2005). Such strategies advocate concentrating on the abilities of parents to provide a nurturing parenting style. An evaluation of the Webster Stratton Parents and Children Series group parenting programme, led by trained and supervised health visitors, also found significant improvement in reducing child behaviour problems and improved mental health at immediate and 6-month follow-ups (Reading 2004). However, at 1 year the differences between intervention and control groups were not significant, even though qualitative responses from parents indicated the programme had improved both parental mental health and parent–child relationships. Reading concluded that whilst parenting programmes have the potential to promote mental health and reduce social inequalities, further work is required to improve any long-term gain.

Parenting programmes as a whole have been used to treat parents already involved in the child protection system and have shown limited benefits. Further, family centres usually work mainly with mothers, even though they aspire to working with families (Joseph Rowntree Foundation 2005). Sanders *et al.* (2003) argued for the importance of community-wide support structures to promote positive parenting in order to reduce the prevalence of child abuse and neglect. This is much in line with the neighbourhood mapping approach advocated by Nelson and Baldwin (2005). Sanders *et al.* (2003) outlined the criteria required to make parenting programmes really effective:

- knowledge of current prevalence rates for the targeted child outcomes
- knowledge of prevalence rates of parenting and family risk factors
- evidence that changing family risk factors reduces prevalence
- availability of culturally appropriate, cost-effective, evidence-based and accessible interventions.

The new *National Service Framework for Children, Young People and Maternity Services* (DoH/DfES 2004) insists that primary care trusts and local authorities have available evidence-based parenting training programmes, focused on child behaviour management and delivered by specifically trained professionals (Ramchandani & McConachie 2005). However, we must be careful of picking interventions off the shelf: even rigorously conducted studies often do not describe fully the interventions used, such as context, and it is difficult to know if they will work in a different culture (Petticrew & Roberts 2004).

A recent review of integrated services by family centres and new community schools suggested they may benefit families in the long term; however, such benefits may not be quantifiable and at the moment are not captured by standardised evaluation measures (Joseph Rowntree Foundation 2005). Whilst the evidence is still a little ambiguous, there is an overall agreement that family support, through structured parenting programmes, should be available for vulnerable families.

Sure Start

Sure Start initiatives are widely considered to provide a solid start to vulnerable children in their early years. Nurses, midwives and health visitors are a crucial element in the delivery of such multidisciplinary initiatives, and the evidence base in support of *Sure Start* continues to grow.

At government policy level it has been stated explicitly that the development of *Sure Start* draws heavily on the experience of the American *Head Start* programme (Glass 2000, 2001). *Head Start* was established in the 1960s throughout the USA and has been researched extensively through randomised controlled trials. *Head Start* programmes focused on provision of pre-school education with active parental involvement. In addition to the educational component, family support was also provided. *Head Start* was targeted at families living below the poverty threshold and trials showed promising educational benefit for the children involved. In the medium term these educational effects were less significant, but longer-term follow-up showed that the benefits of *Head Start* re-emerged at high school. It is now recognised by researchers (if not by politicians!) however, that early intervention alone cannot be expected to produce outstanding long-term benefits without ongoing support for children throughout their childhood (Macdonald & Roberts 1995).

There is a strong emerging evidence base for early family support projects such as *Sure Start*. Yoshikawa (1994) presented a comprehensive review of early family support projects and concluded that the most beneficial programmes shared the following features:

- the programmes provided support for children in both peer group and family settings
- the programmes had a home visiting component
- the programmes included education and/or day care
- support was both home and pre-school/centre based.

Consideration should be given to the training needs of teams working with vulnerable families. All team members should be in receipt of regular updates on child protection issues: it is not enough to say that child protection cases are not included or are referred elsewhere. The recommendations from the Climbié Inquiry emphasise the need for robust procedures, collaboration and communication (Laming Report 2003). Central to this is the identification and use of an appropriate framework to guide practitioners in the assessment process of families with young children.

Teams can fail because of reliance on strong individuals who may leave or become absent. Training should therefore be offered regarding the development and succession of roles and responsibilities in such teams. It is also important to note that *Sure Start* initiatives are not a uniform package of interventions and whilst they are intended to work across vulnerable communities, it is not always easy to identify these reliably. Thus it might be worth considering auditing referrals in terms of socio-economic status and ethnicity to ensure consistency and true representation across the community. Given the low visibility of some people in the community, it is important to involve the services of specialist organisations within the community; for example, the specialist health visitor for travelling people or local ethnic minority community leaders. In addition, since *Sure Start* projects provide a range of services that interact with and perhaps overlap other services, it is important to identify clear boundary definitions for team members and statutory services.

It is encouraging that the guidance for development of *Sure Start* programmes in the UK seems to be founded on evidence-based principles. *Sure Start* is very much based on the ideology of early interventions, of working with families when children are at their most vulnerable. Indeed there is a plethora of evidence to show that children are given a much better start in life if their needs are met early (Macdonald & Roberts 1995).

Children in hospital

Given that about one and a half million children a year spend time away from home in hospital, hospitals have a duty of care to provide a safe and secure environment to a doubly vulnerable group (vulnerable by virtue of being children and being hospitalised for whatever reason). In the early 1990s, following the case of Beverley Allitt, the Clothier Report (Clothier 1994) led to a review of security within paediatric units. Despite occasional high profile scandals (such as Allitt), there is little evidence to suggest that children are abused in hospital, in contrast to children's residential homes (Chesson & Chisholm 1995). Even so, there is a potential risk, not just from direct physical or sexual abuse, but from wider institutional, programme and system abuse (see Butler, Chapter 10, in this volume).

In their exploration of safeguarding children from abuse in hospital, Kendrick and Taylor (2000) emphasised three crucial aspects for all health practitioners.

- Listening to children: There must be accessible ways for children to voice their concerns, and partnership and family involvement in care is another aspect of the protection of children (Utting *et al.* 1997).
- Selection, training and support: The quality of staff and carers is crucial. Major reviews have shown discrepancies in recruitment and selection processes. It is unlikely that, however rigorous, screening processes will prevent all abusers from entering the system (Rae *et al.* 1997). Therefore it is important to ensure that dangerous practice is avoided, rather than assuming that all dangerous people have been screened out (Stark *et al.* 1997). It is also crucial that staff are appropriately educated and skilled in awareness of all the needs of children.
- Inspection, monitoring and standards: Residential care placements for children are subject to statutory reviews and inspections. Children's services in hospital are not yet uniformly inspected, however, nor is there always a child protection policy in place. The responsibilities of professional registering bodies such as the GMC and the NMC to remove individuals from the professional register where there is cause for concern have not always been as responsive or as tightly controlled as would be always in the public interest (Long 1992).

Kendrick and Taylor (2000) concluded:

While we would be the first to praise the positive work of nurses, doctors and other medical staff in children's health services, it is vitally important that the issue of the abuse of children in hospital settings is addressed openly and honestly. It is crucial that an holistic and integrated approach to the care and protection of children and young people in hospital is adopted and the current agenda of quality care in the NHS must address the particular needs of children. (p. 572)

Multiprofessional approaches

High profile inquiries have galvanised the government into developing a better coordinated approach to children's services. It is apparent that many of the recommendations made by Lord Laming and others are now being translated into policy initiatives and in turn these should filter down to have an impact at the practitioner–child/family interface. There are three crucial factors in this:

1. the need for high quality information to be recorded and to be available to whomever, whenever it is needed
2. the need to provide training and education for all workers involved with vulnerable children
3. the need to develop multiprofessional, cross-agency methods of working.

As can be seen from the above, there is clearly a need for a more joined-up coordinated approach in safeguarding vulnerable children.

The aim of multiprofessional working is to be applauded, but the reality is difficult to achieve. Multiprofessional working and collaboration has been promoted as the best way forward, not only within child protection, but also in general in the provision of services (e.g. Scottish Executive 2000, DoH 2002c). It is often said that such an approach will improve outcomes for the client – but will it? Although there is literature available that discusses successful collaborative projects (e.g. Stepans *et al.* 2002), to date there is a significant lack of empirical evidence demonstrating that collaborative working improves client outcomes. Indeed, the reverse seems to be the case, with much literature citing the difficulties and barriers to engaging in truly collaborative approaches (Loxley 1997, Leathard 2003). Mutual respect and non-hierarchical relationships are the foundations of successful collaborative working (Kenny 2002).

It has to be questioned, however, how realistic is such an aim. Health practitioners are not a homogeneous group and there continue to be difficulties in achieving collaboration in the provision of services in a field which, by tradition, has a pecking order deeply rooted in the superiority of the medical profession. Achieving collaboration across the organisational and professional boundaries with others responsible for the care of people therefore seems likely to be even more difficult. Major stumbling blocks include the organisational culture in which individuals are working, differing professional values and methods of professional socialisation, issues of power, and the continuing absence of any research that can clearly demonstrate a link between collaboration and improved client outcomes.

A number of challenges therefore face health practitioners who may be involved in working with vulnerable children and their families, not least because the whole arena of child protection within health care has changed rapidly within recent years. High profile public inquiries have resulted in a radical overhaul of the way in which children and young people are safeguarded, resulting in a tremendous drive in policy development that has major implications for health professionals. Health practitioners' roles in child protection may be observational, forensic, investigative and/or therapeutic. Making these truly effective, however, and ensuring that all health practitioners are aware of their responsibilities and enabling them to play their full part in multiprofessional practice, still requires more work.

Key points and messages for practice

- Child protection and the safeguarding of children is everybody's business – not just the health visitor and the midwife. Health professionals who may not be working directly with children have an important part to play through their work with vulnerable parents and carers.

- The ability to prevent or detect child abuse – whether physical, psychological or emotional – requires confidence and skill. This can only be gained through appropriate education, training, supervision and continual updating.

- There is a need to develop multiprofessional, or more particularly interprofessional, ways of working which put the child and family, rather than the professional or service, at the centre of care delivery. This can only be achieved if hostilities and professional rivalries can be suspended and a genuine commitment to working together fostered.

- There needs to be better communication between professionals and with children and with families. There needs to be better recording of this communication and the information it generates. Whilst the new Information Strategy will go some way to improving information sharing, the quality of that information is still dependent on the practitioner.

Annotated further reading

Crisp B R, Lister P G 2004 Child protection and public health: nurses' responsibilities. Journal of Advanced Nursing 47:656–663
This study investigates the work of nurses involved in child protection issues. The authors discuss the lack of consensus regarding what this involvement should entail and make a case for nurses, other than just health visitors, to have a role in child protection.

Department for Education and Skills 2005 Common core of skills for the children's workforce. DfES, London
This document sets out six key skills and knowledge areas that practitioners working with children will be required to have and explains what will be required within each of these in detail. This document will shape the way in which practitioners will be trained and the way in which services for children and young people will be provided in the future.

Department of Health 2004 The Chief Nursing Officer's review of the nursing, midwifery and health visiting contribution to vulnerable children and young people. DoH, London
Produced in response to a recommendation within Every Child Matters, *this review considers the requirements of children with a wide range of needs and how these can be met by nurses, midwives and health visitors across all work settings. It provides useful advice to service commissioners, managers and agencies on how to develop and support an appropriately skilled workforce to meet the needs of children and young people.*

Commission for Social Care Inspection 2005 Safeguarding children. The second joint Chief Inspectors' Report on arrangements to safeguard children. CSCI, London
This second report draws together the conclusions of inspection activity carried out by a range of agencies across England, reporting on progress already made and work still needing to be done to safeguard vulnerable children.

Rouse S 2002 Protecting children: the role of the health visitor. In: Wilson K, James A (eds) The child protection handbook, 2nd edn. Baillière Tindall, Edinburgh, pp. 305–318
This chapter provides a comprehensive overview of the historical and political context of health visiting in relation to child protection and discusses the role of the health visitor at three strategic levels.

Sammons P, Power S, Robertson P, Elliot K, Campbell C, Whitty G 2002 National evaluation of the new community schools pilot programme in Scotland: phase 1: interim findings. Scottish Executive, Edinburgh
Health practitioners have an important role in schools. New community schools, integrated schools, full service schools and health promoting schools have received much political attention for the early opportunities they afford children and families (e.g. breakfast clubs). A useful account is provided by the authors of this document.

Hall D M B, Elliman D 2003 Health for all children, 4th edn. Oxford University Press, Oxford
Also known as Hall 4, the fourth edition sets out proposals for preventative health care, health promotion and an effective community-based response to the needs of children, families and young people.

Taylor J, Daniel B 2005 Child neglect: practice issues for health and social care. Jessica Kingsley, London
Neglect is now recognised as leading to significantly poor outcomes for children in the short and long term. Children who are neglected are not likely to seek help in their own right and are highly dependent on professionals such as health visitors identifying and responding to their needs for support and protection.

Useful addresses

Children's National Skills Framework Team
526 Wellington House
133–155 Waterloo Road
London SE1 8UG

Commission for Social Care Inspection
33 Greycoat Street
London SW1P 2QF

Department of Health
PO Box 777
London SE1 6XH

NHS 24
Delta House, 50 West Nile Street
Glasgow G1 2NP

Useful websites
Child Health Specialist Library – useful resource for professionals and lay people involved with children: http://rms.nelh.nhs.uk/childhealth

Department for Education and Skills – useful for publications, reports and statistics (all DfES documents cited in this chapter can be viewed here): www.dfes.gov.uk

Department of Health – useful for publications, reports and statistics (all DoH documents cited in this chapter can be viewed here); also contains a practical guide to the law relating to child protection: www.dh.gov.uk

Gateway to search NHS services in England: www.nhs.uk

Access to the Safeguarding Children publications: www.safeguardingchildren.org.uk

Sure Start: www.surestart.gov.uk

UNICEF, the charity working to protect children across the world: www.unicef.org/protection

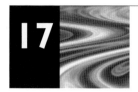

17 Safeguarding children in education

Mary Baginsky and Jo Green

INTRODUCTION

It has long been accepted that schools are well placed to play a part in a holistic approach to children's welfare. The history of schooling, while also containing stories of barbaric and inappropriate treatment, reflects a shift towards society's growing awareness of and responsibility for children. Thus, as the twentieth century saw an increasing awareness of child abuse and an increased role for government in devising relevant policies, a more formal role for schools in protecting children also developed. Although there is no empirical evidence to support it, there was a belief in some quarters that teachers did not think child protection was their concern. If there were teachers who thought like that – and there were probably some – the next generation has embraced the responsibilities willingly and define themselves as central to the process of safeguarding children (Baginsky 2003a).

From Plowden to Cleveland

Over the past 40 years there has been a more concerted attempt to develop systematic strategies and programmes designed to help address the issue of child protection, although the fact that new legislation in the form of the Children Act 2004 has now been deemed necessary implies a failure of that which preceded it. The emphasis on agencies working together was evident as long ago as the 1945 Inquiry into the death of Dennis O'Neill (Home Office 1945), the Curtis Report (Curtis 1946) and the Children Act 1948. These references continued in reports issued over the following years, becoming more evident and specific in the 1960s in the Central Advisory Council for Education Report (Plowden Report) in 1967 and Committee on Local Authority and Allied Personal Social Services Report (Seebohm Report) in 1968.

However, a new impetus followed the death of Maria Colwell and the subsequent Inquiry (DHSS 1974b). As a result, a *Memorandum on Non-Accidental Injury to Children* (DHSS 1974c) was issued to Area Health Authorities and Directors of Social Services and copied to the Schools Section of the Department of Education and Science (DES). The *Memorandum* recommended that the Director of Education be one of the local authority representatives on Area Review Committees. It identified the professionals who should attend case conferences and recommended that persons with statutory responsibility for the continuing care of the child should be present, alongside those responsible for the provision of services. Teachers were included in the list of those who could be invited as appropriate, along with police surgeons and representatives of the housing department and other agencies that may have information about the child and family.

The *Memorandum* also dealt with the training of those who worked with young children and their families in order to familiarise them with all aspects of the problem, particularly the early warning signs. It recommended that the Area Review Committees monitor training and develop a training plan designed to increase knowledge, awareness and vigilance amongst various groups. One of these groups was staff in schools, particularly those in nursery and primary schools, and education welfare officers. It was recognised, then as now, that:

In the long run it is through training and preventative work that there are real prospects of reducing the incidence of non-accidental injury to children.

(DHSS 1974c, p. 5)

However, there is little evidence of a specific 'education voice' in the years that followed. Even though the intention remained to ensure inter-agency (and inter-professional) cooperation and coordination, there was a steady growth in the level of concern and dissatisfaction with the professional response to such issues, as demonstrated in the Cleveland Inquiry (Butler-Sloss 1988) into child abuse and inquiries into the deaths of children at the hands of their carers.

Some of the Inquiry Reports did, however, refer specifically to schools and to teachers. The Chairman's report on the Lucie Gates Inquiry (London Borough of Bexley 1982) referred to the importance of teachers being able to recognise indicators of abuse. In the same year, the Richard Fraser Inquiry (London Borough of Lambeth *et al.* 1982) criticised the failure of school staff to understand the correct procedures to follow in the case of suspected non-accidental injuries. A few years later the report of the Inquiry into the death of Jasmine Beckford (London Borough of Brent 1985) commented on the divide that existed between social workers and schools, which was a barrier to collaboration. The Inquiry emphasised a teacher's essential role in monitoring children by acknowledging that no other adult, with the exception of the child's parents or carers, 'enjoys such an intense, continuous, consistent and private relationship with a child' (p. 10).

The Children Act 1989 and what accompanied it

Although there had been a growing demand to increase cooperation across agencies, there was little guidance on how to achieve this until the Children Act 1989. The Act, described by the then Lord Chancellor, Lord Mackay of Clashfern, as 'the most comprehensive and far-reaching reform of child law which has come before Parliament in living memory' (Hansard 1988), was built on an assumption that there should be a coordinated approach to disadvantaged and vulnerable children. It brought education within the net by placing specific duties on local education authorities (LEAs) to assist local authority social services departments acting on behalf of children in need or investigating allegations of abuse. The guidance that accompanied the implementation of the *Working Together Under the Children Act 1989* (Home Office *et al.* 1991) identified specific tasks for teachers and school nurses and set the context for joint working between schools and social services departments.

Just prior to the passage of the 1989 Children Act, Circular 4/88 (DES 1988) recommended that a senior member of an LEA's staff should act as a child protection coordinator and, similarly, that schools should identify a member of staff to take responsibility for child protection. Seven years later, Circular 10/95 (DfEE 1995) further clarified the responsibility for child protection issues within education departments, schools and colleges and gave guidance on links with other agencies involved in the protection of children. Each LEA was directed to appoint a senior official to have overall responsibility for the coordination of policy, procedures and training and for making sure that procedures were set out in authority-wide documentation. The guidelines reinforced the recommendation that all schools should have a senior member of staff as the designated and named child protection liaison teacher/coordinator and that this person should have received adequate training.

From guidance to practice

Even by the late 1990s, however, there were few UK texts that examined the role of schools and education in child protection, Maher (1987) and David (1993, 1994) being the most significant exceptions. *Child Abuse: The Educational Perspective* (Maher 1987) grew out of a seminar on child abuse which had taken place at Stoke Rochford in 1985. The issues discussed at the seminar and in the book are as relevant today as they were in the mid 1980s, including the need for more training for teachers in the subject and a more informed understanding by all the relevant professions of each other's practice. While Maher speculated that abuse was an issue likely to be affecting a significant minority of children, another contributor to the 1985 conference (Creighton) quoted the rate of reported abuse* as being then 0.73 cases per 1000 children and from this extrapolated that an average teacher in an average school would come across an abused child once every 30 years.

Twelve years later the National Society for the Prevention of Cruelty to Children (NSPCC) claimed that at least two children in every class suffered serious abuse at some point in their lives†, which seems to reflect both a greater awareness of the incidence and prevalence of abuse as well as a shift in definition. One of the most significant themes throughout the book was that teachers tended to underestimate the importance of their role in multi-agency networks. With hindsight, it is a shame that in the years that followed, more emphasis was not placed on Maher's conclusion that teachers' perception of their lack of expertise needed to be addressed by raising their confidence, as such an apprehension may have accounted for their failure to engage with other agencies and been interpreted as a lack of interest.

Similarly, David (1993, 1994) was the first to define the role of the teacher within the multi-agency framework, following the Children Act 1989, from the perspective of a teacher. Although writing specifically within the context of early years education, she raised issues that have not been explored to any great extent in the intervening years within the UK context, such as the impact of curricular changes, the time this work requires, and the difficulties of bringing people together with very different understandings and prejudices about abuse. In the later edited work by David (1994), both Braun and Schonveld (1994) and Goodyear (1994) explore the challenges to be faced in training students and qualified teachers in child protection. They claimed that while teachers do care a great deal about child protection issues there were obstacles to their further participation. One of the most important challenges was for teachers to become absolutely clear and confident about their role before they could be expected to contribute to work across agency boundaries. It is interesting that one of the few non-educationalists to have attempted to set out training priorities for teachers did so without any reference to LEA or school policies or context (Pugh 1992).

---

* Creighton pointed out that all knowledge about the extent of abuse was based on reported cases.
† BBC interview with Mary Marsh, Chief Executive of the NSPCC, on 19 November 2000 discussing findings of the prevalence study, *Child Maltreatment in the United Kingdom* (Cawson *et al.* 2000).

There are few research studies examining the way in which teachers and schools in the UK have dealt with these issues; far more attention had been paid to it in the USA. For the most part, those that did exist drew on specific case studies or were based on limited samples or specific authorities. One of most influential studies was reported by Hallett and Birchall (1992; see also Hallett 1995). In attempting to identify the factors that might impact on inter-professional collaboration over child protection they surveyed GPs, health visitors, paediatricians, specialist police, social workers and teachers. Social workers, police and paediatricians were identified as the key network figures. Teachers and general practitioners headed the list of those whose role was very unclear to other professionals. Only a minority of workers believed the system was working smoothly, with many instances of inter-agency and inter-professional friction and confusion being identified. However, it has to be remembered that the research was taking place at a time when the schools and LEAs were just beginning to make a significant response to the Children Act 1989.

Informal reports, followed by research evidence (Baginsky 2000a), indicated that not only were schools appointing designated teachers for child protection in line with DES and subsequently DfEE* guidance (DES 1988, DfEE 1995), but that more of them (and possibly other teachers as well) were also receiving training related to the post. Many LEAs began to keep lists of the designated teachers in their schools and record the training they received. In 1995 and 1997, specific funds were made available for child protection training through Grants for Education Support and Training (GEST) funding. This supported the development of existing and new training programmes and enabled many designated teachers to receive training. In many cases the LEA rather than the Area Child Protection Committee (ACPC) provided the training. The numbers in many authorities would have overwhelmed the ACPC training provision. In most cases there was close liaison between the LEA and the ACPC, with the latter often providing multi-agency training that enabled teachers to join other professionals to examine how and why agencies worked together on child protection.

LEAs had been concerned that they would not be able to sustain the level of training when GEST support disappeared but in fact the actual provision, if not attendance, increased slightly between 1998 and 2002 (Baginsky 2003a). The biggest challenges came from two sources: the volume of training needed and the ability of schools to release teachers. Not only did they have to train new designated teachers in addition to maintaining training updates for existing ones, LEAs also had to raise the level of child protection awareness of all teachers, usually by providing training sessions after school or during in-service training days. In most authorities, even with a dedicated child protection officer, it would have taken years to cover all schools. Although the number had increased, many authorities did not have a dedicated officer and the post-holder was also responsible for a range of issues in addition to child protection. The second challenge – that of teachers being free to attend – was a reflection of the pressures on schools as well as the shortage and cost of supply teachers. In most cases, priority was given to releasing designated teachers for initial training, but it was more difficult for a senior member of staff or a headteacher to be out of school for multi-agency training, which often took 2–3 days. LEAs and ACPCs were in agreement that teachers did not attend these courses in sufficient numbers and were most likely to have to cancel their places.

---

* The Department of Education and Science (DES) changed to the Department for Education (DFE) on 6 July 1992, to the Department for Education and Employment (DfEE) on 4 July 1995 and to the Department for Education and Skills (DfES) in June 2001.

There were other factors that got in the way of working effectively with other agencies, some more obvious than others. As noted above, there was a push to engage schools more closely in child protection procedures in the late 1980s and early 1990s; however, from the mid 1980s onwards, schools were under the pressure of almost constant change with the introduction of the national curriculum, new inspection regimes and both increased accountability and autonomy. LEAs were also assuming responsibilities in relation to both the Children Act 1989 and the DES (and subsequently DfEE) guidance at a time when their future was in some doubt: although a great deal of power had effectively resided with LEAs since they came into existence in 1902, the fraught relationships between the government and certain LEAs made the role of the LEA a manifesto issue in the 1987 general election. From then on, government policy was to reduce the powers of LEAs and give greater autonomy to schools by the delegation of budgets to schools, and the introduction of grant-maintained status with the option for schools to remove themselves from LEA control.

These steps, combined with the limitations and reductions placed on local government funding and expenditures by the Education Reform Act 1988 and successive legislation, left LEAs with responsibility for the:

servicing, monitoring and management of local education. They also dissolve the essential notion that the schools of a local authority form a 'system'.

(Radnor & Ball 1996, p. 54)

As far as their responsibilities for child protection and inter-agency collaboration were concerned, the dissolution of that 'system' was at best a disadvantage and at worst a significant impediment to how effective an LEA could be in ensuring that schools conformed. So while LEAs have been active in supporting schools over policies and training it has not usually been regarded as a key function of the LEA and was not prioritised in terms of seniority of staff or resources.

Although it is impossible to judge the precise impact of the negative press that social workers have received over the years, and particularly at that time, it seems likely that it had some impact on the willingness of other professionals to work with them or to trust their judgements. At the very time when schools were being brought more formally into child protection procedures, social workers were being condemned for acting too slowly in cases such as that of Kimberly Carlile (London Borough of Greenwich 1987) and Tara Henry (London Borough of Lambeth 1987), and too hastily in removing children in Cleveland.

From observing the child protection training that many designated teachers received it was clear that the emphasis was on the signs that might indicate a child was suffering abuse and on the reporting of concerns to the social worker. The terms 'significant harm' and 'child in need' are fundamental to the Children Act 1989 but were rarely explored or explained in training. Within the Children Act 1989, there is no definition of risk; child protection is constructed in terms of 'significant harm'. There are no absolute criteria on which to rely in judging what constitutes significant harm and it is dependent on an assessment of risk. Within a child protection context, thresholds have been defined as:

the point at which behaviour is defined as abusive. Furthermore they represent the point beyond which one set of actions relevant to one stage of the child protection process is superseded by those of a successive stage.

(Little 1997, p. 28)

In other words, they represent the point at which there will be the next level of intervention: the decisions to accept a child abuse report, then to conduct an investigation, and then to substantiate maltreatment. All too often, however, there was no discussion of what might happen when the referral reached social services or of the thresholds that might then apply. This is not to deny the difficulties of providing training in a complex area using short and bolted-on courses (see Baginsky 2000b): such training is of questionable value, however, if it fails to deal with the complexities that face teachers in practice. In a study of the interface between schools and social services over child protection referrals (Baginsky forthcoming), it was evident that some social service departments were applying inappropriately high thresholds in responding to child protection referrals, usually because of the pressures on limited resources. When schools did not receive an appropriate response (or sometimes no response) following their referral of a child because of their concerns, it led to frustration, bemusement and disengagement. Relationships between social services and schools are then put under strain.

The second Joint Chief Inspectors' report (Commission for Social Care Inspection 2005a) noted, just as its predecessor had, that in most areas there were serious concerns amongst staff of all agencies about the thresholds that social services were applying in their children's services and the adequacy of guidance, advice and support when they raised concerns about the welfare of particular children or young people. While the report stresses that many of these difficulties were explained by staff shortages within children's teams in social services, the Inspectors found that the effect was to produce a reluctance on the part of schools to refer concerns. This is an issue that has been identified in many Ofsted reports on local education authorities (Baginsky 2003b). Similarly, Ofsted reports have repeatedly commented on the fact that while managers in education and social care often work well together, this has not always been reflected in the relationship between schools and social service teams.

The research on the interface between the two agencies also found that social workers expressed frustrations both over many of the referrals they received from schools and over their lack of awareness of current procedures and practice. On occasions they complained about schools' failure to make timely referrals and to hang onto concerns for too long; more frequently, however, they referred to schools making too many inappropriate referrals. Schools were anxious to play their part in a collaborative approach to safeguarding children but were too often confused by the threshold for action by social services and by the definition of what constituted 'at risk of significant harm' and 'a child in need'. Social workers wondered why schools did not make direct referrals to services in the community which might be able to help families, while schools were unaware of when they could make such a referral and usually did not have knowledge of available providers.

So while schools accepted their responsibilities to report concerns, they were less proactive than some social workers may have wanted, especially with the shift towards prevention and support rather than investigation, following the publication of *Child Protection: Messages from Research* (DoH 1995a). This summarised the results of a number of research projects which had been sponsored by the Department of Health and concluded that risk and investigation dominated social work with children to the exclusion of assessing and providing services to children in need. The document suggested that many vulnerable children were falling through the net because of a failure to employ a holistic assessment.

New guidance on how agencies should work together – *Working Together to Safeguard Children** (DoH *et al.* 1999) and the *Framework for the Assessment of*

---

* The most up-to-date version of this document was published by HM Government in 2006. For a full discussion of this, see Chapter 11.

Children in Need and their Families (DoH *et al.* 2000) – was therefore introduced in an attempt to remedy this. The Framework sought to change the way in which social workers approached assessment and intervention by helping them to 'take a more holistic approach to family assessment and consider the wider environment and its influence on family functioning' (Hamilton & Browne 2002, p. 40). But even though the DfEE was a co-signatory to both these documents, the Department failed to publicise their implications for education in general and schools specifically, nor did it provide guidance on implementation. Consequently, there was a low awareness of their existence and significance in schools, and frustration amongst social workers.

The shortage of social workers has impacted not only on decisions over whether or not to take any action but also on available time for face-to-face discussions between the professions. If two professionals have the opportunity to discuss cases and concerns directly, it is more likely that they will be able to reach agreement as well as reaching a better understanding of each other's domain and decision making. Although it is not inevitable, experience suggests that where teachers and social workers are able to establish contact, learn about each other's work and priorities, and access each other's expertise and knowledge, many of the barriers and frustrations dissipate, along with any stereotyping. Sometimes this happens when schools and social service teams are geographically close or where local services have agreed to meet regularly to review practice. Experience has also shown, however, that while schools nearly always welcomed the opportunity to have direct contact with social workers, they were frustrated by having to go through call centres and discuss cases with administrative staff over the telephone.

Recent developments

After a late amendment to the Education Bill 2002, s.157 and s.175 became part of the Education Act which received Royal Assent in the summer of 2002. S.175 states:

1. A local education authority shall make arrangements for ensuring that the functions conferred on them in their capacity as a local education authority are exercised with a view to safeguarding and promoting the welfare of children.
2. The governing body of a maintained school shall make arrangements for ensuring that their functions relating to the conduct of the school are exercised with a view to safeguarding and promoting the welfare of children who are pupils at the school.

Although s.175 did not come into force until June 2004, s.157 of the 2002 Act, along with the Education (Independent Schools) Regulations 2003, came into force on 1 September 2003, and placed the same duties on the proprietors of independent schools.

The amendments to the Bill were a direct result of the death of Lauren Wright in May 2000. Although the Inquiry into her death (Norfolk Health Authority 2002) found other agencies to be culpable, the child protection arrangements in Lauren's school were deemed to be wholly inadequate. One of the main concerns was that although staff at Lauren's school had failed her in every way by not following guidelines, these guidelines had no force in law and it was this issue that the late amendment sought to redress. They did not introduce new functions but upgraded to requirements functions that were previously only recommendations.

During the passage of the legislation, concern was expressed by some teachers' associations that it would lead to private actions against individuals, but this was not the intention of the amendment. Rather, the purpose of s.157 and s.175 of the Act was to add further safeguards for children by placing the duty to make child protection arrangements on a statutory basis. It gives grounds to the governing body, or the employing authority in the case of local authority staff, to give proper consideration to possible disciplinary action against an individual employee.

In September 2004, government guidance (*Safeguarding Children in Education*, DfES 2004f) was issued to local authorities, governing bodies of maintained schools and non-maintained special schools, further education institutions and proprietors of independent schools, as well as head teachers of all schools and principals of Further Education Institutions. It replaced the existing education child protection guidance (Circular 10/95, DfEE 1995) and was issued with the status of 'strongly recommended'. The new guidance sets out the specific duty to safeguard and promote the welfare of children. In this respect, it emphasises the need for all staff within education services to share the view that the safeguarding of children may best be undertaken by proactively making detailed arrangements to provide a safe environment within educational settings.

The guidance also makes clear that, within the wider remit of safeguarding and promoting the welfare of *all* children, there remains a need for education staff to identify those *individual* children who are suffering or may be likely to suffer significant harm and for appropriate action to be taken. It does not, however, go into the detail of what such appropriate action should be. Rather it notes that staff working with children across the agencies should be familiar with the practice guidance contained within *What to Do If You're Worried a Child is Being Abused* produced by the Department of Health in June 2003 (DoH 2003b) in response to the Laming Inquiry following the death of Victoria Climbié, who died in February 2000, just 3 months before Lauren Wright. She had not been registered at a school and therefore the opportunity for education staff to have identified her as suffering from the ill-treatment which eventually led to her death was lost. This opportunity was available to the staff at the school which Lauren Wright attended but it had been missed. It is vital, therefore, that while schools and local authorities embrace the wider implications of minimising the risk of harm for all their pupils, they do not lose sight of the core responsibility for reacting to concerns about individual children who may be suffering harm.

These two aspects of the duty placed upon education staff – to safeguard all children and to protect individual children from harm – are coterminous. The shift towards a preventative model for education staff provides the opportunity to embed within schools an ethos of responsibility for safety and care which permeates all school policies and practices and affords the opportunity for staff to make their own specific contribution to the objective of keeping children safe, an objective shared by colleagues in other professions.

In the summer of 2003 two further child deaths occurred. Holly Wells and Jessica Chapman, pupils at a school in Cambridgeshire, were murdered by the caretaker of a neighbouring school. These deaths tragically highlighted the need for more to be done to ensure that children were protected from unsuitable people who might try to gain access to children through their employment. As a result of an Inquiry into the deaths of the two girls, Sir Michael Bichard made 31 recommendations including that headteachers and school governors should receive training to ensure that the process of appointing staff reflected the importance of safeguarding children (Bichard Inquiry Report 2004). The DfES responded to this recommendation in the summer of 2005 by commissioning the National College for School Leadership to provide online training (www.ncsl.org.uk/saferrecruitment) and by writing guidance for all educational establishments and businesses that provide staff to schools – *Safeguarding Children: Safer Recruitment and Selection in Education Settings* (DfES 2005j). This guidance supplements *Safeguarding Children in Education* (DfES 2004f) and, as such, complying with it becomes a duty within s.157 and s.175 of the Education Act 2002.

Implementing the *Safeguarding Children in Education* guidance

When local authorities, governors and schools (both maintained and independent), as well as further education institutions, put safeguarding policies in place or update those that exist, they must have regard to any guidance issued to them by the Secretary of State. Herein lie the teeth of the new 'guidance' documents: policies, procedures and all other safeguarding arrangements that are put in place by a school must demonstrate that they are in accordance with the guidance or 'that they achieve the same effect' (DfES 2004f). Any education institution, therefore, which fails to have regard to this, by ignorance or choice, does so at its peril.

The *Safeguarding Children in Education* guidance is not prescriptive in its advice to local authorities and governors, nor is it a comprehensive guide on how schools should safeguard and promote the welfare of their pupils. Rather, it emphasises the importance of schools embracing and embedding safeguarding practices into every aspect of school life. The government's safeguarding agenda contained within *Every Child Matters* (DfES 2004b) emphasises education as a universal service – for the majority of children this means attending school on a daily basis – and school staff are considered, therefore, to be uniquely placed to ensure that all children are provided with the means to stay safe while they are at school. However, in order for the outcome of 'staying safe' to be achieved, school staff will need to consider the effectiveness of their policies and practices in a number of areas. These areas include, for example, how the school deals with bullying and racist behaviour, how school staff support those pupils with specific medical needs, how the school monitors the effectiveness of its security system and how it monitors the safety and welfare of those pupils who are on work experience placements.

The term 'child protection' has sometimes been understood by school staff to mean that their response to concerns about a particular child should be immediate. In practice, this has shaped the training which teachers have received: it has focused on the skills to recognise signs or symptoms of possible harm and the knowledge of how to make an appropriate referral to their colleagues in their local social services department. The training must now embrace the skills that all school staff will need in order to respond to the imperatives covered within 'safeguarding', as well as those needed to recognise the potential for harm, which may appear in many forms that are different from those previously associated with child abuse and neglect. In the light of their increased responsibility to safeguard and promote the welfare of children, teachers and other members of school staff have raised concerns that their commitment to protect their pupils from harm is not matched by opportunities to attend appropriate training. In these circumstances, a school's leadership team should be seeking advice on these matters from their colleagues within the local authority.

The guidance (DfES 2004f) from the Secretary of State makes it clear that local education authorities have strategic, operational and support responsibilities. This means that – in addition to planning and coordinating services, allocating resources and working with other agencies (strategic), and taking responsibility for safeguarding children who are not in school (operational) – they must make sure maintained schools are aware of, and able to fulfil, their responsibilities in this area (support). The guidance sets out what this support role entails. At this level the local authority has to:

- make sure relevant induction training is available for all new staff working in the authority who will work with children, as well as for governors
- make sure that refresher training is available for these members of staff every 3 years
- make sure staff with designated responsibilities in schools receive appropriate training on appointment and that refresher training is available every 2 years
- monitor the performance of schools in this area
- make available to them model policies and procedures
- provide appropriate advice and support.

This means that officers within the local authority who hold a delegated responsibility for safeguarding will have to ensure that all staff working with children in schools are provided with the skills needed to adopt this proactive approach to safeguarding generally, in addition to those skills needed to recognise those pupils who may be suffering abuse or neglect. It is unlikely that multi-professional training provided by the Local Safeguarding Children Boards will be able to provide direct and regular training for all school staff. It will be necessary for education services within the local authority, together with governors and headteachers, to identify ways which will ensure that all school staff are appropriately trained in carrying out their child protection and safeguarding duties.

All schools in the independent and maintained sector must have a designated person for child protection and, equally necessary, all staff must be equipped with an understanding of the role of this designated person so that they can discuss with them any issues of concern. All staff in both sectors must also have both induction training and 3-yearly refresher training. In addition to basic awareness training, the designated person must attend multi-agency training every 2 years in order to enhance and update their understanding of the importance of the role of the school within the multi-agency approach to safeguarding children. Whereas Circular 10/95 (DfEE 1995) referred to a *designated teacher*, the 2004 guidance has introduced the *designated person*. However, it is important that this person has the seniority within the school to carry out the duties of the post, which include advising staff who may express concerns about individual children and committing resources to a variety of child protection and safeguarding matters throughout the school community.

Ultimately, however, it is the responsibility of the governing body to remedy any deficiencies or weaknesses in child protection arrangements. It is therefore essential that the designated person has a clear and overarching view of how effectively all school policies and procedures contribute to the aim of safeguarding children so that they can report to and advise governors accordingly. It is therefore important that the designated person has sufficient resources and time allocated to enable these duties to be carried out, which must include the time needed to take part in interagency discussions and meetings and, additionally, to arrange for similar resources to be in place to enable other staff also to contribute to multi-agency work with individual children where this is appropriate.

With a senior member of staff, experienced and well-trained in all aspects of child welfare, at the helm of all child protection and safeguarding matters within school, an ethos of promoting the welfare of pupils within a safe environment can quickly and thoroughly permeate all aspects of school life.

The voice of the child and the response

When contributing to the government's consultation on their plans for the 'change for children' agenda contained within *Every Child Matters* (DfES 2004b), young people said they wanted to be safe from:

- accidental injury and death
- maltreatment, neglect and sexual exploitation
- exposure to violence
- bullying and discrimination
- crime and antisocial behaviour.

These and other basic rights are enshrined within the UN Convention on the Rights of the Child (Office of the High Commissioner for Human Rights 1989) which was ratified by the United Kingdom in 1991. The following articles are particularly relevant:

Children shall be protected from all forms of physical or mental violence, injury or abuse, neglect or negligent treatment, maltreatment or exploitation, including sexual abuse, while in the care of their parents or of any other person. Child protection should include support for the child and their carers, prevention, identification, reporting, referral, investigation, treatment, judicial involvement, and follow up of instances of child maltreatment. (Article 19)

Any child who is capable of forming his or her own views shall be afforded the right to express those views freely in all matters affecting them. (Article 12)

A school ethos that values and promotes good practice with regard to keeping children safe will have listening to children at its core. All staff in schools should know how to listen to children attempting to raise concerns with a trusted member of staff according to their age, understanding and preferred method of communication.

Such an ethos will encourage children to communicate freely and openly about their concerns or worries, without fear or anxiety, and with a confidence that their concerns will be taken seriously, in an atmosphere of openness and respect. Such an atmosphere is more obvious to children when opportunities for discussion about safe and healthy lifestyles are included within the school curriculum generally, not just as part of the Personal, Social and Health Education curriculum. The elements of 'staying safe', given above, which children themselves have highlighted, can all be brought to the classroom in an appropriate and age-related way. Staff delivering lessons on, for example, the need for children to recognise and avoid situations which may be dangerous, may discuss issues such as domestic violence or abuse; however, they must also then be prepared for children to raise personal concerns about such issues and respond appropriately.

Allegations against a member of staff

All aspects of child protection and safeguarding must be handled sensitively but there is one issue in particular that raises further difficulties for individual members of staff, i.e. when a child makes an allegation against another member of staff. In such circumstances the matter must always be immediately referred to the head-teacher, except when the allegation concerns the headteacher, in which case the matter should be immediately referred to the designated person, who must inform the Chair of Governors. Children cannot be expected to raise their concerns in an atmosphere in which adults are either disbelieving or dismissive. It is important therefore that all staff in a school are aware of their duty to report concerns raised by children and are confident about being able to do so in an appropriate and non-judgemental way. Staff should similarly feel confident and able to report behaviour by colleagues if they see such behaviour as inappropriate or it otherwise causes them concerns.

It is vital that safe recruitment and selection procedures extend to all those working with or who otherwise come into contact with children, whether they are directly employed or working in a voluntary capacity. Governors and headteachers need to be completely satisfied that any person they are selecting to work in their school is fit and suitable to do so. Equally, governors and headteachers need to ensure that, in cases where a person ceases to work at their school and there have been concerns about their suitability to work with, or have contact with, children, or where that person has committed an act of misconduct, the appropriate procedures for sharing information are followed. Specialist support will undoubtedly be needed by schools to manage staff disciplinary matters regarding child protection and safeguarding. The local authority human resources staff or the school's personnel provider will be able to offer such support. The person within the local authority with delegated responsibility for child protection will normally manage the process of an allegation made against a member of education staff and will consult with the headteacher or Chair of Governors, offering support and advice where appropriate.

The vast majority of those who wish to work in schools do so because of a desire and a commitment to enable children to achieve their full potential. It is a sad fact, however, that a small minority of adults abuse the trust that is placed in them and the number of allegations made against teaching and ancillary staff is currently growing. It is impossible to say whether this represents an increase in the level of abuse by education staff or rather is a reflection of children's growing confidence to report such abuse.

In November 2005 the Department for Education and Skills published new guidance for local authorities, governors, headteachers and employment agencies for dealing with allegations of abuse against teachers and other staff. The guidance should be used by all schools, including non-maintained schools, independent schools and academies, as well as further education institutions and all local authorities exercising education functions (DfES 2005k). The guidance seeks to ensure that any allegation of abuse made against a teacher or other member of staff, or volunteer, in an education setting is dealt with fairly, quickly and consistently in a way that provides effective protection for the child and at the same time appropriately supports the person who is the subject of the allegation.

The bigger picture

The changes in relation to the safeguarding responsibilities are taking place within the context of the *Every Child Matters: Change for Children* programme (DfES 2004b) which implements the legislative intentions of the Children Act 2004. Inter-agency governance at a national level was achieved with the coming together of children's services and education in an expanded DfES in 2002. The intention is that this now moves down, through an integrated strategy and processes, to the front line where delivery of services occurs through education, social services and health, and that there should be a focus on safeguarding children, alongside the development of integrated structures and collaborative working. There is, however, no one model and the new arrangements are expected to take several forms. The intention is to have multidisciplinary teams based in accessible settings such as extended schools and children's centres, where designated lead professionals coordinate casework, although there will be many schools that will not be service hubs. Although the intention is that full-service schools will become hubs for coordinated local provision of health, education and social services, there will be very few such schools and it is not clear what the role of schools which are not hubs in this sense will be. While s.157 and s.175 of the Education Act 2002 place a duty on schools to safeguard and promote the welfare of children, they do not place them under a duty to cooperate (s.10 Children Act 2004), and teachers are not named as one of the groups *working with children* that may be part of multidisciplinary teams.

The DfES explained this in terms of the arrangements operating at a strategic level, so the duty to cooperate applies to strategic-level bodies involved in assessing need, developing overarching plans and commissioning services. Four associations representing education and social care leaders issued a joint statement expressing their concerns that, while schools are vital in protecting children, their role had been left unclear in the legislation (Association of Directors of Education and Children's Services *et al.* 2005). The omission was linked in many people's minds with the *Five Year Strategy for Children and Learners* (DfES 2004g) in which plans to devolve further powers to schools, leading to increased disengagement from LEAs, were outlined. The intention is for funding to be directly allocated to schools, with local authorities taking on a 'strategic' role, no longer directly involved with school administration.

Speaking at the Inter-Agency Group Conference in June 2004, Dame Denise Platt, Chair of the Commission for Social Care Inspection, questioned the compatibility of increased devolution of power to schools with increased integration; she also linked the further delegation of budgets to schools with the possibility of reduced resources for children's trusts (Platt 2004). Policy analysts such as Hudson (2005) have commented on how the *Five Year Strategy* and the *Every Child Matters* programme seem to 'pull in different directions' and on the tensions between the imperatives of welfare and attainment. Only time will tell if this is significant but there is a danger that schools under pressure to raise educational performance might not give cooperation with other welfare agencies the required priority.

Key points and messages for practice

- Induction and regular child protection training for school staff is mandatory.
- School staff have a key role in an integrated and multiprofessional approach to safeguarding.
- Listening to children is at the heart of a safeguarding school.
- Robust recruitment and selection procedures help to deter, reject or identify people who might abuse children.

Useful websites

www.teachernet.gov.uk/childprotection – This DfES website contains advice on child protection and offers guidance to schools on the wider issues contained within the duty to safeguard and promote the welfare of children. Model policy documents and guidance on procedures are available to all staff accessing the site and these are regularly updated to keep abreast of the developing agenda.

www.ncsl.org.uk/saferrecruitment – Safer Recruitment is an online training package which has been commissioned by the DfES and developed by the National College for School Leadership in response to recommendation 16 of the Bichard Inquiry Report published in June 2004 which relates to training for headteachers and school governors to ensure that interviews to appoint staff reflect the importance of safeguarding children.

www.everychildmatters.gov.uk – This public website gives a range of news, advice and guidance across the whole of the government's 'change for children' agenda. Information for parents, children and young people as well as professionals is available and it is a useful resource for anyone wishing to keep abreast of new government initiatives.

18 Child protection proceedings in court

Mary Lane

INTRODUCTION

The exhortation in guidance to the Children Act 1989 to engage in partnership with parents has not prevented a steep rise in the number of care proceedings since the Act was implemented in 1991. Involvement in court proceedings has become an everyday and central part of child protection work and it is vital that social workers, health professionals and carers who testify in court have the skills to do so competently: it should not be assumed that, because the welfare of the child is paramount in care and now in adoption proceedings, the judiciary will always follow the professional's view of what is in a child's best interests. Parents are automatically entitled to public funding (previously known as legal aid) to pay for representation in most of these court proceedings and it is inevitable therefore that, at least initially, the vast majority of applications for care and placement orders will be contested. This chapter gives practical and realistic guidance in preparing for and giving evidence in court hearings.

A court will not grant an emergency protection order, care order or placement order unless it is convinced that the threshold criteria are met, i.e. that the child is suffering or is at risk of suffering significant harm attributable to the standard of parental care, and the order is necessary to afford protection to the child or to authorise adoptive placement against parents wishes. (An additional category of significant harm, intended to address situations in which children were witnesses to domestic violence – impairment suffered from seeing or hearing the ill-treatment of another – was inserted into the Children Act 1989 by s.120 of the Adoption and Children Act 2002.)

The court will also require evidence from the local authority to support the validity of the care plan for the child beyond the court proceedings.

When adoption is the care plan, a placement order must be applied for within the care proceedings (Adoption and Children Act 2002, s.21 and s.22). In most local authorities this second application will be made by the looked-after children team social worker who has instigated and given evidence in the application for the care order. The grounds for a placement order include, in most cases, the significant harm threshold already before the court, but local authorities must also convince the court of the reasons for adoption being chosen rather than other options for permanency, and be ready to assist the court in its duty to consider which orders, if any, for contact between the child and birth family will meet the child's needs in the context of an adoption care plan. The complexity of this evidence requires a good knowledge and understanding of adoption and contact issues as well as child protection.

Families often find courts 'frightening and daunting' (Murch & Hooper 1992); many professionals share that view and experience.

The advice in this chapter is based upon the premise that knowing more about what happens in court and why, and how lawyers approach *their* tasks, will better equip witnesses for successful court appearances. It is important, however, to be realistic about the way courts are, rather than to see them as we might want them to be. Despite the pressure for family courts to be 'non-stigmatic responsive institutions employing conciliatory procedures' (Murch & Hooper 1992), courts hearing child welfare matters are not 'user friendly': they are still formal and based upon the adversarial model. Witnesses should therefore acknowledge the particular nature of legal proceedings and adapt behaviour and attitudes accordingly when in the court arena.

Much misunderstanding may be caused between the 'caring' professions and the legal profession because the latter is steeped in tradition and tends to adapt slowly to changes in family life. Judges have traditionally been predominantly white, middle class, middle-aged to elderly men, and most magistrates have conservative life experiences. The judiciary may therefore regard all those who come before them in the light of the usual stereotypes. Women projecting unconventional images of motherhood or femininity may have their evidence devalued, and the discrimination experienced by members of ethnic minorities generally may be present for professionals in court. It is the author's experience, however, that the extensive training given the judiciary in recent years has caused them to bend over backwards to demonstrate rejection of outdated and stereotypical attitudes towards those who appear before them, and court application and response forms now recognise that language and disability issues need to be taken into account to ensure all litigants will be able to participate on an equal basis in court hearings.

Stereotypical attitudes are not necessarily adverse to a witness's credibility – female professional witnesses giving evidence about children may have the advantage of more credibility, at least initially, than their male colleagues, and all witnesses with qualifications and experience will have enhanced status in court, whatever their gender or race, especially if they come across in court as having the qualities consistent with those of credible professionals.

Competence as a witness does not require unthinking collusion with values and methods discordant with those most cherished, but compliance with the procedures and etiquette peculiar to legal fora is necessary. Court is not the place for professionals to challenge with hostile or dismissive behaviour and witnesses should remember that they are not in court on their behalf, but to achieve decisions which protect or enhance the welfare of children. It is therefore important to acknowledge the particular nature of legal proceedings and adapt behaviours (e.g. by dressing appropriately – see below) and attitudes accordingly for the purposes of the court hearing.

Some aspects of litigation in family proceedings are now outlined to assist the reader's understanding. Since barristers and solicitors have rights of audience in family courts, the word 'advocate' is used for both, meaning the lawyer in court.

The Protocol for judicial management of Public Children Act cases

Despite the imperative to avoid delay in the Children Act 1989, care proceedings have taken a very long time to reach resolution, an average of 1 year. The Protocol was implemented on 1 November 2003 with the objective of completing all care proceedings within 40 weeks or less (save in unforeseen or exceptional circumstances).

Core elements of the Protocol include judicial continuity (the same judge for the same child at every hearing), consistency of approach to procedural issues such as

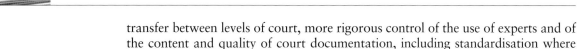

transfer between levels of court, more rigorous control of the use of experts and of the content and quality of court documentation, including standardisation where possible.

The Protocol's success in achieving reductions in delay, in the teeth of intractable problems such as shortages of social workers, experts and judges, is patchy, but it is an inescapable and significant part of child care litigation and professional witnesses should be familiar with its requirements and terminology.

The adversarial method

A social work academic has written of courts as 'a context in which winning is more important than an exploration of all possibilities and options. Social workers seek to have their plans ratified on the basis of selected and selective evidence' (Ryburn 1992). However, the partisan approach this deplores is not a matter of choice when courts are asked to resolve disputes. Professionals may find it hard to accept that their 'non-judgemental' approach may have to give way to taking sides and that, on occasion, the partisan approach requires them to say things in court about others, in their presence, which compassion would otherwise leave unspoken. The conduct of the court process has its foundation in the adversarial method whereby justice is arrived at through a verbal contest between two or more parties, with advocates as their 'champions', according to formal rules designed to achieve a fair hearing for all of them, with each challenging the other's version of events and presenting their own in the best light in order to persuade independent arbitrators to decide in their favour. Adversarial hearings are most ferocious in criminal courts and whilst some legal decisions and procedural methods have tempered the combatant nature of family court proceedings (e.g. relaxed rules of evidence), they have not destroyed it. Whilst care proceedings are adversarial, efforts are usually made to conduct hearings in a less adversarial way.

There are, however, developments stemming from the Human Rights Act 1998 which have slowed the erosion of the adversarial method in family proceedings in order to protect the right under Article 6 to a fair trial for *all* parties, especially the birth parents (see Lyon, Chapter 11, in this volume). Once in court, witnesses may find their own experience less adversarial than anticipated, but it is still necessary to prepare, psychologically and evidentially, for combat, especially in relation to challenging cross-examination.

The power of oral evidence

In family courts, disclosure of each witness's evidence is required in advance of the hearing. Detailed knowledge of what will be said in court does not, however, make the outcome of hearings certain – in contested hearings the judiciary make their decision *after* witnesses have been seen and heard. Oral evidence can be more powerful than written, because the judiciary has much more than words on paper available to them. They can take into account witnesses' demeanour, appearance and attitudes in assessing the value and credibility of their evidence. For the same reason, oral evidence can weaken or even destroy a witness's credibility. In other words, convincing testimony is a matter not only of the evidence given, but also the *way in which* it is given.

Taking instructions

Solicitors accept their clients' instructions, but not uncritically – they should identify weaknesses in cases, give realistic appraisals of the likelihood of success, or suggest viable alternatives. In first meetings between solicitor and witness, the history of the case is discussed if not already known by the solicitor. Witnesses should give their solicitors as much detailed information as possible, including, where appropriate:

- *Family tree*, a diagram of the members of the family, their names, dates of birth, and relationship to each other
- *Chronology* in date order, of significant events, including the beginning (and end) of the witness's involvement with the case. Solicitors will value witnesses' expertise about the emotional or medical impact of events (e.g. repeated admissions to care, shaking a young baby, etc.) and may need help in linking facts to theory (e.g. the effects of abuse, known risk factors, etc.)
- *Names and addresses of other potential witnesses*, e.g. previous health visitors, or the colleague who witnesses a crucial incident, and if possible an opinion as to their likely attitude to giving evidence.

It is also the case that to be forewarned is to be forearmed. Sometimes procedural or practice errors, omissions, etc. occur prior to court proceedings, even in the most professionally conducted cases. Since they may be used by opposing advocates to attack witnesses, it is vitally important that in the privacy of interviews with their own solicitors, witnesses raise these, so that they can be taken into account, and their potential to damage evidence defused.

Preparing evidence

The adversarial method is the basis of the approach taken by lawyers to the preparation and presentation of evidence. A legal textbook has the story of a judge, exasperated by constant interruptions from advocates, asking, 'Am I never to hear the truth in this matter?' – the answer came back from one of them, 'No, my Lord, you will hear the evidence'. Advocates must not lie or mislead the court but do select and shape the information provided by their clients into evidence, presenting the court with that which is persuasive in their favour, and dissembling what is not, rather than giving an all-inclusive exposition.

Turning information into evidence

Teachers of advocacy skills suggest that evidence is prepared by concentrating on six or seven of the strongest and most crucial points arising from the information – the 'pillars' on which the case is constructed – and discarding points which are weak or peripheral. The next exercise is to play 'devil's advocate', often with the help of the future witnesses, by trying to predict the points and arguments which might be advanced from the other side to demolish these pillars, what their pillars might be and how they can be demolished. Witnesses might puzzle at the omissions or the emphasis placed on particular aspects of evidence by the advocate but there comes a time, after all the thought and preparation before court, when witnesses must rely on advocates' skills and judgement.

Leave of court for expert advice

Expert witnesses are those whom the court (judge or magistrates) decides are experts. Formal qualifications are not always necessary. For example, a person with lengthy experience of fostering can give expert evidence about foster care. All professional witnesses have some expertise, but in consultation with their solicitors should consider whether the effective presentation of a particular case in court requires support from those having more; for example, sufficient practice experience to give valid evidence about the prospects of an adoptive placement for a boy of 7.

The usual practice is for the 'expert witnesses' to be agreed amongst the parties, and approved by the court. The expert is then usually instructed by all parties, although this does not prevent the commissioning of further experts by one or more party if the court is persuaded of the need.

The Protocol (see above) requires much closer scrutiny by the judiciary of applications to bring in 'expert witnesses', and this has led in some hearings to a reduction in their use, a consequent decrease in the length of proceedings, and a growing recognition of the value of the knowledge and expertise of social workers and other professionals and carers already involved in the case (described by one children's guardian as expertise 'from stock').

Court rules require permission from the court for experts to examine children for the purposes of giving their expert evidence. Without leave, the evidence may be excluded by the rules of evidence.

Research evidence

Research-based evidence backing up a witness's views will be welcome by advocates, but any research offering alternative views should also be mentioned. A witness intending to use research in evidence should be able to quote chapter and verse and to answer questions about it, as well as deal with contradictory research with which a cross-examiner might challenge the witness. A good advocate becomes an instant expert on any subject!

Evidence of what children have said

Social work witnesses giving evidence about what children have said may be challenged about their familiarity with the two documents (as far as lawyers are concerned) most relevant to interviewing children about abuse – the 'Cleveland' Report (Butler-Sloss 1988) – even if the issue before the court is not *sexual* abuse – and the guidelines to video-recorded interviews with children. Whilst these are principally about children's evidence in criminal proceedings, they should be complied with whenever children are interviewed about alleged abuse (see Williams, Chapter 20, in this volume). Cleveland is usually raised by advocates as an example of (alleged) over-zealous intervention in family life in the hope of introducing doubt in the judiciary's minds about a social worker's case.

Witness statements

Rules of court and the Protocol require that written statements of the evidence to be given by all witnesses are prepared and submitted to court in advance of the final hearing. The intention is to ensure that as much evidence as possible can be agreed, that oral evidence is given on contentious matters only, and to enable each party to prepare their case in the knowledge of what they have to challenge or counter. Statements are either prepared by the solicitor or the witness, who should ask the solicitor to check them. The statement is signed by the witness after carefully ensuring, even though the wording may not quite be their own style, that the contents are true. The sanction of perjury applies to untruthful or misleading statements.

Witnesses should be aware of, and prepare their evidence in the light of where their evidence 'fits in' with the other evidence to be given. This can be ascertained from advocates and by reading other witness statements, bearing in mind whether they are the principal witness setting out the case for a care order, in a supporting role giving evidence about a crucial incident, or an expert witness on a particular point. This will be especially important if the witness is not in court throughout the hearing and therefore does not hear the evidence given before theirs. The Department of Health handbook *Reporting to Court under the Children Act 1989* (Plotnikoff & Woolfson 1996) gives valuable and easily accessed guidance to writing statements.

After witness statements have been submitted to court, new evidence can only be given with the leave of the court. The solicitor should be informed immediately of any significant developments in the case after submission of statements so that the other parties can be informed as soon as possible and are not 'ambushed' in court.

Directions hearings

These are relatively informal court hearings, held in the weeks or months before the final hearing, to identify evidence which is agreed or remains in dispute as statements and reports become available, and to decide procedural matters. These include obtaining leave for expert evidence, timetabling – establishing when all the evidence will be ready, all witnesses available – and setting a date for the final hearing. It is unusual for witnesses to give oral evidence at directions hearings, but the crucial parties should attend so that they can give instructions to their advocates on the directions being requested and check dates being suggested in their diaries.

Personal preparations for court

Do not underestimate the importance of dress and appearance. For example, some inexperienced professional witnesses seem to believe that if they dress casually for court, they can make the proceedings more relaxed. However, this simply does not work – it might be interpreted as disrespect and is also more likely to make witnesses feel uncomfortable when surrounded by others who are formally dressed. Dress should be smart and 'sober', the kind of clothes worn to an important interview. Formal clothes may also increase witnesses' confidence and sense of occasion. Keep makeup and jewellery toned down. Badges, whatever worthy causes they espouse, risk damage to witnesses' credibility because of the possibility that the judiciary assessing the witness may hold different views.

Witnesses should read over their evidence the night before court but not burn the midnight oil. They should also get to court at least half an hour before the start of the hearing. Witnesses will need time to compose themselves and ensure they are comfortable. Witnesses who are unavoidably delayed on the morning of court should ensure their advocates are notified so that an adjournment can be requested. An advocate will not start a hearing with vital witnesses absent.

Viewing the courtroom

Another good reason for arriving early is to have a look at the courtroom before the hearing starts. The object is to become familiar with the layout; for example, where you will be sitting, where the witness box is, and the distance between the witness box and where the judiciary is sitting (important for adjusting the loudness of the voice). Ushers (black gown or badge and clipboard) will usually oblige by showing witnesses around whilst the courtroom is empty. Nervousness is an occupational hazard of court witnesses but, up to a reasonable level, it is conducive to good performance. Nerves are also a reassuring sign that the witness's physiology is normal – adrenalin is pumping around the body to produce alertness. Witnesses who are not nervous may perform badly because they are too blasé or over-confident. Take whatever stress-reducing measures are available, except alcohol and other mood changing substances. It may be reassuring to know that even the most experienced advocates are frequently anxious before court, but most have developed ways of concealing it in public.

Outside the courtroom

The time immediately before going into court is valuable for negotiations between advocates. Sometimes the reality of actually being at the court door focuses minds positively on compromises that might avoid or shorten the battle ahead and your advocate will need your instructions. If the advocates go into 'huddles', which exclude key professional witnesses and seem to be making 'deals', join in to ensure your views are part of the debate, so that you, and not the advocates, are giving the instructions. However, beware of being overheard – valuable clues to your strategy can be picked up this way.

It frequently happens, for a number of reasons, that on the morning of the hearing, all is suddenly agreed at the court door, or there is an unexpected adjournment. Whilst this means a day or more of unpleasantness is avoided, it can be experienced as a huge and uncomfortable anticlimax. If this happens, take advantage of the opportunity of unexpected free time to do something relaxing and pleasant, to recharge batteries and come back down to earth.

The court hearing

In family courts, all witnesses will usually be allowed to remain in court throughout the proceedings, both before and after giving evidence.

Order of examination of witnesses

The applicant for the order that is the substance of the court case is the first to call witnesses to give their evidence and all the applicant's witnesses are examined at this stage. Each witness is examined 'in-chief', first by their own advocate, and then cross-examined by the advocate(s) for other parties. They are then re-examined by their own advocate. Those challenging the application call their witnesses next and all their witnesses are examined at this stage. Children's evidence is usually last to be heard – children's guardians (CAFCASS or Welsh assembly officers) and all their witnesses (and/or occasionally the children) are examined at this stage.

If witnesses have not finished giving their evidence when there is a break in the hearing (e.g. at lunch or at the end of the day), they are forbidden by rules of evidence from speaking to their own advocates or other witnesses about any aspect of the evidence and may be asked questions when next in the witness box to check compliance with this rule.

Giving oral evidence

Witnesses can make a good start to their 'performance' by walking confidently and purposefully into the witness box. All eyes, including those of advocates for other parties, will be on the witness at that point and a lot can be revealed about them. The impression should be of a witness at ease with the evidence they are about to give.

Using written evidence in court

Giving oral evidence is not a test of memory. In most court hearings, a bundle of all the documents filed in the proceedings will be available in the witness box, including all the witness statements. This bundle should be paginated so that when a particular statement is the subject of examination the witness is referred to it by the page number. At the same time as the witness turns to the document, so will the judge and advocates, so there is no need for undue haste in looking for the right page.

Witnesses may be asked about dates or events which are not in their statement or anywhere in the bundle. This is usually a diversionary tactic by the cross-examiner, an attempt to fluster or weaken credibility by demonstrating that a witness cannot remember a certain date or the exact words used at a particular time. Whilst witnesses should always bring their files to court, they should not take them to the witness box because of the rule of evidence about 'memory-refreshing documents', i.e. if used *in the witness* box, files or other records must, at the request of opposing advocates, be submitted to their scrutiny. However, if the *judge or magistrates* regard the information requested by the cross-examiner as necessary, and if witnesses cannot give it without looking at their file, they may direct a brief adjournment so that a professional colleague of the witness in court, or the advocate for the witness, can extract it from the file. Copies of the relevant record must then be made available to all the advocates.

Taking the oath or affirmation

Every witness promises to speak the truth, by religious oath or non-religious affirmation. This is the judiciary's first encounter with the witness and first impressions count. The oath or affirmation should be un-rushed, pronounced with sincerity and solemnity, looking at the judiciary. Since affirming is still relatively unusual, the usher or clerk should be warned in advance of the witness going into the box so that the correct card is readily available, or better still, the witness should memorise the words so that the card is not needed. The impression of competence in a witness might be diminished by jarring the smooth administration of the affirmation if the card has to be hunted for round the courtroom.

Christian oath

Taking the Bible/New Testament in the right hand:

I swear before Almighty God that the evidence I shall give shall be the truth, the whole truth and nothing but the truth.

Affirmation

This needs practice, as the phrasing is awkward:

I do solemnly and sincerely and truly declare and affirm that the evidence I shall give shall be the truth, the whole truth and nothing but the truth.

Non-Christian oath

If the witness's religion demands a non-Christian religious form of oath or other ceremony which the court is unlikely to know, the usher or clerk should be told before court starts so that the necessary book or equipment can be obtained – or witnesses could bring their own.

Sit or stand?

After the oath/affirmation, the judge or magistrates may invite the witness to sit – do not do so until invited. Thereafter, it is for each witness to decide which feels right in that particular setting. Witnesses of short stature or having quiet voices should, when giving evidence in the high-sided witness boxes in some formal courts, stand so that they can be seen and heard and to maximise their 'presence' in the court! Whether sitting or standing, however, avoid slouching and be upright and alert.

Addressing the judiciary

Witnesses are giving evidence to magistrates or judges only – it is they who must be convinced by it. Witnesses may look at the advocates when listening to questions, but should look at the judiciary when giving the answers. This breaks the normal rules of conversation and seems alien at first, but witnesses should remember that although evidence is given to the court by way of questions and answers, it is not conversation (more about this later). Eye contact with the judiciary should be maximised, within reason, to increase credibility. The occasional smile – in an appropriate place – is a good way of establishing rapport. It is important to speak clearly and pace the reply to take account of the fact that most judges and magistrates make their own notes of the evidence – watch the pen or keyboard! Judges or magistrates should be addressed as follows:

The Family Proceedings (Magistrates) Court – 'Your Worships', 'Sir' or 'Ma'm'
County Court – 'Your Honour'
High Court – 'My Lord/Lady' or 'Your Lordship/Ladyship'.

There are times during oral evidence when witnesses may need to create a pause, or emphasise some particular aspect of their evidence, especially when a cross-examiner is making damaging inroads or causing the witness to fluster. The witness who looks the judiciary in the eyes and says, 'Your Worship (Honour etc.) I would like to say,' guarantees that for the next few minutes the questions stop, and the judiciary give the witness their full attention.

Qualifications and experience

If a brief account of their present occupation, professional address, qualifications and experience is not in their statement, this is the first the court will hear about professional witnesses. These details should be stated briefly but clearly. Prepare a succinct CV in advance – every professional witness should know how many years they have been a social worker or health visitor without having to count them up in the witness box! Witnesses should also give the full name of their qualifications, not just the initials 'CQSW' or 'RSN'. If employed in an unusual capacity or by an organisation with which the judiciary may not be familiar, the witness should give a short explanation (e.g. community link worker, family centre staff). Modesty about being a manager is out of place in court – the witness is aiming to impress the judiciary with their knowledge, experience and seniority.

Examination-in-chief

The first evidence witnesses give is via questioning by the advocate acting for them. The purpose of evidence-in-chief is to put before the judiciary the evidence in support of the case. In essence, evidence-in-chief is an oral repetition of a witness's statement and this stage is often dispensed with to save time.

However, giving some evidence-in-chief allows witnesses the opportunity to add power to the written word with colour and detail; for example, the statement referring to concerns about domestic hygiene can be brought to life with graphic details! In addition, in this earlier stage of giving evidence via a friendly advocate asking the questions, witnesses can show confidence and competence, thereby establishing credibility with the court and 'settle into' the role of giving evidence before coming under attack in cross-examination.

The technique of evidence-in-chief

Evidence-in-chief should be a relaxed exchange between witness and advocate, with the flow of questions and answers easy and rhythmic, like a long rally in tennis or the movement of a metronome, and *seem* like conversation. Advocates use their skills to ask questions in a way that allows the evidence to be brought out with convincing impact on the court, emphasising the facts and details that are essential to proving the case. Witnesses give answers to the judiciary, but occasional eye contact with the advocate will maintain the teamwork between advocate and witness.

Leading questions

A leading question has only one answer. For example, if a crucial piece of evidence is that a child told the witness they did not want to see their father again, a leading question would be, 'Did she tell you she did not want to see her father?' Rules of evidence prohibit the witness's own advocate asking leading questions during examination-in-chief. Hence the need for careful preparation, so that witnesses will know in which direction their advocates are going if questions sound obscure, or several questions are needed to reach the same point that leading questions get to directly! The clue to the answer to a non-leading question may lie in key words; for example, 'Did she *say* anything to you about her *father?*' Although witness and advocate know the answer, no leading questions have been asked.

In family courts, the rule excluding leading questions in evidence-in-chief is often relaxed to the point of being ignored, but that will not become apparent until the actual hearing and the witness should be aware of it as part of their preparation for evidence-in-chief.

Leading questions can be asked in cross-examination, however, and frequently *are* in order to try to put words into the witness's mouth.

Cross-examination

This is without doubt the aspect of giving evidence that causes greatest apprehension. Curiously, many 'helping' professionals seem to regard cross-examination as an experience which must be suffered passively, but there is no rule that witnesses must endure it without defending themselves and their evidence. Indeed, a witness on behalf of a child has a duty to defend their evidence under challenge in cross-examination, although at all times remaining polite and dignified.

Psychologist Rhona Flin argues that 'torturing' witnesses by cross-examination is not an effective way to ensure truth emerges (Flin & Spencer 1990), but cross-examination is a time-honoured and central element of the adversarial method. Cross-examination is verbal chess – it can be intellectually stimulating and even exciting but a few survival techniques can make it an experience in which the witness is victor, not victim.

The purpose of cross-examination

Cross-examination is the vehicle used by advocates to destroy or weaken the evidence given 'in-chief' by attacking or undermining it, or the credibility of witnesses, and introducing evidence favourable to their case – usually in the form of alternative explanations or re-interpretations of what the witness has said.

In family courts, cross-examination is likely to be less ferocious than in criminal courts, and the bullying advocate who reduces the witness to tears risks alienating the judiciary and giving witnesses the 'sympathy vote'. However, if aggressive cross-examination is successfully denting the credibility of witness or evidence, a court may allow it to continue. Cross-examiners try to devalue or negate any aspect of witnesses or evidence, which include qualifications, experience, memory and attempts to demonstrate witness bias or misunderstanding. Cross-examiners may try to make witnesses muddled or lose confidence, or contradict themselves, and although it may *feel* like a personal attack, it is not. Goading witnesses into losing emotional control, getting angry or upset, is part of an advocate's tactics. Seeing it as such, and maintaining professional dignity, will help witnesses rise above it.

Surviving cross-examination

Survival depends on preparation begun long before the court hearing. Witnesses who have done their work competently, and made adequate recordings, should have little to fear when faced with searching questions about their work. Having well-organised evidence, thoroughly prepared, with the potential weaknesses covered in work with the solicitor, with the main points of evidence in their statements, will also help witnesses to avoid being flustered or thrown off balance. Witnesses who have mastered all the facts and know the main pillars of their cases will be hard to undermine. Giving evidence-in-chief with confidence and panache may assist survival in cross-examination because advocates watch witnesses during this stage and make their own assessments of their strengths and weaknesses. Witnesses who appear vulnerable may attract more challenge than strong ones. Body language should be just as calm and confident in the witness under cross-examination as during evidence-in-chief. Backing away into the farthest corner of the witness box or losing eye contact with the judiciary will help the cross-examiner by signalling that the witness is feeling threatened.

In evidence-in-chief, the witness and advocate work together to establish an easy flow and rhythm to the questions and answers. In cross-examination, witnesses should try not to allow the advocate to set the pace or establish a rhythm, because the advocate thereby gains control of the encounter and is able to push and pull witnesses in dangerous directions. Interrupt the rhythm by giving long answers when short ones are expected (and vice versa), ask for questions to be repeated, or drink a glass of water.

Witnesses are not obliged to give the exact answers the cross-examination questions require. Again, it is not conversation. Anyone who has observed some politicians being quizzed by journalists could learn from their technique of giving answers *they* want, whatever the questions! If an advocate insists on a simple 'yes' or 'no' answer, the witness could give it, and then add elaboration or explanation, weakening the impact of the first answer, just as the cross-examiner is about to move on to the next question. Alternatively, witnesses, facing the judiciary, could say that in their opinion, a simple 'yes' or 'no' answer is inadequate and go on to give the appropriate answer. Witnesses should look at the judiciary to give their answers. In fact, *it is not necessary to look at the cross-examiner at all.* Witnesses feeling threatened by advocates can help themselves by not looking in their direction even during the questions. Not only does this prevent intimidation by cross-examiners' body language, it also conveys an unspoken message to the judiciary that the cross-examiner is of no importance.

Whenever possible in answer to cross-examination questions, witnesses should take opportunities to restate to the court the main points of their evidence-in-chief, so that the court's attention is drawn to that, rather than the cross-examiner's distortion of it.

Multiple cross-examination

In each court hearing, the advocate for the witness will conduct the examination-in-chief and re-examination, but all the other advocates representing other parties in the case are entitled to cross-examine that witness. This could mean three or more cross-examinations! This may not be the nightmare it seems at first because, in reality, some of the advocates in a multi-party case (e.g. the children's guardian) may support the witness's case. In preparing for court, witnesses should ascertain from their own advocates, and from reading witness statements, which of the other advocates is in support or opposed on all or some of the issues or evidence.

Witnesses can then take advantage of the rule permitting leading questions in cross-examination by allowing themselves to be 'led' by the supportive advocate, in the knowledge that the interests of the cross-examiner and the witness coincide.

Re-examination

When cross-examination has finished, witnesses may be tempted to relax and let down their guard. They should, however, remain alert. The next questions will be from their own advocate in re-examination.

The purpose of re-examination is to repeat parts of the witness's evidence and/or repair damage to it sustained in cross-examination. For example, if during cross-examination witnesses became confused, or their credibility was shaken, questions in re-examination will be directed at untangling the confusion, correcting misunderstandings and putting the evidence 'back on the rails'. Alternatively, advocates may want their witnesses to remind the judiciary of some important points so that the last words they hear are a restatement of the witness's evidence-in-chief in case this has been dented by cross-examination.

Leading questions cannot be asked in re-examination, so questions from one's own advocates may again be indirect, or long-winded. Witnesses should re-establish eye contact with their advocate to facilitate the communication and teamwork.

After giving evidence

Witnesses will usually be permitted to remain in court after giving their testimony but if they have other demands on their time, the judiciary should be asked by their advocates to 'release' them. This request is usually granted if all parties agree.

Witnesses remaining in court can assist their advocates by making notes of other witnesses' evidence when their own advocate is cross-examining and giving further instructions to their advocates as other evidence unfolds, by passing notes or whispering. This should not be done with such frequency that it causes irritation or distraction, or creates the impression that advocates were poorly instructed in the first place. When listening to other evidence, witnesses should sit in an impassive but respectful manner, not agreeing or making disapproving noises or expressions of shock or amazement.

Final speeches

When all the witnesses have been heard, advocates may give a summary and overview of their case to the judiciary.

Announcing the decision

The magistrates or judge may give their decision and their reasons at the end of the hearing, or 'retire', giving their decision an hour or two later. Judgement can also be reserved to another day.

After the decision

When the magistrates or judge have given judgement, professional witnesses should take the news calmly and with dignity, whatever the outcome. Witnesses should expect to feel tired and sad after a court hearing, even if they get the decision they wanted. This is partly because of the adrenalin draining away – but mostly because child protection decisions inevitably involve loss to one party or more. This is the time to seek supportive debriefing from trusted colleagues.

Like most things that are worthwhile, developing skills and confidence as a witness in court takes practice and experience. A respect for, and acceptance of, the unique rules and procedures of the judicial process are a good beginning. Whilst social workers and health professionals have different training and often different values from lawyers, there is no reason teamwork cannot be achieved, with roles and skills being complementary, ensuring that the right decisions are made for children who need the protection of the courts.

Key points and messages for practice

- Be realistic about the way courts are, rather than seeing them as you might want them to be.
- Dress appropriately for your appearance in court.
- Know your own evidence well.
- Don't take cross-examination personally.

The work of the children's guardian

Ann Head

INTRODUCTION

The decision of a local authority to institute care proceedings is clearly a very serious one, which may result in a child's compulsory removal from their family. In addition to the measures to protect children's interests described in previous chapters, however, there is a further safeguard for the child in the court's appointment of a children's guardian (previously guardian *ad litem*), a person independent of the local authority, whose prime duty is to safeguard the interests of the child. The appointment of guardians *ad litem* and their duties under the Children Act 1989 are matters dealt with under s.41 of the Act and in the Rules of Court. The assumption is that a guardian *ad litem* (now children's guardian) will be appointed in the great majority of public law cases.

> For the purpose of any specified proceedings the court shall appoint a guardian *ad litem* for the child unless satisfied that it is not necessary to do so in order to safeguard his interests.
>
> (Children Act 1989, s.41(1))

The term guardian *ad litem* was altered to children's guardian from 2001 when the Criminal Justice and Court Services Act 2000 was implemented. This Act dealt, amongst other matters, with the creation of a new service, the Children and Families Court Advisory and Support Service (CAFCASS), originally established as a non-departmental public body accountable to the Lord Chancellor but subsequently made accountable to Parliament through the Department for Education and Skills. The new service took on the roles and responsibilities previously covered by:

- the Family Court Welfare Service (that branch of the Probation Service reporting to the civil courts on the welfare and care of children post divorce and separation)
- the Guardian *ad litem* and Reporting Officer Service (comprising employed and self-employed appointees, working for a countrywide number of Panels, governed by Panel Committees but ultimately the responsibility of local authorities)
- that part of the Official Solicitor's Department dealing with the welfare of children, which had been the responsibility of the Lord Chancellor's Department.

Hunt *et al.* (2002) summarise the differences between the three previous services in terms of management structure, the qualifications and employment status of practitioners, and throughput of cases. The authors also refer to an earlier paper by Hunt and Lawson (1999):

> The three services differed greatly in particular roles, spheres of operation, organisational structure and ethos. Integration was therefore bound to be challenging. Managing the guardian element, however, was likely to present particular difficulties because of its strong traditions of practitioner autonomy.
>
> (Hunt *et al.* 2002, p. 1)

The history of the role of the children's guardian has its roots in the Adoption Act 1958. The guardian *ad litem* (GAL) was designated by this Act to be the person appointed by the court to safeguard the interests of the child in adoption proceedings. The extension of the concept to the field of public law resulted from a need for the child in care proceedings to be represented by a voice independent of the local authority bringing the proceedings and of the child's parents.

This need was highlighted by the Field Fisher inquiry into the death of Maria Colwell (DHSS) (1974b), a child who had been returned from foster care with relatives to her mother and stepfather and who subsequently died at the hands of her stepfather. The Inquiry Report concluded that an independent social worker's views of Maria's best interests and of her own feelings in the matter would have been helpful to the court deciding her future. A further pressure to secure an independent voice came from David Owen's Children Bill 1974, which directed attention to the need for independent legal representation for children:

In any proceedings relating to a minor in any court, separate representation should be considered and, if appropriate, the child should be made (if not already so) a party of the proceedings.

(Children Bill 1974, clause 42)

The Children Act 1975 reflected all these needs and also the views of the Houghton Committee (1972) on adoption, in making provision for courts to appoint GALs in care proceedings, working with solicitors who would represent the child's views and position in court (subsequently known as the 'tandem method of representation').

Full implementation of the provisions of the 1975 Act had to wait until 27 May 1984, when it became mandatory for local authorities to establish panels of GALs and reporting officers (whose task is to interview parents whose consent is required for an adoption order and to advise the court whether that consent is given freely and with full understanding of its implications), who would be able to act in the full range of care and related proceedings, as well as in adoption and freeing for adoption cases.

Early studies (e.g. Murch & Bader 1984) of the work of GALs drew attention to the wide variations in the number of appointments in care and related proceedings, consequent upon the degree of discretion allowed in the 1975 Act. The Children Act 1989 addressed this issue by requiring the appointment of a GAL 'unless the court is satisfied that it is not necessary to do so in order to safeguard the child's interests' (Children Act 1989, s.41(1)) and it extended the range of work to be encompassed by GALs. The duties which fell to the GAL after the enactment of the 1989 Act were set out in the *Manual of Practice Guidance for Guardians ad litem and Reporting Officers* (DoH 1992b), which has not yet been superseded.

The role of the children's guardian is to report to the court on the following matters (DoH 1992b):

1. Whether the child is of sufficient understanding for any purpose, including the child's refusal to submit to a medical or psychiatric examination, or other assessment that the court has power to require.
2. The wishes of the child in respect of any matter relevant to the proceedings, including the child's attendance at court.
3. The appropriate forum for the proceedings, basing the criteria for the transfer of cases on:
   i. exceptional complexity, importance or gravity
   ii. the need to consolidate with other proceedings (e.g. adoption and contact proceedings)
   iii. urgency.

4. The appropriate timetabling of the proceedings, or any part of them, always bearing in mind the dictates of the Children Act, s.1(2) regarding the avoidance of delay.
5. The options available to the court in respect of the child and the suitability of each such option, including what order should be made in determining the application.
6. Any other matter on which the Justices' Clerk or the court seeks the guardian's advice, or concerning which the guardian considers that the Justices' Clerk or the court should be informed.

In practice, the guardian's duties involve appointing a solicitor for the child, unless one has already been appointed by the court because of a delay in appointing a children's guardian (Family Proceedings Court Rules 1991, rule II (a)); identifying to the court any person whose party status in the proceedings would help to safeguard the child's interests (rule II (6)); accepting documents on behalf of the child (rule II (8)); conducting a full investigation of all the circumstances of the case (rule II (9)) which will lead to a written report (rule II (7)); and making recommendations as to the course of action which will best promote the child's interests. The guardian is bound by the court's obligation to reduce delay and to have regard to the matters set out in the welfare checklist (see Chapters 9, 15 and 17, in this volume).

In more general terms, the principal functions of the new service, as provided now by CAFCASS and set out in the Criminal Justice and Court Services Act 2000 (Chapter 43, Part I), are stated to be:

- to safeguard and promote the welfare of the children
- to give advice to any court about any application made to it in such proceedings
- to make provision for the children to be represented in such proceedings
- to provide information, advice and other support for children and their families.

These general duties refer, of course, to all the tasks now taken on by CAFCASS and not uniquely to the role of the children's guardian.

CAFCASS employees are now called Family Court Advisers, whether they are appointed in public or private law proceedings. Other titles in the organisation refer to the actual work carried out; for example, children's guardian, reporting officer and family court reporter (taking the role of the former court welfare officer). Those children's guardians who are self-employed are referred to as 'contractors' for CAFCASS.

CAFCASS has a legal department which provides legal advice to the organisation and takes on the functions of that part of the Official Solicitor's Department which was involved in cases involving children, mainly in the High Court. Thus far this has not affected 'tandem representation' for children in care and related proceedings, whereby children's guardians appoint solicitors from private practice to represent the children in court.

The role

The duties of the children's guardian are many and varied but the main tasks can be grouped as follows.

Practical

The Rules of Court set out above delineate the practical tasks. There has been an increasing stress on the 'case management' responsibilities of the children's guardian, however, who is required to attend all directions hearings with a view to advising the court on any matters which may affect the child and to avoid delay in the proceedings.

In June 2003 the President of the Family Division and the Lord Chancellor introduced the Protocol for Judicial Case Management in Public Law Children Act Cases, which sets out clearly the responsibilities of all those involved in court proceedings concerning children, in terms of minimising delay. Six stages in the proceedings are identified, from the application by the local authority for an order to the final hearing, the completion of which should take no longer than 40 weeks from application; clear time limits are set for the completion of each stage. The children's guardian is to be appointed within 3 days of the application or an indication given by CAFCASS as to when an appointment will be made. If the appointment of the guardian is to be delayed, the court must consider on Day 3 of the application whether to appoint a solicitor to represent the child in the (temporary) absence of a guardian.

The children's guardian must, with the other parties to the proceedings, contribute to a Case Management Conference between 15 and 60 days from the application, by which time the issues in the case have to have been identified and narrowed and other case management matters considered.

The Protocol covers the issue of the appointment of any experts and makes provision for an Experts Discussion/Meeting within 10 days of the filing of reports. The solicitor for the child, or other professional directed by the court, has the responsibility for chairing such a meeting, which must produce a Statement of Agreement and Disagreement to be served and filed within 5 days of the meeting. In practice, this sometimes onerous task is usually undertaken by the children's guardian and solicitor, who decide together which of them will chair, minute and write up such a meeting. In cases of high (often medical) complexity the court can direct that these tasks be undertaken by an expert in the field.

The Protocol has undoubtedly been helpful in setting out the key tasks which have to be addressed and in devising a tight timetable for their completion. The children's guardian continues to have a key role in contributing to the process and advising the court of any factors which may cause the timetable to drift. Unfortunately, the difficult areas of court availability (in terms of judicial personnel, pressure of cases and building space), crises in the availability of suitably qualified social workers, delays in some parts of the country in the appointment of a children's guardian and the availability of experts who can assess and report within the court timetable all continue to militate against the speedy hearing of cases.

Investigative

Investigation entails gaining a full picture of the case from documentation and from those involved, both professionally and privately, with the child. Professional scrutiny will involve the guardian assuring themselves that the child and family have received, and are receiving, those services and interventions necessary to promote the child's welfare.

From contacts with the child, the family and others intimately involved, the guardian will seek to evaluate the problems that have led to court proceedings. This is an opportunity for a reappraisal of the issues and for mediation in relationships, private and professional, which may have become entrenched in the build up to an application for a court order.

In the large majority of cases, the children's guardian will not differ from the local authority in the final order recommended to the court. That final agreement, however, may come at the end of protracted negotiations: it may involve substantial alterations to the local authority's original care plan and it may come with the previously withheld cooperation of parents and others, if they have been able to engage with the guardian in reconsidering the issues. Recent research on practice prior to CAFCASS considers the different aspects of the guardian role in some detail (Hunt *et al.* 2002, 2003).

The Case Management Checklist (Appendix A/3 in the Protocol) referred to above specifically refers to the duty of the children's guardian to scrutinise the local authority files and to confirm that they contain no other relevant documents and that no application for specific disclosure is necessary.

Analytical

Analysis involves testing out the issues arising from conflicting arguments and reaching reasoned conclusions based on experience, research findings, expert advice and a detailed consideration of the facts of each case. As well as reaching conclusions about the order that is most appropriate for the child, the children's guardian has a duty to appraise the detail of the local authority's care plan and indicate whether this is the plan most likely to promote the child's welfare.

Case law has established that the children's guardian may be required to produce notes of interviews and meetings to support the conclusions reached in reports and as reasonable material for cross-examination in highly contested cases (*Re R*, summarised in *Family Law*, April 2002, p. 253).

Representational

The children's guardian must seek to promote the child's best interests, as perceived by the guardian, taking account of the child's wishes and feelings, and must defend their conclusions in the face of challenges by other parties. The duties of the guardian in this respect have been well set out by Timmis, an experienced children's guardian, based on research amongst children who have been the subject of court proceedings. These include (Timmis 2001, 2005):

- child provided with *information* relating to the proceedings
- child *consulted* over the possible outcomes
- views and best interests *advocated for* (practitioner standing *up* for the child)
- child *represented* as a party to the proceedings (practitioner standing *in* for the child).

The tension between the requirements to represent the child's wishes and feelings and to comment on the child's best interests has, however, been the subject of much professional debate. Those coming from a child protection perspective have stressed the need to protect the child from taking adult responsibilities when, by reason of immaturity, they are unable to visualise the long-term consequences of choices made at a young age. Those coming from a children's rights perspective, however, have tended to stress the right of children to be fully involved in decisions about their own lives, whilst rejecting 'paternalistic' attitudes of those with a welfare/child protection perspective. As Head argues:

The central dilemma in the role of the guardian *ad litem* is to reconcile the child's wishes and feelings with a professional assessment of the child's best interests. This echoes the divide between the perspective of the state as protector of children and intervenor in family life and the state as supporter of children's rights and the privacy and self-sufficiency of the family, reflected in statute which has swung from one perspective to the other.

(Head 1998, p. 193)

CAFCASS has had to battle with this issue in both public and private law and an advantage of the new organisation should be the cross-fertilisation of ideas between formerly separate groups of practitioners about this and other key matters concerning the rights and responsibilities of children and their parents.

The Human Rights Act 1998 has heightened the intensity of debates on these issues and particularly about the right to respect for private and family life (Article 8), a right which is sometimes in conflict with the right of the child for protection from harm. The UN Convention on the Rights of the Child has also been influential in the debate, particularly Article 12, which concerns the views of the child (see Masson & Winn Oakley 1999, especially Chapter 2).

There is also a connected debate about the relative merits of child advocacy and negotiation in the context of the guardian's representation of the child. There is currently a strong emphasis on the benefits of negotiation, to prevent child care cases being fought out in court, often to the detriment of family relationships, to save money and to produce a settlement that all parties can live with. Anxiety has been expressed, however, that the weakest party, arguably the child, may have their wishes overlooked or marginalised in this process, from which they are excluded. Masson and Winn Oakley (1999) make various recommendations about how the representation of children could be improved, arguing that in spite of their party status, the representation of children and young people in these proceedings is largely based on shielding them from the process rather than assisting them to participate. They conclude on the basis of their study that children often feel they do not know enough about what is going on and that the system appears to exist for adults rather than children.

The major upheaval of the reorganisation of the guardian service and the heavy stress on negotiation in the court may have militated against the greater involvement of children and young people in the process of their representation. The children's guardian is in a key position, however, to explore ways in which the process can be made more child friendly and to balance the need to involve children and young people where they wish it, with the need to protect those who need adult support and understanding because their wishes and feelings are so confused, painful and difficult to articulate.

Explanatory

The children's guardian will be involved in interpreting the process of investigation to the child, since the advancement of the child's understanding of their situation is a legitimate aim of the children's guardian's (Schofield & Thoburn 1996).

Ruegger (2000), however, following her interviews with children who had been contacted by a children's guardian, concluded that a number were unhappy that their wishes and feelings had been transmitted to the other parties in the case through the guardian's report, since it had not been made clear that this might happen. Clearly it needs to be explained to children the use that will be made of the information they give, even if this restricts what they are willing to share. Timmis (2001) has made helpful suggestions as to how the Welfare Checklist (Children Act 1989, s.1(3)) can be made more accessible to children.

In 2001, as an aid to explaining the process to children, 'Power Pack' booklets were produced by CAFCASS and the NSPCC in collaboration with the Rights of Children Group and the Warwick Law School. Experience of the use of these has been mixed: predictably, while some children find them useful and entertaining, others do not want to engage with them at all. They are, however, an asset to children's guardians as a tool, which may be helpful in increasing the understanding of children and young people of the process in which they are involved. The booklets helpfully draw the attention of children and young people to a website (www.carelaw.org.uk) designed especially for them. As with all such aids, the key to their effectiveness is in how they are used by the individual children's guardian, or not used when they are inappropriate for a particular child.

Research and development

The role of children's guardian is a relatively new one, although comparable systems in Scotland (the curator *ad litem*) and in the USA pre-dated the setting up of panels in the UK.

Early studies of the work of guardian *ad litem* panels focused on the wide variations between local authorities in the size of the panels, the personnel appointed and the use made of the service by the courts. The advent of CAFCASS in 2001 brought substantial changes to the new workforce, however, including a reduction of self-employed practitioners and a move towards the harmonisation of the different roles of the CAFCASS workforce. CAFCASS inherited a mixed workforce but has increasingly appointed new staff who will take on cases in both public and private law. Thus relatively few children's guardians now work solely on public law cases and there have been concerns that their expertise in this area, accumulated during the years of guardian *ad litem* panels, may be diluted or lost.

The gradual loss of self-employed children's guardians now seems inevitable, however, despite the outcome of a Judicial Review in 2003, which directed that the self-employed should not be disadvantaged by the new arrangements. At the end of 2001, self-employed guardians made up 87% of the workforce. By May 2005, figures quoted by the Chief Executive (CAFCASS@smartgroups.com) suggested that self-employed staff made up only approximately 17% of the total workforce (including administrative and managerial staff). One of the purposes of reorganisation, however, was to harmonise welfare services across public and private law cases and the success of CAFCASS may ultimately be judged on the degree to which the new organisation has been able to harness the best practice from the previous areas of specialism and the extent to which the encouraged cross-fertilisation of ideas has been achieved.

Does this change in personnel make any difference to the quality of service given to children in the difficult area of public law proceedings? Those advocating the benefits of a largely self-employed workforce point to the advantages of using experienced practitioners who are unfettered by the bureaucracy of a large organisation and who can respond to the peaks and troughs of demand. Those convinced of the benefits of a largely employed workforce point to the need to have a uniform service across the country, to the safeguards offered by a managed service and to the advantages of an integrated court welfare system.

In their large scale study of the work of the former guardian *ad litem* panels. Hunt *et al.* (2003) highlight the complexities of the role and the consistency with which case-related factors (e.g. length of judicial process, number of children, level of court, number of parties) influenced the number of hours worked by children's guardians pre CAFCASS. They were not in a position to make satisfactory direct comparisons between employed and self-employed practitioners when the research was undertaken but they do lay down independent criteria against which the performance of a future CAFCASS workforce could be measured. A second study using the same data points to the need for the securing of minimum standards in CAFCASS work nationally and a professional debate about best practice:

> One important theme in the research has been the multi-faceted and dynamic nature of the guardian's role. The elements in the guardian's role which are not about investigation, reporting and representation, in particular the centrality of the guardian's function as facilitator and agent of change, need to be more fully recognised and the implications explored.
>
> (Hunt *et al.* 2003, p. 12)

Consistent with the recommendation in the Green Paper *Every Child Matters* (DfES 2003b) for the greater inclusion of children in matters which affect their lives, children's participation is central to the work of CAFCASS, which is encouraging the development of a service that is responsive to the needs and rights of children. In the light of research findings (e.g. Masson & Winn Oakley 1999, Ruegger 2000, Timmis 2001, 2005, James *et al.* 2004), materials are being developed which encourage the participation of children in court proceedings and the inclusion of children in interviewing procedures for new staff are examples of initiatives in this area.

Independence

A key quality of the GAL system, as envisaged in the 1970s, was independence. It was seen as essential that the GAL should be independent of the social services department bringing proceedings, and of the child's parents or other relatives. It was regarded by every early study of the service (see Coyle 1987) as a major flaw that, prior to 2001, the GAL service was the responsibility of social services departments, albeit that the service was at 'arm's length'.

Similarly, Independent Representation for Children in Need (IRCHIN) argued that panel members had to be free from outside pressures and constraints if they were to work, and were seen to be working, independently, which was difficult for as long as panels were funded and administered by the local authorities (IRCHIN 1985a, 1985b).

Following the implementation of the Children Act 1989, attempts were made to distance the administration of GALRO panels from the managerial structure of social services departments by the appointment of panel managers working with advisory committees, with independent representation and by the setting up of complaints boards, again with independent representation. This was only a partial answer to the question of visible independence from the other parties in care and related proceedings.

In November 1991, Cornwall GALs took the issue of budgetary independence to Judicial Review, following an attempt by the Director of Social Services to impose time limits on the amount of time that could be done by a GAL on a particular case (*R v Cornwall County Council* [1992]). The then President of the Family Division, Sir Stephen Brown, found in favour of the GALs, a finding that underlined the importance of guardians as officers of the court whose decisions should not be constrained by social services departments.

The advent of CAFCASS has addressed these difficulties by clearly establishing the independence of the children's guardian from local authorities. However, the budgetary constraints on the new organisation have raised fears about how the guardian's role may be limited in future. In addition, the children's guardian must also demonstrate independence from parents when protecting the child's interests.

The establishment of CAFCASS was generally welcomed as an opportunity to demonstrate the independence of guardians, whether self-employed and contracted to work for CAFCASS or employed as Family Court Advisors. Hopes are that this relatively new organisation will be able to speak in a powerful way for children who are the subject of court proceedings and be as challenging to local authority practice, where necessary, as the former panels sought to be. Fears are, however, that a large bureaucracy will encourage loyalty to itself and standardise procedures, such that the independent voice for the child will be put at risk.

Resources and financial constraints

GALs in the past, and children's guardians today working within CAFCASS, have been criticised for making unrealistic recommendations about the plans which should be made for children, suggesting the use of resources that are not available, thereby either causing dissatisfaction and disappointment to children and their families or favouring some children and families with resources to which others are not able to gain access. Although this is a contentious issue, it is arguable that it is the professional responsibility of the children's guardian to consider all the options for the child, discussing the merits and disadvantages of each, and making it clear why certain options may not be viable. It is only by making clear statements about the absence of necessary resources that children's guardians will be able to contribute to the wider debate about the long-term effects on children and families of the absence of essential provisions. There is arguably also a responsibility on CAFCASS to collate such information and to be pressing the government and local authorities for the provision of appropriate services to meet children's needs.

Budgetary constraints for CAFCASS have assumed considerable importance in the first years of the organisation's existence. Previously, overspends had to be absorbed by the responsible local authorities. It has been made clear by government, however, that CAFCASS must function within its allotted budget and it therefore places considerable emphasis on the efficient use of staff time. This is illustrated by the joint statement issued by the Chief Executive of CAFCASS and the President of the Family Division about opportunities for efficiency savings (Memorandum, 9 March 2005). The suggestion in the memorandum that children's guardians might not need to attend every court hearing was immediately challenged by practitioners, who feared that the child's voice in the proceedings would thereby be minimised and accorded less importance than the voices of the other parties. No doubt there will be many such debates in future when budgetary constraints are in conflict with professional views about the best interests of children.

CAFCASS is also competing for staff resources in a market where skilled and experienced practitioners are scarce. The inheritance of a 'mixed economy' of employed and self-employed staff poses some additional problems for the efficient use of resources. Clearly the organisation needs to have its employed workforce operating at maximum efficiency and there have therefore been directives that new work should be allocated in preference to employed Family Court Advisors.

However, self-employed contractors have urged the benefits of freelance personnel in terms of a flexible response to the peaks and troughs of work, which had already been underlined by the Social Services Inspectorate report of 1990. This reported the marked growth in the number of freelance members who were a previously untapped source of skilled labour, which has been useful in meeting the uneven demand for the service.

In the current climate it is likely that all qualified and experienced staff will be able to access work in this area, whether in a self-employed or an employed capacity; however, as already stated, self-employed personnel are becoming an increasingly small percentage of the total CAFCASS workforce. A recent trend for the increased employment of independent social workers in family proceedings, who are often previous or current children's guardians, is doubtless being monitored by government and by the Legal Services Commission; it remains to be seen whether this development is related directly to the shortfalls perceived in the service offered by CAFCASS and, in particular, to the diminishing number of freelance children's guardians in the organisation's workforce.

Causes of delay

One of the earliest concerns about the appointment of GALs in care proceedings was that this would lead to delays in completing child care cases coming before the courts. Murch and Bader (1984), in an early survey, reported the concerns of many Justices' Clerks about the length of time taken by cases chosen for GAL reports, a view echoed in the Social Services Inspectorate report published 6 years later in 1990.

There is a danger, however, in assuming that all delay is harmful to the child. Clearly there are some cases where an adjournment of the final hearing for a specific purpose – for example to allow a piece of intensive work to be undertaken with parents or to allow a child to build a link with an absent relative – can be very beneficial to the child. However, delays in the completion of children's cases for reasons of inefficiency, lack of resources, non-availability of court time, changes of personnel, etc. are not acceptable and risk causing as much harm as the circumstances which provoked them.

Delays in appointing a children's guardian were also a problem in some parts of the country before the inception of CAFCASS in 2001. The Cleveland Inquiry drew attention to the unwarranted delay in some of the cases examined, caused by the need to appoint a guardian *ad litem* (Butler-Sloss 1988), a concern that was echoed by the Social Services Inspectorate report (1990).

CAFCASS has also had problems in allocating cases to children's guardians. The House of Commons Select Committee reporting on CAFCASS was highly critical of the delays in appointment some 2 years after its inception (House of Commons 2003). In some areas large waiting lists have developed and guidance has been issued to solicitors working in such cases as to how to proceed in the absence of a guardian. It is a priority for CAFCASS to clear the backlogs of all its work and some progress is being made in this respect. A target for 2003/04 was to be able to allocate cases within 7 days. By the fourth quarter of that year 72.6% of cases were allocated within the period of 7 days (CAFCASS 2004).

It has been a matter of concern nationally that court proceedings concerning children have taken too long to resolve. The former President of the Family Division, Dame Elizabeth Butler-Sloss has, with consultation, issued a Protocol for the efficient conduct of care and related proceedings, which has been described above. A review of the working of the Protocol and its effect in reducing delay is awaited. CAFCASS is striving to meet the requirement that a children's guardian should be allocated to a case within 2 days of the issuing of proceedings. The target for 2004/2005 was to be able to allocate 70% of cases within this time frame (CAFCASS 2004).

The implementation of the Human Rights Act in 1998 has encouraged those who act as legal representatives for parents to pursue arguments relating to Article 6, the right to a fair trial, and Article 8, the right to respect for family and private life, to the ultimate extent. This can result in very protracted proceedings whilst expert and residential assessments are conducted following on from the examination of Human Rights Act issues. It is clearly proper that such arguments should be expertly and forcefully put on behalf of parents but it is equally important that those conducting the case for the children should be robust in putting a separate case for the child, where delays of this kind may be causing irreversible damage to the child.

The United Nations Convention on the Rights of the Child was ratified by the UK in 1991 although the UN Committee, reporting in 1994:

> seemed to consider that the UK was complacent about its compliance with the Convention and required to take a more critical look at the actual state of children's rights.
>
> (Marshall 1997, p. 29)

Marshall's consideration of children's rights, as accorded in a range of countries and as measured against the UN Convention, sets high standards for the involvement of children in decision making, suggesting the following elements (Marshall 1997, p. 108):

- accessible and comprehensible initial advice for children
- a person to help them speak, but not speak for them
- a person to help them write their own reports
- a person to safeguard their interests
- a person to advocate their views
- provision of advocacy in a broader sense, not restricted to proceedings.

It may seem that these suggestions are a long way removed from the conception of the role of the children's guardian in care proceedings. However, there is an increasing stress on the rights of children and the principles enshrined in the UN Convention and the appointment in the UK of a Minister for Children suggest that CAFCASS will have to be constantly alert as to whether its policies and practice take sufficient heed of children's rights.

Children's guardians can be very helpful to the court in setting out the wider context of the proceedings by summarising the evidence given by the other parties and by setting out succinctly the options for the court and the likely consequences of each for the child. Sometimes the successful fulfilment of this function and the introduction of a neutral (as between the adult parties) professional into highly contested proceedings can provide a conduit to the settlement of the case without the need for lengthy court proceedings.

Children's guardians and others involved in the process have been slow, however, to direct the attention of those controlling budgets to the cost-saving benefits of such interventions. Hunt *et al.*'s research (2002), cited above, helpfully draws attention to this aspect of the guardian's role. It is to be hoped that the added attention being given to mediation in private law disputes will help to inform and underline the benefits which can accrue from the intervention of a skilled children's guardian in a protracted public law dispute. Workers in both areas will also have to be alive to the dangers of underplaying risks to the child in the anxiety to reach settlement and again CAFCASS should provide a good umbrella for workers from the previous disciplines to learn from each other's practice.

Practice issues and new developments

CAFCASS as an organisation is committed to giving a voice to children in all court proceedings affecting their welfare. That service is to be given in such a way as to respect the ethnicity, family background, religion, gender and any disability of the children or parents concerned:

> Diversity and equality of opportunity will be valued and promoted through anti-discriminatory practice.
>
> (CAFCASS 2003, p. 10)

Key documents such as the one above are available in Welsh, Gujarati, Punjabi, Hindi, Bengali, Urdu, Chinese, Arabic, Mirpuri, Portuguese and Turkish and explanatory leaflets on the work of CAFCASS are also available in a number of different languages.

The details of the race equality scheme devised by CAFCASS are available on the organisation's website (see Useful websites, p. 361).

There have been objections from the initial setting up of panels of GALs that practitioners were overwhelmingly white, female and middle class. Efforts have been made to recruit practitioners from other ethnic backgrounds and from different gender and age groups, bearing in mind the need for guardians to have a sufficient breadth of professional experience to be credible witnesses in court.

The Smart Group organised by NAGALRO, the organisation representing the interests of children's guardians and independent social workers, testifies to the lengths that individual workers regularly go to in order to seek out professional colleagues who are of particular ethnic and linguistic backgrounds, in order that the child's racial and cultural heritage is fully taken into account in any decisions made.

There are always improvements to be made in this area, but there have been noticeable advances in how court proceedings are now conducted (as opposed to 20 years ago) with respect to the use of interpreters, the taking of proceedings at a slower pace for those with a learning disability or other special need (e.g. deafness) and the respect accorded to those of different racial and religious backgrounds. Dr Julia Brophy from Oxford University has conducted a number of studies into the exposure to care proceedings of parents from ethnic minority backgrounds (see Brophy *et al.* 2003b).

Children's guardians, whether employed by CAFCASS or self-employed, operate in an ever-changing social and political scene. Issues come to the fore, receive public and private debate and sometimes result in fresh legislation. Sometimes issues which have been the subject of huge debate disappear from the public eye and fresh issues command attention from government, press and public. Examples of issues which are in the public eye in the early years of the twenty-first century and which affect the work of children's guardians are domestic violence, the roles of men and women in family life, scientific developments in the area of human fertilisation and embryology, the discrediting of certain forms of expert evidence in proceedings affecting children (e.g. Munchausen syndrome by proxy, 'shaken baby' syndrome and cot death), the privacy of family proceedings and the role of the state in family life.

Section 9 of the Asylum and Immigration Act 2004 also promises to result in very real dilemmas for those seeking to protect children in that it will empower government to withdraw benefits from families who have failed in their bid to gain asylum. There is a clear risk that children will be taken into local authority care because their parents are unable to support them and, if that step cannot be taken with parental consent, such cases may well result in care proceedings. The application of the Welfare Checklist (Children Act 1989, s.1) in such situations and the relevant clauses of the Human Rights Act 1998 and UN Convention on the Rights of the Child will ensure that such cases will be fiercely debated and children's guardians will have to take a view on the best interests of children in particularly difficult circumstances.

CAFCASS, as a new organisation, is in a unique position, having brought together expertise and experience from three previous organisations, to address some of these issues. Courts will continue to be assisted in making difficult decisions by children's guardians who can offer well-informed and impartial advice as to the effects on children of the numerous life stresses to which they can be subjected. This demands that those taking on the work are experienced, well trained and supported, and are open to expand both their experience and their training by keeping up to date with ever-changing information and opinion.

The role of the children's guardian has changed considerably since the coming into being of the role in 1985. The Children Act 1989 gave additional scope to the work, and GALs, as they then were, were key players in the enacting of the principles and changed practices espoused in that legislation. A growing area for the practice of children's guardians has been in relation to appointments under Rule 9(5) of the Family Proceedings Rules 1991. This rule enables the court to appoint a GAL for the child in private law proceedings if a decision has been made that the child needs party status in the case and is not of the age and understanding to participate in the proceedings without an intermediary. The ground for such an appointment involves a 'best interests' test:

if in any family proceedings it appears to the court that it is in the best interests of any child to be made a party to the proceedings.

(Family Proceedings Rules 1991)

It was predicted, after the enactment of the Human Rights Act in 1998, that GAL appointments would increase in private law proceedings if children's interests were not judged to be receiving proper protection from a Family Court Reporter (formerly court welfare officer: see *Re A* (Contact: Separate Representation) [2001] 1 FLR 715). Judges can appoint a GAL (the old form is still current in these circumstances, although the President's Practice Direction envisages that the Latin term will in time be made redundant and she uses the term guardian in her Direction [Her Majesty's Court Service 2004]) if they feel that children's interests demand that they should be parties in proceedings to resolve disputed matters of residence and contact.

In such cases, the guardian (*ad litem*) may be an officer of CAFCASS, the Official Solicitor (if he consents) or (if he consents) 'some other proper person' – for example, a representative of the National Youth Advocacy Service. There has been the predicted increase in these appointments which, in the main, have been to officers of CAFCASS. The President's guidance, referred to above, indicates that appointments under this rule should be made only in exceptional circumstances:

Making a child a party to the proceedings is a step that will be taken only in cases which involve an issue of significant difficulty and consequently will occur only in a minority of cases … It must be recognised that separate representation of the child may result in delay in the resolution of the proceedings. When deciding whether to direct that a child be made a party, the court will take into account the risk of delay or other factors which might be adverse to the welfare of the child.

(Her Majesty's Court Service 2004)

There is a useful discussion about appointments under Rule 9(5) in an article by a solicitor in *Seen and Heard* (Dawson 2004).

It was hoped that the advent of CAFCASS would even out the discrepancies in time and attention given to children in need in private law disputes, as compared with children coming before the courts in public law applications. Although successful Rule 9(5) appointments are going some way to redress the balance, it remains to be seen whether budgetary restrictions will limit the use made of these appointments. There remains much to be done to identify those children in both public and private law who need a 'Rolls Royce service' (to coin an often-used phrase) as opposed to those whose needs can be more swiftly and inexpensively diagnosed and met.

The Adoption and Children Act 2002 will have an effect on the identification of children in private law disputes who have a special need for services, in that the definition of significant harm (Children Act 1989, s.31(9)) will be amended to read:

'Harm' means ill-treatment or the impairment of health or development including, for example, impairment suffered from seeing or hearing the ill treatment of another.

This will put an additional responsibility on local authorities to consider child protection procedures in relation to children suffering harm through domestic violence or protracted parental disputes and, in some circumstances, courts will have recourse to making the children parties to the private law proceedings under the Act, without the need to use their powers to make Rule 9(5) appointments.

A further section of the Adoption and Children Act which will affect the role of children's guardians is s.122, which provides for an extension to the list of 'specified proceedings' in which the court may appoint a guardian for the child (Children Act 1989, s.41). 'Specified proceedings' are now to include:

- an application to make or discharge a placement order
- s.8 proceedings (Children Act 1989), in certain circumstances.

It is envisaged that the Lord Chancellor may make rules for the separate representation of children in the above proceedings but these have yet to be published at the time of writing.

In relation to placement orders, which will replace current arrangements for the adoption of children who are subject to or meet the grounds for a care order, children's guardians will be appointed and will have the opportunity to comment on the local authority's detailed plans for the placement of a child, which has often not been possible under the 1989 Children Act, when care proceedings could terminate with the local authority's untested plan for a particular type of placement. The guardian might be reappointed in adoption proceedings for the same child, but this is a very late stage at which to be commenting on the appropriateness of the placement in relation to the child's needs.

As far as s.8 proceedings are concerned, it seems likely that a guardian may well be appointed for a child in disputed proceedings about residence, contact or, more rarely, 'prohibited steps' or 'specific issues'. Considering the example given above of a guardian appointment under Rule 9(5), it seems likely, in the light of s.122 of the new Act, that such children will be made parties to private law proceedings in the future, provided that CAFCASS is able to budget for such proceedings.

The judiciary and others have commented that it would be helpful if the children's guardian were able to review the operation of the care plan after a care order has been made. This suggestion has often been made when subsequent court proceedings have revealed that the agreed plan was never implemented. There has been considerable resistance to such an extension of the guardian's role. The Adoption and Children Act 2002 has brought into being Independent Reviewing Officers whose task is to review local authority care plans and refer cases on to the relevant authority if it appears that the plans have not been put into effect. Early experience of the new role has revealed that no referrals have been made to CAFCASS and there are thus some doubts as to whether the IRO is likely to bring care plan failures to the attention of the court.

Training

Children's guardians have traditionally been trained and experienced social workers, with an understanding of the policies and practices of local authority departments, a knowledge of the law in relation to children and families, and a commitment to working with children.

CAFCASS has inherited both a workforce of children's guardians and a large number of experienced family court welfare officers, many of them trained in the Probation Service and with a strong emphasis on achieving conciliation between adults whose relationships have broken down, and many of them skilled at interviewing the children caught up in these conflicts.

The task for CAFCASS is to maximise the use of the skills whilst moving gradually towards a harmonised workforce. This can only be achieved through training. Induction courses have been set up to orientate new workers to the tasks of the organisation and their role within it. Much work has also been put into devising modular courses in which existing start members can participate, in order to fill gaps in their knowledge or to update themselves in respect of new developments.

NAGALRO, the professional organisation for children's guardians (and now independent social workers as well) has a long and respected record for organising training tailored to the needs of children's guardians and it is to be hoped that this input can continue and will be valued.

There is, as yet, no recognised qualification specifically for those taking on the role of children's guardian. Prior to the advent of CAFCASS many guardians sought out post-qualifying courses which would enhance their knowledge and standing in the court arena. Many were awarded the Advanced Award in Social Work or undertook Master's degrees in particular aspects of the work.

If children's guardians, whether freelance or employed by CAFCASS as Family Court Advisors, are to be able to assist courts in understanding the wishes and feelings of children and are to comment on the best interests of those children – challenging, if necessary, the views of local authorities and parents – their training needs must be answered and their training seen by others to be rigorous. CAFCASS still has some way to go in this area.

Summary and conclusion

The role of guardian *ad litem* came into being with the establishment of panels set up by local authorities in 1984 (see Head in James & Wilson 1988). A further consideration of the role 7 years later commented on the changes since its inception and looked forward to the increasing influence of the child's wishes and best interests in family proceedings. It was hoped that panels of guardians *ad litem* would be removed from the control of local authorities (see Head in Wilson & James 1995).

This chapter considers some of the changes brought about by the setting up of CAFCASS in 2001, bringing together the three services concerned with reporting to courts on the best interests of children: the former Guardian *ad litem* and Reporting Officer panels, the former Probation organised court welfare service and that part of the Official Solicitor's department concerned with the welfare of children.

The role of the children's guardian, governed as it is by statute, has not changed but the influence of the organisational change on the carrying out of the role has been dramatic. Children's guardians are now part of a large organisation covering the welfare of children in public and private law situations; some continue to be self-employed and 'contractors' to CAFCASS. The majority are now employed practitioners, many of them taking on different roles within public and private law proceedings, with the majority requiring significant training.

It has been widely acknowledged that the new organisation was inadequately funded and its early years have been dogged by the difficulties of welding together staff from different professional backgrounds and managing backlogs of work, which, in some areas, have caused unacceptable delays for children waiting for courts to make decisions about their futures.

CAFCASS has an opportunity to ensure that children have a significant voice in proceedings which concern their lives. Its advent has ensured that children's guardians can comment on local authority practice without being constrained by being under local authority control and it has the opportunity to effect a cross-fertilisation of ideas between those who have traditionally looked at issues of domestic violence, communication with children, contact issues and many others from within the previous boundaries of public or private law.

Whether the new organisation can manage its finite resources successfully and carry its key staff with it in making changes will influence the degree to which, in future, those fulfilling the role of children's guardian can effectively elicit and communicate the wishes and feelings of children and reach an informed view about their best interests.

- The essentials of the safeguarding role of the children's guardian remain the same following the creation of CAFCASS. There is a substantial task for CAFCASS in respect of the harmonisation of staff and the promotion of high professional standards and appropriate training.

- Ongoing research is required to monitor the performance of the new organisation and its progress in meeting the needs of children caught up in public and private law proceedings.

- *Every Child Matters* has emphasised the need for the greater inclusion of children in matters which affect their lives. A priority for CAFCASS is to devise policies and encourage practices that maximise the involvement of children.

- There is a priority to consider the needs of those suffering emotional harm as a result of witnessing domestic violence and the intractable disputes between their parents.

Annotated further reading

Adcock M, White R, Hollows A 1991 Significant harm: its management and outcome. Significant Publications, Croydon
　　This collection of papers focuses on the assessment of harm against the background of the Children Act 1989. The contribution of Dr David P H Jones on the effectiveness of intervention is particularly helpful to children's guardians in deciding whether rehabilitation of an abused child to their family is likely to be viable; there is also a useful chapter by Annie Lau on cultural and ethnic perspectives.

British Association for Adoption and Fostering (BAAF) leaflets for using with children can be very helpful to children's guardians in communicating with children in particular situations, for example:
- *Argent H 2004 'What is contact? A guide for children.*
- *Byrne S, Chambers L 1997 Nadia and Rashid's story. Living with a new family. Jack's story. Hoping for the best. Nathan's story. Belonging doesn't mean forgetting.*
- *Byrne S, Chambers L 1998 Jo's story. Joining together. Tina's story. Feeling safe.*

Cooper A, Hetherington R, Katz I 2003 The risk factor. Making the child protection system work for children. Demos, London
　　This short book has a great deal to say about the unsatisfactory nature of risk management in the current child protection system. It makes recommendations for changes in the system and its consideration of 'closed' and 'open' models has considerable applicability to the organisation of family court welfare services.

Hetherington R, Cooper A, Smith P, Wilford G 1997 Protecting children: messages from Europe. The Stationery Office, London
　　A book which sets child protection issues in a European context and challenges assumptions by presenting alternative visions of how children can best be protected.

Horvath J (ed) 2001 The child's world. Assessing children in need. DoH with NSPCC, University of Sheffield. Jessica Kingsley, London
　　Contributions from a number of experts in the field of making assessments of children's needs. It includes chapters on attachment, the assessment of positive factors (resilience), assessing parental capacity and implementing the Framework for Assessment.

King P, Young I 1992 The child as client. Family Law, Bristol
　　Although written specifically for solicitors who represent children, this book covers the principles that must govern the work of a GAL, and deals in considerable detail with the partnership between the GAL and the solicitor. The book discusses the practical steps that are necessary in order to ensure that the child's case is properly put, and also covers ethical issues and problems of communication and assessment.

Masson J, Winn Oakley M 1999 Out of hearing: representing children in care proceedings. Wiley, Chichester
　　This comprehensive picture of representation for children is based on interviews with older children who were involved in court proceedings and on the views of professionals seeking to assist them.

NSPCC with Triangle 2002 How it is. An image vocabulary for children about feelings, rights and safety, personal care and sexuality. NSPCC, London
　　This large collection of cartoon faces and drawings is particularly designed for helping children who have a learning or communication difficulty to explain their wishes and feelings. It can also be a useful tool for children's guardians seeking to understand children who find it difficult to express themselves.

Plotnikoff J, Woolfson R (eds) 1996 Reporting to court under the Children Act 1989. HMSO, London
　　This handbook is primarily intended for social workers and other local authority personnel who are submitting written evidence to the court. It provides a useful checklist for children's guardians as to what to expect in a well-presented case.

Reder P, Lucey C (eds) 1995 Assessment of parenting: psychiatric and psychological contributions. Routledge, London
　　A useful compilation of contributions from experts in the field of parenting and risk assessment.

Westcott H, Davies G, Bull H 2001 Children's testimony. A handbook of psychological research and forensic practice. Wiley, Chichester
　　Although addressing mainly situations where children are giving testimony in criminal proceedings, this book presents a wealth of useful information about children's development, memory and suggestibility, which is invaluable when trying to make sense of what children say during care and related proceedings.

Useful websites

A guide to the law for young people in care: www.carelaw.org.uk
British Association for Adoption and Fostering: www.baaf.org.uk
Children and Families Court Advisory and Support Service (CAFCASS): www.cafcass.gov.uk
Every Child Matters: www.everychildmatters.gov.uk
Law Society Good Practice Guide: www.lawsociety.org.uk/productsandservices/publicationsandgifts.law
NAGALRO: www.nagalro.com
National Youth Advocacy Service (NYAS): www.nyas.net
The Hideout (site for children who are experiencing domestic violence): www.thehideout.org.uk
Views of younger children on *Every Child Matters*: www.rights4me.org
Voice (Voice for the Child in Care): www.vcc-uk.org

Acts of parliament, reports, directions, protocols

Adoption and Children Act 2002
ADSS/ACC/AMA (Association of Directors of Social Services, Association of County Councils and Association of Metropolitan Authorities) Report, April 1986
Asylum and Immigration Act 2004
CAFCASS Business Plan 2004/2005
CAFCASS Service Principles and Standards 2003
CAFCASS/Social Services Inspectorate Report 1990 House of Commons Committee on the Lord Chancellor's Department. CAFCASS 2003 Vol. 1, para. 62. The Stationery Office, London
Children Act 1975
Children Act 1989
Criminal Justice and Court Services Act 2000
Every Child Matters, Green Paper, DfES 2003
Family Proceedings Rules 1991
Human Rights Act 1998
Joint Memorandum from President of Family Division and Anthony Douglas, 9th March 2005
Protocol for Judicial Case Management 2003 Lord Chancellor's Department, made compulsory by Practice Direction issued by the President of the Family Division of the High Court. Practice Direction on Rule 9(5) of the Family Proceedings Rules 1991, President of the Family Division, 5 April 2004
UN Convention on the Rights of the Child

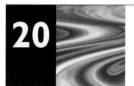

Child protection and the criminal justice system

John Williams

INTRODUCTION

Article 19 of the United Nations Convention on the Rights of the Child imposes on signatory states the following obligations:

1. States Parties shall take all appropriate legislative, administrative, social and educational measures to protect the child from all forms of physical or mental violence, injury or abuse, neglect or negligent treatment, maltreatment or exploitation, including sexual abuse, while in the care of parent(s), legal guardian(s) or any other person who has the care of the child.
2. Such protective measures should, as appropriate, include effective procedures for the establishment of social programmes to provide necessary support for the child and for those who have the care of the child, as well as for other forms of prevention and for identification, reporting, referral, investigation, treatment and follow-up of instances of child maltreatment described heretofore, and, as appropriate, for judicial involvement.

An important part of the protection given to children under this article relates to the potential use of the criminal justice system and the criminal courts. The use of civil law child protection procedures is considered elsewhere in this volume (see Lyon, Chapter 11) but the relationship between the civil law and the criminal justice system in relation to child protection is a complex one. It assumes the involvement and cooperation of a number of different agencies including social services, health, education, the police, the Crown Prosecution Service and the courts: therefore the argument for inter-agency collaboration is as compelling in this area of child protection as in therapeutic work.

There are, however, potential conflicts between the criminal and civil justice systems since, in some respects, they have different objectives and have different rules, procedures and processes. Most notably, the standard of proof required differs significantly: in criminal proceedings the prosecution have to prove the case 'beyond all reasonable doubt', whereas in civil proceedings the standard of proof is 'on a balance of probabilities'. To some extent the House of Lords in *Re H (minors) (Sexual Abuse: standard of proof)* ([1996] AC 563) blurred this distinction in relation to the standard of proof in care proceedings involving sexual abuse. Lord Nicholls was of the view that built into the balance of probabilities standard 'is a serious degree of flexibility in respect of the seriousness of the allegation'. He argues that this does not mean that the standard of proof is higher in more serious cases; the inherent probability of an event happening should be taken into account in deciding whether, on balance, it occurred. Fortin is sceptical of the claim that a higher standard is not being sought, however, stating it bears 'all the hallmarks of casuistry' (Fortin 2003, p. 472).

An issue that arises at the civil/criminal interface is the importance of providing therapeutic support for children, pending criminal proceedings. There is a risk that therapeutic support could be used as a basis for undermining the child's evidence; allegations of coaching or rehearsing the child could, if proven, be fatal to the prosecution. However, it is unacceptable to deny the child in need of it the right to access therapeutic support until the trial is over. The Home Office *et al.* (2001) have therefore issued guidance on the provisions of therapy, *Provision of Therapy for Child Witnesses Prior to a Criminal Trial: Practice Guidance*, and it is essential that this guidance be adhered to.

Two broad categories of therapeutic work undertaken prior to a trial are identified:

- Counselling addresses issues such as the impact of the abuse upon the child, improving the confidence and self-esteem of the child, and providing information to enable them to seek out assistance from a trusted adult if they feel unsafe at some time in the future.
- Psychotherapy addresses issues such as treatment of emotional and behavioural disturbance and treatment of a child who has been highly traumatised and shows symptoms that give rise to concern for their mental health (see Home Office *et al.* 2001, paras 2.4.1 and 2.4.2).

Courts have found, however, that discussions prior to a trial give rise to the possibility of witnesses giving inconsistent statements, or inadvertent or deliberate fabrication (Home Office *et al.* 2001, para. 3.3). The potential need for early therapy is therefore a critical part of the decision on whether to prosecute an alleged abuser and the Crown Prosecution Service must identify the impact of therapeutic work with the child on the criminal trial, although it must not be assumed that therapeutic work will always be prejudicial to the criminal trial.

When assessing the potential impact of therapeutic work, however, two factors must be noted. First, the 'best interests' of the child is the paramount consideration. In some cases this may lead to a prosecution being abandoned in favour of early therapeutic intervention, although delaying therapy until after the trial may be beneficial for the child as it avoids the benefit of the therapy being undone by the experience of the trial. Second, the decision on therapeutic work is not a decision solely for the Police or the Crown Prosecution Service. It has to be an interdisciplinary decision that takes into consideration social services, health and education perspectives, as well as the views of the carers and (very importantly) the views of a child of sufficient age and understanding (see Home Office *et al.* 2001, paras 4.1–4.6).

Another crucial difference between the two systems is the significance of the welfare of the child. Section 1 of the Children Act 1989 states that the welfare of the child is the 'paramount consideration'; this has implications not only for the civil courts, but also for practitioners when making decisions in respect of an individual child. The 'welfare principle' as such does not, however, apply within the criminal justice system: under s.44 Children and Young Persons Act 1933, a criminal court, when dealing with a child or young person 'brought before it as an offender or otherwise, shall *have regard* to the welfare of the child or young person'. This is somewhat less exacting than the civil law approach and the criminal courts must, as discussed below, seek the correct balance between the rights of the witness and of the accused (see Deering case 1997: *R* v *Highbury Corner Magistrates ex parte Deering* [1997] 1 FLR 683).

Review of recent literature and research: an analysis of the policy issues

Are children at a disadvantage when giving evidence in criminal courts via traditional means when compared with non-vulnerable adults? If they are, is it 'fair' to depart from established procedures in order to address any inequalities? If so, are we satisfied that such amended procedures produce reliable evidence and do not prejudice the accused? The answers to these questions need to have regard to the heterogeneous nature of that cohort that we casually refer to as 'children and young people'. In addition, the Human Rights Act 1998 and the European Convention on Human Rights (ECHR) have implications for the child witness and for the accused. As always, therefore, it is necessary to balance competing interests, both in devising policies, procedures and guidance, and very importantly in their day-to-day operation.

Research reveals that children are disturbed by the experience of giving evidence in court. In 1989, Pigot pointed to the confrontation with the accused, the stress, embarrassment, fear of speaking in public, cross-examination, courtroom formalities and the problems induced by delays as factors that contribute to this. Arguably, other witnesses will have the same experience and in that sense children are no different. Although this argument is not without merit, it ignores the fact that children are generally less emotionally and intellectually developed than adults and less able to understand the context within which the criminal justice system operates. For them, the experience is damaging and long term (Pigot, 1989, para. 2.10).

Of course, adults who are vulnerable may also be at a disadvantage and the law now recognises that they also may have special needs within the system. Goodman *et al.* undertook a study in America to examine the effects of the use of closed circuit television on the testimony of children and the jurors' perceptions (Goodman *et al.* 1998). American use of technology (in particular the use of pre-recorded videos) is affected by the Constitutional Right under the Sixth Amendment to face-to-face confrontation. The study was broadly based and identified a number of issues; however, for current purposes two are worthy of note: first, the use of closed circuit technology led to a decrease in suggestibility in younger children; second, testifying in open court was associated with children experiencing greater pre-trial anxiety.

Cashmore and Bussey found that children's concerns about going to court related to three aspects of the process: the reason for going to court, what actually happens in court, and the consequences of their involvement. Children's perceptions of the process included a fear of being punished (e.g. being sent to prison), nervousness about speaking in front of people, being implicated in a crime, retaliation by the defendant and attributing responsibility to themselves for the outcome of the trial (Cashmore & Bussey 1996, pp. 182–183). The Vulnerable Witness Survey (Kitchen & Elliott 2001) found that, of the 49 witnesses who used the live video link, all but three found it helpful.

However, the criminal justice system may be less understanding of the impact of giving evidence in court and more concerned about the quality of evidence. Is evidence given in open court (assuming that the case gets to court and is not screened out because of the effect on the child) the 'best evidence', or is evidence given by pre-recorded video or live link likely to be better evidence?

Ellison reminds us that the 'principle of orality is the foundation of the adversarial trial' (Ellison 2003, p. 10). The perceived strength of this oral tradition is that it exposes evidence to cross-examination, which will assist in exposing inconsistency, inaccuracy and fabrication; face-to-face confrontation is again perceived of as an important element of this process. Ho identifies the basis of the concerns of removing face-to-face confrontation: the rule is based on the two related ideas of fairness, i.e. the unfairness to the opponent of assuming that the absent witness would have been convincing if appearing before the court, and the unfairness of prejudicing the defendant by producing evidence without having the opportunity to erase that prejudice (Ho 1999).

The European Court does not recognise a Convention right to have the witness physically present in courts, however. In *Doorson* v *Netherlands* ([1966] 22 EHRR 330) it said:

> It is true that Article 6 does not explicitly require the interests of witnesses in general, and those of victims called upon to testify in particular, to be taken into consideration. However, their life, liberty or security of person may be at stake, as many interests coming generally within the ambit of Article 8 of the Convention ... Against this background, principles of fair trial also require that in appropriate cases the interests of the defence are balanced against those of witnesses or victims called upon to testify.
>
> (Doorson [1966], para. 70; see also Bates 1999)

The introduction of special measures under the Youth Justice and Criminal Evidence Act 1999 (YJCEA 1999) has given rise to discussion on their compatibility with the ECHR, in particular Article 6, which provides that in determining civil rights and obligations or any criminal charge, 'everyone is entitled to a fair and public hearing'. Special measures are discussed in more detail below; for present purposes, however, they are measures available to children to enable them to give best evidence, the use of a pre-recorded video interview and cross-examination perhaps being the most contentious measure. In one sense, the argument that special measures infringe Article 6 is relatively straightforward. For example, the defendant in *R v Smellie* ([1919] 14 Cr App R 128) was charged with assaulting, ill-treating and neglecting his 11-year-old daughter. When she was called to give evidence at his trial, the court ordered that he should sit on the steps leading to the dock so that he was out of sight of his daughter. He appealed against his conviction and argued, *inter alia*, that a prisoner was entitled at common law to be within the sight and hearing of the witness throughout the trial, and that on a charge of this kind the effect on the jury of his removal from the dock would be incalculable. However, both arguments were rejected on appeal by Lord Coleridge J. He said:

> If the judge considers that the presence of the prisoner will intimidate a witness there is nothing to prevent him from securing the ends of justice by removing the former from the presence of the latter. (p. 130)

Although Smellie is still good law, it needs to be tempered by a recognition that the defendant's right to communicate with their lawyer must not be restricted. Such a right is an integral part of the right to a fair trial within Article 6 ECHR.

In *R v X, Y and Z* ([1990] 91 Cr App R 36) the defendants argued that the use of screens around the witness box was unfair and prejudicial, even though the judge had warned the jury against this. On appeal it was held that the judge had a duty to see that justice is done and that the system operates fairly, not only to the accused but also the prosecution and the witnesses. In this case the trial judge correctly concluded that the necessity of ensuring that the children gave evidence outweighed any possible prejudice to the defendants. (See also the European Commission of Human Rights in *X v UK* ([1993] 15 EHRR CD 113) where the use of screens did not interfere with the defendant's right to a fair trial as the defendant's lawyers were able to see the witness and question him.)

The impact of the Human Rights Act 1998 was discussed by the House of Lords in the case of *R (on the application of D) v Camberwell Green Youth Court; R (on the application of the Director of Public Prosecutions)* v *Camberwell Green Youth Court* ([2005] UKHL 4, [2005] 1 All ER 999, 169 JP 105). The House of Lords had to consider the compatibility of Article 6 ECHR with s.21(5) YJCEA 1999, which removes any discretion to disapply the use of special measures for children in need of special protection (see below). The defendants in these cases argued that the trials were unfair as the child witnesses were not required to face the defendant in open court, but rather present their evidence by pre-recorded video or by a live video link. The House of Lords considered whether the exclusion by s.21(5) YJCEA 1999 of individualised consideration of each case was a breach of the right to a fair trial as it allowed them to be used whether or not the child witness needed them.

Lord Brown of Eaton-under-Heywood stated that the hearing did not cease to be a public one merely because the witness gave evidence by pre-recorded video or live link. On the lack of individual consideration point he concluded that it was unnecessary to justify the use of special measures in each individual case. He said:

> Parliament was perfectly entitled to conclude that the interests of justice generally would be better served by introducing an almost invariable rule such as will not merely in the vast majority of cases maximise the quality of child witnesses' evidence but will also encourage their full co-operation with the criminal justice system, than by retaining the maximum opportunity for face to face confrontation with child witnesses at trial.

Similarly, Baroness Hale of Richmond felt that defendants would not be disadvantaged by the provisions of s.21(5) YJCEA 1999. By limiting the circumstances in which the primary rule can be disapplied, Parliament intended to deny the defendants the argument that special measures were a departure from normal procedures in criminal trials. Unlike the Redbridge case under the previous law (*R (on the application of the Director of Public Prosecutions)* v *Redbridge Youth Court*; *R (on the application of L)* v *Bicester Youth Court* ([2001] 3 FCR 615) at p. 16), the fact that there is no reason to think that a child will be upset, traumatised or intimidated by giving evidence in court does not make it unjust to use the pre-recorded video or live video link. The court must always start from the statutory presumption that there is nothing intrinsically unfair about the child being allowed to give evidence in this way. Article 6 was not violated as all the evidence is produced at the trial in front of the accused, albeit some of it in pre-recorded form or by live video transmission, and the accused may challenge and question the witnesses during the trial. Furthermore, the ECHR does not guarantee a right to face-to-face confrontation.

The European Court of Human Rights in *SN* v *Sweden* ([2004] 39 E.H.R.R. 13) considered whether denying the defendant the ability put questions directly to the witness at the trial was a violation of Article 6(1) and (3)(d) ECHR. It emphasised that the admissibility of evidence was primarily a matter for domestic law. The function of the ECHR and the Convention organs was to ensure that the proceedings in their entirety were fair – this included the way in which the evidence was taken. In making this assessment, regard had to be given to the right of the perceived victim to a private life. It was accepted by the court that 'in criminal proceedings concerning sexual abuse certain measures may be taken for the purpose of protecting the victim, provided that such measures can be reconciled with an adequate and effective exercise of the rights of the defence' (para. 47).

In the UK courts, an attempt was made in *R* v *ex parte D (a minor) (By his Mother and Litigation Friend)* ([2005] WL 62251) to argue that the ECHR gave the defendant the right to be confronted with the witnesses against them and to look them in the eye when giving evidence. The argument is that witnesses may act differently if they had to repeat their story looking at the person whose liberty and reputation may depend upon the veracity of their evidence. This draws upon the right under the Sixth Amendment to the American Constitution that supports the idea of a 'look them in the eye' right. Lord Rodgers of Earlsferry in the Camberwell Green Youth Court case did not disparage that idea, but concluded that there was no corresponding requirement in English law.

There are limits to the extent to which child witnesses can benefit from special provision, however, as there comes a point when such measures are unduly prejudicial to the defendant. In *PS v Germany* ([2003] 36 E.H.R.R. 61), the court noted that the right to a fair trial required that the interests of the defendant be balanced against those of the witness or victim, especially when life, liberty or security of person are concerned, or interests generally coming within Article 8 ECHR. The apparent victim did not provide evidence; instead, the court heard evidence by the girl's mother and a police officer who had interviewed her, and from an expert who commented on her credibility. As the accused did not have the opportunity to cross-examine the person who had made the depositions relied on by the domestic courts, the European Court found that rights of the defendant had been restricted to a degree that was incompatible with Article 6 ECHR (PS v Germany [2003], paras 23–26).

Section 32 YJCEA 1999 provides that on a trial on indictment, the judge should give a jury such warning as they consider necessary to ensure that the fact that a special measures direction has been given must not prejudice the accused.

Implications for practitioners

Practitioners need to be aware of the sensitivities that arise in working at the interface of the criminal and civil justice systems, and social care workers who are involved in investigations of abuse must accept that their role changes from that of providing therapeutic support to that of being involved in forensic work. Preserving the evidence is essential, otherwise the criminal law will cease to be an option; this is particularly important when using pre-recorded video statements. A video-recorded interview with a child serves a number of purposes. The primary purpose is gathering evidence for use in criminal proceedings and as an examination-in-chief of the child. It may also be useful, however, in informing any s.47 Children Act 1989 investigation and in civil child protection proceedings (Home Office *et al.* 2002, paras 2.1–2.2).

Such interviews need very careful and individual planning and their format will depend upon a number of factors, including whether the child is a victim or witness, whether concurrent child protection procedures are being pursued, whether the child is known or suspected of having been abused previously, and the attributes of the particular child (Home Office *et al.* 2002, paras 2.47–2.77). The *Guidance* states:

Thorough planning is essential to a successful investigation and interview. Even if concerns about the child's safety necessitate an early interview, an appropriate planning session is required which identifies key issues and objectives. Time spent covering and anticipating issues early in the criminal investigation will be rewarded by an improved interview later on. It is important that, as far as possible, the case be thoroughly reviewed before an interview is embarked upon to ensure that all issues are covered and key questions asked, since the opportunity to do this will in most cases be lost once the interviews have been concluded.

(Home Office *et al.* 2002, p. 9)

Family and background are also important. Appendix C of the *Guidance* contains an assessment framework which can be used when considering the child in the family context. Parenting capacity, family and environmental factors and the child's developmental needs form the bases of such an assessment.

The Youth Justice and Criminal Evidence Act 1999 builds on the experience of ss.32 and 32A of the Criminal Justice Act 1988. The 1988 Act enabled children to give evidence-in-chief (see Lane, Chapter 18, in this volume) by means of a pre-recorded video interview and to be cross-examined by means of a live television link. It was based in part on the recommendations made in the Pigot Report (Pigot 1989). These reforms were broadly welcomed as a way of enabling children to give evidence and thus providing them with the full protection of the criminal justice system. However, the reforms did not fully implement the recommendation of the Pigot Report, which had recommended that children falling within the ambit of its proposals should never be required to appear in public as witnesses whether in open court, protected by screens, or through closed circuit television, unless they wanted to (para. 2.26).

The ability to pre-record a cross-examination (see Lane, Chapter 18, in this volume) was a serious omission from the 1988 Act and represented 'half Pigot' rather than 'full Pigot' (see Hoyano 2000, p. 265). A review of the working of the 1998 Act (Home Office 1998) made a number of recommendations regarding child witnesses. It proposed that child witnesses should automatically be entitled to the provision of special measures and that for these purposes 'child' should be defined as anybody under the age of 17 years (Home Office 1998, recs 64 and 65). Very importantly, the report also recommended that the provisions should be available in the magistrates' courts, in addition to the youth courts and the Crown Court: the lack of such provision under the old law produced perverse decisions regarding the mode of trial (Home Office 1998, rec. 66).

Under the YJCEA 1999, two basic questions have to be answered: is the witness eligible for consideration and, if so, what special measures should be made available? An application can be made by any party to the proceedings for a special measures direction; the court also has the power to make one of its own motion (s.19(1) YJCEA 1999). All children under the age of 17 years at the time of the hearing are deemed eligible for a direction (s.16(1)(a) YJCEA 1999); no distinction is made between children and young persons. Unlike vulnerable adults, it does not have to be shown that the quality of the witness's evidence would be diminished in order to determine eligibility. Special provisions apply to witnesses who were under 17 years when the video interview took place, but have reached the age of 17 at the time of the hearing (s.22(1)(a) – see below). Before proceeding any further, the Secretary of State must confirm that relevant arrangements may be made available in the area within which the hearing will take place (s.18(2) and (3) YJCEA 1999). Once this is confirmed, the next stage of the process is to determine what special measures should be made available. It is here that we encounter what is known as the 'primary rule' and the distinction between children in need of special protection and those who are not.

Under ss.21 and 35 YJCEA 1999 a child will be deemed to be in need of special protection if the offence is one of the following:

i.   Any offence under the Protection of Children Act 1978 or Part 1 of the Sexual Offences Act 2003
ii. Kidnapping, false imprisonment or an offence under ss.1 or 2 Child Abduction Act 1984
iii. Any offence under s.1 Children and Young Persons Act 1933.

For other offences, the child is deemed not to be in need of special protection.

The primary rule states that for all child witnesses the court must make a special measures direction, which provides for the admission of video-recorded evidence-in-chief under s.27 YJCEA 1999 (see below). Under s.27(2) YJCEA 1999 the video recording, or part of it, may be excluded if the court thinks that the interests of justice require withholding it. This emphasises the importance of ensuring that the video interview is conducted in accordance with the laws of evidence and good practice. However, for the child deemed not to be in need of special protection a caveat applies. The rule will not apply if the court is satisfied that compliance with it 'would not be likely to maximise the quality of the witness's evidence so far as is practicable' (see s.21(4)(c) YJCEA 1999). In such a case, other special measures will still be available if appropriate.

The next stage is to consider cross-examination and re-examination. The YJCEA 1999 distinguishes between sex offences (those included under (i) above) and non-sex offences. If the offence is a sex offence under the Protection of Children Act 1978 or Part 1 of the Sexual Offences Act 2003, then there is a provision for a mandatory video-recorded cross-examination under s.28 YJCEA 1999. However, this does not apply if the facility is not available, or where the witness does not want to use the facility (see s.21 (6) and (7) YJCEA 1999). Unfortunately, s.28 has not yet been implemented. The official line is that implementation is being delayed because a review of the 'workability of this measure in the context of a review of child evidence' is underway (see Home Office 2005c). Cooper is less sanguine and concludes that it 'seems highly likely that s.28 as it currently stands will never fully come into force' (Cooper 2005, p. 458). The failure to implement s.28 YJCEA 1999 means that the live video link should be used.

The failure to introduce video-recorded cross-examination represents a retreat from Pigot who, as noted above, recommended that children should never appear in court unless they wanted to. The failure to implement the 'full Pigot' is disturbing. The many justifications for the use of video-recorded evidence-in-chief apply with equal force to cross-examination. The effect of the lapse of time on recall, the stress of waiting for the trial and the giving of evidence, and the impact on pre-trial decision making by prosecution and defence are equally applicable to cross-examination (see Hoyano 2000, p. 255, and Ellison 2001, pp. 57–59). However, it is interesting to note that, in Scotland, the possibility of pre-recorded cross-examination was excluded from the Vulnerable Witnesses (Scotland) Act 2004.

If the offence is not a sex offence, then a mandatory live link must be used for any testimony not given in a pre-recorded video. However, in these circumstances the court has an option to order video cross-examination under s.28 YJCEA 1999. This provision is subject to the implementation of s.28 YJCEA 1999 (see ss.21(3)(b) and 21(4)(a) YJCEA 1999).

As noted above, the special measures apply to those under the age of 17 years at the time of the hearing. If the witness was 17 years at the time of the hearing, but was under 17 years when the video evidence-in-chief was recorded, they become a 'qualifying witness', although the YJCEA 1999 still provides some protection for such witnesses. The video evidence must be admitted, subject to availability and to any editing or exclusion in the interests of justice (s.22(2)(a) YJCEA 1999). A qualifying witness will be deemed to be in need of special protection if the offence is a sex or violence offence. If it is a sex offence, videoed cross-examination is mandatory; if the facilities are unavailable (as is the case at present), then a live video link must be used unless the witness declined to do so (s.21(7)(b) YJCEA 1999).

Special measures

The YJCEA 1999 makes provision for the following special measures.

Screens or other arrangements to shield the witness from the defendant – s.23 YJCEA 1999

This provision reflects the common law on screens and other arrangements. As noted above, the use of screens was sanctioned by the court in *R v X, Y and Z* [1990]. Similarly, in *R v Smellie* [1919], the court's action in requiring the defendant to sit on the steps leading to the dock out of sight of the witness was upheld on appeal. Arrangements made must not interfere with the right of the accused person to communicate with their lawyer. If communication is impeded, then this may amount to a violation of the Article 6 ECHR right to a fair trial (Home Office *et al.* 2002, para. 5.46). The purpose of the s.23 provision is to prevent the witness from seeing the accused. However, the section provides that the witness must be able to see, and be seen by, the judge, justices and jury, the legal representatives and any interpreter or other person appointed to assist the witness (s.23(2)(a)–(c) YJCEA 1999). In *R v Brown and Grant* ([2004] EWCA Crim 1620 (Transcript: Smith Bernal) 21 May 2004), the Court of Appeal held that the judge should convey to a jury the essential matters involved in using screens and the conclusions they should draw and not draw from it. Any warning need not be repeated in the summing up; indeed it may be more effective if outlined at the time the evidence is given than if it is formalistically repeated during the summing up. Screens are fully available in the Crown Court and the magistrates' courts.

Evidence by live link – s.24 YJCEA 1999

As noted above, a court may direct that a child gives evidence by means of a live link or other arrangements allowing the witness to be absent from the courtroom, but they must be able to see and hear, and be seen and heard by, the judge or justice, legal representatives and any interpreter or person appointed to assist the witness. Facilities are available in full in the Crown Court and the magistrates' courts. Where such a direction is made, the child may not give evidence in any other way without the permission of the court. Permission will only be granted if it is in the interests of justice and, where an application is made by one of the parties, there has been a material change of circumstances since the time when the direction was given.

The use of a live link has been assessed in a number of studies. Murray (1995) based her study on 49 children giving evidence by live link in Scotland and 17 who gave evidence in the courtroom. The findings were encouraging. Very importantly, the use of a live TV link appeared to reduce the extreme fear and distress felt by some child witnesses and gave them a more positive impression of fairness in the legal process. In addition, the use of the video link did not appear to make much difference to the quality of the evidence. However, some of the children would not have testified without it. Lawyers were concerned that the use of the link interfered with witness rapport, made cross-examination more difficult, distorted the impact and import of the evidence, and could detract from the jury's ability to assess the witness's demeanour. Most of the judges approved of the use of live TV links, however, as it alleviated the ordeal of testifying for some child witnesses and helped to secure a more coherent account (Murray 1995, Ellison 2003, pp. 43–45).

Evidence given in private – s.23 YJCEA 1999

The public nature of criminal trials is an important part of the criminal justice process; evidence should normally be given in open court and the whole process open to public view. This includes press coverage of trials. However, the openness of the process may also add to the stress of the child witness and provide the opportunity for them to be intimidated by people in the public gallery. Section 25 YJCEA 1999 allows for a special measures direction to exclude the public from the court during the giving of the witness's evidence. This measure is available in sexual offences proceedings, and if it appears that there are reasonable grounds for believing that somebody other than the accused will intimidate the witness.

The accused, lawyers acting in the case and anybody who is an interprcter or person appointed to assist the witness cannot be excluded under this provision. Members of the media may be excluded, although s.25(3) YJCEA 1999 does allow for one journalist who has been nominated by their peers to remain in the court.

Removal of wigs and gowns – s.26 YJCEA 1999

This seemingly trivial concession may help to make the courtroom more children-friendly. In practice this has been done for many years in cases involving children giving evidence; the statutory provision is of more relevance to vulnerable adult witnesses.

Video-recorded evidence-in-chief – s.27 YJCEA 1999

The ability to video-record an interview with a child and for it to be used subsequently as the child's evidence-in-chief goes some way towards meeting the objectives of Pigot in seeking to remove the need for children to appear in court as witnesses. Detailed guidance on the conduct of such interviews is contained in the Appendix E of the *Guidance*. The general rule is that the interview should be conducted, so far as is possible, in accordance with the rules of evidence that would apply in court (E1.4). The penalty for getting it wrong is that the recording will be inadmissible and the child will have to give evidence in person. The *Guidance* identifies a number of key legal rules that must be adhered to, as outlined in Table 20.1.

Decisions on admissibility are complex and appropriate legal advice should be sought if there is any doubt. The important point for practitioners to consider is that fundamental flaws in the video evidence may lead to the prosecution of the alleged perpetrator being dropped.

Video-recorded cross-examination – s.28 YJCEA 1999

As noted above, s.28 YJCEA 1999 makes provision for pre-recorded cross-examinations to be admitted where a pre-recorded video evidence-in-chief is admitted as evidence-in-chief under s.27 YJCEA 1999. As with pre-recorded evidence-in-chief, cross-examinations admitted under s.28 may be excluded if they fail to follow the rule of the court dealing with cross-examination (see Home Office *et al.* 2002, pp. 122–123). It is regrettable that there has been a retreat from the Pigot view that children should never appear in court and the failure to implement pre-recorded cross-examination evidence is a major weakness in the current arrangements for child witnesses.

Examination of the witness through an intermediary – s.29 YJCEA 1999

The primary role of the intermediary is to facilitate communication between the child and the court. They may be used in video-recorded interviews, live link interviews or where the child chooses to appear in open court. Section 29(2)(a) and (b)

Table 20.1
Guidance on video-recorded evidence-in-chief

Rule	Explanation	Exceptions
The child must not be asked leading questions	A leading question is one that suggests the answer, e.g. 'X got into bed with you, didn't he?' (On the format of questions, see Home Office *et al.* 2002, pp. 42–47)	1. Warming up questions, e.g. 'Do you live at …?' 2. In some instances it may be impractical to ban leading questions, e.g. if a young witness may not be able to understand the question without some prompting
Previous statements: a court would normally prevent a witness from giving evidence of what they had previously said, or what was said to them by another person	The rationale for this rule is that consistency does not necessarily show that the witness is reliable, and also the courts are reluctant to accept statements that are not made in court and subject to cross-examination	1. Previous statements showing consistency in the case of statements made by the witness soon after the offence took place, and also when a witness has previously made a positive identification of the accused, e.g. at an identification parade 2. There is a good reason for proving that the words were spoken, e.g. somebody reports that the child said, 'Dad taught me to fuck' – this may be used as evidence of the child's age-inappropriate use of language, but not as evidence to prove that the father sexually abused the child
Character of the accused	Evidence of any previous convictions or statements relating to the bad character of the accused is not normally admissible Interviewers should avoid eliciting such evidence from the interviewee	An exception may be made where evidence of one offence is so closely connected or similar (e.g. an unusual modus operandi) that its probative value outweighs any prejudicial effect

Adapted from Home Office *et al.* 2002, pp. 139–143.

YJCEA 1999 identifies the functions of an intermediary as first, to communicate to the witness in an appropriate way any questions that may be put to them, and second, to communicate to the court the answers given by the witness. The intermediary can explain, so far as is necessary, the questions or the answers to ensure that there is effective communication. Anybody acting as an intermediary must sign a declaration that they will 'faithfully perform the function' (s.29(5) YJCEA 1999). The presence of an intermediary does not remove the responsibility of the magistrate or judge to ensure that questions put to the witness are proper and appropriate to the child's level of understanding (Home Office *et al.* 2002, p. 124).

Aids to communication – s.30 YJCEA 1999

A special measures direction may arrange for the witness to be provided with an aid to communication if they have a communication impairment. These may include sign and symbol boards.

Conclusion

The interface between civil law protection of children and the criminal justice system raises some complex issues. However, these must be resolved, as child victims cannot be denied the protection of the criminal law. For that reason, procedural changes have sought to accommodate the special needs of children and other vulnerable witnesses. At all times, however, practitioners must recognise the need to achieve an appropriate balance between the interests of the defendant, the witness and more generally the interests of justice. The ECHR seeks to achieve and work within such a balanced approach. One important aspect of this is the need to ensure that proper regard is had to the demands of the criminal justice system. Evidence must be collected in accordance with the well-established rules that operate within traditional courtroom settings. Practitioners involved in investigations must recognise that their role changes from a therapeutic one to a forensic one, with all that this entails.

Close interdisciplinary working and an understanding of the roles and contributions of different professional groups are also essential. The *Guidance* (Home Office *et al.* 2002) provides a comprehensive and accessible resource and should be familiar to all of those involved in the process. Everything must be done correctly the first time as there is little if any opportunity to correct errors at a later stage. The State is under a positive duty to protect children from inhuman and degrading treatment and special measures are one way in which this obligation is discharged. However, whether the UK system, with its heavy reliance on oral evidence, has achieved the proper balance between the defendant and the child witness is, as McEwan (1999) suggests, something that the European Court on Human Rights may wish to revisit in a future challenge by an aggrieved defendant.

Key points and messages for practice

- Practitioners must recognise that their role will change from a therapeutic one to a forensic one. It is essential to recognise this and to avoid trying to combine the two roles.

- Practitioners must have a clear understanding of the *Guidance* (Home Office *et al.* 2002) and of the importance of ensuring that investigations and interviews are conducted in accordance with its detailed advice.

- The inter-relationship between the criminal justice and civil systems is complex and the courts will endeavour to strike the appropriate balance between the interests of the vulnerable witness and that of the accused.

- Listen to the child and ensure that they are informed in an appropriate manner of what is happening.

Annotated further reading

Ellison L 2003 The adversarial process and the vulnerable witness. Oxford University Press, Oxford

There is a considerable literature on the treatment of child and other vulnerable witnesses in the criminal justice system. This monograph is a comprehensive and critical account of recent developments in the treatment of such witnesses in which Ellison considers the ethical, cultural and psychological issues that arise and places them in the context of the changes brought about by the Youth Justice and Criminal Evidence Act 1999. In her conclusion, she states that the true test of the government's commitment to meeting the needs of such witnesses 'will be a preparedness to move beyond the straightjacket of established trial procedure in the search for solutions' (p. 160). She is not sanguine that this will come about.

Home Office 1998 Speaking up for justice. Report of the Interdepartmental Working Group on the treatment of vulnerable or intimidated witnesses in the criminal justice system. Home Office, London

This document outlines the case for the changes in the law and is a valuable research and practice resource.

Home Office, Lord Chancellor, Crown Prosecution Service, Department of Health, The National Assembly of Wales 2002 Achieving best evidence in criminal proceedings: guidance for vulnerable or intimidated witnesses, including children. Home Office Communications, London

Crucial reading for practitioners working in this area, the Guidance *covers planning and conducting interviews with children, witness support and preparation, witnesses at court and a useful set of Appendices dealing with issues such as legal constraints on conducting video interviews, identification parades and technical guidance.*

Home Office, Department of Health and Crown Prosecution Service 2001 Provision of therapy for child witnesses prior to a criminal trial: practice guidance. CPS Communications Branch, Bolton. Online. Available: www.dfes.gov.uk/qualityprotects/pdfs/therapy.pdf

Essential reading for those working with children who may be called upon to give evidence in criminal proceedings arising out of alleged abuse. Although designed primarily for therapists and lawyers, it is valuable reading for all of those working with children who are the victims of abuse.

De Than C 2003 Positive obligations under the European Convention on Human Rights: towards the human rights of victims and vulnerable witnesses. Journal of Criminal Law 67:165

This useful article considers the positive obligations under the European Convention on Human Rights (ECHR) towards vulnerable witnesses, arguing that the ECHR creates positive obligations on states to protect vulnerable witnesses. De Than argues that, as the rights already exist (albeit in partial form), the focus of the current debate should be how these rights can be upheld and extended.

McEwan J 1999 In defence of vulnerable witnesses: the Youth Justice and Criminal Evidence Act 1999. International Journal of Evidence and Proof 4(1)

Jenny McEwan considers in detail the provisions in the YJCEA 1999. She predicts that defendants will probably express considerable disquiet if some witnesses make use of special measures. She points out that European Court of Human Rights case law, which is generally supportive of special measures, may not be appropriate for the British system with its heavy reliance on orality and the use of cross-examination. The effect of special measures may be more prejudicial to the defendant in the British system than in, for example, the German one.

Bates P 1999 New legislation: the Youth Justice and Criminal Evidence Act – the evidence of children and vulnerable adults. Child and Family Law Quarterly 11(8):289–303

Bates recognises that, however sensitively handled, criminal proceedings are likely to be distressing for children, but the provision of special measures is an important step in the greater recognition of their interests in the criminal justice system.

Useful websites

Achieving best evidence in criminal proceedings: guidance for vulnerable or intimidated witnesses, including children: www.cps.gov.uk/publications/prosecution/bestevidencevol1.html

ChildLine: www.childline.org.uk/extra/campaigns-childwitnesses.asp

Children's Legal Centre – Promoting Children's Rights: www.childrenslegalcentre.com/Templates/Topic.asp?NodeID=90730

NSPCC: www.nspcc.org.uk/html/home/newsandcampaigns/caringforchildrenincourt.htm

The Criminal Justice System (Department of Constitutional Affairs): www.cjsonline.gov.uk

The Liberty Guide to Human Rights: www.yourrights.org.uk/your-rights/chapters/the-rights-of-victims-and-witnesses-of-crime/if-the-victim-is-young/index.shtml

Youth Justice and Criminal Evidence Act 1999: www.opsi.gov.uk/acts/acts1999/19990023.htm

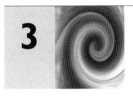
INTERVENTION IN SAFEGUARDING CHILDREN

21 Partnership with parents

Stephanie Petrie

INTRODUCTION

This chapter deals with the key issue of working in partnership with parents in child protection work, which became increasingly important in the 1990s. The context for professionals now working in child protection, however, has changed significantly. Fundamental shifts in policies, legislation and practices, designed to change professional approaches to the identification and assessment of 'children in need' and the way in which services are provided and by whom, have taken place since the late 1990s. The increased emphasis on family support, greater recognition of the rights of children and young people and the reconfiguration of children's services brought about by the *Every Child Matters* (DfES 2003b) agenda and the Children Act 2004 have affected both the concept and practice approaches to partnership with parents. This chapter will first consider the nature of partnership before critically examining policies and practices in their historical context until the present day. A review of relevant research findings on the effectiveness of partnership and service-user perspectives will follow. Finally, a discussion of the implications for professionals with child protection responsibilities will precede a summary of the chapter.

The nature of partnership

The word 'partnership' is now commonly used in health and social care to describe the relationship between clients, patients or service users and professionals. 'Partnership', however, is neither mentioned in statute applicable to the UK nor clearly defined in associated policies and guidance. Is 'partnership', therefore, a legitimate way to describe the interaction between professionals and those on the receiving end of their interventions? Debates as to the characteristics of interactions between the citizen and the professional acting on behalf of the liberal state have taken place for many decades and it has been argued that it is the distribution of power between the key players that determines the nature of the relationship. In the US in the 1960s, for example, those engaged in community and urban development and anti-poverty programmes were concerned with citizen participation. Arnstein (1969) suggested a continuum for understanding that partnership involves a relatively high degree of power sharing that goes well beyond helping, informing, consulting and cooperating activities. Twenty years later in the UK, at a time when the concept of partnership with parents was emerging as an important principle in social work/social care, Jordan (1988) also argued that a high degree of power sharing was necessary:

Partnership ... implies a good deal more than cooperation. It implies a kind of pooling of resources, and fairly close integration of roles, as in the marital relationship, or in a commercial firm. It implies trust, and a good deal of potential or actual agreement on common goals, and the means of achieving them. (p. 30)

These definitions of partnership describe a relatively stable and trusting relationship with shared goals, yet this has always been difficult to achieve in child protection work. Since the primary focus is on the child, one barrier to partnership has often been conflicting perspectives between family adults and professional workers as to the issues of risk and care, which are, in any case, contested concepts (Parton 1998). Indeed, child abuse itself is a contested concept and, as Wattam (1999) points out, 'Perhaps the greatest impediment to the prevention of significant harm is the contested arena of what child abuse should be' (p. 327). Social workers also carry with them into child protection investigations extensive legal and administrative powers and, as discussed below, families are acutely aware of these. Finally, partnership is not usually considered in relation to children since, in practice, and in spite of the provisions of the UNCRC, they are rarely perceived to be citizens or service users. Despite UK and European legislation during the last 20 years, our responses to children have changed little, as Al Aynsley-Green, the newly-appointed Children's Commissioner for England, pointed out at a recent conference: 'The fundamental issue in this country is that children and young people aren't seen as citizens. We have this extraordinary attitude that they are owned by their parents' (CommunityCare.co.uk 2005). These dichotomies affect the way in which professionals, parents and children interact in child protection processes.

More recently it has been argued that the notion of partnership with parents in child protection is in any case inherently flawed and serves practitioners and agencies more than service users (Holland & Scourfield 2004). By providing a semblance of fairness and transparency about power interests, often in written contractual form, it can appear that there is a level of empowerment for the service user: 'Carole Smith has argued that "rights-talk" provides an element of certainty in late modern risk society, and that such talk eclipses value-based talk in contemporary social work discourse' (Holland & Scourfield 2004, p. 30). In a society that is as culturally and ethnically diverse as the UK, notions of partnership derived from a Western concept of 'rights' may not always be understood by or helpful to families. Embarking on forms of 'participation' primarily to meet agency expectations, rather than engaging in individualised and dynamic relationships with children and their families, merely offers tokenistic 'partnerships' that can be experienced by service users as unhelpful (Dale 2004).

As will be shown, the formal aspects of partnership have little impact on the recipients of child protection interventions: it is the quality of the parents' relationship with the worker involved that is important and empowering. The central importance of the quality of the 'helping' relationship is a finding that has emerged consistently in therapeutic effectiveness studies from the early work of Truax and Carkhuff in 1967. User-perspective studies on all aspects of child protection also reveal the critical importance of the worker/client relationship (see below). In the 1990s, government guidance (DoH 1995b) recognised that partnership with parents in child protection was a relationship to be aimed for rather than a right of parents upheld by legislation. It may be, therefore, that the possibility of partnership with parents in the current context will require further emphasis on the centrality of 'relationship' in child protection work, whatever the professional identity of the practitioner involved.

Partnership with parents: policies and practices

The care and control functions of those engaged in child welfare activities have been a matter of debate since their earliest manifestation in the nineteenth century. Parton (1998) suggests that ambiguity is inevitable, and perhaps essential, because the social space occupied by what he terms social technologists is also ambiguous and contested:

The 'social' discourse developed as a hybrid in the space identified between the private sphere of the household and the public sphere of the state and society. It operated in an intermediary zone. It produced and was reproduced by new relations between the law, administration, medicine, the school and the family. (p. 9)

Not surprisingly, therefore, the place of parents in child welfare decision making has had a long and varied history: attempts both to involve parents and exclude them have fluctuated according to the dominant welfare discourse of the time. The nature of welfare provision in the latter half of the nineteenth century, for example, worked against any form of partnership since the parents of needy children were believed to be a pernicious influence on their offspring (Holman 1988). By the late nineteenth and early twentieth centuries, however, things had changed somewhat. Inspectors from the National Society for the Prevention of Cruelty to Children (NSPCC) were greatly aware of the need not to alienate parents and communities in their efforts to protect children (Ferguson 1990). It is since the establishment of the Welfare State in 1948, however, that these shifts in public and professional attitudes towards child welfare and the involvement of parents are of greatest relevance when considering partnership in child protection practice.

Post-war welfarism

The period immediately after the Second World War saw a significant change of attitudes towards poor parents. This shift was attributable to several key developments:

- the insights into the undernourished and underdeveloped state of poor children evacuated from inner cities to the countryside
- the development of ideas about the emotional ill-effects on children of separation from their parents, particularly by John Bowlby (1951)
- concerns about the standards of care provided by the state for children highlighted by the Dennis O'Neill Inquiry (Home Office 1945)
- a broad, although not unanimous, post-war social consensus that a more liberal and humane welfare system was desirable (see Frost & Stein 1989).

As a result of these concerns, a specialist child care service was set up following the passing of the Children Act 1948, which had a particular remit to provide more child-sensitive services to children and families where breakdown was imminent or evident. The focus until the end of the 1950s was largely on providing good standard substitute care, but increasingly it was recognised that more resources needed to be deployed to prevent family breakdown.

Consequently, the Children and Young Persons Act 1963 empowered local authorities to give assistance in kind to families, for the first time in cash, and to prevent children coming into care by provision of social work support. At this time there was a general consensus that the best place, certainly for younger children, was with their parents and that reception into care should be a last resort. Kinship ties (Fox Harding 1991) were believed to be all important and 'maternal' deprivation (Bowlby 1951) was perceived to be at the root of a wide range of personal and emotional problems and a key factor in the causation of juvenile delinquency. During this period, despite increased recognition of the importance of the link between children and their families, professionals functioned as experts (Yellolly 1980), parents were rarely involved in decision making and the number of children in care did not reduce. Partnership with parents was not on the professional agenda since there was an acceptance that, in effect, the expert knew best.

The 1970s to late 1990s

In the 1970s, the social and economic context changed dramatically. The welfarist approach to poorer families was coming under challenge from right-wing groups and theories about cycles of disadvantage and the need for targeting resources more effectively were being developed (Parton 1979). The welfare state was also under attack from feminists and anti-racists, who argued that welfare provision was not universal in its organisation or services (Williams F 1995). The consensus in relation to child welfare therefore began to shift as public and professional attitudes changed and conflicting perspectives emerged. One strand of professional practice was in the direction of generic and community-based services, which were primarily family focused and aimed at keeping children out of care. In contrast, those who wanted to retain a more specialist child care approach were questioning the predominance of 'kinship ties', particularly where this led to children languishing in care (Goldstein *et al.* 1973, Rowe & Lambert 1973). Perhaps the most important factor in questioning the hegemony of 'kinship ties' was that of the growing awareness, in the US and the UK, about what was termed 'baby battering' (Kempe *et al.* 1962), which led to developments in forensic approaches to the detection of non-accidental injury to children. The Maria Colwell inquiry (DHSS 1974b) also revealed the potential dangerousness of some families for children and the inability of welfare-oriented professionals to provide adequate protection for them was high-lighted, leading to the establishment of a more structured system for dealing with child abuse.

The subsequent Children Act 1975 reflected a considerable shift away from the broader family support approach which had characterised child care work since 1948. The focus was now clearly on the needs of children living with their parents to be protected from abuse. A series of inquiries into child deaths in the 1980s (DoH 1991a) were significant in reinforcing the need for a greater child protective stance which paid less attention to the broader family needs than before. This approach has been termed the 'child rescue' model and 'risk assessment' began to emerge in child protection work and eventually came to dominate child welfare (DoH 1995a). To some degree, however, this approach was contrary to the requirements of other developments taking place in the child care field: both the 1984 Short Report (House of Commons 1984) and a review of research published by central government (DHSS 1985b) pointed to practice that did not sufficiently take into account parents' views and rights. However, it was not until the end of the 1980s that these criticisms found full voice, following allegations of heavy-handed and inappropriate intervention into cases of intrafamilial sexual abuse in Cleveland. The resulting Inquiry Report (Butler-Sloss 1988) condemned the treatment of parents during these investigations and recommendations were made about how they should be involved.

The Children Act 1989 was drafted to deal with the tension that exists between the rights of children to be protected and the rights of children and their parents to their own family life. Local authorities were given increased powers attached to orders, but at the same time their powers were curtailed through strict time limits and more rights of challenge. Although the Children Act 1989 pointed to the need for greater involvement of parents than before in all court processes, including child protection proceedings, it did not greatly clarify the appropriate level of parental involvement in the provision of child protection services. The Department of Health, however, issued new guidelines for agencies involved in child protection investigations (DoH 1991f) that stressed that parental (and child) attendance at case conferences should be the norm. These guidelines were far more positive about the notion of involving parents in the child protection process than those issued in 1986, which expressly prohibited the attendance of parents at case conferences (DHSS 1986).

Other factors emerging in the 1990s also began to impact on the nature of partnerships in child protection work. The market paradigm for health and social care initiated by the National Health Service and Community Care Act 1990 led many local authorities to restructure their services for children along similar purchaser/provider lines. There are additional implications for professional/service user partnerships in 'market' transactions (Petrie & Wilson 1999). The 'client' or 'patient' has been transformed into the 'service user' or 'consumer' and whilst it is possible to imagine how professional power can be regulated through the interplay of supply and demand when the service user has real purchasing power, this is rarely the case for welfare recipients. One example of a genuine element of choice in the decision-making process is the Community Care (Direct Payments) Act 1996 that enables disabled adults to be budget holders for their own care. In these situations, professionals are expected to work alongside service users who are able not only to state their preferences but also take control of the decision-making process. In child protection interventions, however, parents are often unwilling consumers with no purchasing power, and children and young people are even more disempowered. Practice guidance (DoH 1995b) nevertheless identified three steps in the process towards partnership: providing information, involvement and participation. It was acknowledged that these approaches were not sequential and were likely to fluctuate over time. Furthermore, it was stressed that partnership was not an end in itself, but a means by which children were to be protected and their welfare promoted. By the mid 1990s, therefore, the main focus was on the involvement of parents and (to a lesser extent) children in child protection conferences. This was seen as the main arena for partnership in practice and although government child welfare policies and professional practice promoted working in 'partnership with parents', it was acknowledged that real sharing of power in child protection work, particularly in the early investigative stages, was difficult to achieve.

Late 1990s to date

By the time of the first New Labour government in 1997, concern about the impact on children of the dramatic rise in poverty since the mid 1970s was high on political and professional agendas (Bennett 2005). Government-commissioned research (DoH 1995a) had shown that the bulk of child care referrals did not involve serious allegations of abuse but resulted from concerns about low standards of care, often in poor families experiencing a range of pressures. The updated *Working Together to Safeguard Children** (DoH *et al.* 1999), the *Framework for the Assessment of Children in Need and their Families* (DoH, DfEE, HO 2000e) and associated practice guidance (DoH 2000c) aimed to change professional decision making in relation to child protection by reducing stigma and directing more resources to meet the needs of children. This change of emphasis was called the 'refocusing' initiative (Platt 2005): broad-based assessments and interventions, provided in partnership with children and their families, were expected to be more appropriate for most families than child protection investigations under s.47 of the Children Act 1989. Child abuse was now understood in eco-systemic terms and assessments therefore

---

* The most up-to-date version of this document was published by HM Government in 2006. For a full discussion of this, see Chapter 11.

needed to be more holistic, taking into account buffers (i.e. protective factors) as well as risks (Sidebotham *et al.* 2001). *Working Together* (DoH *et al.* 1999) therefore has a specific section on partnership working in child protection (pp. 75–77), reproducing earlier practice guidance on partnership as a process (DoH 1995b) and also addressing the issue of involving children. Family Group Conferences are also recommended as part of a partnership approach in some situations (p. 78).

The horrific death of Victoria Climbié in 2000 and subsequent inquiry (Laming Report 2003) revealed, however, that it was still possible for the sufferings of children to be unrecognised when agencies and workers focused on adults and overlooked the child. Concentrating on family adults at the expense of the child had been identified in most child death inquiries from Maria Colwell onwards and one of the most significant findings of the Laming Inquiry was the number of agencies that had been involved with Victoria whose workers failed to notice her abuse and failed to even speak with her alone: '[N]o manager realized that Victoria had not been seen alone by any professional or given any opportunity to tell her story' (Laming Report 2003, p. 5). Ignorance about ethnic and cultural norms was also a significant factor: inappropriate assumptions were made about how 'African' children related to their elders and consequently Victoria's withdrawn demeanour was interpreted as a form of respect, rather than an indicator of the fear she undoubtedly felt. Another key finding was the impact of organisational dysfunction on front-line services. Organisational failure had been mentioned in many earlier inquiries (Dingwall 1986, DoH 1991a, Parton 1991) but never so prominently. Laming was clear that the ability of practitioners to work satisfactorily had been undermined by lack of resources, including staffing shortfalls, untrained and unqualified staff, ineffective management and lack of adequate supervision:

Whilst the standard of work done by those with direct contact with her was generally of very poor quality, the greatest failure rests with the managers and senior members of the authorities whose task it was to ensure that services for children, like Victoria, were properly financed, staffed, and able to deliver good quality support to children and families.

(Laming Report 2003, p. 5)

Of perhaps greatest concern was the way in which local authorities were using s.17 of the Children Act 1989 to restrict eligibility for family support services: children who were not on the child protection register rarely received services and Victoria Climbié received neither services nor protection. Her death revealed the fragile state of children's services in local and health authorities and trusts. Once more the focus of debate was on how to balance protection and prevention, a concern that has been a feature of child welfare legislation, policies and practice since the middle of the twentieth century.

The radical reforms initiated by the *Every Child Matters* (DfES 2003b) agenda, the Children Act 2004 and the *National Service Framework for Children, Young People and Maternity Services* (DoH/DfES 2004) aim to rationalise and improve services for all children and bring together two important child welfare policy strands: better protection and specialist services targeting the most vulnerable children, and increased 'evidence-based' preventative services in the community for all children. These reforms are to be carried out through Children's Services Authorities that draw together Education and Social Services, although there is the possibility of integrating services for children still further through the establishment of children's trust pathfinder authorities, of which there are 35 currently being evaluated. The Children Act 2004 places increased requirements to share information and work together on all agencies who might be involved with children, in order to safeguard and promote their welfare: multi-agency and multidisciplinary teams and services are expected to be the norm.

Those working in services described as universal are expected to use the Common Assessment Framework (CAF) (DfES 2003b) to assess the needs of children. CAFs are to inform initial assessments (DoH *et al.* 2000e) if they are necessary, and must be conducted by qualified social workers. A lead professional, who could come from any agency involved with children, will act as a single point of contact and will coordinate interventions and services. As child protection concerns may emerge at any time, leading to s.47 (Children Act 1989) enquiries, there will be some families already receiving support services who will have established relationships with workers providing these. It is likely, therefore, that some professionals will be involved in ongoing child protection work more closely than before, since it is the needs of the child and family that will determine who the lead professional should be, not the agency for which they work. Any member of the children's workforce – including social care, health, education and voluntary sector professionals – could fulfil this role, depending on the skills and knowledge needed.

Consultation is underway on a new draft of *Working Together to Safeguard Children** (HM Government 2005a) and although the term partnership is not specifically mentioned, Chapter 9 outlines in some detail the principles underlying work with children and their families where there are concerns about possible maltreatment:

[T]hose working together should agree a common understanding in each case, and at each stage of work, of how children and families will be involved in the safeguarding children processes, and what information is shared with them. There should be a presumption of openness, joint decision-making, and a willingness to listen to families and capitalize on their strengths, but the overarching principle should always be to act in the best interests of the child.
(HM Government 2005a, p. 150)

The bulk of this very lengthy guidance document is directed towards all agencies that might have involvement in child protection activities and outlines in detail procedures and timescales. It is important, therefore, to understand what those at the receiving end of professional interventions experience as effective partnership in order to recognise and retain 'best' practice at a time of major change.

Partnership with parents: research findings

1970s to late 1990s

Prior to the 1970s, there was little research into adults' experiences of being at the receiving end of child welfare interventions, let alone those of children and young people. One of the earliest studies, undertaken by Mayer and Timms (1970), revealed that social workers and their 'clients' had quite different views of the nature of their relationship. Although workers perceived themselves as emotionally neutral and professionally helpful, their 'clients' often experienced punitive and contemptuous interactions. Even when the intervention was valued and helpful, perceptions sometimes differed. 'Clients' compared the helpful relationship to a friendship, implying a connection of equals; workers, on the other hand, withheld 'self' from these interactions, since engaging in a more equitable relationship was felt to be unprofessional. Rees (1978) found considerable evidence of confusion,

---

* The most up-to-date version of this document was published by HM Government in 2006. For a full discussion of this, see Chapter 11.

uncertainty and even fear felt by clients in their contacts with social workers. Sainsbury *et al.* (1982) found that workers and their clients frequently had different agendas, which was particularly apparent where issues of social control predominated, a finding supported by Rees and Wallace's (1982) research review, which drew attention to the fact that suspicion or fear was common amongst people with child care difficulties.

In contrast, studies by Sainsbury (1975) and Fisher *et al.* (1986) described practice that was experienced as helpful by family adults, even when the social control function was paramount. In the first study, practical help, genuineness and straight talking were valued by service users. Interventions were most effective when parents were involved in decision making in order to identify their own needs and how these and the needs of their children could best be met. In the latter study, most appreciated were 'a "cards on the table" business-like approach, a consistent showing of concern and an exhibited desire for their involvement in the decisions and activities of care' (DHSS 1985b, p. 29).

Until the studies sponsored by the Department of Health following the Cleveland Inquiry (1995a), there was little research into parents' views about being at the receiving end of child protection investigations. Small-scale studies by Brown (1984) and Corby (1987) were among the few that sought parents' perspectives in child abuse investigations in this period. Most parents felt that the process was stigmatising and painful, and most felt ill-informed about the process and their rights within it (Prosser 1992). Lewis *et al.* (1992) reviewed several studies of parental participation at child protection case conferences: some found that both professionals and parents considered the arrangements beneficial; others that, from the parents' viewpoint, participation was minimal. Corby *et al.* (1996) and Corby and Millar (1997) sought the views of a small number of parents about their involvement in the child protection system over an 18-month period following investigation, finding that parents who felt alienated in the early stages of the process were still unhappy at this later stage, thus confirming the findings of Farmer and Owen (1995).

This lack of knowledge of parents' perspectives was transformed by the research commissioned by the Department of Health in the wake of the Cleveland Inquiry and the controversies there, which, not surprisingly, placed great reliance on parents' (and children's) views. In all, 20 studies were initiated and published individually, being summarised in *Child Protection: Messages from Research* (DoH 1995a). Two of the key findings specifically related to working in partnership with parents: that involving parents did not place children at greater risk, and that the quality of the interaction between professionals and families during the early stages of intervention was critical to the quality of later work. Of greatest importance were findings that most children subject to child abuse inquiries were from poor families. Bebbington and Miles (1989) had revealed how indicators of poverty, deprivation and ethnicity were highly correlated with the entry of children into local authority care. Children of mixed ethnic background, for example, were two and a half times more likely to enter care than white children. Although social workers believed they were applying similar practice judgements in all situations, it was clear that some children were at greater risk of coming into care than others. It was becoming apparent that living in care could also expose children and young people to significant harm (Utting *et al.* 1997). It was argued that there should be a shift in focus towards meeting needs rather than identifying deeds, and that professionals needed to adopt a more engaging and supportive approach, with the emphasis on working with parents to enhance the development of their children rather than initiating what were considered to be heavy-handed child protection investigations that were both unnecessary and costly.

By the late 1990s therefore, the child protection system itself was under attack. Partnership with parents was not only absent in most child protection processes but also the system, it was argued, made it difficult for professionals and parents to work together to safeguard and promote the welfare of children because of the narrow focus of assessments and the inappropriate use of s.47 (Children Act 1989) enquiries. The policy objective was to 'refocus' local authority resources (Spratt & Callan 2004, Platt 2006) away from unnecessary child protection investigations so that the families of vulnerable children in the community received more services designed to support and enhance their parenting capacity. It was expected that the number of child protection investigations would reduce and family support services would be developed and provided, with the involvement of service users in partnership.

Late 1990s to date

The 2000s have been characterised by increasing central government surveillance and regulation of local government welfare practices through management by performance indicators and inspections. In relation to child welfare, including child protection, performance indicators have been derived from a range of indices of need, while local authority performance has been tied to central government funding and, if judged unsatisfactory, to punitive action such as special measures. Although there has been a great deal of criticism of this approach in health, welfare and education (e.g. Jones & Novak 1999), consideration of this issue is beyond the scope of this chapter. What is relevant, however, is that evaluations of services, including the seeking of service-user perspectives and increasingly those of children and young people, have become characteristic of this type of regulation. From the late 1990s, government funding programmes widened and extended service provision in the community for young children and their families, especially those identified as vulnerable. The intention was to offer preventative services that parents could access on a voluntary basis (Glass 1999). Consequently, alongside changes in child protection approaches, government made more resources available through more than 500 *Sure Start* local programmes. Evaluation was a requirement for all *Sure Start* programmes and, in addition, a national evaluation was commissioned. It is worth pointing out that whilst practitioners are urged to engage in evidence-based practice, government initiates major shifts in policy without waiting for findings from the studies they have commissioned. As Tunstill *et al.* wryly point out, government policy on *Sure Start* had changed before the National Evaluation of *Sure Start* finished:

[G]iven the current emphasis on an evidence based approach (Cabinet Office 1999) the implications of the commissioning of the National Evaluation were that future policy development would draw on its subsequent findings. Perhaps unsurprisingly … government policy in respect of children and families has continued to develop, in advance of conclusive research findings to emanate from NESS.

(Tunstill *et al.* 2005, pp. 165–166)

Initial findings from this and other studies suggest that parents are more likely to engage and remain involved with services that address their wider life concerns rather than simply their parenting. Few programmes, however, have successfully reached minority ethnic families or those who are most marginalised (Statham 2004, Foster 2005, Tunstill *et al.* 2005).

At the point at which all services for children are facing further major change in the context of *Every Child Matters* (DfES 2003b), evidence is emerging about the effectiveness of the systems and processes initiated by the Children Act 1989, the refocusing initiatives of the late 1990s, and the *Framework* (DoH *et al.* 2000e). The evidence is somewhat contradictory, however. On the one hand, it has been stated that the Children Act achieved its main aims (DoH 2001b, Thoburn 2001) whilst on the other, it has been argued that, far from achieving its objectives, the Children Act 1989 has failed in some significant areas. In particular, despite the rhetoric of partnership, the number of care orders and length of court proceedings have increased (McKeigue & Beckett 2004). There are similar conflicts in findings from a number of studies examining the impact of the 'refocusing' initiative and the *Framework* (DoH *et al.* 2000e). Some commentators (e.g. Cleaver & Walker 2004), albeit acknowledging a lack of objectivity because of their role in the development of the approach, claim that the involvement of parents and children in the assessment process has been strengthened. This has been largely supported by other small-scale studies (e.g. Spratt & Callan 2004, Platt 2004).

Other research, however, reveals a more equivocal response from parents (Dale 2004) in relation to their experiences of child protection processes. Nevertheless, all studies concur that where relationships were formed that family adults regarded as helpful (even if the outcome was not as they wished), the key factor was the style and skill of the practitioner. As mentioned earlier, this has been a consistent finding of studies on interventions and service-user satisfaction since the late 1960s, although there are as yet no studies on the perspectives of children involved in child protection processes, despite the increased emphasis on the rights of children and young people. As Holland and Scourfield (2004) point out:

We have gained some headway, we believe in listening to children who are looked after, but child protection investigation and assessment is still often an adult-to-adult affair. (p. 33)

Notwithstanding the support for family group conferences in guidance since the early 1990s, findings suggest that the approach remains on the margins of practice in the UK (Brown 2003), even though there is substantial evidence of their effectiveness elsewhere (Connolly 2006). What is not yet clear is how family support services and child protection interventions will integrate in a way that supports families to care for their own children without leaving them unprotected from significant harm.

Implications for professionals

The helping relationship

Research has therefore shown consistently that those at the receiving end of child protection interventions appreciate professionals' understanding of their point of view and honesty about the nature of the power relationship. This is crucially important in cases where there are serious concerns about a child's welfare, as the notion of sharing power with parents at this early stage may be unachievable. A consistent theme of many inquiries into cases where children have suffered significant harm, often resulting in death (DoH 1991a, Laming Report 2003, Social Work Inspection Agency 2005), has been the inability of workers to acknowledge and exercise their authority because partnership with parents sometimes became confused with avoiding conflict with family adults at all cost, in some cases because the workers were also fearful. Although there may sometimes be considerable conflict and resistance to intervention, it is always possible to acknowledge different family perspectives, to be honest about the power dynamics, and to ensure families can challenge State intervention, with the support of advocates when necessary. The focus must remain on the child and the child's welfare, however, and workers may need to exercise their authority in a way that precludes any power sharing with parents whilst being open and honest about this and, of course, open to challenge. It is also important to be aware that the interaction between service users and child protection professionals at this stage can have an important effect on work at later stages (Farmer & Owen 1995). It should be stressed that working openly and supportively in these early stages of intervention (particularly where serious abuse is involved) depends considerably on the strength of inter-professional effectiveness and communication.

There are some additional factors that are likely to affect how partnership in practice can be approached. When identifying family partners, it is important to be alert to power imbalances within the immediate family, particularly in situations involving domestic violence. Professionals may need, on occasion, to form an open, partisan partnership with one parent in order to safeguard the welfare of the child, rather than adopting an even-handed approach. In cases where it is clear who has abused the child, for example, the child's protection needs are often best served by working closely with the 'non-abusing' parent (but see Featherstone, Chapter 6, in this volume). It must be appreciated that in some situations, such as those involving serious intrafamilial sexual abuse, it cannot be assumed that the non-abusing parent (usually the mother) will immediately believe her child (Hooper 1992). This does not indicate a lack of care or concern in most cases but is rather an indicator of the degree of psychological stress experienced and highlights the need for careful therapeutic responses: there is a balance to be struck between minimising delay and allowing enough time for children and family adults to move past initial trauma. There are programmes for 'non-abusing' parents that integrate therapeutic interventions and partnership approaches with some degree of success (Hill 2005).

Since the Children Act 1989, children are increasingly placed in the care of relatives. In most cases such placements are beneficial (Broad 2001). However, the inspection into the lives of the children of Eilean Siar (Social Work Inspection Agency 2005), like the Tyra Henry inquiry many decades earlier (London Borough of Lambeth 1987), highlights the dangers of over-reliance on relatives without careful assessments. Nevertheless, it is essential that children's actual family relationships are acknowledged and that partnership work is not solely restricted to biological parents but also involves significant others: a sibling or grandparent may be the safest and most important person to a child, for example. Assumptions cannot be made about how many partners there will be, or even if there will be more than one partnership simultaneously or sequentially.

As outlined earlier, research shows that interventions are likely to have successful outcomes if parents are able to identify their own needs and how their needs and those of their children can best be met. This entails involving parents in the decision-making process. Although there was growing interest in family group conferences (FGC) based on the New Zealand model (Connolly 1994) in the 1990s (Marsh & Crow 1998), these have not commonly been used (Brown 2003). It has been suggested that one reason for this 'is the very procedural approach to dealing with children deemed to be at risk' (Brown 2003, p. 338) in the UK but a review of recent research suggests that FGCs have a good record in relation to child safety, even with most children remaining in their families of origin (Merkel-Holguin *et al.* 2003), and that families generally feel positive about involvement and subsequent plans. In the UK, however, families involved in FGCs tended to receive less support and resources than families involved in traditional case conferences and less than a quarter of promised resources are provided (Marsh & Crow 1998). This is perhaps indicative of the fact that, despite the rhetoric of partnership, family contributions to deciding how best to safeguard and promote their child's welfare are valued less than those of professionals. More thought must now be given to how children and young people subject to child protection interventions can be involved and heard in decision making. This is now perhaps the greatest challenge facing all professionals involved in child protection work.

Multi-agency working

The current radical overhaul of children's services is designed to ensure that safeguarding and promoting the welfare of children is accepted as a wider social responsibility and not just delegated to child protection social workers. Child abuse can be conceptualised as a spectrum: at one end are families in which there are situational harms to children that are unlikely to reoccur if stressors are removed; at the other are families involved with pathological cruelties from which children must be protected. The difficulty is that 'at the time these two kinds of families may not appear very differently from one another' (Bridge Child Care Consultancy Service 1991, p. 2). There is now a great deal of evidence about the aetiology of many forms of child harm (see Chapters 2–4 in this volume) and it is important that this knowledge is accessible to all those working with children. The previous preoccupation with risk assessments has, however, masked the importance of individual judgements:

> [D]espite increasing sophistication in the design and evaluation of risk assessment tools, the variables for assessing children in the contexts of their families are so complex that professional judgements underpinned by theory and research still remains the cornerstone of best practice.
>
> (DoH 2001b, p. 12)

Lead professionals may be establishing helping relationships and coordinating services for families where there are child protection concerns and, in effect, taking the lead role in partnership work; however, a child protection investigation may alter that relationship considerably, and for some time. Nevertheless, all those working with children need to be able to work honestly and openly with family adults, even if difficult issues arise. It is in everyone's interest to be clear about the abuse issues: children must be protected from harm; parents have rights to information so that they can, if they wish, challenge decisions; and professionals must be clear about their accountability, roles and tasks. Consequently, although it is important to ensure that professional identity and expertise are not devalued, ongoing *multiprofessional* child protection training must become a permanent feature of children's services.

There has been a tendency for senior managers, however, to become focused primarily on structural issues at the expense of human resource considerations at times of change (Laming Report 2003). Although there is no evidence that organisational structure *per se* has an impact on the quality of service provision (Axford & Little 2004), restructuring can seduce managers into believing that positive changes have been made. Each time child protection networks are disrupted, however, effective communication between professionals, and between professionals and families, is likely to be impaired. The quality of communication as outlined above is a consistent factor in determining both child protection outcomes and service-user satisfaction. Axford and Little (2004) point out that the most important organisational challenge is to ensure accurate and ongoing data collection of local need and a sufficiently flexible structure that enables services and approaches to be developed or discarded as needs arise or diminish. Indeed, it has recently been argued that quality child protection practice is as dependent on organisational effectiveness as it is on worker competence (Johnson & Petrie 2004, Munro 2005b). Adequate resources including numbers, experience and expertise of staff are critical. Effective management and the availability of appropriate supervision have also been found to be important.

Perhaps the most significant factor, however, is the organisational culture. Where this was characterised by communication pathways that flowed up, down and sideways and a 'no-blame' culture that enabled staff to share learning from the 'near-misses' as well as success stories, the number of unexpected disasters reduced (Johnson & Petrie 2004). Child protection work has been bedevilled by a 'naming and shaming' culture since the early 1970s and it may be that widening responsibility for safeguarding and promoting the welfare of children and a strengthened multiprofessional approach (DfES 2003b) may herald a change in climate. If this does not happen, there is a real danger that the reluctance of many professionals to remain in child protection work will lead to it becoming 'a second-class option for newly qualified and agency staff' (Holland & Scourfield 2004, p. 29). Effective partnerships with parents in child protection interventions are dependent on experienced practitioners and effective partnerships between agencies and professionals (see Luckock, Chapter 14, in this volume).

Summary

Partnership implies a sharing of power between those involved but the extent to which parents (and more recently children) are involved in decision making in child protection has fluctuated since the middle of the twentieth century as social attitudes about child welfare have changed. Research has shown consistently that involving parents secures better outcomes for children and that effective partnership work is dependent on the quality of the helping relationships. Children's services have been reconfigured on a multi-agency, multiprofessional basis to ensure that children are safeguarded and their welfare promoted. Current policies for 'children in need', including children at risk of significant harm, reflect elements of the 'universalism' of the welfare state and the targeting approach of welfare markets. These sometimes conflicting demands and societal expectations are critical factors when implementing partnership with parents in practice. Safeguarding and promoting the welfare of children through effective partnerships with parents depends on competent and confident professionals and organisational effectiveness. Particular attention must be given to preserving networks and communication pathways at a time of significant change and attracting and retaining experienced practitioners from all professions to child protection work.

Acknowledgement

The author wishes to acknowledge Adrian James' and Brian Corby's contributions to earlier editions of this chapter that have informed this revised version.

Key points and messages for practice

- Partnership implies a sharing of power between those involved yet this is not always possible in child protection work, especially in the early investigative stages.
- Involving parents secures better outcomes for children and effective partnership work is dependent on the quality of the helping relationships.
- Safeguarding and promoting the welfare of children through effective partnerships with parents depends on competent and confident professionals and organisational effectiveness.
- In the current context particular attention must be given to preserving networks and communication pathways at a time of significant change and attracting and retaining experienced practitioners from all professions to child protection work.

Annotated further reading

Beckett C 2006 Essential theory for social work practice. Sage, London
Although aimed at social workers, this text details practice theories for intervention including cognitive–behavioural and Rogerian approaches that are used by many other professionals. The theories are presented in ways that show how to maximise power sharing with those on the receiving end of interventions whilst recognising real constraints and ambiguities in the current welfare context.

Horwath J (ed) 2001 The child's world. Jessica Kingsley, London
This edited collection was issued to support the Framework for the Assessment of Children in Need and their Families *(DoH 2000e) and was based on training materials aimed at practitioners, managers and trainers. There are some useful 'how to' chapters on undertaking assessments in partnership with children and families, especially Shemming on how to empower those involved, Banks on working with minority ethnic groups and Marchant on assessing children with complex needs.*

Scott J, Ward H 2005 Safeguarding and promoting the well-being of children, families and communities. Jessica Kingsley, London
There are two particular strengths of this text: first, contributors come from the US and Canada as well as the UK which enables practitioners here to consider longstanding successful programmes and projects that have emerged in societies similar to our own; second, the concept of vulnerable children and families is considered in its widest sense. The focus is on effective interventions rather than policies and procedures.

Useful websites

All professionals should go to the websites for the Laming Report and *Every Child Matters* (listed with the references) and consider the implications for their own agencies/specialisms. In addition, the following websites offer some insight into the perspectives of children, young people and family adults, including those who have experienced professional interventions.
Children's Commissioner for England: www.childrenscommissioner.org
Children's Commissioner for Wales: www.childcom.org.uk/english
Family Rights Group: http://www.frg.org.uk/index.asp
Northern Ireland Commissioner for Children and Young People: www.niccy.org
Scotland's Commissioner for Children and Young People: www.cypcommissioner.org
Voices from Care Cymru: www.voicesfromcarecymru.org.uk/main.htm

Individual work with children

Margaret Crompton

INTRODUCTION

You are mistaken if you think we have to lower ourselves to communicate with children. On the contrary, we have to reach up to their feelings, stretch, stand on our tiptoes.

(Korczak 1925; in Lifton 1989, p. 172)

Attention to the 'wishes and feelings of children' in all decision making, as a requirement of the Children Act 1989, followed the findings of the Cleveland Inquiry (Butler-Sloss 1988) which had given a salutary reminder about the importance of treating children as people, not objects. Maintenance of 'that perspective of the child as client' requires development of 'skills in communicating directly and honestly with children, young people and adults, recognising the need to take time and not to compel ... clients to talk' was emphasised in the Guidance Notes for Diploma in Social Work courses (CCETSW 1991, p. 18).

Subsequent documents have restated principles of good practice fundamental to direct work with children and young people. The *Every Child Matters: Change for Children* strategy policy briefing, for example, refers to the Children Act 2004 and includes in the changes necessary to achieve the 'five outcomes ... which are the key to well-being' 'listening to children, young people/their families in planning provision' (TEN 2004, p. 3). The importance of cooperation between individual practitioners and agencies is stated and restated. As each new abuse disaster makes sensational news and stimulates yet another expensive court case, inquiry and report, followed by repetition of instructions to really attend to children, it is tempting to wonder how it is that practitioners seem to ignore what must be the basis of their work. Consultations undertaken in preparation for this revision demonstrates that, far from ignoring the need to work directly with children, many practitioners are focusing on and developing this practice, contributing to a long tradition. Practitioners need not to be instructed to work with children, but to receive training (initial and ongoing), recognition, respect, resources – including time and support. Fundamental is permission and encouragement to work directly with children. Those whom I consulted spoke particularly highly of the importance of meeting together.

The implications of regarding the child as a client and of direct, honest and unpressured interaction must form the base of any work with children, together with avoidance of labelling by symptom. Only attention to the whole, individual child by the whole, individual worker can lead to communication. Whatever the agency and context of the interaction, it is essential to respect children and to be clear about the purpose of contact for each child.

The Utting Report (Utting *et al.* 1997) found that 'Looking after [children living away from home] would be easier and much more effective if we really heard and understood what they have to tell us' (p. 7). Ensuring that children are heard and understood requires practitioners really to listen, and not to substitute mechanistic procedures (Smedley 1999, p. 114).

Di Ashton Dent, a nursery nurse in an NSPCC Family Centre, summarised thus:

> If you centre on the whole child she goes away from the sessions as a stronger person with increased confidence because she knows what's going on. If you centre totally on the abuse, on what actually happened, where is the rest of the child? You can give the child the impression that only the abuse is important.
>
> (Crompton 1980, p. 12)

Fifteen years after that interview, Di is a Children's Services Practitioner, still with the same agency, having achieved qualifications in social work (including the Advanced Award), non-directive play therapy and transactional analysis. Although she has studied and gained experience, her basic philosophy is unchanged. Her former colleague, Marian Taylor, is now manager of two innovatory Social Services Department Family Centres. Penny Turner, a senior family support worker, spoke of her passion for her work. Practitioners at a combined staff meeting discussed a wide range of communication methods and materials, and described their experience of working with children. The commitment, initiatives and positive, informed approach of all these practitioners more than balances the discouragement inherent in the highly publicised examples of poor practice and negatively critical reports that have beset children's services for so long.

There are many kinds of abuse and many reasons for referral. The observable scars of children who have been subject to physical abuse (including neglect and sexual assault) are accompanied by wounds to the emotions, mind and spirit. Children also suffer invisible assault, unaccompanied by visible clues but nonetheless desperately needing careful attention from adults. Physical and sexual abuse attract far more attention than cognitive, emotional and spiritual abuse.

The main focus of this chapter is an introduction to some ways of communicating with children, including an account of work with a 10-year-old boy. Although some material is drawn from texts focusing on work with children who have been referred to agencies because of observed abuse, the aim is to discuss work with children who have, as part of their whole experience of life, suffered abuse, as distinct from 'abused children'.

Emphasis is on straightforward, uncluttered, simple methods and approaches. Children and workers have neither time nor energy for elaboration and the most effective interactions are those in which child and adult meet, with minimal accessories, material or verbal. This is exemplified by the work of Madge Bray (cofounder of Sexual Abuse: Child Consultancy Service (SACCS)) who describes the essence of her approach as 'simplicity':

> It is based on a willingness to receive, at the child's own pace, whatever it is that the child wishes to impart. As the adult she listens, responds and sets the boundaries ... She sits on the floor with a toybox and creates an environment where play is the natural medium of communication.
>
> (Boyle 1997, p. x)

The chapter is organised in three sections:

1. Children and practitioners
2. Communication: time, space and contact; art; music; stories; drama; spiritual well-being
3. Being with Mark: work with a 10-year-old boy.

Children and practitioners

The idea of working with, and not only on behalf of, children is far from new. Kastell (1962), Winnicott (1964) and Holgate (1972) were among influential writers and teachers in the UK, while in the USA the texts of Axline and Oaklander were first published in 1947 and 1964, and 1969 (new edition in 1978), respectively. Practitioners in day, field and residential agencies understand the importance of play and the skills of listening, seeing, waiting and communicating. Stevenson (1991) emphasises the need for continuing efforts towards good practice, not least because of deficiencies in social work training which has lacked rigour and placed too little emphasis on 'knowledge and well-researched evidence ... Because a social work qualification is a licence to practise measurable standards should be set and adhered to' (p. 5). Decisions about individual work regarding philosophy, models of human development and intervention, and efficacy of such intervention, should be well-founded (CCETSW 1991, p. 10).

Initial and post-qualification training should be a respected specialisation, with academic and practical work on many aspects of childhood, including the history of politics and philosophy in the legislation of education, employment, religion, health and social welfare, together with the day-to-day culture of school, leisure, fashion, family and peer group. Students should spend time in playgrounds and discos and read teen magazines and children's literature (Crompton 1992, pp. 5–6). Study should include a range of models of development and behaviour, and of approaches to helping.

Ongoing in-service training is also essential. Lincolnshire Social Services Department, for example, has a training strategy for staff from all areas of the service which includes a core skills training plan for all staff, a training plan for services for looked-after children and family placement staff, and a training plan for children with disabilities teams and for residential staff. There is also in place a robust Lincolnshire Area Child Protection Committee Multi-agency Training Plan. The training plan reflects current legislation and government guidance, including *Every Child Matters* (DfES 2003b) recommendations, common core of skills and the Children Act 2004. The programme includes a 3-day course, 'Communicating with Children'. The core skills training is for staff across the children's services, including residential, fostering, adoption, domiciliary and other social care workers. The nine objectives include recognising why practitioners need to communicate with children; identifying processes that facilitate communication; practice skills/techniques in communicating with children; considering the needs of children who have experienced abuse, and of black or disabled children; considering motives for working with young people. Opportunities are provided for staff to undertake training in NVQ, BASW Distance Learning and post-qualification programmes. Barbara Simpson (Senior Training Officer) notes:

Training is progressive with staff completing the LACPC Foundation training in Child Protection. This then leads to clusters of other training. There is an ever changing agenda which we try to keep abreast of. However, we also continually re-visit core skills and social work principles to ensure we continue to work effectively and sensitively with children and their families.

Communicating with children requires professional rigour, including clear definition of the purpose and aims of every interaction. Stevenson's comment, 'Prompted in particular by concern about sexual abuse, social workers have rushed to observe children's play with little open discussion of the justification for the inferences drawn' (1991, p. 6), illustrates the confusion of undertaking action without a sound philosophical grounding.

The decision to offer helping interaction to an individual child requires careful thought, understanding of what such interaction might entail, and commitment by both worker and agency, before the offer is made. O'Hagan (1989) is anxious that focusing on the individual may 'exacerbate the crisis generated by the disclosure' (p. 116) and Furniss (1991) points out that seeing children individually is not automatically synonymous with individual counselling or therapy. Disciplined definition is required, with an understanding of possible difficulties for workers (Stone 1990).

Moore (1992), whose down-to-earth chapter 'Face-to-face work with the abused child' emphasises that 'An abused child has the right to be the primary client, to be facilitated in a face-to-face way, to make sense of what has happened', advises practitioners to offer children 'warm, friendly, personal help' and 'reassurance that they are understood and respected' (pp. 127, 130–131).

It is essential to recognise the whole person in the real world, where the 'actual situation' and the problems of life have to be met again and again. The most important aim is to develop strength with which to face and manage challenges and suffering.

Glaser and Frosh (1988) note that individual work may accompany, replace or succeed time-limited group experience and comprise contact with 'a professional, usually their social worker, teacher or counsellor' (p. 146). Decisions about what kind of help can be offered depend not only on an assessment of what should be available, but also of agency resources, and may be quite arbitrary. Workers should be clear about constraints.

The purpose of providing opportunities for communication directly between children and professionally caring adults may be simply defined as *assessment* and *help*. It is important to be clear about the primary purpose of interaction, particularly when considering such communicative activities as those reviewed in the second part of this chapter. *Assessment* includes, for example, all activities leading to writing reports, making recommendations to courts and planning for future accommodation. Tasks include gathering information, communicating to children information about possibilities and constraints, learning about feelings, perceptions, preferences and plans. *Help* comprises provision of an environment conducive to developing self-awareness, confidence, self-esteem and the ability to trust wisely, to make realistic plans and decisions, and to form relationships that contribute to the well-being of all involved. Tasks include helping children to recognise and manage external realities (past events, present accommodation, future relationships) and inward experiences (memories, perceptions, feelings), and to cooperate in forming realistic plans. The implications of such concepts as self-esteem need analysis (see Roberts 1993). Trust, too, should be carefully considered (Crompton 1990).

Another word used frequently and loosely is 'therapy'. It is not always clear whether practitioners and authors associate 'therapy/therapist' with their original connotations of disease and healing. More important is the need to be clear about the distinction between 'therapeutically informed intervention' by social workers and long-term therapeutic work which requires more specialist skills. Therapy within social work interactions should not be confused with psychotherapy (Glaser & Frosh 1988). A distinction should also be made between this and such specialisations as art, drama, music and play therapies. Wilson *et al.* (1992) differentiate between 'the use of play in play therapy and in activities … which are used by an adult to explain, clarify, prepare or for other purposes work on an area which the adult has identified as one of concern', defined as 'play-related communication' (p. 13).

Professional rigour requires semantic and conceptual precision. If individual, group or family-based help is available, the reason for choosing one approach rather than another should be clear. The exclusive attention of one adult offers the best chance of a peaceful, private and relaxed period, away from the immediate pressures of family relationships or identification in a group with a label, and the child can use this kind of interaction freely.

Workers' principal skills must be *really* to *see* and to *listen*. This necessitates leaving all fears and assumptions behind and endeavouring to engage with the world of the child, both internal and external. Smedley (1999) considers that 'We will not reach children unless we can convey to them our openness to understanding their deep hurt, and we cannot do this if we deny our own pain' (p. 114). Moore (1992) advises: 'Communication is a reciprocal giving and receiving of thoughts and feelings. The worker's body posture and tone of voice must convey empathy and understanding' (p. 132). Mearns and Thorne (1988), following the Rogers person-centred model (Rogers 1951), define *empathy* as 'a continuing process whereby the counsellor lays aside her own way of experiencing and perceiving reality, preferring to sense and respond to the experiences and perceptions of her client' (p. 39). *Empathy* is a popular and overused word. The concept is useful but should be approached with care. It is easy, for example, to confuse it with sympathy or with recognition of a similar experience in the worker's own life, or to become dangerously immersed in the child's feelings (see also Crompton 1992).

Adam, for example, felt so much pain, hopelessness and fear during a session that he 'stood up, wanting to throw himself through the window to the conservatory glass roof beneath'. The practitioner 'felt his fear and reflected this. I stayed seated, and quietly talked to him about how I wanted him to be safe'. Adam could later give clear advice about interviewing someone who was suicidal, including, 'you listen to him, try to do what he says, do your best. If you can't do it, explain why ... make sure he's safe ... remember the kid is scared, nervous' (Smedley 1999, p. 122).

Failure really to attend to children may lead to serious consequences. Di (NSPCC Children's Services Practitioner) worked with 15-year-old 'Imogen' whose many problems included learning difficulties and neglect. When Imogen alleged that she had been sexually abused by a family member, the court case was dismissed because her assertion that the assault had occurred on a Sunday was apparently nullified by a witness testifying that the girl had been seen wearing school uniform on the day which, it was reasoned, could therefore not have been a Sunday. However, when Di later asked 'what was Sunday about it?' Imogen explained that her mother had been at home and prepared a meal which was eaten by the whole family together. Since in Imogen's experience this happened only on Sunday, '*Sunday*' described the day. But on the weekday in question, her mother had unusually been at home. As Imogen had no concept of time, '*Sunday*' was associated with events, not dates.

An important element of individual work with children is providing opportunities to relax, escape for a while from the pain, hopelessness and fear described by Adam, and from other pressures and anxieties. A Family Centre Support Worker bought a kite for children whose lives contained great and constant stress; worker and children ran around, laughing together. The relaxing, energetic activity gave the children permission to have fun when they could 'be who they really were in that moment'. At their request, he gave the children the kite which they valued and looked after.

The endeavour to engage so intimately with children's inner lives carries with it the danger of intruding on their privacy. Care should be taken to avoid 'pressing the bruise' or expecting too much response (if any). Even when respecting the right not to speak, it is easy to stimulate thoughts and feelings that are difficult and painful and that continue to have an impact long after the end of immediate contact between child and worker (Crompton 1991).

Children often give clues that they do not wish to pursue a particular line or activity: moving to another toy, running around, changing the conversation. This is in itself a form of communication. Workers should notice the triggers to withdrawal and judge whether the reaction is to the particular topic or activity, perhaps associated with some memory, or to a communication by the worker.

Pressing too hard for overt responses may lead to distortion, even lying. Conversely, apparent failure to respond may mask unexpressed internal activity or alterations of behaviour elsewhere. Dorfman (1951) writes of an aggressive and abusing 13-year-old boy who spent most of his regular and protected hour ignoring her. After 10 sessions, he was told that although the hour was saved for him, he need not continue to attend. His response was, 'Whaddya mean, not come any more? I'll come till the cows come home!' His behaviour outside the worker's room had greatly improved. Only to the worker did he give no overt hint of the positive use to which he put the unpressured hour with her (pp. 244–245).

Respect for *privacy* and non-intrusion is essential but Doyle (1990) notes that avoidance of discussing abusive activities may result from the inability of adults to tolerate children's pain. Interviews may remain superficial and 'the child left feeling that he or she has been involved in something so dreadful that it cannot be discussed. Children should be allowed to talk about the abuse and examine what it has meant for them' (p. 34). Only real attention to individual children, including *waiting* for their own timing, enables them to respond as they wish.

An aspect of privacy demanding special care is *confidentiality*, which cannot be guaranteed, perhaps because a worker fears that the child client, or other children, may be in danger. Some authorities suggest that confidentiality may represent a potential danger, mirroring the secrecy that characterises child sexual abuse cases (Glaser & Frosh 1988). It is most important to give children clear information about limits to confidentiality, including, for example, whether any other staff member knows about interactions between child and worker and, if the worker should be unavailable at any time or leave the agency, whether colleagues know about the child's situation, feelings and attitudes. Such clarity can offer good experiences of honesty and plain dealing by the worker, and opportunities to exercise choice and control about speaking and keeping silent.

Danger, or at least confusion, may be represented by the physical privacy of one-to-one work for children whose experience of private engagements with adults has entailed abuse. Some writers suggest that workers risk seductive behaviour and allegations of abuse by children.

Nonetheless, common sense, good training, professional discipline and efficient agency organisation should ensure that such problems, confusions and dangers are prevented, and that every child for whom it is appropriate has the opportunity for individual, protected, private contact with a worker.

Smedley (1999), discussing transcripts of interviews with children, 'found the same message for social workers … in all stages of child protection work', articulated by Lisa: 'Social workers should try to understand what children are really trying to say, explain any questions the children have, and if they feel left out they should be made to feel important, wanted and loved'. Adam praised his satisfactorily listening social worker – 'I've got big shields around me now' (pp. 117, 118).

Communication

This discussion is necessarily selective and brief. No reference is made to such electronic aids as videos and computers, and the main focus is on work with the minimal material facilities usually available to workers, including drawing and writing equipment, books and a car. The most important constituents of communication are the individual people concerned, within time and space dedicated to the child. Direct work is not confined to any one agency or specialisation. Indeed, cooperation within and between both agencies and individual practitioners is essential to ensure the highest quality of service to children and families, and maximum use of resources. Examples in this chapter are offered as models, not representative of the whole range of practice, and are intended to stimulate readers to develop their own ideas and practice.

Choice of activity and equipment is negotiated between child and worker, having regard to both preferences and explained, understandable constraints. For example, when working with a 10-year-old boy, without access to any room, my age and abilities precluded football or swimming but we were able to share simple art work and walking. Equipment was kept in a carrying box which I took to every meeting and gave him at the end of our contact. Shelter was provided by a café and my car. Cooperation in developing an activity may help to increase self-confidence and, thus, strength in managing everyday life.

Although some reference is made to 'therapy', examples illustrate activities which may be undertaken by non-specialist (but trained) workers. For example, a chapter on play therapy follows but there are innumerable ways in which play, interpreted very broadly, can be used as both a vehicle and an environment for communication by non-specialist practitioners.

Bannister is one of many writers to stress that workers should not seek to interpret the process and/or product of children's creative activity, for not only may such interpretation 'be incorrect or irrelevant' but also, most importantly, 'the child has expressed feeling and, may be, found a solution' (1989, p. 84; see also Oaklander 1978, Crompton 1992, West 1996).

Although 'face-to-face with children' is sometimes used of direct work, play activities essentially provide opportunities for interaction without being face-to-face, so that eye contact need not be sought or forced, and verbal conversation may play only a small role.

Agencies sometimes produce packs of ideas for play activities. However, such material can be useful only as a reference base to stimulate creative development by individual practitioners and children. Family Centre staff recommended worksheets from several sources (see Annotated further reading).

Time, space and contact

A satisfactory physical and psychic environment, including safety and privacy, is essential. Whether meetings take place in playrooms or cafés, hospital wards or cars, workers are themselves part of the environment. For example, clothes should be appropriate for sitting on the floor, painting or walking. It is important not to insult children by dressing in a slovenly fashion: dress should reflect care and respect. It may even be possible to avoid wearing colours which are known to be particularly disliked by an individual child.

Anxiety about laddering tights or creasing trousers may be regarded by children as anxiety about being with them, for workers' feelings also contribute to the environment of the interaction. If adults are exhausted, anxious, unhappy, angry, depressed or ill, energy available for the children is limited and they may sense the emotionally charged or depleted atmosphere. Similarly, if adults are fit and fully able to concentrate on the children, the emotional environment will be clearer and more spacious.

Workers with abused children may communicate their feelings about the abuse too; for example, anger towards the abusers, horror about the events and sympathy with the children. It may at times be preferable to postpone a contact than to expose a child to the worker's feelings.

Yet postponement itself can be perceived as rejection or evidence of the child's lack of worth. Meticulous courtesy and attention to punctuality and reliability are essential aspects of the total environment and the messages given and received. Children should not be kept waiting or let down because 'something has come up'. Khadija Rouf (1989) writes that she:

> got a social worker, Sue. She was okay but because our family had gone past crisis point she never came round. That is to do with big caseloads, I know, but we did *all* need someone to talk to … [Workers should] remember that a lot of children are on their own. Don't let them down. If you arrange to go out, then go out. If you say you'll be in court, then for God's sake be there. Abused children have been let down enough. (pp. 9–10)

Attention should be given to the duration of interactions. Respect for the whole child includes recognition that life continues outside the playroom. The child may have other appointments, friends waiting or a favourite television show which will be missed if workers do not honour agreed stopping as well as starting times.

Enthusiastic work with a boy led to extended hours spent in the sitting room of the foster home. In one case, belated recognition that this delayed teatime and kept the family from the television led to better discipline and timekeeping by the worker. Beginnings and endings of not only individual sessions but also the entire period of contact are especially important (Crompton 1990).

Contacts should never be interrupted by telephone calls or enquiries from colleagues. Discussions with the agency director or court appearances would not be interrupted for the worker to take a message. Working with children requires concentration and continuity.

The physical environment is in itself a form of communication, indicating to children attention to their welfare. Some agencies provide well-stocked playrooms where workers may ensure a period of uninterrupted ownership of protected space. Many workers create defended space, for example, in 'empty broom-closets and in the back of gymnasiums' (Shapiro 1984, p. v).

It may help children's sense of being individual and cared-about if workers keep their materials in separate, particular bags, indicating that they are not just other 'cases'. Attention to materials is important; for example, folders used for life story books could be chosen in the child's favourite colours. Shopping together is not always possible, so care shown by a worker in demonstrating choice on behalf of the child is beneficial.

A personal set of coloured pencils, which only the child has a right to use or not to use, may offer some sense of control. If the favourite colours are constantly used, while others are neglected, children can see how their own choices affect the world, even in the form of only one coloured pencil. No other child is interfering and workers can protect this aspect of the child's environment by keeping the containers and equipment themselves and bringing them, regularly and intact, to appointments, thus indicating that the individual child is remembered and respected during the intervals between contacts. Similarly, children may keep their own equipment. This offers opportunities for them to demonstrate control and the ability to protect important possessions. The equipment can become a symbol of the continuity and reliability of contacts with workers.

Protecting and respecting material property that children share with workers indicates respect for, instead of abuse of, children. It helps to establish wise trust and encourages children to feel that, through those material extensions of themselves, they have worth.

Much important communication occurs indirectly through such aspects of everyday life as clothing and food (Crompton 1990). Respect for a child's personal preferences and cultural traditions (e.g. dietary and clothing requirements) is essential and lack of such respect can be a form of abuse (Ahmed *et al.* 1986, Gardner 1987, Crompton 1998).

A nurse, for example, expressed exasperation that she was expected to obtain a special meal for a Muslim baby whose religion forbade her to eat pork. The nurse considered it to be acceptable to feed the child pork because, 'since the food was mashed up, the parents would not know what she had eaten, and the baby would certainly be unaware of the contents of her dinner' (Crompton 1998, p. 163).

Kenward (1989) illustrates the powerful symbolism of food for Anna (8 years old): the availability of food had 'been dependent upon her being sexually cooperative'. When her foster mother offered her food, Anna said: 'I'm hungry and I want it. I can't make my hand take it.' The foster family helped, partly by giving Anna control of serving food. Offering, receiving and sharing food can provide opportunities for children to exercise choice and control, and to experience ordinary routines of social interaction (see also Crompton 1990, Chapter 10).

Anxiety can be raised in a child who feels unable to conform to adult expectations of everyday behaviour. Kenward (1989) quotes John (11 years old) following a visit to new foster parents: 'I liked them very much but they didn't know how I am inside … I don't know what they want me to do or how to do it and I'm afraid in case I make them angry and they hurt me' (p. 32). Such clear expression of inner confusion is rare and illuminating.

Whatever the physical environment and activity, workers themselves define the immediate environment. On a walk, for example, the adult provides a boundary within which the child may choose the path, the speed, whether to stop and look down a rabbit hole or run across a field, leaving the worker behind. The child's freedom is safely within the context of the contact with the worker. Such freedom is not abandonment or lack of caring and boundaries are not arbitrary obstacles. Workers are the providers of space, time and interest. They set limits and ensure that doors are safely closed, so that there will be no interruptions. The environment must be non-threatening and safe, offering opportunities for choice, control, stimulus and peace.

Art

Workers do not have to be skilled artists to share artistic activity with children. Inadequacy may even be helpful if a child can discover and demonstrate greater competence than an adult, perhaps taking the superior role of teacher. Simple, cheap materials are easily transported for spontaneous use. Drawing, painting and modelling provide opportunities for absorbing and relaxing activity. Children who have been subject to the stresses of abuse and investigation may find respite in a holiday from words, within space and time provided by a non-pressurising adult. Clues about feelings may be implied through choice of subject, colour, materials, use of space, concentration and response to making a mess, and it is interesting to note what is done with the product. For example, a picture may be given to the worker, taken home to a parent, treasured or destroyed.

Materials need not be used for obviously creative purposes. A nursery nurse noted that a 5-year-old used clay to dunk in a bowl of water, saying, 'I'm drowning the clay', soon after her sister had been accidentally drowned in her presence (Crompton 1990, p. 42).

Sharing artistic activity may help to relieve tension; for example, when awaiting a court appearance or on a journey.

Drawing may be included in making life story books with children. An artistically unskilled worker may manage at least matchstick people or may be able to draw simple outlines to be coloured in, at will, by the child, or the child may draw all the pictures. Shapes of houses, people, animals, cars and so on can easily be cut from sheets of coloured paper and stuck onto paper or card. Very young children can be fully involved in choosing colours, gumming, choosing the position for shapes, and older children can also draw and cut. Pictures can be cut from magazines but young children may not appreciate the difference between photographs of models and of themselves: an attempt to teach a young boy about his life as a baby, using a photograph from an advertisement, led to confusion as he thought the picture was of himself.

Working with a bereaved child, a Family Centre Worker used playdough as a 'stress buster', to emerge from the deep places of the centre of the session to achieve a relaxed ending. Practitioner and child rolled the dough out on a table, both enjoying the shared physical activity and fun.

A colleague, working with 'Gill' (10 years old) who had been sexually abused, started making a tree with sturdy trunk and roots going into the ground; Gill said 'the trunk looks like me, upright, not bending' and also wrote a fairy tale about herself.

Another found that *The Huge Bag of Worries* helped 'Kelly', an adolescent girl with learning difficulties and poor attention span, who had, it was thought, been sexually abused. The materials were used during meetings over 6 weeks; Kelly could relate pictures to her own life and worries, and encouraged her to draw herself and her own house, for example (Ironside 1999). Another practitioner noted the paucity of appropriate materials designed for children with learning difficulties.

These practitioners emphasised the importance of finding the right 'key' by attending to the clues children give.

Ross (teacher and art therapist) associates 'an art therapy approach' with developing children's self-esteem. She appreciates that: 'Many people feel unconfident about their art ability. Cutting out magazines to make pictures (collages) can be a great "leveller" and encourage even very unconfident children to join in.' Working with a variety of materials can aid expression of a range of emotions and 'the act of manipulating clay or smearing pastels or brushing paint … can be a healing experience'. She notes that 'children are the "experts" of their own images' and warns that their 'privacy needs to be safeguarded. No child should ever be encouraged to reveal more than they do of their own accord. It must be left to each individual to decide at what level they wish to enter into the activity' (1997, pp. 17–18, 14).

Allan (1988), Bannister (1989), Jones (1992) and Hagood (2001) discuss drawing by children who have been sexually abused, including illustrations (pictorial and narrative) and analysis of method.

Music

Music may be overlooked as a communicative activity, especially when workers are shy about their own abilities. Musical instruments may be too large to transport but equipment in playrooms and residential units could include percussion, piano or keyboard, recorders and guitars, and a cassette/record player. Many cars are equipped with radios and cassette players.

Music may contribute to the total communicative environment; for example, children or workers may choose some recorded music to accompany an activity. Workers should be aware of the impact of such choices. A child might use a very noisy CD to overwhelm or distract the worker, or might respond with distress to the worker's choice of some melody intended to be calming. A piece of music or a sound may have important resonances which stir memories (possibly disturbing). A child who has suffered abuse may respond with anxiety to a record which was popular during the period of abuse or a favourite of the abuser, or even played during sexual or violent episodes and/or assaults on the emotions and spirit. Choice of background music offers children some control and a ground for negotiation about duration and volume.

Children may like to play instruments alone, perhaps finding relief and release in pounding a drum or piano, or finding relaxation in devising apparently formless, meditative melodies. The presence of the worker is important, protecting space, time and activity, and demonstrating acceptance and attention.

Playing an instrument or singing may be shared by child and worker and can bring relaxation and enjoyment, also providing opportunities for children to demonstrate abilities which can attract praise and encouragement for further development, invaluable when self-respect has been demolished.

Listening to music together can demonstrate the worker's ability to attend to the child, without pressure on the child to buy that attention with words (answering questions, offering revelations) or actions (collusion in abusive acts).

Words may be included in the form of songs, composed by the child or in the form of recorded or sung music, offering a clue to the child's feelings. Laurel, after confinement in a secure unit for unruly behaviour, chose to play again and again a record with words of loss and bewilderment. She did not seek to converse with the quietly attentive adult but recognition of the presence of that adult suggested that the choice of record was made partly in order to express something about herself (Crompton 1992).

Dance offers opportunities for relaxation, expression of feeling, concentration on the music or shared enjoyment and a break from the need for speech. Further discussion of music may be found in Crompton (1980, Chapter 6; 1992, Chapter 10) and Oldfield in Milner and Carolin (1999, pp. 188–199).

Stories

Telling a story can provide an environment of comfort, particularly if the child can be cuddled. The child, too, may be the storyteller. Luke (6 years old) would lie on the settee in his foster home. While not very articulate, at these times he would tell a story about a recent experience, the words tumbling out with great feeling as he relaxed. When these stories were carefully written out, his rapidly spoken words and lively tales helped Luke gain a sense of himself existing in some relationship to the past, present and future. Also, he learned that the stories were of enough value for an adult to listen, write out between sessions and return to him. Joint illustrations used matchstick figures and outlines which Luke could colour in, as well as his own drawings (Crompton 1992).

Bray includes the whole of 'Jessica's Story', beginning, as all good stories do, 'Once upon a time …'. She sets the scene for writing the story, sitting with Jessica on her knee. (Practitioners need to be clear about agency policy regarding touching and holding children.)

Jessica says:

'Do you want to write? Do you like to write me a story?'
'Yes, I do.'
'But how will you know it's me?'
'I'll try to get it as close as I can.'
Jessica nodded pensively.
'I don't cry, do I, Madge? Will I cry in my story? I haven't cried, ever.'
'No, then probably you won't cry in your story.'

(Bray 1997, p. 168; the story is on pp. 169–184)

Bray concludes: 'I have often written stories for children which paralleled their own life experience in order to help them make sense of distortion in their lives' (p. 184).

While life story books have many uses, it is important to guard against, for example, imposing a boring and unimaginative activity; making such a book is a creative adventure, shared by child and practitioner. However, crucially, the eventual story, in whatever form, belongs to the child; practitioners should beware of becoming attached to such products. Crompton discusses communication through both life stories and other forms of narrative (1980, 1992). Oaklander (1978) includes sections on writing, poetry and books. Allan (1988) describes serial story writing with a physically abused adolescent (pp. 199–211).

Printed books may be useful as aids to communication but, as with any pre-packaged material, there are difficulties. Non-fiction books about feelings or experiences may be dull and/or confusing. Reading a story about experiences similar to the child's own may be reassuring, demonstrating that the child is not unique and that feelings about such experiences are known to other people. However, published stories usually have neat plots and endings, whereas real experience is continuing and complex. Adults should not expect 'identification' with fictional characters.

The most influential books are usually those chosen by the individual child and it is useful to be aware of children's favourite and least favourite texts. Responses may be very different from those expected by adults. As a child, I avoided looking at illustrations of a menacing genie, an exploding witch and a little naked boy floating down a stream alone. These represented terrifying power and powerlessness to the child but to adults they were only illustrations of charming stories.

Published material may most usefully form an aid to relaxation and to learning about ways of managing challenges However, a programme of planned and guided reading may be devised, aiming to give support and modify behaviour, and known as *bibliotherapy*. Bibliographies of focused texts are sometimes produced by libraries.

Particularly interesting and potent aspects of story telling are found in myths, legends and fairy tales. Apparently simple stories may hold different meanings for different individuals. Leroy, an 8-year-old black American gleefully told me about 'Missy Red Riding Hood', wagging an admonitory finger. Polish students found the message of that story and of *Snow White* to be that they should not trust people. Yet for Julia (8 years old) who had suffered from severe neglect by her mother, 'Snow White provided an opportunity to enact the part of the wicked (step)mother, "Only in this story, she doesn't win", Snow White is queen' (Hunter 1987, p. 28). *Rapunzel* represented comfort and security to an American 5-year-old when he learnt that his grandmother, who often cared for him, was to enter hospital. Bettelheim (1976) suggests that he learnt, 'That one's own body can provide a lifeline', just as Rapunzel's hair was used as a ladder: 'if necessary, he would find in his own body the source of his security' (p. 17). A girl who had problems with body images was helped through *The Ugly Duckling* (Bannister 1989).

Janusz Korczak regularly told the children in his orphanage (many of whom had been abused by physical and/or emotional assault or neglect and, in pre-war Warsaw, were certainly socially abused and religiously oppressed) such old tales as *Puss in Boots*. He considered that, 'children who feel worthless in a society that doesn't value them, who feel angry and powerless because their parents ... can no longer protect them, need to believe that there are magic forces that can help them overcome their difficulties'. (Nazi occupation is far from being the only condition necessary for children to feel unvalued, angry and powerless.) Such traditional tales, full of difficulties and obstacles requiring perseverance and strength of will, were 'close to life' (Lifton 1989, p. 74). (Further discussion of myths and stories may be found in Crompton 1992, Chapter 7; Crompton 1998, Chapter 15.)

Narratives may recount an imagined story, remembered 'real' experience or a combination – a dream. Mallon (2002) quotes Linda (10 years old) who had recurrent nightmares from the age of five: 'There is a man, a devil, taking me away. Then there are people coming after me to kill me.' Linda's current dreams are also terrifying: 'There is man and a lady. I was crying. Catapulted into a lady's garden. Then a man is chasing me. He chopped me up.' At five, Linda had been sexually abused by a stranger, subsequently imprisoned. Mallon advises: 'Sometimes our dreams are far wiser than we know' and encourages practitioners to listen to children's accounts of their dreams (pp. 83, 60).

Allanson (a sculptor and play therapist with experience from Family Service Units and the NSPCC) describes the narratives of Lisa, an 18-year-old girl with learning difficulties who had suffered sexual abuse by her stepfather, rejection and disbelief by her mother, and subsequent sexual and racist abuse from foster carers:

Stories provided her with the dramatic distancing that fiction can provide and enabled her to describe tragedy, abandonment, love and sometimes resolution. She interwove elements of her own life story with the stories she told.

I cannot remember how she came to tell her first story, just the excitement as the words came flowing out of her mouth, the mouth of a woman who had been labelled as learning disabled throughout her education. She started to illustrate her stories with small pencil drawings and the stories just continued to flow.

(Allanson 2002, p. 59)

Cattanach (2001) comments that stories told by both children and adults are:

not often direct narrations of life events but concern imaginary lives. These imaginative stories contain similar life changes to the reality worlds of children and adults. Complex life events cannot always be understood through talking about what happened in reality talk, because the full impact can only be described and contained through metaphor, imagery, myth and story, or sometimes play without words. (p. 8)

Drama

Drama (including role play) is perhaps one of the most difficult and potentially dangerous methods and should not be used without consultation. The feelings and memories stimulated may have repercussions for both child and worker. For example, the experience of wielding power when playing a role may be frightening for a powerless child, and new ideas about family relationships may be stimulated but not expressed, leaving a child in a state of bewilderment.

Bannister (drama therapist, psychodramatist and social worker), writing of work with sexually abused children, describes how Michelle (7 years old) whose father had died, revealed that he had sexually abused her. Through acting based on *The Lion, the Witch and the Wardrobe* (Lewis 1950), she began to gain strength and autonomy. She took the parts of, first, a child who rescues the Lion, and then the Witch, 'a very powerful person who had control over everyone'. After this, she could take the role with which she really identified – the Lion, whom she played as 'strong and brave and able to help others'. When his friends had rescued him, 'they thanked him for allowing himself to be caught because this protected them' and they 'admired Michelle's strength and power and also her kindness. The Witch was dead so the Lion dug a hole and buried her. Michelle's healing had begun' (Bannister 1989, p. 94; see also Bannister 1998).

This recalls the *Snow White* theme explored by Julia with psychotherapist Margaret Hunter. Julia could explore aspects of her feelings and history by enacting roles from the story, including that of the stepmother (Hunter 1987).

A toy may provide a third ear and voice through which child and worker may communicate. May (6 years old) wanted to name a large glove puppet 'May' but was dissuaded by her social worker, who felt that three-way conversations in which two participants had the same name would be confusing. May then chose her own second name and the puppet became 'Jessie'. Jessie became a regular participant in conversations, was always physically, even if silently, present, and at times behaved in such ways that May accused her of being naughty and put her outside the door. The worker sometimes felt in danger of losing control and noted, 'don't let materials run away with you – I felt the glove puppet begin to take me over, began to lose focus on the child and to enjoy the game too much' (Crompton 1990, p. 97).

A nursery nurse, Elaine, also recorded that role-playing interaction was difficult and disturbing. Selma (6 years old) attended a voluntary agency weekly, with the aim of learning strategies for coping with her bizarre and neglecting mother. Although doing well at school and in good physical health, Selma appeared to be emotionally abused. During the fourth session, she began to act as mother to a doll and Elaine took the role of Selma, who then 'became' her own mother. They walked to a pile of teddies at one end of the playroom:

Selma/mother had been very aggressive but now she changed her whole voice and manner and asked Elaine/Selma 'Would you like a present?' in a very soft stroking way. She gave Elaine/Selma all the teddies, then took her to the other end of the room to give another, enormous bear. Elaine/Selma said, 'I can't carry it'. Selma/mother immediately became annoyed: 'You will have it. I've bought it for you.'

Elaine/Selma found the difficulty was in coping with the 'gentle mum'. She felt frightened and puzzled: 'What have I done that's made her nice?' She waited for aggression to return, to be punished for the Selma/mother's being 'nice'.

Selma did not want to leave the role of mother and had enjoyed the power and control. Both she and Elaine 'needed a great deal of debriefing and cuddling'. Elaine wondered whether it had been a good idea to give her that taste of control, and she was also aware that 'Selma had let Elaine in on her world and feelings but then had to go home again to all the real stresses' (Crompton 1990, pp. 12–13). Elaine was well supported by a colleague with whom she could share such anxieties. Such work should not be undertaken unless consultation is available. (See also Ryan and Wilson (2000a), who describe the way in which a young girl, Diane, devises during therapy a series of role plays to explore her difficult experiences with her birth family. They include a section on practice issues in responding to these spontaneous role plays.)

Spiritual well-being and communication

An important element of communicating with children who are in any way associated with abuse (including as perpetrators) is attention to spiritual well-being. This may be associated with religious beliefs and observances. However, for many other people who are not adherents of any religious tradition, the concept of the whole person comprises not only body, mind and emotions but also spirit. It is therefore essential to recognise the importance of spiritual and/or religious elements of children's lives and experiences.

In order to communicate effectively, practitioners need to be clear about, and respect, both their own and other people's concepts and beliefs. These notes briefly introduce some aspects of a practice focus which is developing both within the UK and internationally and about which a number of texts are available.

Article 27 of the UN Convention on the Rights of the Child (Office of the High Commissioner for Human Rights 1989) establishes 'the right of every child to a standard of living adequate for the child's physical, mental, spiritual, moral and social development'. Neglect and abuse are inimical to ensuring adequacy in every aspect of children's standard of living. Smedley (1999) considers that a frequent consequence of abuse is impairment of children's cognitive, emotional and spiritual development (p. 114).

Crompton (1998) devotes a substantial section of *Children, Spirituality, Religion and Social Work* to discussion of 'Spirituality, religion, abuse and neglect', including material on 'Abuse associated with religious and ritual practices' (pp. 139–178). She considers that all abuse includes abuse of the spirit, however this is defined. An NSPCC practitioner, for example, suggested that 'the spirit can be abused if ... children are constantly "put down", their fantasies rejected or adults are intent on making them pliable and obedient'. She visualised the body language of children who have been abused as 'dragged down, slumping, exuberance crushed' (p. 144).

Abuse, and thus impairment of spiritual well-being, may sometimes be directly associated with religious beliefs and observances. For example, if children are:

- compelled to engage in religious practices which they have not chosen
- deprived of freedom and encouragement to worship according to their chosen religions (including fasts and festivals)
- oppressed, bullied and persecuted because of association with religion
- sexually abused within the context of a religious organisation (e.g. by a priest) (Crompton 2001, pp. 67–80).

At the time of writing, concern is expressed about children apparently illegally brought from Africa for involvement in religious rituals; it is thought that some have been assaulted, even killed. There are also investigations into allegations that some children are regarded as being witches and/or possessed by demons. While this matter cannot be discussed here, practitioners need to be alert to, and informed about, beliefs and practices which may entail harm to children.

Language associated with religious belief may be confusing and distressing. 'Religious language often depends on a positive view of the value and trust placed in fathers, parents and family ... which may have an effect on the child's spiritual life.' For example, if the deity is represented as a father, yet the child's own father commits incest or other forms of abuse, the concept of a divine father is fraught with problems. If the physical father commits abuse, may not the divine father similarly bring harm? Or, why has the divine father failed to protect the child? 'The child may be frightened to acknowledge these feelings but may need help in understanding the role of such language' (Armstrong 1991, pp. 20–21; Crompton 2001, pp. 68–69).

Anxiety about or hostility towards religious beliefs and affiliations can hinder communication between practitioners and children. Kate, a social worker and

Christian, was with a colleague when a girl told them that she had become a Christian. The colleague later confided: 'I'm glad you were there – I wouldn't have known how to respond.' Since practitioners must constantly be prepared to respond appropriately to information about appalling and distressing experiences, how is it more difficult to 'know how to respond' to material about religious belief and spiritual well-being? (Crompton 1998, p. 152).

The Barnardo's publication *Who am I?* (Crompton 2001) includes in Section 4 'Nurturing spiritual well-being in practice', a Unit on 'Children who have been abused or neglected'. Among questions for practitioners are:

- Are any children you know crushed' or 'dis-spirited'? How is this shown, for example, in body language, withdrawal, lack of energy?
- How can children whose spiritual well-being has been impaired be helped to regain health and wholeness? (Crompton 2001, p. 68).

Spiritual well-being is nurtured by attention to all aspects of life and needs no special skills or activities. Most important is, as in all communication, really listening and responding to every kind of message, in noise or silence, aggression or withdrawal, words or actions.

The wisdom of religious traditions can strengthen and inform practice. For example, Aliya Haeri bases her counselling process for recovery from abuse 'on a model of self according to the Qur'an, Islam and Sufism'. The five-stage recovery process includes 'Affirming the child's innocence', 'Release by re-living the experience', 'Healing the whole person', 'Empowering the client to see justice done' and 'Liberation through unity'. Crucially, 'It is not enough to counsel the client through the trauma alone, but also to treat her at the same time on the levels of the body, emotions, mind, soul and spirit as a unified human being'. The client is helped to 'visualise herself as whole and in well-being. By taking this decision, she takes responsibility for her healing and creates her own reality' (Haeri 1998, pp. 98, 99).

Attachment to a religious organisation can contribute to development of confidence and self-esteem. A girl who had been sexually abused by a family member later chose to be baptised into a Church and said that she had never expected to feel so loved again. She was realising that the abuse had not been her fault, and that God and other Christians could love her (Crompton 1998, p. 152).

Di (NSPCC) and 'Roy' (13 years old) visited, by chance, a school display of architecture associated with worldwide religious traditions. Fascinated by both the buildings themselves and their significance, Roy began to talk about needing something important in his life, something constant to hold onto, which was lacking in his experience of both family and education. Whatever the later outcome, sharing the experience of the display and discussing the significance of the exhibits enabled Roy to pursue and reveal deep feelings and new ideas. It was essential that Di received Roy's insights with respect; she was not afraid of a conversation about religion, but neither did she over-encourage him. Roy's spiritual well-being was enhanced by the environment created by the practitioner, the experience of the exhibition which was both relaxing and stimulating, and the safe opportunity to make discoveries about himself which were received with respect.

Children's spiritual well-being is nurtured by creative activity, imagination and interaction with trustworthy, attentive adults. Whether or not associated with religious belief and observance, it is an essential element of individual work and communication (for examples of communication methods, see Crompton 1998, 2001, and Crompton & Jackson 2004).

Being with Mark: work with a 10-year-old boy

This account of work with 10-year-old Mark illustrates some of the ideas mentioned above.

Mark was a member of a family in which sexual abuse had taken place and had been placed in a series of short-term foster homes. I was employed as an 'extra' social worker to help him emerge from the 'fog' in which he seemed to live, learn about the events that had brought about the break-up of his home and prepare for a so-called 'forever' home. Although not the direct victim of physical abuse, as a sibling, his life was irrevocably changed, for example, because of his removal from home. I was engaged to offer intensive, weekly, time-limited contact, in cooperation with the regular social worker. Contacts were substantial, usually about 90–120 minutes.

My aims were to offer Mark a structure of protected and reliable space and peacefulness, time that was all his own and interactions in which he had my whole attention. I hoped that we could really *meet* each other and that he could show me how, if at all, I could help him. There was no reason why he should like or trust me, or even give me his time. There was no reason why I should be able to make contact with him. My one guideline was *wait*, combating the urge to be seen to be successful within a short period of time (in the same way that workers are beset by pressures to produce results within set times by managers, case conferences and court schedules).

Since most of our meetings were after school, when Mark was tired, it was particularly important to find ways in which we could be relaxed and have a place of our own. We had no access to an office or playroom but found a hospitable café. When Mark moved to yet another short-stay foster home, we found a river bank where we could park in privacy and he could choose one of several walks and activities. He could either walk with me or run ahead, he could share his discoveries, we could watch a ship together or walk peacefully apart.

Mark was never greedy. In the café he never asked for extra food or drink but relished his two weekly milkshakes. He had choice and (with money I gave him) ordered the refreshments – an opportunity to gain social confidence too.

We worked hard. Every week, Mark dictated a story about recent events and I wrote, fast and illegibly. Then he drew an illustration, demonstrating ability and enjoyment. He taught me to draw such impossible objects as a bicycle, enjoying both his own achievements and the satisfaction of his superior skill (particularly important for a child with poor self-image). This pattern emerged from our first meeting when, on a walk, we had an adventure with a goose which became an excellent story and illustration when we next met. We thus immediately had shared experience and continuity.

Between meetings, I wrote out the week's story very carefully, using coloured pens or the computer. My care and the continued existence of the story demonstrated that Mark himself had continued to exist for and with me and that his words had substance and were worthy of my time. With his own pictures, the stories built into a book recording the important events of his life. Finding a beautiful feather, getting lost, visiting a park – everyday events which had been important in themselves – became the focus for communication between us and were records of his past.

Darker aspects were regarded in the same way. When Mark wanted to discuss the abuse events and the reasons for his own removal from home, he asked his regular social worker for an explanation. At our next meeting, we wrote down this part of his story. Remembering that children should not feel defined by abuse or any other event or symptom, writing the story demonstrated that Mark's life included, but was not confined to, this aspect of his history.

His scattered parents and siblings could be gathered with stories, descriptions and drawings, helping Mark to decide how he foresaw his future, whether to be placed with a sibling or alone, and in what kind of family and place.

A whole day was spent visiting the scenes of his early life, including the maternity hospital and court. When a site on which he had loved to play and of which he had vivid memories was found to have been tarmacked and fenced by high wire, he asked: 'Why do things have to change?' We called at the museum to which Mark had gone on a recent school outing, and the castle, where he bought presents for his foster family and himself – his own choice was a cuddly toy (which, with a similar gift from his mother, became both a useful focus for and the medium of discussion of painful subjects, and a comforter). Writing, drawing, meals, silence and fun contributed to this important day.

Mark and I looked forward to seeing each other. I think he gained confidence, control, a sense of continuity and of himself. However, I felt that I failed him. The social services department did not provide a 'forever' home during my period of contact. I had been asked to visit weekly but, after 5 months, mileage for a return journey of 80 miles was abruptly axed. When telling Mark that I could no longer visit him, I selfishly allowed my own anger and frustration to show and Mark, not understanding that my feelings were not directed at him, withdrew and asked, 'Can I go now?' If I had realised and controlled my self-absorption, it might have been better to have ended the day's contact early than to give Mark his full time, but spoil it. I would have valued support for myself, but I worked from home and did not wish to bother Mark's busy social worker.

We said goodbye in McDonald's, Mark's choice. I gave him all the materials we had used during our meetings and a strong carrying case, demonstrating that I had kept his possessions safe and that those aspects of his life which they represented were now in his own keeping. I had taught him to trust me and to enjoy being himself. It was important that in parting he should not feel abandoned, lest all my care become only another form of abuse.

We used physical activity, storytelling, writing, drawing, sending and collecting postcards, food, drink, car rides, toys, visiting places, conversation, explanation and silence. I tried to respect Mark's privacy and to be sensitive to his non-verbal messages, to be clear, straightforward and honest, and to give Mark opportunities for choice, control and the development of self-confidence. I was concerned for every aspect of his well-being – cognitive, emotional, physical, social and spiritual. Everything was important for its own sake and I was (usually) careful to avoid interpretation traps.

It was frustrating that I could not complete the work for which I had been contracted. Mark had been abused at second hand by his family, and in effect by the failure of the department to provide appropriate care (within the period of my contract). The financial cost was a small price for the attempt to help a hurt and bewildered child and more resources should have been available routinely (including, perhaps, the use of part-time, experienced specialist workers to undertake this kind of intensive time-limited contract). Working with Mark was not a luxury but there are still many 'Marks' for whom no such help is available.

Conclusion

This survey of individual work with children has, of necessity, been swift and superficial. It is hoped that readers will consider the questions raised, slowly and in depth.

One of the main strands has been the importance of achieving and maintaining good standards of practice based on well-focused, substantial training, and supported within equally well-focused agencies. Clarity of thought, demonstrated through, for example, precision of language, definition of role and task, and self-knowledge, is combined with loving care for every individual child.

Children must not be labelled by symptom or experience. Effective help can be offered only by a whole, individual worker to a whole, individual child, taking into account the whole life of the child, together with the resources and constraints of the agency.

Really *meeting* a child may be helped through many kinds of communicative activity but no materials or techniques can produce communication if the worker has no wish, or skill, to engage in such interactions.

Shared activities can offer opportunities for children to develop strength, confidence and self-esteem, to experience achievement, choice and control, and to share unstressed time with an adult who does not threaten or pressure and who gives reliable and courteous attention.

To achieve the commitment and skills discussed in this chapter, practitioners need training (initial and ongoing), recognition, respect, resources – including time, support, and, fundamentally, permission and encouragement to work directly with children.

Acknowledgement

For generous and invaluable advice, information and help I thank Di Ashton Dent (Lincoln NSPCC Family Centre) and staff of Lincolnshire Social Services Department: Katie Prince (Development Manager) and colleagues at Child and Adolescent Mental Health Service; Barbara Simpson (Senior Training Officer Children's Services); Marian Taylor (formerly NSPCC), Sylvia Morgan, Penny Turner and colleagues at SSD Family Centres.

Key points and messages for practice

- Respect every child as a whole individual.
- Attend to each child's unique forms of communication.
- Respond appropriately and creatively, using methods comfortable for both child and practitioner.
- Cooperate with and learn from colleagues.
- Training, both for initial and advanced qualifications, and in-service, should include substantial focus on all aspects of children's lives (e.g. development, communication, legislation, rights).
- Practitioners should be respected and encouraged within and outside their employing agencies; the often low level of respect for practitioners reflects attitudes to the children whom they seek to serve. It is easy, and negative, to cast blame after a failure but approval for good (or 'good enough') practice is infinitely more useful to both practitioners and children.
- Agencies should, as priority, provide resources (e.g. protected space, materials, training, consultation, time and above all staff) for direct work with children.
- Practitioners from different agencies (e.g. education, health, police, welfare) should meet to share ideas and experience about e.g. methods of communication, spiritual well-being, etc. in order to develop inter- and intra-agency trust and enhance practice when practitioners need to cooperate about individual children.

Annotated further reading

This list includes most of, and adds to, texts noted in the second edition. Some especially recommended by practitioners are indicated **RP**.

Aldridge M, Wood J 1998 Interviewing children: a guide for child care and forensic practitioners. Wiley, Chichester

While this text focuses on interviewing children during investigation of alleged abuse, the material has relevance to wider contexts of working with children. The authors (specialists in language acquisition and disorders) discuss children's language development with chapters on, e.g.:

- *'Asking questions' (pp. 107–145)*
- *'Children's language and development' (pp. 146–187)*
- *'Interviewing children with special needs' (pp. 188–217).*

Armstrong H (ed) 1991, 1997 Taking care: a church response to adults, children and abuse. National Children's Bureau, London

A practical guide to helping non-professionals to develop awareness of, and ways of responding to, abuse in various manifestations.

Bannister A (ed) 1998 From hearing to healing: working with the aftermath of child sexual abuse, 2nd edn. Wiley (with NSPCC), Chichester

A collection of papers focusing on some unusual aspects of working with children, e.g.:

- *'"To all the flickering candles": dramatherapy with sexually abused children', Di Grimshaw (pp. 35–54)*
- *'Young children who exhibit sexually abusive behaviour', Carol Day and Bobbie Print (pp. 118–141)*
- *'Therapeutic issues in working with young sexually aggressive children', Anne Bannister (pp. 142–151).*

Brandon M, Schofield G, Trinder L (with Stone N) 1998 Social work with children. Macmillan, Basingstoke

A useful general text introducing numerous aspects of working with children, e.g. child care policy, children's rights and the Children Act 1989, and the developmental framework. Three chapters are of particular relevance to practice with children who have been abused:

- *Chapter 3: 'The Voice of the Child in Practice', which introduces 'Key factors: Legal context; Agency context; A place to work; Knowledge; Skills; Relationship; Honesty; Genuineness, warmth and empathy' (pp. 69–73).*
- *Chapter 4: 'Working with Children in Need and in need of Protection' (pp. 95–117), which includes a summary of 'Principles underpinning work' (pp. 103–105) based on guidance in Department of Health publications Working Together (1991) and The Challenge of Partnership (1994). Emphasis is on 'Children as active participants' (pp. 100–102), advising that 'Children and young people … need to be fully informed and involved without bearing additional responsibility' (p. 111).*
- *Chapter 6 'Children looked after by the Local Authority' (pp. 141–165) including, e.g. 'Making sense of the past and the present' (pp. 153–162); 'Participation in decision-making' (pp. 162–165).*

Bray M 1997 Sexual abuse: the child's voice: poppies on the rubbish heap, 2nd edn. Jessica Kingsley, London

The author, a social worker, trainer and therapist, co-founded SACCS (Sexual Abuse: Child Consultancy Service) and 'Leaps and Bounds', which comprises five houses and two smaller units providing for 30 children. Her book, first published in 1991, comprises powerful accounts of work with children in the form of stories that 'honour and celebrate the remarkableness of each child's capacity for survival and healing' and explore 'the meaning of these discoveries' (p. xx). The author's own experience and beliefs enrich both the immediacy and depth of this essential reading.

Burch M 1992 I want to make a life story book. Department of Social Policy and Professional Studies, University of Hull, Hull

The author has drawn on her experience as mother to five adopted children and 30 years fostering to produce a guide which includes a model for such a book, photographs, stories and other ideas.

Butler I, Robert G 2004 Social work with children and their families: getting into practice, 2nd edn. Jessica Kingsley, London

Students' textbook comprising practice focus units including: Course text, Exercises, Study texts, Points to consider, Notes and self-assessment, Recommended reading, Trainers' notes, Web resources. Unit 6 Child abuse.

Clarke J I 1998 Self-esteem: a family affair, 2nd edn. Hazelden, MN **RP**

Transactional analysis applied to seven family situations, focusing on developing positive self-esteem in all family members, and developmental stages (e.g. infant, 3–6 years, 7-12 years), including worksheets and exercises. Analyses '4 ways of parenting' and associated messages: 'Nurturing, Structuring and protecting, Marshmallowing, Criticizing' and offers useful comments on age-appropriate vocabulary. A–Z of 'Things to do instead of hitting', e.g. L. Do an angry dance; T. Play angry notes on a piano; Y. Decide to think. Resolve the issues about which you are angry' (p. 145). Clear, accessible, practical.

Crompton M 1998 Children, spirituality, religion and social work. Ashgate, Aldershot

This text introduces numerous aspects of spirituality and religion in relation to children/young people, including rights, day-to-day implications of religious observances, spiritual well-being and distress. Of particular relevance to working with children who have been abused are:

- *'Spirituality, religion, abuse and neglect' (pp. 141–180).*
- *Chapter 11: 'Abuse and neglect' (pp. 141–155) 'explores associations between abuse/neglect and spiritual well-being' in the context of the UN Convention on the Rights of the Child (1989); reference is made to, e.g. 'Responses to religious teaching'.*
- *Chapter 12: 'Abuse associated with religious and ritual practices' (pp. 157–180) introduces ideas about 'Intentional abuse', 'Abuse informally associated with religious organisations', 'Oppression, persecution and sectarianism', 'Abuse intentionally associated with ritual practices', 'The needs of practitioners'.*
- *Chapter 15 offers ideas about communication through 'Stories, myths and legends' (pp. 217–234).*

Crompton M 2001 Who am I? Promoting children's spiritual well-being in everyday life: a guide for all who care for children. Barnardo's, Barkingside, Ilford

This resource includes material on nurturing spiritual well-being in everyday practice, with a section on children who have been abused or neglected. Developed from the CCETSW training pack Children, Spirituality and Religion *(1997), this guide is intended for practical use by all practitioners concerned with children's social and/or health care. While material focuses on spiritual well-being, all ideas, references, questions and suggestions are relevant to individual work. Material includes:*

- *Rights and legislation*
- *Ideas about the meaning of spiritual well-being*
- *Communication (storytelling, talking, creativity/imagination)*
- *Practice units (abuse/neglect, living away from birth parents, bereavement/death, learning disability, offending).*

Doyle C 1997 Working with abused children, 2nd edn. Macmillan Education, Basingstoke

Clear, straightforward ideas and advice to practitioners includes: Section 3 'Individual work with children' (pp. 41–62) with numerous subsections, e.g. 'The helping process' (pp. 53–62) which includes 'The expression of emotion', 'Positive messages', 'Protective work', 'Ending individual work'.

Hagood M M 2001 The use of art in counselling child and adult survivors of sexual abuse. Jessica Kingsley, London

Foreword (Marian Liebmann): 'This book demonstrates how most of the ways of "reading" children's pictures are based on psychoanalytic views which are derived from adult work, which may not apply to children. [It] provides another dimension often missing from studies of children's pictures: the huge body of work done on developmental aspects of children's drawings' (pp. 9–10). Numerous case and pictorial illustrations. Note especially Chapters 2, 3, 4 and 9 on aspects of the use of art in counselling sexually abused children.'

Kennedy M 1995 Submission to the National Commission of Inquiry into the Prevention of Child Abuse. Christian Survivors of Sexual Abuse (CSSA), London

This report provides invaluable material about children who have been abused within a religious context (e.g. by ministers of religion) or when children abused by their fathers have been taught that God is a loving Father. Many responses by survivors are supplemented by comments on, for example, fear, forgiveness and guilt, and there are ideas for expressing their pain, anger and hurt to the deity in the form of special liturgies and worship (p. 26).

Mallon B 2002 Dream time with children: learning to dream, dreaming to learn. Jessica Kingsley, London

An introduction to 'dream sharing', stimulus and ideas about attending to and communicating with children; illustrated with children's pictures and accounts of dreams, including:

Part 1 The basics
- *Chapter 2: Ages and stages*
- *Chapter 3: Dream sharing: practical guide*

- *Chapter 4: The Dreams of Harry Potter*

  Part 2 Dream themes
- *Chapter 6: Nightmare taming*
- *Chapter 7: Creative dreaming*
- *Sleep and dreams: Books for children (under 5/5–9/11+).*

Milner P, Carolin B (eds) 1999 Time to listen to children: personal and professional communication. Routledge, London

This thoughtful collection of papers illustrates how the authors, drawn from a wide range of settings, 'use time to listen to children on matters that concern them and decisions that affect them … to enable children to learn an understanding, respect and responsibility for themselves, plus a respect and understanding for others' (p. 2).

- *Part III: 'At work with children', includes 'Child protection: facing up to fear' (Chapter 7) by Barbara Smedley (pp. 112–125) in which perceptions of, and work with, several children who have been abused are described.*
- *Part IV: 'Listening creatively', introduces different modes of communication, including practice examples:*
  - *Chapter 10: ' "I'm going to do magic …" said Tracey: working with children using person-centred art therapy', Heather Giles and Micky Mendelson (pp. 161–174).*
  - *Chapter 11: 'Listening to children through play', Carol Dasgupta (pp. 175–187).*
  - *Chapter 12: 'Listening: the first step toward communicating through music', Amelia Oldfield (pp. 188–199).*

Nash M, Stewart B (eds) 2004 Spirituality and social care: contributing to personal and community well-being. Jessica Kingsley, London

This interesting collection of papers originates in New Zealand. Judith Morris (social work consultant/play therapist) contributes 'Heroes' journeys: children's expression of spirituality through play therapy' (pp. 189–213); illustrated, discusses application of attachment theory, case example 'Daniel in residential care following neglect and sexual abuse' (pp. 200–203).

Plummer D 2001 Helping children to build self-esteem: a photocopiable activities book. Jessica Kingsley, London **RP**

Focus on feeling, imagination: 'Providing children with the means to foster creative use of their imagination can help them to build a unified sense of their inner and outer worlds; can enable them to see events, problems and challenges from a different viewpoint, and can help them to find the way forward that is most appropriate for their individual needs' (p. 14). Substantial A4 format, including:

- *Part 1 Theoretical background: (elements of self-esteem – self-knowledge, self and others, self-acceptance, self-reliance, self-expression, self-confidence)*
- *Part 2 Instructions for self-esteem activities*
- *Part 3 Activity worksheets (for activities in Part 2)*
- *Appendix B Signs of possible low self-esteem and/or anxiety*
- *Appendix C Adult behaviour that supports self-esteem in children*
- *Appendix D Building your own self-esteem*
- *Appendix E Relaxation script*
- *Appendix F Children's storybooks to read (6–8 year olds).*

Also by Deborah Plummer:

Plummer D 2004 Helping adolescents and adults to build self-esteem, a photocopiable resource book. Jessica Kingsley, London

Ross C 1997 Something to draw on: activities and interventions using an art therapy approach. Jessica Kingsley, London

Clear, concise, practical collection of ideas and examples, illustrated with children's pictures and wise advice. Some examples directed at work with age-specific school classes, others relate to work with individual children, transferable to communication in other settings.

- *Example 9. Upper junior. Individual art therapy sessions with a year 6 pupil. Focus of concern: 'L was extremely withdrawn with occasional outbursts. He appeared to have very low self-esteem and was ostracised by most other children, who said he smelled bad. (He soiled himself on occasion.)' Aims of the intervention include diagnostic appraisal, providing space for L to talk and be listened to, raising confidence and self-esteem, liaising with teacher. Focus and outcomes summarised with examples of artwork (pp. 106–110).*

Sinason V (ed) 1994 Treating survivors of Satanist abuse. Routledge, London

This book of papers by practitioners in a range of fields explores many aspects of a controversial subject. One paper with particular relevance to practice with children is: 'Fostering a ritually abused child', Chapter 10, by Mary Kelsall. Russell had been severely physically abused and later described horrific experiences of ritual abuse. With the help of a psychotherapist, his foster parents hold on to the deeply disturbed boy (pp. 94–99).

Stone M K 1995 Don't just sit there, do something: developing children's spiritual awareness. RMEP, Norwich

From long experience in education, the author offers straightforward ideas about and examples of helping children 'to reflect upon experience, to explore feelings as well as ideas, to develop imagination as well as the memory, to engage the whole of a child's being' (p. 5). The attractive A4 format, illustrated with photographs and children's drawings, contains many examples of children's thoughts and responses, useful for all communication, whether or not directly associated with spiritual development.

West J 1996 Child centred play therapy, 2nd edn. Arnold, London **RP**

RP Practitioners recommend materials are available from:

Reconstruct Ltd. Training, Direct Work With Children, 9A High Street, West Drayton, Middlesex UB7 7QG. tel. 01895 443632, fax. 01895 431696. Email: reconstruct@cix.co.uk

Women's Aid Federation England (WAFE) 1994 All children should be safe: workbook. PO Box 391, Bristol BS99 7WS

Also

Hindman J A 1983 A very touching book: for little people and for big people. McClure-Hindman, Durke, OR

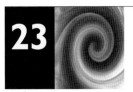

23 Non-directive play therapy with children and adolescents who have been maltreated

Virginia Ryan

INTRODUCTION

Current professional interest in play therapy has been heightened by recognition of the seriousness of many maltreated children's and young people's emotional difficulties. It also is due to play therapy's effectiveness as an intervention for those who require therapeutic help. One particular approach, non-directive play therapy, is a viable and non-intrusive method of working with children and adolescents who have been maltreated (West 1996, Ryan & Wilson 2000a, Wilson & Ryan 2005).

This chapter will give an overview of this method of play therapy and then discuss the relevance of non-directive therapy within statutory settings. Child protection concerns, care decisions and court proceedings – including children as witnesses – are all important considerations at referral for therapy and during therapeutic interventions and will be referred to briefly. The last part of this chapter will present a case example of non-directive play therapy with a 13-year-old girl who was sexually abused. It will illustrate the ways in which her therapist, carers and social worker all worked within their specified roles to meet the emotional needs of this young person.

An overview

The most significant way in which non-directive play therapy differs from other play interventions and therapies is in its non-directive nature. The choice of issues and the choice of play contents and actions in the playroom are determined by children themselves, rather than by their therapists or other adults. Non-directive therapists are trained to establish certain basic limits to behaviour in the playroom, yet the atmosphere in the playroom is intended to be relaxed and non-threatening. Therapists have adult responsibility for physical and emotional safety, for care of the materials and the room, and for time limits. With children and young people who have been maltreated, it is even more important that limits are set clearly and consistently, and that therapists themselves recognise and respond appropriately to the changing emotional needs of each child they help during therapy.

Non-directive play therapists assume that children and young people will instigate therapeutic changes and achieve therapeutic insights for themselves. Therapists facilitate these changes without overt directions, suggestions or interpretations. Instead, therapists develop close helping relationships in which children's feelings and thoughts are reflected and responded to empathically. Therapists also are trained to use their own feelings and thoughts within relationships they develop with children in therapeutic ways. Children and young people can therefore use both the playroom environment and their therapists to resolve their chosen emotional difficulties at their own pace and in their own manner. Some children may choose to use dramatic play as their primary means of communication and change in the playroom, other children may use the clay, cars or toy soldiers. Still other children and young people may choose to primarily talk and sit quietly with their therapists. In particular cases, for example with children who have serious attachment difficulties, it may be helpful to include their carers directly in play therapy sessions. In other cases, sibling pairs or group therapy may be the preferred option. More recently, filial therapy – a well-researched combination of family therapy and play therapy where carers are trained as therapeutic change agents for their own children – has been offered in the UK (Ryan forthcoming).

Historically, non-directive play therapy was developed in North America by Axline (1971, 1987), who adapted Rogerian client-centred therapy with adults to child therapy (Rogers 1951). Children's play had already been established in psychodynamic practice by Klein and A Freud as the primary medium for therapeutic help with children (Wolff 1996). Axline, and to a lesser extent other practitioners (e.g. Moustakas 1953, 1959, Ginott 1961), relied heavily on clinical examples to explain the practice of non-directive play therapy. They did not specify its procedures or develop its theoretical underpinnings rigorously. This aprocedural and atheoretical stance was deliberate. Early practitioners believed this stance was needed to counteract what they saw as the rigid and convoluted theorising of psychoanalytically trained child analysts and the simplistic and prescriptive stance of behavioural therapists. Non-directive play therapy did not evolve into a major, recognised school of therapy with closely specified techniques during this period. Currently, non-directive play therapy as a method of intervention has been evolving further in North America, most notably by Guerney (1984) and Landreth (2002), and in Britain by the author of this chapter and by one of the editors of this book, Kate Wilson (e.g. Ryan & Wilson 2000a, Wilson & Ryan 2005).

Approved training programmes for play therapists, including training to be a non-directive play therapist, are offered in a few countries, most notably in the US and the UK. The most well-established professional organisation for play therapists is in North America, the Association for Play Therapy, Inc; it offers training, international membership and conferences. Within the UK play therapy has developed into an accredited profession during the last decade, with the British Association of Play Therapists (BAPT) accrediting university training programmes leading to a nationally recognised professional qualification and establishing a professional register and code of ethics (see website and contact details at the end of this chapter for further details).

Until the establishment of the BAPT, non-directive play therapy in the UK was practised in relative isolation at child guidance and child treatment centres by a variety of professionals. There was a tendency to drift into other therapeutic techniques and into direct work with children, while attempting to remain 'child-focused'. The practice of non-directive play therapy is now well defined, with the well-established postgraduate Diploma and MA in non-directive play therapy at the University of York (followed by a further period of academic study for a PhD for qualified students) (see end of chapter for address of the University of York course). Three other play therapy courses have been approved by the BAPT and offer child-centred training.

In my writing with Kate Wilson on non-directive play therapy, we have further developed non-directive play therapy theoretically by setting it within the context of current child development theory and research, including the ways in which symbolic play serves an adaptive function in normal development (Ryan & Wilson 2000a, Wilson & Ryan 2005, Chapter 2). Using a broadly adaptive model, play is conceptualised as serving the function of assimilating personally important experiences for normally developing children into their existing mental structures, called schemas. With troubled and abused children these schemas are likely to be poorly developed and/or distorted. Therapy aims to help these children develop more adaptive, flexible ways of organising their mental representations of personal experiences.

We have also updated non-directive play therapy practice:

1. We have looked at the place of individual child treatment within a wider systemic framework (e.g. Wilson & Ryan 2005). In addition, filial therapy has been advocated as a very successful systemic intervention (Hutton 2004, Ryan 2004, forthcoming).
2. We have discussed the role of non-directive therapy within statutory work, including the usefulness of therapeutic assessments in identifying children's needs, wishes and feelings in civil court proceedings (Ryan & Wilson 2000a, 2000b). We have also argued that non-directive play therapy, by remaining within children's metaphors and issues, is suitable for pre-trial interventions with child witnesses in criminal courts (Ryan & Wilson 1995a).
3. We have demonstrated that other therapeutic techniques (e.g. structured exercises and certain psychodynamic and cognitive/behavioural techniques) can be modified and incorporated into a non-directive play therapy approach (Ryan & Wilson 1995b, Cigno & Ryan 1998, Wilson & Ryan 2005).

Research in play therapy is well established in North America, but only beginning to be carried out with UK populations. Empirically based research studies in non-directive play therapy from the US are increasing and are reported most frequently in the *International Journal of Play Therapy*. US research reported in this journal ranges from practice issues, such as therapists' opinions on limit setting, to training issues and to process issues within therapy sessions themselves with children and adolescents. The most important research to date is US meta-research findings of outcomes of play therapy. These meta-analyses have demonstrated that overall play therapy is effective with a variety of populations (LeBlanc & Ritchie 2001, Bratton *et al.* 2005). In addition, empirical support for filial therapy is beginning to be well documented (Ryan, VanFleet *et al.* 2005). These studies generally do not incorporate earlier research in play therapy because this research generally did not have tightly specified process and outcome measures, a difficulty held in common with the earlier, general child therapy research literature (Guerney 1984). Research in child therapy, including play therapy, now focuses on more carefully defined subgroups within clinical populations, such as children with conduct disorders (Herschell & McNeil 2005) and on evaluating specific interventions and outcomes for such groups (e.g. Kazdin *et al.* 1990, Reddy *et al.* 2005).

Further research is needed, particularly in the UK. Of particular concern for this chapter, definitive process and outcome research on non-directive play therapy for children and adolescents within statutory settings remains scant. Within the play therapy literature with this population, filial therapy has the most relevant outcome research base for empirically based practice (see Ryan). Encouragingly, UK research in play therapy and filial therapy now is underway.

Broader policy considerations

Non-directive play therapy allows children and young people to address issues of their choice and to restructure their internal mental schemas at their own pace, within the relaxed environment of the playroom. It is a more comprehensive approach to therapy than other more limited interventions, such as programmes on the enhancement of self-esteem or behavioural programmes. Non-directive therapists do not target specific maladaptive behaviours, but assume that children choose for themselves to focus on the issues troubling them. For this reason it seems highly suitable for children within statutory settings, who often have multiple emotional difficulties.

Another strength of the non-directive approach is that it enhances choice within the playroom, and thus serves as an antidote to maltreated children's experiences in which abusers removed age-appropriate choices from the children they abused. In addition, by staying within children's play metaphors and communications, children who often have had multiple professional relationships that focused on verbal exchanges (e.g. investigative interviews, discussions about moving with their social workers) are allowed the freedom to choose to play rather than being required to talk through their emotional difficulties with adults.

All therapeutic interventions with maltreated children, including non-directive play therapy, must be practised alongside consideration of child protection issues. Individual therapy with children cannot protect them adequately if their environments are currently abusive. Indeed, in such cases, therapy is contraindicated and child protection issues must take priority. There are several reasons for this:

- Children who are already scapegoated or identified as the sole problem in abusing families may be further scapegoated by being singled out for an intervention.
- Children may be unable to make substantial therapeutic changes because their emotional energy needs to be channelled primarily into emotional and physical survival.
- If children do make therapeutic changes, despite these obstacles – say by becoming overtly angry when abusing parents make unreasonable demands on them – children may put themselves at greater risk of harm in an already abusing environment.
- Children will often compare their therapist and therapeutic relationship with other significant relationships.

If children's intimate relationships with their carers are already seriously inadequate and cannot meet their needs, or if the relationships are unsafe, children may become overly and unrealistically attached to their therapists. Their therapeutic relationships will then tend to be misused by children to fulfil needs which can only be adequately met for them on a daily, long-term basis by carers (Glaser 1991, Wilson & Ryan 2005). Therefore, for individual therapy to be safe and productive, children's environments must, at the very least, be minimally stable and adequate for the fulfilment of their physical and emotional needs.

The practice of non-directive play therapy also has relevance for care decisions and court proceedings concerning children. Often it is through individual sessions that are utilised freely, rather than in sessions directed by an adult's agenda, that children's current concerns and the intensity of these concerns are discovered. This information is of great importance in making care decisions and in presenting evidence in court based on the Children Act 1989. Evidence from non-directive play therapy sessions can be quite different from, but as equally valid as, evidence derived from other means, such as direct questioning and family assessments (Ryan & Wilson 1995a, 2000a, 2000b). While the contents of play therapy sessions must be kept as confidential as possible, important themes emerging in these sessions will usefully inform care decisions concerning children. Evidence of further abuse of already abused children may also emerge in non-directive play therapy sessions (see 'Non-directive play therapy with maltreated adolescents' below). This in turn will further inform care decisions and the necessary protection of these children.

Finally, professional issues about the conflict between meeting the therapeutic needs of children when court proceedings require that children give evidence in court, and simultaneously meeting legal requirements for non-contamination of children's evidential statements have been set out in detail (Home Office *et al.* 2001) The grave legal concern over contamination of evidence by professionals' suggestions and interpretations, especially in sexual abuse cases where children are often the only other witnesses to events besides the accused, is addressed most helpfully by non-directive play therapy. In contrast to psychodynamic and directive approaches, it does not use interpretation in its practice. Therapists instead keep to the metaphors and symbols used by children to reflect their ongoing feelings. Furthermore, non-directive therapists employ therapeutic suggestion in a much more curtailed and circumspect way than other therapeutic methods (Ryan & Wilson 1995a).

Most importantly for children's therapeutic needs, this method – more than any other therapeutic method – enables children to set their own pace for examining painful current material and memories. As well as addressing children's best interests by providing therapeutic help as soon as possible, research also seems to demonstrate that children who have been traumatised by damaging personal experiences make better witnesses if they have been able to examine and work through on an emotional level their 'worst moments' prior to giving evidence concerning these events (Pynoos & Eth 1984). Non-directive play therapy therefore offers the advantage of preserving children's own perceptions of these traumatic events; children's evidence in court is not invalidated by undue therapeutic suggestion, directions or interpretations.

Child abuse and non-directive play therapy

As well as the advantages of employing non-directive play therapy in statutory settings described above, non-directive play therapy is effective with maltreated children and adolescents because it is directed at the underlying emotional damage they have sustained. The short- and long-term emotional effects of abuse on children and adolescents within a family context have already been discussed in an earlier chapter (see Hanks and Stratton, Chapter 5, in this volume). Although these effects will vary, and even though a number of maltreated children do seem to recover from their abusive experiences (Finkelhor 1992, Hall & Lloyd 1993), the experiences themselves are inevitably emotionally damaging to children's development (Wilson & Ryan 2005). Also, it is generally recognised that children who have been abused need increased levels of care either from their own families or from their new caregivers (Downes 1992, Sinclair *et al.* 2005a; see also Thoburn, Chapter 27, in this volume). These increased levels of care often extend to children's relationships with professionals in positions of authority, such as teachers and social workers. Maltreated children often make greater demands on professionals' as well as carers' capacities for limit setting, appropriate physical and emotional closeness, and individual attention, even after the abuse has stopped.

Maltreated children frequently develop damaged, overly accommodating, emotional responses to abusive experiences – responses such as passivity, peer aggression and regression to less mature levels of functioning, to name a few. This is because children's responses to ongoing abusive experiences seem to result in relatively permanent adaptations in their mental functioning. These adaptations can be conceptualised as changes in mental organisation, with this organisation viewed as made up of mental schemas that are at one experientially, but conceptually can be divided up into several levels of functioning: cognitive, perceptual, motor and emotional/social. These schemas mentally represent not only children's carers, but simultaneously represent internally the most fundamental aspects of children's own schemas about the self as well. This conceptualisation of mental functioning is well documented in the attachment literature. Personally significant interactions always involve the development of schemas concerning the self *and* significant others (see Wilson & Ryan 2005, Chapter 2, for a fuller account).

Maltreated children have of necessity overly accommodated their behaviour and mental responses to their abusive relationships within their environments. These accommodations will necessarily involve disturbed personal schemas concerning both the self and carers. Repeated abusive experiences, or even one traumatic experience, may lead children to develop strongly negative or conflicting personal schemas about themselves and significant others. A highly compensatory environment, after removal from an abusive one, may not be sufficient to enable children who have been maltreated to abandon their previously adaptive, persistent mental schemas, or to transform them into more positive ones. Children often need an intensive, corrective experience such as non-directive play therapy in order to re-enact their emotionally damaging experiences on this mental level. Both the imaginative play materials and activities in the play therapy room and the therapist's skill in developing a helping relationship which suits each individual child may be needed to supplement this safer environment.

Children and adolescents who have been sexually abused, for example, may have developed a mental schema which contains strong feelings of fear and anger towards their carer along with other positive feelings of trust and affection. The cognitive component of this schema may also contain discrepancies concerning parents who treat their child as an adult sexual partner and yet restrict that child's freedom in taking on a parental role in other ways. Relatively permanent cognitive explanations – usually deliberately fostered by the abusing adult (see Wyre 1991) – such as 'I am unusually sexy, that's why my father/mother can't help being sexually attracted to me' may develop. Motor level conflicts are also common: sexual abuse involves parts of children's bodies, usually both children's intimate body parts as well as body parts such as the hands and mouth which are normally involved in non-sexual activities. Children will have difficulty assimilating their abnormal, sexually abusive, bodily sensations and motor responses into existing motor schemas involving normal motor experiences. Take a motor schema related to physical care: a child having their hair brushed by their carer, for instance, would usually have developed a motor schema for hair-brushing associated with feelings and personal experiences of nurturance; however, in sexual abuse, hair-brushing for some children may have emotionally powerful, sexual connotations as well.

Non-directive play therapy is of particular value for maltreated children and adolescents who have sustained this kind of emotional damage. Non-directive play therapy gives them the time and privacy to address these deeper mental levels of personal experiences using symbolic (or imaginative) play, accompanied by their therapists' focus on reflecting children's ongoing feelings. Symbolic play, as stated above, is a natural vehicle children use to assimilate and express their personal experiences. Abused children actively direct their own process of symbolic re-enactment of personally meaningful experiences, thus automatically individualising and personalising the play therapy sessions for themselves.

Another feature of abuse – its coexistence with other forms of abuse – is also addressed in this way. Very often the separate effects of neglect and emotional, sexual and physical abuse may be difficult to unravel (see Hanks and Stratton, Chapter 5, in this volume). Because of its highly individualised approach, non-directive play therapy can readily adapt to whatever additional issues emerge during therapy for children. Besides the possibility of other forms of abuse, it is likely that children will also be able to symbolically recreate and explore the 'worst moments' in their traumatically abusive experiences (Pynoos & Eth 1986). These personally traumatic experiences may include their experience of, as in one case, sudden, inexplicable abandonment during a special, happy outing arranged by their neglectful parent, or in another case, a child finding out that the abusing parent had lied to the child about the child's much valued toy being stolen when, in fact, the parent had deliberately sold the toy and kept the money herself. Furthermore, because children often understate the extent of their abuse initially, the extent of their abusive experiences may be discovered in non-directive play therapy. (The implications for child protection issues when further abuse is disclosed in therapy are discussed in the section 'Non-directive play therapy with maltreated adolescents', below, and in Wilson & Ryan 2005.)

Returning to symbolic play, this type of play necessarily involves all the cognitive, perceptual, motor and emotional/social levels of functioning for children, thus enabling them to integrate and rework all these levels of their abusive experiences. Furthermore, besides immediate play symbols that children are consciously aware of, there may be many more remote or more threatening meanings to mental symbols of which they are unaware. Because children determine the contents and issues of play therapy sessions, they are able to give symbolic expression to thoughts and experiences which are less threatening to them, but which also connect with and activate more threatening schemas. In this way, non-directive play therapy does not raise children's anxiety by dealing directly with highly self-threatening experiences or by dealing directly with the coping mechanisms children have developed to protect themselves from anxiety, such as denial, dissociation or displacement. Children break down their own barriers to self-threatening experiences with the help of their therapists' reflections, using the natural and fundamentally non-threatening activity of play.

Non-directive play therapy, therefore, is based on real choices of content and issues which are made by children rather than by their therapists. This feature of the non-directive method is especially important in work with children who have been abused. Control over these children's important personal experiences has been exercised abusively by their carers to meet adults' emotional needs for power, aggression or sexual gratification, and not to fulfil these children's own needs. By the reintroduction of choice over personally meaningful experiences in non-directive play therapy, the lack of choice and their previous experiences of adult coercion are directly counteracted. When maltreated children and adolescents have control over the content of their sessions and the pace of therapeutic change, this seems to reduce their compliant or reactive mental schemas, and the overt, disturbed behaviour that accompanies these schemas, that were originally developed in response to adult demands. As a result, children's awareness of their own personal thoughts, feelings and responses is enhanced. Additionally, because therapists follow children's activities, thoughts and feelings, and reflect these back, children begin to realise that their own external and internal actions during play therapy sessions are of importance to their therapists and, therefore, become of more value internally to themselves as well.

In practising non-directive play therapy, therapists are trained to subordinate their own needs and emotions to those of the children they work with. But therapists are also trained to be consciously aware of their internal emotions, especially those generated by specific interactions with particular children. These emotional reactions, which must be separated from personal, private emotions by therapists, are then used by them to help clarify and give primacy to children's expressed feelings.

This general subordination of personal emotions, thoughts and needs by therapists is a necessary part of the practice of non-directive play therapy and particularly necessary when working with maltreated children. This caregiving function of therapists can be conceptualised as an artificial enhancement of normal adult–child nurturing relationships (Heard & Lake 1997). In normal development, the subordination of adult needs to those of children (e.g. an adult waiting to eat until a hungry child has been fed) is made workable because the parent's primary emotional need is to care for their children (Erikson 1963). However, a recurring feature of abusive experiences for children is that this normal adult–child relationship pattern has been damaged, and adults have put the fulfilment of their own emotional and physical needs before those of their children. This helps account for the extreme adaptations and vacillations observed in maltreated children's emotional reactions. In normal development, children's needs are adequately met and they gradually learn to wait and to subordinate some of their own needs to others' needs. But maltreated children often over-subordinate their own needs to others, or else become desperate and frantically out of control in an attempt to force adults to meet their needs. Even when these children's needs then begin to be met in a more appropriate manner in a non-abusive environment, they often retain a learned fear that their needs will not be met consistently or fully.

Non-directive play therapists therefore participate in sessions at children's own pace and under their direction with great predictability, thus subordinating their own adult needs but at the same time maintaining their adult, guiding role. Therapists need to respond congruently with appropriate, healthy adult responses to maltreated children's expressed behaviour, thoughts and feelings. For example, if a child who has been sexually abused attempts to thrust some playdough down the front of a therapist's trousers, that therapist is responding congruently and helpfully by saying he does not feel comfortable because that place is private, stopping the child's actions. At the same time, however, therapists need to help maltreated children express their difficult feelings and perhaps perform these actions in a more socially acceptable way, say to a doll, when children indicate they need to re-enact and rework their abusive and traumatic experiences in therapy.

The above example illustrates that although the overall emphasis in non-directive play therapy is permissive and child-centred, it is essential that therapeutic limits are established by therapists in their adult role. Indeed, both therapeutic limits and emotionally healthy adult responses are an essential component of this approach. In these adult interactions with children, therapists enable children to develop emotionally healthy responses to necessary adult limits on their behaviour. More generally, these responses in therapists also make normal adult–child interactions more understandable and predictable to maltreated children (Ryan & Wilson 1995b). During these therapeutic encounters, children are able to correct in non-threatening ways previously self-destructive and antisocial adaptations they developed in response to abusive experiences.

The practice of non-directive play therapy, as implied above, entails creating an enhanced play environment in which the toys and materials provided are conducive to symbolic play (see Wilson & Ryan 2005 for a further discussion of the appropriate setting and equipment). This equipment remains the same for each session. The sessions themselves take place at the same time each week and usually last for an hour. We have suggested that a short-term, time-limited intervention, say 10 sessions to begin with, with a review and the possibility of 10 more sessions is a workable arrangement. (Again, see Wilson & Ryan 2005 for an extended discussion of preparation and planning issues.) For more seriously damaged children and adolescents, more sessions may be required. Often, too, these very damaged children may need therapeutic input at key future points in their lives, say during adolescence or when changing schools, or when moving from a shorter-term foster placement to a permanent home.

This regularity of time and place is adhered to in order to promote emotionally troubled children's relaxation and confidence in a new environment. More important still, therapists themselves, in addition to the playroom environment, must convey familiarity easily to children in their initial sessions. Therapists need to communicate appropriate responsiveness to children they meet through their friendly, yet non-directive and non-intrusive, stance during each session (Ryan & Wilson 1995b).

In summary, the practice of non-directive play therapy entails:

- careful preparation and planning to promote children's confidence in trusting themselves to therapy
- the development of a trusting, accepting relationship with children
- empathy and reflection of children's feelings by therapists in a non-threatening manner
- therapists using their own feelings congruently to reflect back to children appropriate responses to their expressed behaviour and feelings
- establishing appropriate therapeutic boundaries.

Working therapeutically within statutory settings

An important consideration in setting up and engaging in play therapy with maltreated children and adolescents is ensuring that all those involved in their care work together to provide a milieu that enables therapeutic progress. Often birth parents, foster carers and residential workers, if children and adolescents are in local authority care, and the key social worker are important figures in supporting therapeutic interventions. This chapter has already argued that children in abusive home environments may be put at further risk if therapy is offered under those conditions. Highly unstable and/or unsuitable care arrangements were also discussed as inappropriate for a referral for therapy. Play therapy cannot insulate children from abusive care. Nor, sadly, can it compensate for inadequate and emotionally neglectful care environments (Ryan *et al.* 1995).

As well as needing a relatively stable and emotionally available attachment figure for their emotional well-being, children and adolescents referred for therapy have additional emotional needs. They often become worried about the unfamiliar relationship they are expected to develop with their therapists, a normal reaction to beginning therapy. In addition, abused and neglected children's anxiety is heightened considerably due to maladaptive parent–child relationships stemming from their previous care history. Acutely troubling thoughts and feelings may emerge during the course of play therapy sessions, and children's and adolescents' behaviour may deteriorate in the shorter term when emotionally difficult issues are being addressed. Patience and hope are required by experienced and sensitive carers at these points in therapy (Ryan & Wilson 1995b, 2000a).

Children and adolescents may also begin to change emotionally by making small changes in their behaviour and self-concept at home and at school. Understanding the significance of such changes, and being responsive to small but meaningful changes, are essential from carers in order to promote therapeutic progress. Carers therefore need emotional flexibility and often deeper levels of understanding of underlying emotional issues of children and adolescents in their care. Social workers and therapists can further help carers understand their essential role in caring for children during therapy sessions. Carers in turn will give valuable information and insight from their own relationships with children to their social workers and therapists. Regular meetings to review progress and to inform one another of key themes emerging in therapy, while respecting confidentiality, are crucial. Therapists and social workers also rely on carers to inform them of key events in children's everyday lives.

Carers – whether birth parents, foster carers or residential workers – may all need additional support, not only from the children's therapist and key social worker, but also from other professionals such as managers, workers from voluntary agencies and fostering social workers, in order to take an active, participatory role in therapeutic change, rather than being passive observers (Ryan & Wilson 2000a). Carers may also be asked to take on a more direct role in the play therapy sessions, either by taking the role of co-therapist or, as mentioned above, by being trained in filial therapy. These options are particularly relevant when young and traumatised children need play therapy, or when children and adolescents exhibit serious attachment problems (Ryan 1999, 2004).

We have argued elsewhere that all adults need to be clear about their different roles and tasks:

[The social worker] retains the overall management of the case … The therapist is there to help resolve conflicts, create understanding and lessen fears; [the carer is the] attachment figure to enable the child to establish and maintain a sense of identity and well-being by providing stability, affirmation of self and a sense of belonging.

(Ryan *et al.* 1995, p. 134)

Social workers may themselves work therapeutically with various family members, such as parental couples in children's birth families. They also may offer appropriate direct work to children in coordination with therapists who are conducting play therapy sessions. There may be a need for increased practical support from social workers, including arranging transport to therapy for children and carers, and increased guidance to carers on behaviour management and on promotion of therapeutic changes.

Therapists initially help carers and social workers at referral to understand their therapeutic role and the aims and practice of non-directive play therapy. For carers and social workers unfamiliar with play therapy, visual material in conjunction with explanations from therapists may be beneficial (see details on a training video at the end of this chapter). Therapists also provide help with therapy-related issues in children's and adolescents' homes and help both the carers and the social workers integrate children's needs and new responses expressed during therapy into everyday life. In addition, school environments need both increased input from children's social workers and direct contact with children's therapists in order to provide children with sensitive care within school and to help children implement therapeutic changes with peers and school staff alike. For some children, school settings can be optimal settings for play therapy sessions, since schools are well placed within families' immediate neighbourhoods and can often be used as community resources (Drewe *et al.* 2001).

Non-directive play therapy with maltreated adolescents

Before illustrating the practice of non-directive play therapy in a statutory setting with a 13-year-old girl who had been sexually abused, the appropriateness of this technique with adolescents will be discussed. Some practitioners state that children aged 12 and over of normal intelligence are unsuitable for non-directive play therapy. The suitability of non-directive play therapy for older pre-adolescent children has also been questioned and a different, more realistic set of games and activities is often made available by play therapists for this age group (Guerney 1984, West 1996).

However, case studies with adolescents are beginning to be documented in the play therapy literature; this approach seems to have advantages over a purely adult counselling relationship (Wilson & Ryan 2002, Gallo-Lopez & Schaefer 2005). We have argued elsewhere that non-directive play therapy is both an effective and theoretically justifiable therapeutic method with troubled adolescents. Briefly, non-directive play therapy can help adolescents integrate earlier childhood experiences, present concerns and future, more adult concerns into their developing sense of unique personal identity. Children and adolescents who have been abused have particular problems in integrating experiences that have been abusive into an emotionally healthy sense of self, as discussed above. When their personal mental schemas have been arrested or distorted, adolescents who have been maltreated find it difficult to rework schemas of their childhood selves and apply them to emotionally healthy ways of functioning in more adult relationships. Not only will their earlier emotional development have been damaging, and parental role models been unhealthy ones, but maltreated adolescents may also have developed difficulties in peer relationships and difficulties in their desire and ability to integrate into wider adult society in an emotionally healthy manner.

Non-directive play therapy can be used to help these adolescents integrate emotionally damaging experiences into their current identities. In order to work effectively with this age group, however, certain practice issues must be considered throughout. While a few more highly structured materials may be desirable for this age group, most materials should still lend themselves to unstructured symbolic activities and play. As with younger age groups, materials (such as art materials, puppets and staging) should be selected that can be used at the highest potential level of adolescent functioning, as well as selecting materials that can be used for much younger, regressive play. Both types of material should be made freely available for adolescents' use. Adult-sized furniture also immediately demonstrates to adolescents that the room is used by a range of ages in which to both sit and talk and to play. These preparations are needed for adolescents because their therapists need to be aware of adolescents' heightened sensitivity and negative reaction to being treated 'only as a child'. At the same time, as with younger children, therapists must enable adolescents to feel a sense of permissiveness in the room which extends to whatever thoughts, activities (or non-activities) and materials adolescents themselves choose. Older children and adolescents can be given the choice of attending progress meetings and therapists can offer to outline the themes they intend to discuss beforehand, during their play therapy sessions, and ask adolescents if they wish to address issues either for themselves or with their therapists' help during these meetings.

Furthermore, concerns over privacy and confidentiality are often greater for adolescents than for younger children. A private room without any outside interruptions and which is not overlooked is particularly necessary for adolescents, who may be more self-conscious of others' reactions to their sessions and will only manage to engage freely with the materials and therapist in private. Another related area of concern to adolescents may be anxiety about peers' and other outside adults' interest in therapy sessions, and others' possible misuse of this information by getting teased or being labelled as different or deranged. Again, therapists must be sensitive to arranging sessions at times which minimise potential intrusions (e.g. lunch-time or after school). With children and adolescents who have been maltreated, privacy may be an even more sensitive issue. Too much privacy in one-to-one interactions may be reminiscent of abusive experiences, or this intimacy may direct adolescents' attention too painfully to gaps and discrepancies in their other significant adult relationships. In these cases, individual therapeutic interventions may not be possible, and other interventions may be more appropriate initially, such as group work or family work.

Another important related concern is the extent to which therapists can assure adolescents that the content of sessions will remain private. It is essential, however, that children and adolescents who have been maltreated are given permission explicitly by their therapists to reveal whatever contents of sessions children and adolescents choose to others in close relationships. Otherwise, again, therapeutic relationships may too closely mirror previously abusive ones. Of course, it is impossible, and indeed misleading, for therapists to guarantee complete confidentiality. All therapists must consider issues of confidentiality in light of their professional obligation to report disclosures of abuse made within therapy sessions. Added considerations for therapists working in statutory settings include the kind of communication to be established with carers, the type of information from sessions which will be shared with referring agencies through case conferences and reports, and the level of detail to reveal in court proceedings (Ryan & Wilson 1995a, Wilson & Ryan 2005).

While younger children may have more difficulty understanding the circumstances under which therapists must discuss their sessions with others, adolescents are usually able to understand these issues. However, adolescents may also feel a heightened need for confidentiality from their therapists, compared with younger children. In particular, children and adolescents who have been maltreated may want complete confidentiality, having often been previously subjected to different forms of threats and coercions by abusing adults to ensure the secrecy of the abuse, and thus the abuser's freedom from detection and punishment. This need for security and exclusivity can be generalised to any close relationship with an adult, including individual therapy. In addition, abuse often engenders feelings of shame and guilt, both feelings that can be heightened when others learn of their difficulties stemming from abuse.

It is imperative, therefore, that therapists discuss confidentiality issues and recording procedures with adolescents (and with young children, in keeping within their understanding) at the beginning of their time together. If this discussion is omitted, adolescents may falsely believe, in keeping with their needs, that their therapists are offering complete confidentiality. Adolescents may then be less guarded and, justifiably, feel betrayed when their therapists must report general sessional themes or specific abusive incidents to others. With abused adolescents (and children), mistrust of adults or overly trusting responses are already likely to be a crucial feature of their emotional difficulties. Their therapists will be likely to increase this emotional damage if issues of confidentiality are not addressed honestly and sensitively from the start.

Using non-directive play therapy with an adolescent who had been sexually abused

Patricia was 13 years old at the time of referral for play therapy sessions. Her initial appearance was of a self-assured, verbally aggressive and articulate older adolescent. She was physically mature, attractive and careful about her appearance. Patricia had disclosed sexual abuse by her uncle and later by her stepfather as well, but she was disbelieved and blamed for the resulting investigation by her family, which included her mother, stepfather, 16-year-old sister and 6-year-old half-brother. Patricia's extended family had already been investigated for sexual abuse. From the case notes on file, the atmosphere in these related families seemed to be highly sexualised, with a blurring of adult–child role boundaries and a failure to maintain sexual boundaries between generations.

When Patricia began to attend play therapy sessions, which took place for an hour once a week over a 3-month period (15 sessions altogether), she had been separated from her family and placed in foster care because of the continuing risk to her of sexual abuse. Several key themes which were important to Patricia emotionally emerged during her play therapy sessions. These themes illustrate many of the points raised earlier about the value of non-directive play therapy in working with adolescents and children who have been maltreated. The way in which therapists work within statutory settings will also be illustrated in this case example of Patricia. Two important themes for Patricia in her sessions, to be discussed below, include her therapist's trustworthiness and her reworking of childhood memories and distortions of bodily image arising from sexual abuse. (For a more extended discussion of these themes, see Ryan & Wilson 2000a.)

Theme one: her therapist's trustworthiness

A key theme for Patricia throughout her sessions was whether her therapist was a trustworthy and reliable adult. This issue seemed to have strong emotional salience for her because of her emotional development within an abusive family atmosphere. She shared her family's mistrust of and anger with any professional in a role of authority and was particularly vehement about social services' interventions which investigated sexual abuse. Patricia repeatedly blamed social services for removing her from home, yet she also began to express surprise during her sessions that her statements about sexual abuse had been believed by professionals despite her family's denials. Another conflict for Patricia was that while she desperately wanted to return home, and later in therapy expressed a longing to return to her pre-school existence within her family, she was at the same time deeply hurt by her family's rejection of her. In the process of therapy, Patricia began to consciously acknowledge to herself that her family often distorted information given to her, to other family members and to professionals, as well as keeping secret from her much about the extended family's complicated and disturbed relationships. Patricia's growing ability to examine her family's attitudes was made possible not only by the permissive atmosphere of her therapy sessions, but also by her therapist's predictable and caring responses to Patricia's verbal statements and reflection of her quickly changing and conflicting feelings. Patricia seemed to use her therapist increasingly as an anchor for thinking about her family and herself.

Confidentiality was an important, recurring theme for Patricia and an important element in the development of a trusting relationship with her therapist. Patricia tested out with her therapist the level of confidentiality of her sessions with other professionals, often aggressively challenging her therapist on whether her social worker would be informed of what she was doing in the sessions. Towards the end of their sessions together, when Patricia's level of trust in her therapist had increased, she confided that she had not told her therapist earlier about several of the dangerous games she had been playing with peers because she had enjoyed having secrets from her therapist. Besides, she was certain that her therapist would have told her social worker or the police. Her therapist reflected Patricia's feelings, that it was fun to feel more powerful early on by having secrets from adults who were trying to know just about everything about you. Her therapist also acknowledged that Patricia was right. As an adult with some responsibility for Patricia, her therapist would have tried to prevent Patricia from seriously harming herself and others, and might have had to tell others.

Patricia also spent an inordinate amount of time speculating about other younger children who used the room. While this topic was related to Patricia retrieving her childhood memories, which are discussed below, she also seemed both intrigued and challenged by her therapist's rule of confidentiality regarding other children's use of the playroom. Patricia returned to this topic often, used a variety of persuasive arguments, and even resorted to a younger child's wheedling tone in her attempts to test out her therapist's resolve in keeping this rule. Her therapist said repeatedly that she must maintain confidentiality for other children as well as for Patricia, thus enforcing a necessary therapeutic limit. Her therapist also reflected Patricia's varied feelings, including a genuine interest and concern for the younger children who needed therapy, and a belief that if she was persistent, her therapist would weaken and do something she felt was wrong. Patricia's use of more abstract thinking on this issue allowed her therapist to reflect Patricia's feelings back to her at each occurrence, to subordinate personal feelings of harassment when Patricia adopted manipulative means to weaken her resolve, to state her own position to Patricia clearly and to give reasons for her position that Patricia at 13 years old could understand. Using this non-directive approach, Patricia actively engaged in a process common to normal adolescence, but usually engaged in with lesser intensity. That is, Patricia was examining and understanding her own values and how these differed from both the values of her therapist and the values of her own family. Therefore, for Patricia, her therapist represented the adult world of values in a very direct, interactive sense, with Patricia gradually developing trust in her therapist, albeit somewhat grudgingly.

Theme two: Patricia's reworking of childhood memories and distortions in bodily image resulting from sexual abuse

While the first theme seems to rely heavily on non-directive counselling skills rather than play therapy *per se*, it is important in understanding Patricia's progress in therapy to note that from her first session onwards Patricia was purposeful in choosing an activity to perform with her hands while she talked. Patricia seemed to have no difficulty accepting the play setting or materials as appropriate for her age. (Her initial worries instead centred on her own use of the materials, which she considered to be inept and 'babyish', and on being ridiculed by peers for needing therapy at all.) She decided to use the clay and spent her early sessions, and a few sessions towards the end of her 15 sessions, modelling in this medium. Her early work in clay consisted of forming simple clay figures and using her hands to work them into smooth curves and then squeezing them shapeless again as she concentrated on verbal exchanges with her therapist.

After her initial play with the clay as an adjunct to her conversation, Patricia began to concentrate more intently on her ongoing activity using her hands, and her talking with her therapist lost prominence. Motor activities and sensations became central, and Patricia began to cover her hands completely with smooth wet clay, allowing it to harden before washing it off and restoring her hands to their usual clean, well-manicured condition. Her therapist reflected Patricia's feelings and hypothesised to herself (and not to Patricia, as an insight-oriented therapist may have done) that perhaps Patricia was beginning to rework on a motor and affective level using symbolic means, the abusive masturbatory experiences she had disclosed during her earlier investigative interview. Along with the clay, Patricia also began to use the playdough in the room and to remember several happy times in her earlier childhood when she had enjoyed similar play and felt well looked after by her mother.

Following these play sequences, Patricia began to experiment with finger paints, first covering her hands with bright, vivid colours and then coating them repeatedly with more colours until they turned a sticky, dark brown. This process of covering her hands in thick layers of sticky paint lasted for several sessions, with Patricia using her whole body in a diffuse, sensual way. Her therapist reflected Patricia's feelings of how good the process felt at the beginning; however, it never stopped there. Patricia had to make her hands messier, even though they weren't as nice as at the beginning. Her therapist also reflected Patricia's disgust with her transformed hands by the end of her play, followed by her anxiety over needing to quickly make her hands perfect again.

Patricia's actions became less frantic and of shorter duration during sessions, as she continued to rework what appeared to be her abusive experiences on this symbolic level. Her therapist made occasional reflections, but Patricia, while continuing her activities without constraint, did not herself verbalise her feelings and actions during this time. However, she did verbally express great concern that her therapist would keep the paints ready for her use, for as long as she needed them. After several sessions Patricia finished completely with the finger paints and chose to return to her earlier medium of clay. It is interesting to note that Patricia's intense and prolonged play with finger paints paralleled changes in her appearance. She became more casual in her dress, then decided to change her hairstyle and generally became younger looking and more similar in appearance to other young adolescents. It seemed that by reworking her abusive experiences on a motor and affective level in symbolic play, Patricia had transformed her previously distorted mental schemas involving her body and its actions into more age-appropriate ones.

Statutory considerations in Patricia's therapy

In this chapter, general considerations of the therapist's role in working with other professionals within statutory settings have been outlined. This section illustrates the ways Patricia's therapist worked in partnership with her carers and other professionals involved in her life.

Patricia's social worker, Matthew, had been given leave by the court to release court papers, including chronologies and witness statements, to her therapist before she began therapeutic work. The therapist also received a letter of instructions from the court agreed by all parties involved in ongoing care proceedings to provide a report on Patricia's therapeutic progress and make recommendations for her future therapeutic needs after 10 weekly sessions with her.

Patricia's therapist read the court documents released to her prior to her referral meeting with Matthew. At their meeting she familiarised Matthew with her method of therapy and requested an additional document on an earlier psychiatric assessment of Patricia. They had a preliminary discussion of practical arrangements for therapy, including the time of day suitable to Patricia, her therapist and her foster carers, who would be asked to accompany Patricia to her sessions. Matthew discussed his ongoing involvement with Patricia's family, which currently was of serious concern to him. His numerous attempts to engage Patricia's mother in actively cooperating with him in protecting her children from the possible abusive relationship they had with her partner had, he considered, been largely unsuccessful. Her mother was hostile to him and viewed his requirements of supervised contact by herself and her partner with Patricia as coercive, all described in his court statement.

Matthew had already informed the therapist in their initial referral conversation that Patricia's foster placement was stable, potentially long term, and seemed to be meeting her physical and emotional needs adequately. However, Patricia's future remained uncertain, since it was dependent on the outcome of her care proceedings. Patricia appeared relatively accepting of their care in the shorter term; however, she had repeatedly told him that she wanted to return to her mother's care.

Patricia's therapist clarified her own position: any serious child protection concerns would first of all be raised with Patricia and then reported quickly to Matthew; she would introduce herself to Patricia's mother, foster carers and Patricia herself in the presence of her foster carers in separate meetings prior to beginning her work. Matthew would be an important part of progress meetings with Patricia's carers, and other options of including the school, Patricia's birth mother and Patricia herself at these meetings would be reviewed with Matthew after these introductory meetings (see Wilson & Ryan 2005, Chapter 5, Planning and assessment).

The therapist's initial meeting with Patricia's mother appeared to preclude the development of a cooperative relationship between them at this stage in court proceedings. Her mother stated that she and Patricia were coerced into being involved with the therapist by social services and that it would do no good. It was Patricia's lies and defiance which were the issues, not any emotional problems. Her therapist attempted to redefine Patricia's problems, but her mother was not receptive to this alteration. The therapist also explained her role as external to social services and Patricia's mother forcefully replied that in that case the therapist needed to support her request to social services for unsupervised access to Patricia. When the therapist empathised with the mother's feelings but felt unable to support her request, Patricia's mother refused to consider further meetings.

The foster carers were, on the other hand, very eager to be involved in Patricia's therapy, and immediately understood the need for Patricia to have their emotional support before and after therapy sessions; they were interested in developing their understanding of important emotional issues for Patricia. They also stated that Patricia might want to be included as part of these meetings, but wondered if she would be able to tolerate her social worker's presence. Her therapist planned to discuss this with Patricia during their session prior to the first scheduled progress meeting, and after they had begun to establish an initial therapeutic relationship together.

Patricia's foster carers became an important link for Patricia between her therapy sessions and her day-to-day life. Patricia initially refused to attend progress meetings, but wished to know the exact details of the first meeting. Her therapist and foster carers willingly shared these details with her, as they had agreed at the meeting, and Patricia then chose to attend the later progress meetings. She became able to tolerate the tension engendered in her by Matthew's presence at these meetings with the help of her foster carers and her therapy sessions. The options of including the foster social worker and school in these meetings were not taken up, since the social worker and foster carers felt they were maintaining adequate working partnerships with them. The adults also agreed that Patricia would have found widening the number of adult professionals attending their progress meetings to include school and fostering an added complexity that would be difficult for her to cope with easily.

Summary

Therapeutic work with Patricia was used to illustrate how adolescents in non-directive play therapy commonly combine symbolic play with talking to their therapists, who in turn need to employ non-directive counselling skills more intensively for this older age group. A core skill in working with both children and adolescents is their therapists' ability to reflect children's or adolescents' feelings during sessions in an accurate, yet non-threatening manner. Therapists must also have developed a coherent, personally meaningful and viable theoretical framework for therapeutic practice, as outlined in this chapter, to allow the use of personal feelings congruently in making appropriate, emotionally normal responses to children's and adolescents' expressed behaviour and feelings.

Conclusions

This chapter has argued that non-directive play therapy provides practitioners with a theoretically rich and coherent system of therapy based on developmental principles. This feature, along with its non-coercive and non-intrusive nature, provides the rationale for using non-directive play therapy as a preferred method of therapy with children and adolescents who have been maltreated. While play therapy is evidence based and research shows that in general it is effective for children, more definitive research on process and outcome issues in non-directive play therapy for the UK, particularly in statutory settings, is urgently needed.

It is important that qualified play therapists with active membership in their professional organisation nationally are employed in working with this vulnerable group of clients. In addition to employing skilled and qualified professional play therapists, the effectiveness of such interventions is dependent upon non-abusive, relatively stable and responsive care environments. Professionals and carers all have vital roles to coordinate in play therapy interventions. This chapter also argues that non-directive therapy, by being sensitive to age-related issues, can be an effective intervention for adolescents as well as children. To illustrate this method of therapy for young people within statutory settings, a case example of a young adolescent who had been sexually abused was presented.

Key points and messages for practice

- Non-directive play therapy is a viable and non-intrusive method of working with children and adolescents who have been maltreated. Theory, research and practice show the efficacy and strengths of this therapeutic approach, but more detailed research is needed on therapy with looked-after and adopted children and young people.

- When children have been previously mistreated, distortions in adult–child relationships may arise and be maintained even in non-abusive environments when children have been maltreated previously, indicating the need for therapy.

- Non-directive play therapy addresses children's emotional adaptations developed in abusive environments both directly and indirectly. Children are helped intensively to develop healthier adult–child relationships. In addition, the choice of issues, the pace of change and the choice of play contents and actions in the playroom are determined by children themselves, rather than by their therapists or other adults.

- Non-directive play therapy is a systemic and developmentally sensitive approach to helping children, young people and their families. Carers can be included in either indirect or direct ways in interventions.

- Child protection concerns, care decisions and court proceedings – including children as witnesses – are all important considerations at referral for therapy and during therapeutic interventions.

- Therapists, carers, schools and social workers all need to work within their specified roles to meet the emotional needs of looked-after children and young people. Social workers are key to supporting successful play therapy and will need to maintain involvement in the therapeutic process.

- Social workers should consider play therapy is a viable treatment option for young people on their case load, as well as for children. Adolescents are able to address their concerns experientially as well as verbally during this form of expressive therapy.

- Social workers and their managers need to ensure that play therapists are qualified professionals meeting national professional standards. The British Association of Play Therapists' website and register should be referred to for therapists' qualifications.

Useful addresses and websites (including training information)

British Association of Play Therapists (BAPT)
31 Cedar Drive
Bristol BS31 2TY
Tel/fax: 01179 860390
Email: info@bapt.uk.com
Website: www.bapt.uk.com

Training leading to a professional qualification
MA/Diploma in Non-directive Play Therapy (BAPT approved)
Department of Social Policy and Social Work
University of York
Heslington, York YO10 5DD
Tel: 01904 321 235
Fax: 01904 321 270
Website: www.york.ac.uk/depts/spsw/pt/ptwelcome.htm
(This programme may also lead on to further study and registration for a PhD.)

Annotated further reading

Axline V 1987 Play therapy, revised edn. Ballantine Books, New York
A general introduction to play therapy including Axline's eight principles.

Carroll J 1998 Introduction to therapeutic play. Blackwell Science, Oxford
A well-written and accessible introduction to this topic for professionals interested in the use of play. There is a chapter on non-directive play therapy which gives a general overview of this approach.

Reddy L A, Files-Hall T M, Schaefer C E (eds) 2005 Empirically based play interventions for children. American Psychological Association, Washington, DC
The first book of its kind providing empirically validated play interventions for children and families with emotional difficulties.

Ryan V, Wilson K 2000 Case studies in non-directive play therapy. Jessica Kingsley, London
Non-directive play therapy is explained by the use of cases to illustrate theory and practice.

Ryan V, Wilson K 2000 Playing matters. Department of Social Policy and Social Work, University of York, York
This video is intended for play therapy training and as an aid to carers and professionals in understanding non-directive play therapy, with an accompanying booklet. Illustrations of non-directive techniques with untroubled children and carers are provided.

Wilson K, Ryan V 2005 Play therapy: a non-directive approach for children and adolescents, 2nd edn. Baillère Tindall, Edinburgh
An updated extension of theory and practice in non-directive play therapy, including a chapter on maltreatment and play therapy.

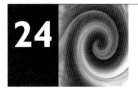

24 Parenting issues and practice in safeguarding children

Brigid Daniel and Catriona Rioch⁻

INTRODUCTION

This is a time of unprecedented change in the development of parenting work. A raft of policy initiatives and legislative changes across the UK both inform and drive this agenda. This is resulting in parenting achieving a high profile in the media as well as in the political arena. In this chapter we give a brief overview of the main policy initiatives, present some of the key research findings relating to parenting and offer some practice suggestions. We include short quotes from parents who took part in a study evaluating parent support projects to illustrate some of the issues (Burgess 2005).

Legislative and policy context

In the UK policy documents set ambitious expectations on behalf of children. So, for England, the policy is that 'children should have the support they need to:

■ be healthy
■ stay safe
■ enjoy and achieve
■ make a positive contribution
■ achieve economic well-being' (DfES 2004b).

These lists of outcomes for children are based on current understanding about children's developmental needs and the assessment framework for England and Wales is structured in such a way as to draw a very clear link between children's developmental needs and parenting capacity to meet them (DoH 2000e). The main 'tasks' of parenting are set out as:

■ Basic care
■ Ensuring safety
■ Emotional warmth
■ Stimulation
■ Guidance and boundaries
■ Stability.

The policy vision is for a continuum of services built upon the firm foundation of support for parents (DfES 2004b). The aspiration is that support should be on offer to assist parents and that the state should only take on more direct responsibility for the well-being of children when parenting falters either because of omission or commission.

The Children Act 1989 and Children (Scotland) Act 1995 form the basis of legislation of work with parents in that they enshrine the main principles:

- that the welfare of the child should be paramount in the context of care and protection of children
- that the concept of parental responsibilities has to be set alongside the concept of parental rights.

The Children Act 2004 and proposals for change in Scotland (Scottish Executive 2005) reflect the government's vision of improving outcomes for children. They contain key messages about improved coordination and joint working between services, early intervention, local accessible services for children and families, greater consultation with service users and increased accountability of agencies to both deliver services and take responsibility for the protection of children. They introduce common or integrated assessment frameworks promoting more effective sharing of information and one plan of action for each child.

The United Nations Statement on the Rights of the Child outlines children's rights in relation to survival, care and protection. It upholds children's right to a family life and places a duty on governments to provide parents with 'material assistance' and relevant support, where needed, to enable them to fulfil their responsibilities to their children. It is important to recognise that children have needs as well as rights, and these include good and consistent basic physical care, affection and security, new experiences which help them to develop, positive guidance and control and increasing responsibility which develops autonomy. These are the things parents need to be able to provide for their children.

Having a clear understanding of what children need from their parents helps to inform when support or intervention is necessary and it is recognised that there is a need to achieve seamless and more effective support for children and their families. A number of legislative and strategic guidance documents such as the Crime and Disorder Act 1998, the Antisocial Behaviour (Scotland) Act 2004 and *Health for all Children* (Hall & Elliman 2003) emphatically promote parenting education as an important contributor to child and family well-being. A number of other legislative and policy initiatives have been put in place to address the support needs of families, promote effective multi-agency working and ensure improvement in the lives of children. These include:

- Sure Start
- National Service Framework for Children, Young People and Maternity Services (DoH/DfES 2004)
- Every Child Matters (DfES 2004b)
- Hidden Harm (Home Office 2003b)
- The Children's Fund
- Children's Trusts
- Child Protection Reform Programme (Scotland)
- Integrated Children's Service Plans (Scotland).

Refocusing of services is at the heart of many recent policy and legislative changes. To that end recent legislative and policy initiatives across the UK are focused on changing the way services are provided to children and families to improve their well-being, to safeguard and promote their welfare, to identify and protect those at risk of significant harm, and to improve accessibility of services by families as well as improving outcomes for children. The Darlington Social Research Unit outlines how services over the last decade have increased attempts to protect children from maltreatment by the provision of family support, while ensuring effective

Table 24.1
Historical refocusing of services

Refocusing from	Refocusing to
Residential care	Family-based foster care
Supporting children away from home	Supporting children in their home environment
Separate services for children at risk of social, health and psychological problems	Mainstreaming services so that they can support all children, including those at risk
Separate processes for child protection and family support	Using family support as a primary mechanism to protect children from harm

(Reproduced with permission from Axford & Little 2004.)

intervention for those harmed by their parents (Axford & Little 2004). The authors clarify that the main theme in *Every Child Matters* is to set out a broader vision for family support. They produced a helpful table outlining this, within the context of the historical refocusing of services (Table 24.1). It should be noted, however, that they clearly argue that in refocusing services acute and restorative services will always be needed.

Such developments support the premise that parenting work should be set within the context of an overarching framework of tiered levels of intervention, including universal, early intervention, treatment and tertiary provision. As parents, children and families have diverse needs, there needs to be a 'menu' of services available which address the key messages as described above. This is also in the spirit of the existing guidelines which emphasise the need to view child protection within the context of family support (DoH *et al.* 1999). The vision, therefore, is for a more measured, focused approach by all agencies to avoid duplication of services and ensure direct work is undertaken with families, is coordinated and will achieve the maximum impact. Above all, it is essential that the main focus of all parenting work has to be on what will achieve the best outcomes for children and young people.

Underpinning the policies and legislation are some key messages:

- the importance of early intervention (not necessarily early in a child's life but at the point of needs emerging)
- the need for integrated working and planning
- all agencies have responsibility to provide accessible services which support parents in their parenting responsibilities
- the need for some refocusing of service provision
- the need for the provision of more accessible services for children and families.

These strands of policy and theory need to be transferred into the strategic planning of parenting services within the context of child protection, the engagement of parents and the implementation of direct practice.

It is important to remember that being a parent is a complex and demanding task requiring a level of understanding about self and others which is not automatic. It requires an evolving repertoire of behaviours that are congruent with children's changing developmental needs. Therefore, it is the case that *all* parents need information, help or support with parenting at some point.

There is a huge amount of variation across services in aim and type of provision. Some services, such as health visiting, have traditionally been offered on a universal basis, but these are increasingly becoming targeted. Most parenting programmes are, to an extent, targeted either geographically (e.g. in areas of multiple deprivation) or on particular groups perceived to be vulnerable (e.g. young parents).

Multiple difficulties in families, which have accrued over time, need planned, assessed and long-term solutions if lasting change is to be made (Sutton *et al.* 2004). For families such as these, who have complex or multifaceted difficulties, parenting support alone may not be sufficient. Some parents will need access to adult support services to meet their own needs and increase their sense of self-efficacy before they can address the parenting task. Where abuse or neglect has been substantiated there has to be a clear protection and support plan that incorporates close attention to the parental issues and sets out how they will be addressed.

Parental views on the most effective services

A number of studies have gathered parental views about what they want from services. This is crucial information since, if the aim is to prevent problems from escalating into abusive or neglectful situations, services must be perceived as accessible and valuable.

Quinton (2004) brought together findings about parent support needs from a number of studies. One of the overarching themes was the message from parents that they wanted services to be practical and professional, to listen to them and take their views seriously, to treat them as partners and to be emotionally supportive. Grimshaw and McGuire (1998) identified some key aspects of parenting programmes that are important for stakeholders, including the need to ensure that there is access for everyone, that parents can all feel included in the group and can share their experiences, and that views of children are attended to.

Ghate and Hazel (2002) focused on the particular adversity of living in poor environments and asked about both semi-formal and formal services. Parents wanted services to be more accessible, for example with extended opening hours and short waiting lists. Accessibility was a big problem for formal services and parents said how difficult it is to get prompt and appropriate help for issues such as children's behaviour problems, truanting and ill-health. Parents especially wanted more information about what to expect as 'normal' behaviour in children, how to deal with behaviour problems, education issues and different types of discipline.

One important message from Ghate and Hazel's study concerns the link between the use of informal, semi-formal and formal services. The study showed that semi-formal and formal services did not tend to be turned to as compensation for lack of informal help. Instead a pattern emerges where 'some parents appear to have relatively high "consumption" levels across all dimensions of social support while others have low consumption levels' (Ghate & Hazel 2002, p. 151). It is the experience of many child care and protection workers that parents who are most in need of assistance often fail to seek it, or to make use of it once it is offered. Baldwin has proposed that parents need 'supports' to enable them to access services and 'bridges' to enable them to move between universal and more targeted services as the level of need fluctuates (Baldwin & Spencer 2005).

I was glad to meet the course leader a couple of times before we started. If I hadn't felt comfortable with her I wouldn't have gone.

(Quote from a parent; Burgess 2005)

Assessment of parenting capacity

The common thread in current understanding about parenting is the centrality of secure attachment relationships (Howe 1996, 2005, Howe *et al.*1999). The bonding between parent and child and subsequent attachment between the child and parent is now recognised as the driver for associated parenting activities. The accumulated evidence makes it clear that secure attachments are promoted if care-givers are sensitive and responsive to babies' emotional cues and if they initiate positive interactions with their babies. There is also evidence that it is very damaging for children to experience parenting that is 'low on warmth and high on criticism' (DoH 1995a). The linked concept of resilience is now also gaining currency as a useful framework for understanding individual differences of developmental trajectories in the context of adversity (Gilligan 2001, Daniel & Wassell 2002). This concept is therefore particularly helpful when considering children who are experiencing the undoubted adversity of abuse or neglect. A main emergent message from a number of empirical studies of resilience is that it is underpinned by the presence of supportive parenting that promotes secure attachments (Luthar & Zelazo 2003). When children lack secure attachment, other factors then become important, including wider community supports and good school experiences.

Beyond the fundamental building block of secure attachment it becomes increasingly difficult to pin down parenting and the associated roles and tasks. Parenting is carried out in many different ways within and across cultures. At the same time, by virtue of their differing temperaments and characteristics, children themselves help to shape the nature of the parenting environment. It is therefore not really possible to identify one agreed set of parenting activities that can be described as 'optimal'. This contributes to a related problem for practitioners. Just as there is no specific template for optimal parenting, there is no specific template for less than optimal parenting. Despite the considerable body of evidence about child development and how development can be promoted, the child protection system struggles to pin down and define the *absence* of an appropriate parenting environment. Careful assessment of each individual child's circumstances is therefore essential.

A comprehensive review of the literature showed that many factors influence parenting (Centre for Community Child Health 2004). These factors include:

- characteristics of parents such as age, gender and experience
- personal adversity such as substance use
- psychological factors such as stress and mental ill-health
- child characteristics such as temperament and disability
- family factors such as family structure and home environment
- cultural and social factors such as poverty and neighbourhood.

Three key areas that are particularly relevant to child care and protection are explored here.

Impact of poverty

The impact of poverty upon parenting is now well documented (Thoburn *et al.* 2000a, Tuck 2000, Golden *et al.* 2003). It has been graphically described by as having a 'corrosive influence' on family functioning (Jack 2001, Spencer & Baldwin 2005). Its very prevalence is perhaps why it can become invisible to practitioners and why they fail to assess properly its impact upon the family. However, if practitioners fail to appreciate the impact of poverty upon parenting their assessments will be flawed (Jack 2001). The exact impact of poverty on parenting is complex. There are large numbers of people rearing children in situations of deprivation without abusing or neglecting them. There is, therefore, a danger of stigmatising poor parents. The current position tends to coalesce around an interactional model whereby poverty is seen to interact with other psychological, social, emotional or interpersonal problems to drag parenting behaviour down.

Ghate and Hazel (2002) found that parents in poor environments were more likely to have physical ill-health than the general population and an elevated tendency towards depression. Parents with poor emotional or mental health were also more likely to have a child with challenging behaviour. Parents faced a range of stressors including low income, poor accommodation, a greater likelihood of lone parenthood and conflict in the home. Parents were worried about hazards and dangers to their children in the wider environment. The risk factors tended to overlap and their effects were cumulative.

Seaman *et al.* (2005) carried out two linked studies to examine parenting in disadvantaged communities in Scotland. One study gathered parents' views about the threats to their children's safety and well-being and how they sought to protect them from the perceived threats. The other study gathered children's views about their perceptions of the community, the risks therein and the ways in which their parents sought to protect them. The studies found a strong degree of concordance between parents and children of the threats in the environment and children understood why parents wanted to keep them safe. Children also relied on friendship networks for protection from perceived risks. Overall the studies found that the parents were no different from other parents in the general population in their aspirations for their children but that they adopted pragmatic tactics to try to protect their children from dangers in the locality.

Factors affecting mental well-being

Schaffer (1998) describes parental psychiatric illness as one of the 'most potent' risk factors for a child. He highlights the dual predicament of the potential hereditary nature of the problem and the direct impact upon a child of inappropriate childhood experiences. Within the general population the evidence suggests that parental mental ill-health is a significant issue. For example, the impact of the problem is indicated by a large scale, longitudinal study into the impact of childhood adversity upon adult personality being carried out in Australia. Information about childhood domestic adversity and current personality was collected from 7485 people in the community (Rosenman & Rodgers 2004). It was found that childhood adversity more than doubled the risk of adult neuroticism, negative affect and behavioural inhibition: 59.5% reported some form of adversity, with 37% experiencing more than one type. The main adversity reported by subjects was maternal psychological ill-health. The authors of this study highlight the importance of recognising the long-term effects of maternal mental ill-health during childhood.

Cleaver *et al.* (1999) have summarised the data from a number of studies of child abuse to show the extent to which parental mental illness and substantiated abuse or neglect of children are associated with child protection concerns (Table 24.2) (Cleaver & Freeman 1995, Farmer & Owen 1995, Gibbons *et al.* 1995b, Falkov 1996, Hunt *et al.* 1999).

As Cleaver *et al.* (1999) have also illustrated, children who enter the child care and protection system also have a probability of experiencing parental alcohol and drug problems and/or domestic violence. Indeed, many of these factors can coexist for a range of reasons and, when they do, can lead to a potentially very damaging environment for children. The extent of such problems may also be underestimated because not all mental health problems are formally diagnosed. Some mental health problems may be masked by substance misuse and domestic violence is often hidden. Between 200 000 and 300 000 children in England and Wales are estimated to have one or both parents with serious drug problems, which represents 2–3% of the child population. In Scotland the figure rises to 4–6% of children (Home Office

Table 24.2
The relationship between the rate of recorded parental problems and the level of social work intervention

Parental problems	Referral stage (%)	First enquiry (%)	Child protection conference (%)	Care proceedings (%)	Serious injury or death (%)
Mental illness	13	20	25	42	33–90
Alcohol/ illness	20	25	25–60	70	
Domestic violence	27	40	35–55	51	

(Reproduced with permission from Cleaver & Freeman 1995.)

2003b). The figures suggest that practitioners in a range of services for adults and for children will encounter parents whose parenting capacity is affected by one of these factors. Although not all the children will be at direct risk of abuse or neglect, and only a proportion of them will need to be subject to formal child protection proceedings, many will be vulnerable and they and their families would benefit from supportive intervention to prevent problems escalating.

Emotional and cognitive factors

A common theme that emerges from a number of different theoretical strands concerns the impact on parenting of psychological factors and, in particular, the emotional and cognitive processes that affect the way people relate to their children.

Inner working models are a concept from attachment theory and describe the templates of attachment relationships that develop as a result of attachment experiences. These inner working models can influence the way that people relate to others, and in particular how they relate to their children. Adults with insecure inner working models, who have not had the chance to reflect upon their own attachment experiences, may apply these unhelpful templates to the relationships with their own children (Howe 2005). Thus a parent with an avoidant attachment pattern can be made to feel anxious by the child's demands and react by distancing themselves and rejecting attachment advances. A parent with an ambivalent pattern tends to be preoccupied with their own needs and may react very inconsistently to the child's needs depending upon how they feel. Parents with a disorganised pattern tend to have unresolved attachment traumas which cause them fear or anger so that they present to the child as frightened or frightening, either of which can be emotionally damaging.

With cognitive processes, attribution theory aims to explain how people make sense of events and their own and other people's actions. The theory, originally developed by Heider (1958), has since been applied to many different human arenas. Essentially it proposes that people process events in terms of whether the causes are:

- internal or external
- stable or unstable
- global or specific.

Seligman and Peterson (1986) have summed up attributions that can be associated with depression as: 'It's my fault, it's going to last forever, and it's going to affect everything I do.' An example of unhelpful attributions with regard to child care and protection would be a parent who attributes the cause of the baby's crying to internal and stable personality characteristics that will apply in all domains, as in: 'She is deliberately winding me up because she is naughty and I will have trouble with her for years.'

Table 24.3 *The makings of an abusive incident: a four-stage process**	Stage 1:	The parent holds unrealistic standards regarding what are appropriate behaviours in children
	Stage 2:	The parent encounters a child behaviour that fails to meet her standards
	Stage 3:	The parent misattributes negative intent to the behaviour and does not question her interpretation or blames herself when her interventions do not change the child's response
	Stage 4:	The parent over-reacts, perhaps after making some poorly skilled effort to change the child's behaviour and punishes the child excessively

*Movement through the stages may feel 'automatised' and the process is more likely to occur under perceived conditions of stress.
(Reproduced with permission from Azar 1997.)

Azar (1997) has specifically applied elements of both attachment theory and attribution theory to develop a cognitive–behavioural approach to the understanding of, and intervention with, parents who physically abuse their children. She proposes that the quality of the parenting environment can be affected by the parent's 'relational schema', i.e. the cognitive structures which are developed to assist with processing information. These schemas influence how a parent interprets the causes of a child's behaviour. With young children especially it is often necessary to infer the child's motivation and this requires parents to work out the reasons for the child's behaviour. Parents can also help to shape and assist development by the way that they interpret children's behaviour and reflect this back to them. The abuse of children can spring from rigid parental schemas and unrealistic expectations of the capacities of children, often incorporating inappropriate expectations that children will meet their needs. The pathway from such schemas to abuse is illustrated in Table 24.3.

Azar's model is congruent with the concept of 'the meaning of the child' developed by Reder and colleagues as a result of their analysis of the reports into fatal or near fatal child abuse (Reder & Duncan 1995, 1999, Reder *et al.* 1993). The model draws on a range of psychological concepts to explain ways in which a child can gain a particular meaning to the parent. In some circumstances the meaning of the child can contribute to the development of abusive or neglectful parenting, especially when children represent unresolved emotions and are seen as the solution to experiences of loss, isolation and distress.

Trying not to get angry and remembering how bad things about my own childhood have stuck with me and had a lasting effect.

(Quote from a parent; Burgess 2005)

Assessment of parental capacity

It is essential to carry out a detailed multidisciplinary assessment of parenting capacity to guide intervention on behalf of children who are abused or neglected. A range of services will have expertise and knowledge on different factors and their impact. For example, a substance misuse worker could have knowledge of the extent of a parent's drug problem and the impact on the family finances. A housing officer may be aware of the state of the home and whether neighbours are concerned about the physical neglect of the immediate environment. A health visitor will have detailed knowledge of whether a young child is meeting their developmental milestones and a school teacher will know how a child presents at school and the nature of the parent–school contact. A psychologist, psychiatrist or social worker may be in the position to observe the quality of attachments and to gauge how the parental role is interpreted and what meaning the child holds for the parent. Any assessment must not only gather information about the factors that may affect parenting capacity, but must also include detailed description of the quality of a range of parenting behaviours, the emotional atmosphere for the child and any signs that a child's development is being or is likely to be impaired.

The Department of Health *Framework for the Assessment of Children in Need and their Families* assesses parenting within the context of the assessment of the child and the wider social and economic context of the family (DoH 2000e). However, Cleaver *et al.* (2004b) found in their study of the implementation of the Framework that there was a lack of guidance on how the three dimensions of the framework should interact. In addition, workers were uncertain and lacked confidence in analysing the information they had collected.

Donald and Jureidini (2004) propose that the central importance of parenting and parenting capacity should be given greater emphasis in child protection assessments and decision making where abuse has been established. They propose that the main emphasis should be on assessing the parents' ability to understand empathically and give priority to their child's needs. They are critical of the more common approach to assessments which focuses on concrete factors such as social supports, parental knowledge about parenting and child development. They argue that 'adequate parenting requires that the parents be able to meet the challenges posed by their particular child's temperament and development (which may be shaped by the abusive experience)' (p. 5) and parents need to be able to accept and address their own characteristics that impact negatively on their parenting. They focus explicitly on the parental capacity for empathy, the ability to recognise and respond to their children's emotional and developmental needs, parental attributions to the abuse and parental understanding of the resultant trauma that may have occurred to the child. If parenting capacity is assessed as inadequate, they argue that reunification should not be pursued. Instead therapeutic work with the parent may need to be the first step in addressing parental blocks to recognition or appreciation of their child's needs, such as the parent's own experiences of being parented, mental illness, etc. whilst other supports are put in place for the child.

It is very important to assess parental ability and motivation to change. Some parents may appear to want to change but in fact their day-to-day behaviour towards the child will be no different (Reder & Duncan 1999). Horwath and Morrison (2001) have developed a very useful model for assessing the extent to which there is genuine motivation to change. They propose that motivation can be charted on the two dimensions of effort and commitment to change:

- high effort and high commitment to change is genuine commitment to change
- high effort and low commitment to change is compliance imitation or approval seeking
- low effort and high commitment to change is tokenism
- low effort and low commitment to change is dissent or avoidance.

The only way to really gauge whether parents are able and willing to change within a timescale that is appropriate for the child is to monitor very closely whether the child's actual lived experience has improved.

Preventive and targeted parenting programmes

Based on an analysis of the data from studies of 60 home visiting programmes, Sweet and Appelbaum (2004) asked the simple question: 'Is home visiting an effective strategy?' They considered a range of parent and child outcomes and concluded that home visiting could help change parenting attitudes and parenting behaviour and could lead to improved cognitive and socio-emotional outcomes for children. However, they could discern no consistent pattern to draw conclusions about what type of home visiting is most effective and concluded that programmes are 'multifaceted and complex' and have many different direct and indirect goals. They did find, however, that programmes with the primary goal of reducing child abuse were associated with less 'potential' for abuse as measured by events (e.g. number of injuries and accidents needing medical treatment).

Guterman's meta-analysis of 19 studies asks whether targeted or universal home visiting is more effective for the prevention of abuse by comparing population-based and screening-based programmes (Guterman 1999). He found that both types showed positive effects, albeit very modest. Population-based approaches tended to show more favourable results. His three suggested reasons for this difference between population-based and screening-based programmes will resonate with child care and protection practitioners. First he implicates the poor predictive accuracy of psychosocial screening. Screening tends to produce a large number of false positives which means that amongst those targeted will be many parents who would never have gone on to harm their children anyway. The second reason paradoxically points to the efficacy of screening in that he suggests that some programmes may screen in families who are simultaneously at risk but also less amenable to change. Finally, he suggests that the families targeted by screening may need a different kind of service from that which is offered in home visiting. In particular, he suggests that home visiting services may not be equipped to deal with entrenched problems such as substance misuse and domestic violence.

Some studies have tried to isolate the most effective theoretical underpinning for parenting programmes. One broad-based systematic review of parent education programmes considered 18 studies and concluded that those based on a behavioural approach were most effective, especially if augmented with problem solving (Barlow 1999). The evidence about the benefits of cognitive–behavioural approaches across a range of services and professions is accumulating.

Cognitive–behavioural approaches to intervention build on the theory that unhelpful feelings and behaviours can spring from the way the world is understood and thought about. As described above, problems with parenting can be linked with underlying thoughts. For example, when a child has a tantrum in a supermarket the parent's automatic thought may be: 'Everyone is looking at me and thinking I am a useless parent and a useless person.' The cognitive–behavioural approach to intervention would help people to identify such thoughts and to replace them with different ones, such as: 'Many of the people who are looking at me are parents themselves and they are feeling empathy with me as they remember all the times their toddler had a tantrum in a supermarket.'

Our relationship is more positive as I am more confident. Before I was worried that I was being bad to him.

(Quote from a parent; Burgess 2005)

These approaches have been incorporated into many parenting programmes. For example, in one 'Mellow Parenting' programme, groups of mothers who are depressed are encouraged to help each other identify such thoughts and think of different ones. Group participants are then asked to do 'homework' in which they are asked to reflect on moments of difficulty in parenting, to write down the feeling and behaviour, to identify the underlying thought and then to imagine what suggestions the group would come up with for a replacement thought (Puckering 2005).

It was good to be in a group. It was a good size and everyone took part and were helpful to each other. We all had similar problems.

(Quote from a parent; Burgess 2005)

The Webster-Stratton programmes are some of the most extensively evaluated. Not only are they underpinned by learning theory, they also incorporate considerable attention to the nature of engagement with the parent (Webster-Stratton 1999). The programmes aim to increase positive and nurturing parenting, while at the same time decreasing negative or harsh parenting using a range of approaches including video-taped vignettes. The basic parenting programme covers issues such as how to play with the child, the art of effective praising, use of rewards, limit setting and handling misbehaviour. The groups aim to help parents to develop problem-solving skills using cognitive–behavioural approaches. For example, parents are helped to reduce their negative attributions about themselves and their children. The collaborative approach that runs through the programmes appears to contribute to the positive outcomes for children's social competence.

We tried the ideas about trying to avoid being angry and letting things escalate. We had homework to do. There were ingenious and relevant ideas.

(Quote from a parent; Burgess 2005)

However, one of the emerging concerns with parenting programmes that are based on a purely behavioural approach is the extent to which behavioural strategies such as 'time-out' and 'ignoring' can be used in the service of abuse by parents who are unable to identify empathetically with their children. In these circumstances, the above behavioural strategies may simply be used to replace shouting and smacking as the medium of abuse (Barlow & Stewart-Brown 2005). Practitioners, therefore, need to be alert to this potential when encouraging parents to take part in such programmes.

Parenting support needs to be available not only for parents of children in the early years, but also throughout primary school and for parents of teenagers; services for parents of older children are, however, in short supply. The challenges of effective parenting change as children develop, with the teenage years usually proving the most difficult, particularly when young people have suffered trauma in their early years. In tackling the maturational tasks of adolescence, feelings and memories of previous abuse or neglect may be reawakened.

It would be good to have follow-up because if you're doing well you get less support. But it can still be difficult so I will need support as he gets older.

(Quote from a parent; Burgess 2005)

There are lessons about working with parents of older children from research in the youth justice field. The Youth Justice Board's Parenting Programme has been evaluated over a period of 3 years, following the introduction of Parenting Orders in England and Wales (Youth Justice Board 2003). The evaluation considered the process of setting up and implementing projects which offered services to parents and measured the outcomes in terms of their impact on parents and young people in 34 out of 42 new parenting projects. At least in the short term, there were positive changes in parenting skills and competencies in:

- improved communication with their child
- improved supervision and monitoring of young people's activities
- reduction in the frequency of conflict with young people and better approaches to handling conflict when it arose

- better relationships, including more praise and approval of their child, and less criticism and loss of temper
- feeling better able to influence young people's behaviour
- feeling better able to cope with parenting in general.

Parents communicated positively about the skills and approach by the workers. Evidence from the evaluation suggested that the combination of a genuinely supportive ethos to the service, staff's skills and parents' real need for support overcame the initial hostility some of the parents felt due to the statutory requirement to attend.

I knew I needed to learn to improve my parenting skills. The girls are important to me. Sometimes it's just easier to lay into them.

(Quote from a parent; Burgess 2005)

Intervention where abuse or neglect has been substantiated

It is not possible to provide comprehensive guidance on intervention with parents when abuse and neglect has been substantiated because of the range of potential circumstances (but see other chapters in this volume, e.g. Ryan, Chapter 23, for further discussion). If the decision is for the child to remain at home, then the focus of work has to be on ensuring that they are provided with the conditions within which to thrive safely. Often such intervention requires a package of support for parents and children. When the plan is to provide intensive support for parents it is vital to ensure that there is careful monitoring of the actual experience of the child because there can be a danger of assuming that intervention with the parents will automatically improve the child's life – this assumption is dangerous.

Howe and colleagues offer extensive guidance for intervention guided by principles of attachment (Howe *et al.* 1999, Howe 2005). First it is important to assess the parent's own relationship history, including their memories of attachment histories and the impact on their thoughts and feelings about attachment. It is then necessary to consider the impact that this attachment history has upon the parenting environment, i.e. the quality and characteristics of the caregiving, including the type of nurturing and discipline patterns. Finally, the child's attachment style can be assessed from the observation of the attachment behaviour in relation to the parent. Intervention with the adult would focus on offering the parent the opportunity to reflect upon their own attachment history so that they can gain some insight into the feelings that the attachment behaviour of the child may provoke. The parent's empathy with the child can be encouraged, with the aim of supporting the parent to develop 'mind-mindedness'. Parents who are mind-minded show an interest in the child's mental states and are sensitive to their internal thoughts and feelings. Parents can be supported to develop such mind-mindedness in the context of a trusting therapeutic relationship.

I did get to understand things from my kids' point of view.

(Quote from a parent; Burgess 2005)

Parental resilience is affected by both personality and environmental factors. Resilience is associated with having a good sense of self-efficacy and self-esteem. In other words, parents need to feel that they can make choices and that they can have some control over the trajectory of their lives. It is also associated with having social support and being able to call on support when needed. As Ghate and Hazel's (2002) study showed, some people appear to be more able to make use of support of all kinds than others. Parents who lack support and are isolated may need to learn how to make use of potential support. Some guidelines for the promotion of resilience are summarised by Luthar and Zelazo (2003). They stress that it is important to maximise user involvement and work alongside informal supports. Intervention should address parental mental health and parent–child relationships. Intervention needs to start early, to continue over the long term and to build the capacity to sustain the changes after intervention.

Cognitive–behavioural approaches

As with the broader cognitive–behavioural approaches incorporated into parenting programmes, the principles can be drawn on in intervention with individual families when abuse and neglect have been substantiated. Azar (1997) describes the process of 'cognitive restructuring' that aims to assist a parent to consider the way that their thoughts are linked with actions and to help them replace those thoughts with ones more attuned to the child's stage of development. One example she gives is the replacement of the thought, 'He knew what he was doing' with 'He's only 2, he doesn't know any better.' Table 24.4 illustrates some of the distorted cognitions that can underlie abuse or neglect and that can be restructured. The intervention is most effective if the parent is encouraged by the kind of questions to work out these processes for themselves.

Table 24.4
Phases in parents' narratives that may signal the need for cognitive work

Phrase	Example statements	Distorted underlying assumption/expectation/ cognitive problem
'He/she knows'	He knew I was tired. He knows his father had a bad day. She knows I don't let her do that.	Assumption of mind reading
A string of personality-based comments	He's a sneak. She's a brat.	Stable negative internal attributions
Evidence of a power struggle	She thinks she's boss! I can't let her get away with this! He thinks he can put one over on me!	Low self-efficacy
Overly personalised explanations of causality with strong language	He knew it would get to me. He knew people were watching, and he did it anyway. She was trying to destroy me.	Misattributions
Self-deprecatory statements	He must think I'm stupid. She must really think I'm dumb!	Negative self-schema
Explanations that are similar to descriptions of others in the parent's life	He's just like his father – no good! She looks at me just like my mother did when I did something wrong. When she does that, she reminds me of me.	Discrimination failure

(Reproduced with permission from Azar 1997.)

I learned that kids pick up on big and tiny things going on in their mum's life and that it affects their behaviour and can put everything up in the air.

(Quote from a parent; Burgess 2005)

The same principles can be used in intervention with the non-offending parents of children who have been sexually abused (Deblinger & Hope Heflin 1996). The response of the non-abusing parent to the sexual abuse of their child can be one of the most important influences on the way the child recovers from the experience. Deblinger and Hope-Heflin's book sets out a comprehensive guide to the use of a cognitive–behavioural approach with the child and the non-offending parent. Briefly, the focus of the work with the non-offending parent (the majority of whom are mothers) is to equip them with the coping skills they need to support their children. The first stage is to establish a trusting therapeutic environment that will allow the mother to express all the feelings she has, including any thoughts of anger towards her child. There follows a joint process of identifying any dysfunctional underlying thoughts. Dysfunctional thoughts can be of two kinds: unproductive or inaccurate. Unproductive thoughts are those that sap energy at the expense of the recovery. For example, whilst anger at the perpetrator is justifiable, a mother can be so consumed by anger that she is unable to assist her child. She can be supported to redirect her energy into the joint therapeutic process. Inaccurate thoughts can be countered by factual information. For example, a mother who blames herself or who cannot understand why her child did not disclose sooner can be assisted by the extensive research information about the extremely cunning tactics used by perpetrators to groom children and ensure secrecy.

Key principles for working with parents

Regardless of the nature of provision and extent of targeting, it is essential to take account of the process of engagement with parents and the importance of developing a good working relationship. Research indicates that there are some features which need to be in place to facilitate engagement and the helping process. Quinton's research (2004) offers some key messages:

- Relationships and support are at the heart of engagement with parents and it is not necessarily about *what* is offered but *how* it is offered that essentially matters.
- There is a need to *empower* parents by building on their strengths, treating them with respect and offering services that are practical and involve them in problem solving.
- Diversity in support provision is important.
- Multiple problems need multiple solutions.

There are a range of practical ways in which engagement with parents can be facilitated.

Empowerment

Especially at the beginning of an intervention it may be useful to agree that the parent and worker write up notes of a session or a visit together. This helps parents realise that their views are important to the practitioner and engenders trust.

Clear philosophy of work

Parenting can be an emotive subject for many people. People can have diverse attitudes and values in relation to parenting. It is the one thing we all have experience of: we have all been parented and some of us are parents ourselves. It is important that practitioners do not presume that because they work together, they share the same philosophy about parenting. Practitioners should develop shared statements about values, child protection and equal opportunities in relation to parenting work so that there is a shared philosophy and an agreed approach. These can be included with project information that is given to parents and professionals.

Attention to literacy skills

It should not be assumed that all parents will have reasonable literacy skills. If offering leaflets, it may be helpful to include audio tapes and it is important to ensure that everything is explained clearly in discussion.

Relationship building

There must be sufficient time for in-depth assessment of needs and to build a relationship prior to intervention or introduction to a parenting programme. For some parents individual work will be needed for a long period of time prior to a group or as the only form of intervention.

Realistic goals

Parents must be involved in agreeing goals that are achievable and realistic for them. Where practitioners and parents disagree on the nature of the assessment, the goals or the plan for intervention, then the difference needs to be openly acknowledged. Wherever possible, practitioners should aim to integrate any plans for the protection of children within a programme that also addresses the parents' stated needs.

Perseverance

It should be assumed that persistence will be needed in finding ways to engage some parents and that there will be some missed appointments. There are strategies to assist with this; for example, the use of reminders such as text messages and phone calls in advance for meetings. Any missed appointments or home visits where no one answered the door must always be followed up.

Nurturing

Many parents need to be reminded that they have to look after themselves in order to have the strength and stamina to cope with their children and begin to effect changes. It is useful to try to find ways to encourage them to do this; for example, by including personal time for them in their action plans, giving small gifts such as bubble bath or chocolate as rewards for their achievements.

Introductions to groups

If the plan for intervention includes attendance at a group, child care and transport arrangements must be in place if needed. Parents' anxiety about attending groups for the first time must not be underestimated and everything must be done to support their attendance, such as accompanying them from home to group. It may be helpful to hold an initial informal meeting of parents before starting the group and, if possible, to use parents who have previously participated to offer encouragement.

Honesty

All practitioners from all agencies must be extremely clear from the start about information sharing with other agencies and procedures for reporting child protection concerns.

Inclusion of fathers and other carers

It is essential to make attempts to include fathers or other substantive carers in the engagement and assessment process. At times this may involve meeting with them separately as well as a couple or family. If a father or other carer is considered to be a risk to the child or practitioner then steps must be taken to ensure that they can be engaged in a safe way.

Working with differences and diversity

It is necessary to pay due attention and respect to differences in culture, ethnicity, religious belief, disability, etc. whilst always remembering that the welfare of the child is paramount. Assessment must take account of any significant personal needs parents may have, such as mental ill-health, medical conditions, disability, etc. which may prevent or impact on their ability to address parenting issues. They may need to be referred to specialist services and may need help with advocating for resources on their behalf.

Implications for supervision and support and training of staff

Supervision and support

Managers from all agencies should consider how they can create opportunities for staff to share experience and knowledge, practice tools and parenting programmes through avenues such as peer or group supervision, external consultants and practitioner groups. Although these should never replace individual supervision, they may add another learning dimension and also encourage networking and multi-agency work. Managers should ensure that regular supervision is in place. Parenting practitioners often address issues such as child protection and domestic abuse. It is vital that staff are allowed to explore their feelings and the impact of this work on them, as well as discussing case management and related tasks. Volunteers as well as sessional workers should also receive supervision.

Training

The following types of training are recommended for staff involved in delivering parenting services:

- Generic training in ways of working effectively with parents.
- Specialist training related to topics that staff are likely to come across in the course of their work, especially in targeted provision in relation to work with

adults, such as mental health, substance misuse, domestic abuse and working with survivors of childhood abuse.

■ Specific parenting and family programmes, including validated programmes such as Webster-Stratton; Triple P; Strengthening Families, Strengthening Communities; Mellow Parenting; Video Interactive Guidance (VIG) and Family Group Conferencing.
■ Child-related training, such as attachment and resilience, child development and child protection.
■ Inter-agency training which aids the process of multidisciplinary working by encouraging networking, a better understanding of the respective roles of other agencies and opportunities to share practice experience.
■ Others, such as adult learning and lifespan development.

The Parenting Education and Support Forum (2004) have developed National Occupation Standards for work with parents which were approved by UK Standards Approval Board in April 2005. Training on these will be available at NVQ and SVQ levels 2–4, and other qualifications will be developed based on these standards. It is anticipated that these will be implemented UK-wide in the near future. The expectation is that all employers and practitioners should evidence how they meet these Standards. The Standards are made up of units and elements of competences and each competence is designed to address an area of responsibility in work with parents. These are (p. 3):

1. Build and maintain effective and positive relationships with parents and others with an interest in working with parents.
2. Create and provide safe, inclusive environments and services that empower parents and support the development of confidence and resilience.
3. Provide parenting programmes in accordance with the values and principles set out in the National Occupation Standards.
4. Update knowledge and reflect on own practice and support the development of others' knowledge and practice.
5. Influence and contribute to policies, strategies and development opportunities for parenting services and projects.
6. Create and sustain a framework for ensuring and maintaining the quality of delivery of parenting.

Conclusion

It will be evident from the scope of this chapter that parenting issues are central to child care and protection practice and that they cover the full spectrum from the need of some parents for some advice to the extreme harm some parents can cause their children. The vast majority of parents want to care for their children and would not knowingly harm them. However, parenting is a highly demanding and complex responsibility that can be undermined by personal and environmental circumstances, and flexible and accessible services can make all the difference when a parent is struggling. There are some parents who abuse and neglect their children and who do not engage willingly with support services. In such circumstances professionals need a very good understanding of parental issues so that they can ensure that their children receive the kind of prompt and nurturing response they need to allow them to experience a safe, healthy and happy childhood.

- Strategic planning of services for parents must take account of the need for a continuum of services that link in a complementary fashion.
- The overwhelming message from the research into parents' views is that parents want services to be accessible before problems can escalate and become entrenched.
- Different parents want and respond to different types of service delivered in different ways and by different statutory and non-statutory organisations and personnel.
- Any type of parenting support or intervention is dependent upon the skills of the practitioners to engage meaningfully with parents.
- Practitioners at all levels of the organisation should be aware of the strategic planning in their locality and should be prepared to contribute to the shaping of local policy.
- All services and all practitioners must be sensitive to both implicit and explicit indications that a parent is in need of some help and must respond in a timely fashion.
- Practitioners must be aware of the range of services on offer and must be skilled in assessing the 'fit' between a parents' expressed need and the nature of service provision.
- Practitioners who offer voluntary support or compulsory intervention with parents must have the opportunity to develop and nurture their skills in engaging with, and maintaining, a therapeutic relationship with service users.

Annotated further reading

Cleaver H, Unell I, Aldgate J 1999 Children's needs – parenting capacity: the impact of parental mental illness, problem alcohol and drug abuse, and domestic violence on children's development. The Stationery Office, London
   Summarises a large body of research literature on the factors that affect parental capacity and the impact upon children.

Deblinger E, Hope Heflin A 1996 Treating sexually abused children and their non-offending parents. Sage Publications, Newbury Park, CA
   Describes cognitive–behavioural intervention with parents and with children in sufficient detail to guide therapeutic work post-abuse.

Howe D 2005 Child abuse and neglect: attachment, development and intervention. Palgrave Macmillan, Houndmills
   This book provides a readable and vivid account of the range of ways in which the parental attachment history can impact upon the parent–child relationship. The book includes comprehensive guidance on attachment-based intervention.

Lloyd E (ed) 1999 Parenting matters: what works in parenting education? Barnardo's, Barkingside, Ilford
   This edited text focuses on the evidence about what works in parent education and as such is a valuable resource for strategic planning.

Quinton D 2004 Supporting parents: messages from research. Jessica Kingsley, London
   This book unpicks the meaning of support and draws on the findings of a range of empirical studies in offering messages for practice.

Useful websites

Aberlour National Parenting Development Project: www.aberlour.org.uk
ChildcareLink: www.childcarelink.gov.uk
Department for Education and Skills: www.dfes.gov.uk
Fathers Direct: www.fathersdirect.com
Mellow Parenting: www.acamh.org.uk
National Family and Parenting Institute: www.nfpi.org; www.e-parents.org.uk (parents' site)
Parenting Education and Support Forum: www.parenting-forum.org.uk
Strengthening Families, Strengthening Communities: www.extension.iastate.edu/store
Triple P: www1.triplep.net
Webster-Stratton Parenting Programme: www.incredibleyears.com
Youth Justice Board: www.youth-justice-board.gov.uk

25 Working with abusing families

Arnon Bentovim

INTRODUCTION

In recent years, family work in child abuse has changed from a focus on providing family therapy to a much clearer concept of family work in a wider systemic context. The relationship between therapeutic work and statutory contexts has been clarified and developed in the work at the Great Ormond Street Hospital for Children, London, in Rochdale and elsewhere (Dale *et al.* 1986a, 1986b, Bentovim *et al.* 1988, 1998, Furniss 1991) and through the work of multisystemic (Brunk *et al.* 1987) and multimodal approaches. Family centres, which traditionally provide little more than a holding environment, can now work in a more structured and goal-orientated manner, stressing aspects of responsibility, self-help, autonomy, strength and resourcefulness of families and family members (Asen *et al.* 1989).

Family work with abusive families is beginning to differentiate between families where there is physical abuse and neglect, and families where sexual abuse has occurred (Crittenden 1988, Stratton & Hanks 1991, Hanks 1993, Kolko 1996). Work with families where children have been emotionally abused is less developed; the focus is still largely on defining the core concepts involved (Crittenden & Ainsworth 1989, Erickson *et al.* 1989, Hobbs *et al.* 1993, Glaser 2002).

This chapter draws on an earlier chapter in the first edition of the *Handbook* by Furniss and Miller.

The chapter begins with a brief review of some of the relevant literature on family violence and abuse and the impact on children living in a climate of adversity. Next, some conceptual and planning issues are considered which relate to working with abusing families. These include:

- the differences between family therapy and consultation
- the distinction between a family approach and a family therapy approach to family work with abuse
- issues of motivation, indicators for involving the whole family and the differing emphasis given to change and growth in work relative to the different forms of abuse and neglect.

A range of practice issues relating to family work and family therapy for all forms of child abuse is then covered, and several family therapy techniques are described which can be useful in work with abusing families.

Family intervention is then considered more specifically. The steps which need to be taken for effective family work are laid out, as well as a range of approaches that can be useful at different stages of work with families.

The final part of the chapter focuses on families where child sexual abuse has taken place. A distinction is made between child sexual abuse and other forms of abuse, highlighting the therapeutic importance of some key aspects of the family work that is required, including the evaluation of suspicion of child sexual abuse and the handling of disclosures, trauma work and work with siblings.

Family violence

A brief review of the literature

In my book *Trauma Organised Systems: Physical and Sexual Abuse in Families* I reviewed the work of Straus and Gelles (1987) who demonstrated the extraordinary extent of violence within the North American family. They demonstrated widespread violence between men and women, parents and children, children and their peers, and the widespread use of physical violence and the use of objects and weapons. I noted similarities in the United Kingdom and Europe and with other studies, which have now been brought together in many parts of the world, reviewed by the WHO. This indicated how widespread is the climate of violence, abuse and neglect, and the evidence of disruption of day-to-day life (Bentovim 1995).

The position taken by Straus and Gelles is not whether the family is a violent institution, but how violent it is and which factors make for more, rather than less, violent interaction. They described a number of factors which, although fostering growth and development for children, can go towards making families prone to violence, abuse and neglect. This includes the following factors:

- *Time at risk*: The more time a family spend together, the more opportunity for conflict. Poor environmental conditions, low income, poverty, unemployment, poor education and isolation are markers for violence.
- *Ranges of activities and interests*: There are striking differences in family members' activities relating to life stage which are inherently conflictual. Abusive parents perceived differences linked to ordinary development as hostile or rebellious behaviour.
- *Intensity of involvement*: Intensity, commitment and involvement in family interactions is considerable. Mutual antagonism, high levels of criticism, threats and shouting are not only evidence of intensity, but can also be abusive. Resentment between younger children and teenagers, boys and girls, men and women can occur. Coercion resolves conflicts, punishments deal with perceived transgression, power-orientated responses can occur.
- *Rights to influence*: Abusive parents may show authoritarian styles – insensitive to children's levels of abilities and needs, use intrusive, assertive techniques – or are neglectful, insensitive and undemanding. This affects children's social and intellectual competence, spontaneity and formation of conscience.
- *Age and sex differences*: The family is a unique arena, made up of different ages and sexes. There is major potential for conflicts between generations, families and sexes. Patriarchal views can pervade the childhood of one or both parents, and women and children may be accepted as appropriate victims of violence and abuse.
- *Ascribed roles and distorted beliefs*: There is an assumption that a woman who has given birth and the man who is the biological father are deemed capable of parenting. Authority and dependent relationships are defined through social construction; the adults have rights to make demands and expect compliance. Parents who are youthful or with limited abilities cannot adapt to the growing needs of children and abusive individuals take advantage of the roles left vacant when a parent leaves.
- *Involuntary membership*: The family is an exclusive organisation, where members are expected to take responsibility for each other. It is not so easy to flee the scene or resign from the group when abuse occurs.

- *Families and stress*: Events from the parents' childhood, the life cycle, birth, maturation of children, ageing and retirement, unemployment, illness and handicap all impact on the family group. Although stressful events can help develop resilience and coping strategies, they can also evoke a violent response.
- *Extensive knowledge of social biographies*: Intimacy and emotional involvement reveal and foster a full range of identities and roles, strengths, vulnerabilities, likes and dislikes which are all known and can be used to protect or attack, and such knowledge fosters beliefs. An attribution of deserving punishment or sexual interest provides meaning and reason for abusive action.

Protective factors

The time the family spends together can also provide the opportunity for support and nurturance. A wide range of activities and interests can help foster talents and strengths, intensity of involvement provides emotional fulfilment and rights to influence can assist children to fulfil their potential. Age and sex differences provide a test-bed for understanding and tolerance. Ascribed roles can also provide strength and identities; involuntary membership ensures that there will be commitment and care for individuals with disability. Coping with trauma, stress and change can lead to resilience, coping and the resources to deal with the inevitable stress of living in the world today, tolerance, continued care and understanding.

Models to account for family violence

There are a number of different theories to account for the development of family violence:

- *Cycle of violence*: This describes the intergenerational transmission of violence, associated with risk and protective factors resulting from the experience of the parents as children.
- *Psychopathological explanations*: These link the inability to control violent impulses and individuals showing a pervasive sense of discontent, anger and irritability – attitudes arising from the impact of mental health factors, alcohol and substance abuse and domestic violence (Cleaver *et al.* 1999).
- *Sociocultural models – ecological explanations*: This argues that human behaviour should be studied in context. Social and economic privation transform predisposed high risk individuals to develop violent means to control stressful events. Parents may be socialised into abusive practices and interactions as a result of cultural, community and family influences, harsh punishment in childhood and patriarchal societal views. Unemployment and limited occupational opportunities are seen as stressors that can provoke abusive action.
- *Social interactional explanation*: Interactional processes between parent and child in the specific familial context occur in the context of larger social structures. This explains why some parents abuse and children grow up in a climate of violence, abuse and neglect. The 'eco-systemic' model is a development of this approach.
- *Cumulative models*: Cumulative models demonstrate that the reinforcement of a number of different areas of stress – biological, genetic and environmental – gives rise to the climate of violence between family members; for example, the work of Dixon *et al.* (2005a) which demonstrated the additive effects of parental abuse in childhood, parenthood under 21, violent partners

and avoidant attachment patterns. The risk of abuse is four times greater if a parent has been abused in childhood, rising to 17 times greater with these additional factors.

The impact of abuse on development

General view of the process of abusive action (Bentovim 1995)

What characterises all forms of family violence, abuse and adversity are the negative interlocking aspects of the relationship between parent and child within a social context. A 'climate of violence' results in negative, emotionally abusive attitudes towards the child or partner – a prerequisite to any form of abuse, whether physical, sexual or emotional.

A protector is absent or potential protectors are neutralised and unavailable. The perpetrator feels overwhelmed by impulses to actions of a physically, sexually or emotionally abusive nature, felt to be beyond control. The cause is attributed to the victim, who is construed as responsible for the victimiser's feelings and intentions. Actions on the victim's part to avoid abuse are interpreted as a further cause for disinhibition of violent action or justification for further sexual or emotional abuse.

A process of silence and dissociation spreads to victim and victimiser and those who could potentially protect. This leads to the delayed recognition of severe abusive patterns in secrecy and silence. Both victim and victimiser minimise experiences, dismiss events and blame themselves or others. As a result of the repeated nature of violent actions, traumatic stressful effects come to organise the reality and the perceptions of those participating – what I have described as a 'trauma organised system' (Bentovim 1995). This includes potential protectors and professionals who become involved in the family situation. There is a pressure not to see, not to hear or not to speak so that identification becomes problematic and complex.

The scenario of family violence, abuse and neglect is like an iceberg with different facets appearing at different stages of the children's development and in different forms.

General effects on development

It is helpful to consider three major areas of children and young people's development to understand the way violence impacts on children (Bentovim *et al.* 1998):

1. The regulation of emotional states (Cicchetti & Toth 1995)
2. The development of attachment (Carlson *et al.* 1989)
3. The developments of an adequate sense of self and relationships (Culp *et al.* 1987).

These three areas reinforce each other, are intertwined and come to underpin the relationship models of the individual child and young person, both within the family and within the social context. Overwhelming stress is characteristic and there is an inter-related biological and psychological response. A child or young person living in a world invaded by fear and anxieties has their perception of themselves and others coloured and directed by such experiences. The greater the exposure to stressful factors, the more likely it is that extreme responses will be shown.

Figure 25.1 describes the responses to contexts that have traumatic effects, i.e. living in a context or climate where the child is exposed to a cumulative set of abusive experiences. It is helpful to think of responses in each significant area as externalising or internalising. The direction of responses is indicative of the coping

Figure 25.1
*Responses to
traumagenic contexts.*

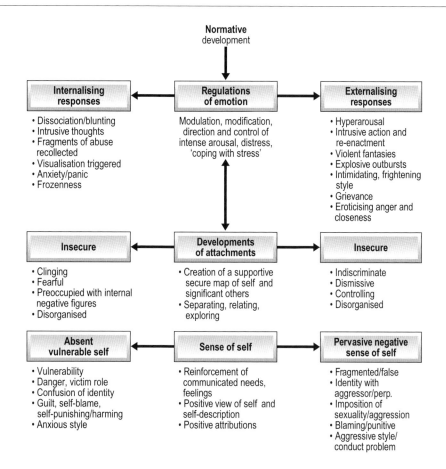

mechanisms used – a general avoidant mode or an active coping response, including responses which can indicate an identity with the aggressor rather than the victim.

Conceptualising these complex interactional factors to make systematic evidence-based assessments and models of intervention

Research approaches in the field of family violence, neglect and abuse during the 1990s (e.g. *Messages From Research*, DoH 1995a) indicated that although a narrow focus on abuse resulted in protection, it does not impact on the complex processes of family life, resulting in the persistent negative emotional and behavioural effects. Subsequently, a new approach was introduced – *Working Together to Safeguard Children** (DoH *et al.* 1999) and the *Framework for the Assessment of Children* (DoH 2000e) – an eco-systemic approach to understanding the relationships between the family and environmental factors, the sort of parenting which this gave rise to, and the impact on children and the way that their needs were met during development (see Fig. 3.4, p. 62).

This was expressed in the triangle which attempted to demonstrate the mutual interaction of family and environment, parenting capacity and how well the needs of children were met. A number of evidence-based approaches were developed to

---

* The most up-to-date version of this document was published by HM Government in 2006. For a full discussion of this, see Chapter 11.

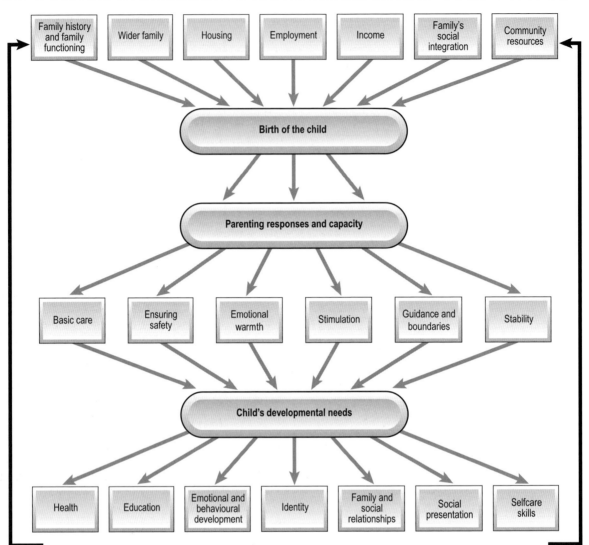

Figure 25.2
Family and environmental factors.

assist professionals in making such complex assessments which helped to meet the needs of children and parents and from which intervention flowed (Cox & Bentovim 2000, Bentovim & Bingley Miller 2001, Cox & Walker 2001).

Figure 25.2 represents the developmental process inherent in this approach by reconfiguring it to demonstrate that family and environmental factors developmentally influence the response of a parent to the birth of a child. Characteristic parenting patterns are evoked to meet infant and young children's needs and these responses in turn influence the child's development. There is always a feedback between the different levels which is demonstrated through the triangular model. The development of the child at different stages impacts on parenting, evoking a variety of parenting responses associated with a parent's own experiences. This in turn impacts on family and environmental factors and the wider family and family functioning, on housing and on employment. It is helpful to assess these different areas in isolation, analysing the mutual influence of these different levels on each other and ultimately on the needs of the children.

Parenting can be relatively efficient in meeting children's needs at one phase of their development, perhaps in infancy when their needs are limited. Meeting the growing needs of a mobile child, children going through particular phases of development, or moving through into adolescence, may be more challenging. Parents who themselves have personal difficulties, learning difficulties or live in an alien, unsupportive context with little family and community support are particularly vulnerable. There are linear 'over time' processes, as well as circular reinforcing processes.

Family assessments – children, parents and families

If it becomes clear from initial assessments that children are growing up in a climate of violence, adversity, abuse and neglect, a detailed 'core' assessment is required which analyses their needs and the nature of parenting, and establishes what family and environmental factors are present. The aim of assessment is to create a profile of children's needs, to understand the way in which those needs have become established and to what extent they require help in their own regard. The capacities of family members to provide parenting, what support and therapeutic help would assist them and whether alternative care is required is also assessed.

The process of assessment begins with the assessment of harm and protective needs established from the initial concern. We know from a variety of sources that a significant number of children live in contexts which are not known to care professionals.

There are a number of assessment steps that should be taken when it has been established that a child needs to be safeguarded as a result of suffering harm. Arriving at a full understanding of the context in which harm occurs and its effect on the child has been likened by Hobbs *et al* (1993) to putting together the pieces of a jigsaw to create a total picture. The steps include the following:

- Stage 1: Phase of identification and protection from harm
- Stage 2: Assessment of children's needs, parenting capacity, family and environmental factors
- Stage 3: Assessing the likelihood of response to professional intervention in the context of the level of the child's needs, the level of parenting capacity and family and environmental difficulties
- Stage 4: Developing a plan of intervention to include therapeutic work in a context of safety and protection from harm
- Stage 5: Rehabilitation of the child to the family when living separately or moving on from a context of protection and support
- Stage 6: New family phase – placement of children in family contexts where rehabilitation is not possible.

Stage 1: Phase of identification and protection from harm

A number of professionals from different disciplines will be involved, through a process of strategy meetings, child protection conferences, core assessments and reviews (DoH *et al.* 1999, DoH 2000e), with action following to protect the child depending on the level of abuse and risk of future harm.

Initially the full extent of abuse of a child is frequently not known, nor is the extent of the trauma (Carlson *et al.* 1989). When one child has been identified as being abused, it is not unusual for other children in the family to be found to have been abused. It may emerge that a parent, who is perceived as protective, may also have been involved or have condoned abusive action. There may be considerable uncertainty about parenting capacity to protect their children or the extent of abuse until further assessments are completed.

Severe extensive abuse in a child, or more than one form of abuse, will make it more likely that there will be major difficulties associated with parenting capacity and family and environmental factors. The emergence of mental health difficulties or substance abuse in parents, or domestic violence that has not been reported (Cleaver *et al.* 1999), indicate a greater level of complexity in the case and will require more extensive professional and agency intervention. It may be necessary to use interventions, supported through child protection conference decisions or a court order, to work with and motivate parents who themselves may have considerable difficulties and require extensive services.

Stage 2: Assessment of children's needs, parenting capacity, family and environmental factors

Decisions about urgent action to protect the child and provision of services require well-coordinated planning between and within agencies. Evidence-based approaches to initial and core assessments are helpful to ensure that there is adequate assessment of all levels of family and environmental factors, parenting capacity and the needs of the child. As families will require longer, more specialist assessment to assist in making longer-term decisions, it is essential that initial and core assessment are sufficiently thorough to assist in determining the level of protection required.

A number of different approaches to carrying out an assessment are required depending on whether children are living away from home with foster carers or in children's homes, whether they are living at home but attending the Family Centre or are being intensively supported by social work intervention. A parent and child(ren) may be living in a refuge or with other family members, but whatever the context of care at the time of assessment, the following elements need to be assessed.

Observation of parenting

It is essential that children are seen in their current context, with whoever is basically providing their day-to-day care. *Home Observation for Measurement of the Environment* (Caldwell & Bradley 2001) provides an excellent evidence-based approach to carrying out detailed assessment of the current parenting and environmental context in which a child is cared for. The approach introduced by Cox and Walker (2001) emphasises the importance of exploring the care of the child in the last 24 hours by whoever is providing that primary care. This establishes not only the quality of care being given to the child, but also the care the child requires at that point. Through home assessment of children in the early years, both infancy (0–3 years) and late toddler stage (3–5 years), as well as children of primary school age (6–10 years), adolescence and children with special needs, an accurate picture can be built up of the current parenting and the child's response to this. Figure 25.3 describes the areas of parenting which emerge from the assessment.

Figure 25.3
Contents of the
HOME inventory.

0–3 years Subscales	3–6 years Subscales	6–10 years Subscales
Responsivity	Learning materials	Responsivity
Acceptance	Language stimulation	Encouragement of maturity
Organisation	Physical environment	Emotional climate
Learning materials	Responsivity	Learning materials and opportunities
Involvement	Academic stimulation	Enrichment
Variety	Modelling	Family companionship
	Variety	Family integration
	Acceptance	Aspects of the physical environment

Cox has emphasised that an hour spent tracking a child's day provides an opportunity to establish a good deal about the child's day-to-day life for observing the child's interaction with the caregiver. The question is not what 'generally' happens but what happened yesterday.

If a child is in alternative care it is important to establish the state of the child at placement in order to understand not only how immediate needs are being met, but also extrapolating since placement, providing information about the state of the child at placement in care and the response to a positive parenting experience.

The home assessment presents an evidence-based view of the quality of parenting provided, and also supplies considerable additional information about parents and children. It is possible in reviewing current needs to obtain information about the child at school, as well as through the child themselves, to establish overall health needs, a picture of the child's social adjustment and a general picture of family relationships and parental health and adjustment.

Establishing the child's needs

It is essential that an *individual interview(s)* takes place with the child to establish their needs. Whether the child is seen alone or with a supportive adult such as a social worker will depend on where the child is living. Depending on the child's age and stage and the nature of their problem, such assessment may take the form of a one-off assessment, or a series of meetings, particularly if the child or young person has shown evidence of considerable levels of disturbance, indicating that there has been significant experience of distress which may not have been reported. It may require a number of meetings to establish a rapport and to enable appropriate sharing. The use of approaches such as questionnaires and scales can establish an overall picture of needs and can form the basis of an interview. The *In My Shoes* computer-assisted interview (Calam *et al.* 2005) can be a valuable approach to such assessments. If a young person is showing evidence of offending behaviour, a set of instruments may also be required which explores areas of self-esteem, sexuality and impulsiveness.

Constructing a profile is a complex task which requires not only individual interview with the child, but also observation of the child with their family and school and reviewing a history of earlier experiences. The child also needs to be seen with parents or parent figures who have played a significant role in providing care, who may have been responsible for harm, failures of care, neglect, and physical and emotional abuse.

Family and environmental factors

Family meetings therefore take place not necessarily with the whole family, but with those members of the family who are perceived to be supportive – this may include a maternal/paternal figure or an extended family member. This means that, in situations of family violence, issues of safety need to be taken into consideration. Couples may be seen together and individually. When an allegation has been made against a particular parent, it is essential that contact is not retraumatising and may need to be delayed. Assessments may well need to take place over a period of time. Various combinations of the family need to be planned, and younger and older children should be seen together and separately, particularly when there have been allegations of abusive action perpetrated against a younger child by an older sibling. There may be a risk of silencing and retraumatisation which would impede the process of assessment of the child's needs.

The family assessment (Bentovim & Bingley Miller 2001)

The various elements of the family assessment have the aim of helping professionals and are integrated to provide both a qualitative and quantitative assessment of the family, including parenting. The assessment includes a number of components, as follows.

1. *A model of family life and relationships* incorporating different dimensions of family life relevant to assessing family relationships and the way the family is meeting the needs of children (Fig. 25.4).
2. *Language is designed to be specific*, focused on behaviour rather than opinion, and as observable as possible. This is to promote building a relatively objective basis for describing and understanding what we see when we encounter families, when we need to make an assessment of parenting.
3. *A set of scales to assess the level of competence, strengths and difficulties* for any particular family we are assessing, which includes parenting, and these are integrated into 'The Family Assessment Recording Form' (see component 5, below).
4. *A range of methods to help families talk about their lives* and to promote family interaction during the assessment process are introduced. A structured set of interview schedules helps the worker to systematically map with the family the concerns or problems bringing them to the assessment and to explore the dimensions of family organisation and family character in the context of family history. A schedule containing family tasks provides an effective way of helping families talk or do things together without an interviewer interrupting the sequence of their interaction.
5. *The Family Assessment Recording Form* takes an assessor through the systematic exploration, description and assessment of a sequence of areas of family life and relationships. The format provides a structured layout for recording, assessing and rating family functioning along the dimensions of family organisation and family character.

Figure 25.4
The family assessment model of family functioning: elements of family organisation and family character.

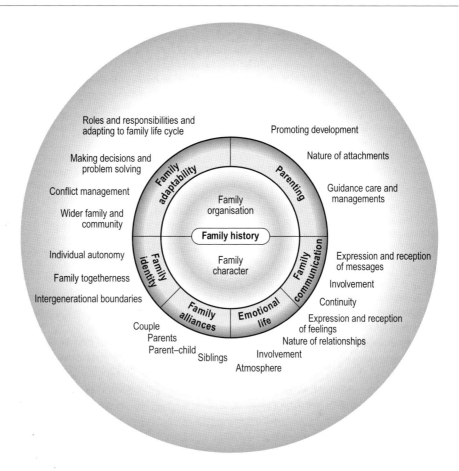

6. *Family organisation* contains the basic notions of the family's adaptability to the needs of the children, and the parenting skills required to meet these needs. The context for this basic aspect of family organisation is the notion of *family character* which looks at the type of communication within the family unit, the emotional life of the family, the nature of the alliances between family members and the identity of the family. We see these components of family character as underpinning the basic organisation of family life, i.e. adaptability to children's and other family members' needs and the capacity to provide adequate parenting (Fig. 25.5).

7. At the end of the Family Assessment Recording Form, a *family profile* allows the assessor to bring together the information gathered during the assessment and to record the views of the family of their own strengths and difficulties and their views of the assessment. It also outlines the outcome in terms of functioning which needs to be addressed.

While the family assessment emphasises family strengths and competence, it is intended to play an important part in assessing the nature and degree of any difficulties which may need to be addressed to ensure that children's needs are being appropriately responded to. Family difficulties may be contributing to possible significant harm, and the family assessment is designed to give professionals a systematic evidence-based approach to providing family assessments and recommendations for children to the courts when this is necessary.

Reasonable strengths	Moderate strengths and difficulties	Considerable difficulties
Emotional warmth conveyed by parents or carers towards children, pattern of stimulation and praise being displayed by parents to children	Some stimulation, emotional warmth and/or encouragement by parents or carers with inconsistencies and evidence of criticism, lack of warmth and inadequate stimulation	Lack of emotional warmth, stimulation or encouragement with evidence of rejection, coldness, little or minimal stimulation and marked critical attitude by parents towards children

As with any assessment, families need to be aware of the purpose for which the family assessment is being used, whether it be to work in partnership with families or in situations where professionals may be required to use appropriate authority to ensure a child is protected from significant harm.

Stage 3: Assessing the likelihood of response to professional intervention in the context of the level of the child's needs, the level of parenting capacity and family and environmental difficulties

Family work needs to be considered in all forms of treatment of child abuse where rehabilitation is being contemplated. Rehabilitation can only be considered when there is a reasonable prospect for change which emerges following an initial phase of assessment. A *hopeful prognosis* (Bentovim *et al.* 1987, Sylvester *et al.* 1995) requires that:

- abuse is not of such severity that rehabilitation would be dangerous or unlikely (e.g. sadistic abuse, multiple injuries, severe neglect)
- parents take adequate responsibility for abusive action
- there is a protective capacity within the family (e.g. a non-abusive parent who is prepared to protect the child over and above their relationship with their partner)
- there is a willingness to work reasonably cooperatively with child care professionals
- parents accept the need for change even if it is with the motivation of maintaining children within the family context
- there is a potential for the development of a reasonable attachment and relationship between the parents and children
- appropriate therapeutic settings be available in the community, a day-care setting or residential resource depending on the severity of abuse, where work including children and families can be planned in a hopeful context.

The *prognosis is hopeless* for family work when none of these criteria is fulfilled. Such family situations may include:

- rejection of the child
- severe forms of abuse
- a failure to take responsibility, needs of parents taking primacy over the needs of the children
- a combative oppositional stance to professionals
- psychopathology in parents – for example, drug abuse, serious marital violence or longstanding personality problems which may not be amenable to therapeutic work or within the child's timeframe

- complete inability or unwillingness to accept that there are problems, or absence of resources for treatment.

Family work has no place in such situations since the child may be persuaded to withdraw their statements or to become part of a process of maintenance of secrecy and denial.

Situations are of *doubtful prognosis* where professionals are not yet clear from the original work with the family whether the situation is hopeful or hopeless. There is uncertainty whether:

- there is adequate taking of responsibility
- parental pathology is changeable
- there is going to be willingness to work with care authorities and therapeutic agencies
- resources will be available to meet the extensiveness of the problem.

A phase of continuing assessment will be required to determine whether a care plan can be formulated, including family work.

The particular approach to work with the family will depend on the assessment of the child. Children who are severely traumatised by physical, emotional or sexual abuse may be retraumatised through contact with an abusive parent, even when that parent is taking responsibility for their abusive action. In such situations it is often essential for the majority of work to be carried out with the child individually, in groups or with a protective parent before any question of contact with the abusive parent is considered.

Family work needs to be at its most intensive when rehabilitation is considered following parental involvement in individual and group work, either as a protective parent or as an abuser dealing with abusive and violent action. Work involving the whole family may then become possible.

Stage 4: Developing a plan of intervention to include therapeutic work in a context of safety and protection from harm

Working with abusing families

Traditional conjoint approaches to working with abusive families have been criticised by feminist thinkers such as Bograd (1988). Potential dangers occur in attempting to work conjointly with families where an abusive family member was organising family life and grooming children to become victims of their perverse interest and abusive action. Secondary victimisation, retaliation and increasing silencing and fear are likely and against the interests of children. Attempts to 'restructure' the relationship between an abusive father and a terrified child are misplaced.

Thus it became essential to focus on the traumatic reality caused by abuse and its impact on individual functioning and relationships. Those who were traumatising the child are part of a system that allowed them to maintain abusive action in secrecy. Other adults in the children's world are also caught in the process and involved in a system of secrecy, denial and blame. In the growing area of trauma therapy, Eth and Pynoos (1985), Figley (1990) and Herman (1992) stressed the need to work with the facts of abuse and the objective reality of traumatising events. Therapeutic work required the tracking of such details for each individual before there could be any possible integration for the family as a whole.

An integrated approach which brings together all aspects of therapeutic work is crucial to effective work with abusing families. Therapists need to help families and individuals deal with the trauma they have experienced, to look at the relationship between the individual traumatic experiences that have evolved and to assess the impact of both on the way family members now relate.

Individuals have to make sense of their own experience and their own psychic sense of causality – the meaning given to that traumatic experience. This 'constructed reality' of individual family members or the family as a whole (e.g. that 'abuse is harmless', 'the child's action evoked an abusive response', 'silence is best', 'don't trust anyone outside the family') will hinder the growth and development or recovery of the family members and will therefore require therapeutic intervention.

Social service and legal systems evaluate the risk to the child and the actual harm resulting from child abuse and neglect, and act on that assessment in their work with abusing families. This may include work to change the relevant patterns of family relationships or to provide alternative care outside the family for the abused or at-risk child.

When a therapist remains neutral and adheres to the concept of circular rather than linear causality, focusing on the interlocking processes between family members, this may blur the issue of individual responsibility. What is required is a process that integrates the legal child care issue and the therapeutic approaches – for example, Bentovim *et al.* (1988), Furniss (1991), Sheinberg (1992), Sheinberg *et al.* (1994), Bentovim (1995) – and this is further developed in this chapter.

Therapeutic work within a legal framework of protection: conceptual and planning issues

Family therapy and consultation

This is a clear distinction between family therapy which occurs as a result of a free contract between the family and the therapist and conditional family work in the context of statutory decision making. Here the basic contract is not between therapist and family, but between therapist and the statutory agency and between the statutory agency and the family. Basic rules of confidentiality do not apply. Therapeutic work with abusive families is an aspect of consultation to statutory agencies and can only take place with close and open cooperation between therapist and statutory worker. This avoids damaging splits in the professional network between the therapist as the 'good person' and the statutory worker as the 'source of all bad things'.

Therapeutic work with abusing families needs to relate to the requirements of decision-making processes by statutory agencies and needs to be made explicit to the family. This can be achieved by having the social worker present during assessment and family sessions or by referring explicitly to the link between therapist and statutory agencies. We might therefore ask: 'What would the social worker/the court say about the change you have achieved so far in these sessions? Do you think they would feel it is safe for your child to live with you again or not?' This reminds the family and therapist that the work is part of consultation and not traditional family therapy.

A family systems theoretical framework helps conceptualise the dysfunctional aspects of abuse at a family level, keeps the family process and the child's needs in mind and opens up the options for different, concurrent forms of therapy in addition to family sessions. It also provides a unifying rationale for a range of protection, care planning and therapeutic tasks whilst attending to the welfare of the abused child and family.

In some less serious abusive situations conjoint family sessions may be the appropriate sole form of therapy. With sexual abuse and serious forms of abuse concurrent forms of therapy are always required. Abusers need individual and/or group work focused on their abusive behaviour and cycles of abuse. Mothers as non-abusing parents need individual help with the crisis of emotional turmoil, loss and practical problems that come with disclosure (Hooper 1992). Group work counteracts the isolation, disempowerment and low self-esteem associated with living in a family system shaped by abusive acts in a context of secrecy (Hildebrand 1988). Research on outcomes of treatment in child sexual abuse (Hyde *et al.* 1996, Monck *et al.* 1996) demonstrates the effectiveness of group intervention with parents and the role of parents supporting children constructing a trauma narrative enhances the therapeutic effect (Cohen *et al.* 2000).

The aim of therapy for the child needs to be the therapeutic transformation from traumatic powerlessness to effectiveness and survival (Furniss 1991, Bentovim 1995). Family sessions break the taboo of silence about abuse but cannot give the child the necessary space to experience adequate privacy and to develop self-worth, self-respect, autonomy and individuation, i.e. to reverse traumatic effects, dysregulation of emotional functioning and insecure attachments. This is achieved by individual or group sessions which provide the individual space for self-experience (Wilson & Ryan 1994). Concurrent family work provides a complementary domain of openness.

Successful outcome depends on the willingness and the quality of cooperation between therapists and on the ability of therapists to conceptualise their own form of therapy as part of a 'holistic' systemic framework incorporated in a multimodal approach to a complex reality.

Issues of motivation

Our skill needs to lie in knowing why abusing families are not motivated to be helped and how we can motivate them to feel that they want help. Frequently families are not primarily self-motivated to seek help because 'secrecy' allows families to function despite the 'hidden' pain. They may be motivated to cooperate because of the danger of family break-up and because of the openly stated preconditions for rehabilitation or for keeping their children at home.

The framework in family work in cases of child abuse needs to be positively reframed by an explicit therapeutic contract which states the required aims and goals of family work. Questions like: 'What do you think needs to change in your attitude and behaviour towards your child in order for social services/the court to be satisfied that it is safe for you to continue living with your child?', or, 'What do you think social services/the court needs to know from you for them to trust your word when you say you are able to understand and satisfy the needs of your child without abusing him/her?' The process of defining the aims for family work can help to motivate family members towards a wish for therapeutic change if they feel co-responsible for the development of explicit, understandable, operationalised and detailed goals for therapy. Motivation can grow with perceived success. The aims of family work are outlined in Box 25.1.

Disruptions of a child's attachment can be repaired through individual and group work. *Individual therapists* need to create a working alliance with the child or young person, to be consistent and reliably available, and to create a sense of safety. *Group work* fosters cohesion, belonging and identity, provides a sense of safety in the group to reverse the fears inherent in family life, and shares support substituting pleasure for pain. *Family work* can foster the development of secure attachments both in the phase of separateness (or as the situation moves to the next phase of separateness) and in the phase of rehabilitation. Connections may be made

Box 25.1
Aims of family work

Assigning responsibility for the abuse

■ At the outset children often blame themselves or parents blame the child; where the parent abuser(s) denies abusive action, the following treatment aims needed to be achieved:
  – father/mother/children acknowledge that abuse was the responsibility of the perpetrator, not the child
  – mother/father acknowledge their own responsibility for abuse or for lack of availability to the child to be protective when applicable
  – there needs to be evidence that the child has resolved traumatic responses and conflicted feelings towards the perpetrator and parents, i.e. instead of justifying the abuse through various distortions and rationalisations, the appropriate attribution of responsibility is taken.

Treatment focused on parenting

■ To foster increasingly secure attachments
■ To establish a capacity to provide adequate basic care
■ To recognise and respond to individual needs, appropriate to age
■ To provide adequate protection from further abuse
■ To develop capacities to foster the development of children.

Treatment focused on family relationships

■ Family members were able to express reasonable anger to each other in an appropriate non-destructive and non-scapegoating manner
■ Family members could develop relationships sufficiently open for painful issues to be confided and shared between child and parents, and between the parents themselves
■ Family allows members space to speak and listen to each other without scapegoating
■ Recognition of appropriate qualities in all family members, including each member recognising positive aspects of themselves
■ Establishment and maintenance of appropriate generational boundaries.

Treatment focused on acknowledging the origins and effects of abuse

■ Recognition of potential and actual emotional damage which might be the result of abuse
■ Parents show a capacity to help the child with actual behavioural effects of abuse
■ Recognition of the effect of their own abusive experiences in their own youth (where relevant)
■ Recognition by adults of the need for help on an individual and couple basis, including specific help with sexual difficulties
■ Ability of the family and professionals to work together cooperatively.

Treatment in a context of safety to help the individual

■ During this phase there needs to be work where the victim is separated from the abusive context, e.g.:
  – the child living with a protective parent/family member
  – the perpetrator living separately
  – the child living in alternative care.

Abuse-focused therapeutic work for victims

■ Whether individually or within group contexts, this is required in order to:
  – repair attachments
  – manage emotional dysregulation
  – develop a healing sense of self.

through a caring parent sharing and comparing their own experiences in their family with the child's experience. Family therapy techniques such as *reframing negative behaviour* and positive connotation (giving apparently negative behaviour a positive meaning) connect children with family scripts and parents' experiences growing up. The process of 'externalising' distances abusive experiences from self and relationships, and strengthens and promotes bonds within the family with a protective parent. Later, the sharing of experiences and understanding with the abusing parent from their own therapeutic work can help the child or young person feel part of the family context, rather than being blamed, excluded and scapegoated.

Therapeutic work with emotional dysregulation is aimed at reducing anxiety, developing a capacity to cope with emotional problems, and to be able to effectively process experiences of abuse by sharing, exposing them and constructing a healing narrative with an individual therapist, the group contexts and eventually with family members. A variety of approaches are helpful to monitor arousal and foster containment. To be involved in such work, a protective parent needs to be able to be open to the experiences of the child, to be able to listen and share, and to contain what may have been an extreme sense of terror, fear and powerlessness at the hands of the abusive parent. Safe family care rituals help to cope with sleeping difficulties and relaxation techniques help to cope with excitement, anger and sexualised behaviour to avoid retraumatisation.

To develop a more *satisfactory sense of themselves*, the child has to be helped to realise that what are defined as problematic (e.g. switching off angry oppositional behaviour, fear and avoidance) are part of a survival script and coping strategy, and are therefore strengths, not weaknesses. Family work needs to be absolutely clear about the origins of blame in order to help the child understand the abuser's attributing abusive action to the victim rather than taking responsibility. Family work requires a carefully planned apology and taking of responsibility for abusive action. This must be more than the often brief acknowledgement which is possible in the earlier phases of work.

Stage 5: Rehabilitation of the child to the family when living separately or moving on from a context of protection and support

Rehabilitation requires that parents themselves confront their abusive behaviour. When both parents have taken part in abusive actions they need to acknowledge the extensiveness of these actions in order to understand their origins and the damaging effect that they have had on the child. The apology session is a valuable component of part of a rehabilitation process. Questions that the child has about what has happened to them, and who is responsible, can be put to the abusive parent(s). Responses can be worked out with the therapists, and a joint meeting established where responsibility can be taken and victims freed from confusion, guilt and blame.

Intensive couple therapy is required to address violence between parents before meetings involving the victim and siblings can be initiated. Family structures are required to maintain protection.

Asen *et al.* (1989) indicate that in about 30% of cases of severe physical abuse and neglect, rehabilitation is not possible. In child sexual abuse in the Great Ormond Street series (Monck *et al.* 1996), 9% of children could be rehabilitated to the family which included the abuser, 52% could live with a protective parent, and a further 39% could not live with any family members because of rejection or disbelief and needed a new family context.

Stage 6: New family phase – placement of children in family contexts where rehabilitation is not possible

When a child cannot return home, intensive family work with a new family is required, planning long-term care, and preparation of a family for a child who has experienced extensive abuse. Physically abused children may be challenging. Sexually abused children have a high level of sexual knowledge and sexualised behaviour. There needs to be planning of protection within the foster family and consideration of the appropriate mode of contact with the original family. Work with the foster family or alternative adoptive family is essential to maintain an appropriate supportive stance and to incorporate the victim into a new family context (Bentovim & Bingley Miller 2001).

Family work in different forms of abuse

The treatment of child physical abuse

A review of the treatment of long-term sequelae of child abuse (Stevenson J 1999) revealed a limited number of studies using a controlled design to evaluate treatment approaches with abusing families characterised by physically abusive actions. Two approaches describe satisfactory results: Kolko (1996) and Brunk *et al.* (1987).

Kolko's study of treatment of physical abuse

Kolko (1996) contrasted cognitive–behavioural treatment with family therapy and community care as a control; both cognitive–behavioural treatment and family therapy were effective.

Cognitive–behavioural treatment focuses on child and parent separately. The work with the parent uses well-developed successful parent training approaches. The aim of the work is to implement parallel protocols addressing cognitive, affective and behavioural repertoires, clarifying family stressors, developing coping and self-control skills, and training in safety, support, planning and relaxation. Parents were trained in interpersonal affective skills, the use of social supports and assertion rather than the use of inappropriate punitive models. Parents' views of violence and physical punishment were clarified, and self-control, anger management and the use of time-out reinforcement were all a part of the approaches used following well-known cognitive–behavioural approaches.

The family therapy approach used an interactional/ecological model, with the aim of enhancing family functioning and relationships. The basic approach was to enhance the cooperation and motivation of all family members by promoting and helping them understand the nature of coercive behaviour, teaching positive communication skills and helping develop problem-solving skills together as a family. There were three phases of work:

1. The *engagement phase*, which assessed structural roles and interactions, used a genogram to help clarify such roles. A variety of family tasks were used, and externalising approaches were used to help separate violent action from the 'real' life of the family. There was reframing of what seemed to be punitive action, or anger, as misplaced attempts to achieve control, togetherness and problem solving. Apparently disruptive behaviour was positively construed as misplaced ways of helping family members pay attention to each other.

2. The *middle phase* of work reviewed the effects of physical force, and what it would mean for there to be a no violence contract for each family member. There was then training to use specific problem-solving skills and communication skills at home, building the capacities and skills of each family member.
3. The *termination phase* required the establishment of problem-solving skills and the development of family routines as an alternative to coercion or physical punishment.

Effectiveness of the approaches

There was significant improvement found both with cognitive–behavioural therapy and family therapy relative to community care; there was significantly less use of force in discipline. Family therapy was associated with the greatest reduction in children reporting their parents being violent towards them and helped identify other significant family difficulties.

Both therapeutic approaches had a greater impact on children's externalising (aggressive) behaviour, the transmission of an aggressive style from parent to child, and on general parental distress. There was improved family cohesion, a marked reduction of conflict, fewer further abusive incidents, children were far less anxious or aggressive, and the incidence of parental depression was very much lower. Cognitive–behavioural work with individual children and adults brought together in a family-focused approach provides the best of both worlds, reflecting the approach advocated in this chapter.

Multisystemic treatment of physical abuse

An approach that links with Kolko's interactional/ecological model is the *multisystemic therapy* approach. Multisystemic therapy has had its major focus with serious juvenile offenders; it has also been applied successfully to maltreating families (Brunk *et al.* 1987). The principles of multisystemic therapy include:

1. understanding the fit between identified problems and the broader systemic context
2. emphasising the positive and using systemic strengths as levers for change
3. developing an atmosphere of mutual trust to promote responsible behaviour and decrease irresponsible behaviour among family members
4. using focused and action-orientated approaches, targeting specific and well-defined problems, defining treatment goals and success
5. targeting sequences of behaviour within or between multiple systems that maintain identified problems
6. encouraging daily or weekly effort by family members, with positive reinforcement given for small gains
7. continuously evaluating effectiveness from multiple perspectives.

This approach is very much in line with the one advocated in this chapter.

The treatment of emotional and physical neglect and abuse and non-organic failure to thrive

Treating physical and emotional neglect and abuse is a challenging task, not least because of the difficulties in defining the entity. Glaser and Prior (2002) point out that neglect and emotional abuse describe interactions which cause harm, rather than the single abusive event associated with physical abuse. Such abusive events usually occur against a background of emotional abuse and neglect.

Glaser and Prior (2002) categorise the different forms of emotional abuse and neglect as:

- emotional unavailability, unresponsiveness and neglect of care
- negative attributions such as rejection, denigration, misperceptions of children's behaviour as hostile and deserving punishment
- inappropriate or inconsistent interactions – expectations beyond capability, or over-protection
- exposure to highly traumatic and damaging events such as domestic violence or disruptive separations
- failure to recognise the individuality of the child
- a failure to promote children's adaptation to social contexts.

Emotional abuse

There is no one approach to intervention with emotional abuse which has been demonstrated to be the preferred option. What is required is a thorough assessment and the application of approaches that have been demonstrated to be successful with emotional and behavioural difficulties of children and families. Stevenson J (1999) reviewed such approaches as well as those demonstrated as helpful in contexts where abuse had occurred.

Iwaniec *et al.* (2002) focus on a particularly severe form of neglect – *non-organic failure to thrive*. This condition is recognised by a serious failure to grow in height or in weight, sometimes associated with small growth of the head and signs of neglect. This can result from emotional abuse and neglect, poor parenting style, inadequate food intake, feeding difficulties and a problematic relationship and interaction between parents and children, insecure attachments and weak bonding. The consequences of such failure to thrive are serious: there can be a poor outcome of mental abilities, poor cognitive development, emotional instability and poor academic attainments. The major therapeutic task is to change unresponsive and often emotionally abusive or neglectful parenting into better-informed and sensitive caregiving. There are two basic categories of intervention:

- immediate – crisis intervention
- longer-term therapeutic work.

Immediate intervention focuses on the child's safety, neglected developmental attainments and urgent family needs. The child's development might be seriously retarded, and therefore there is a requirement for day care or a foster home placement to provide social stimulation, safety and the opportunity to develop mentally and catch up.

When the child and family require considerable *longer term help and support* based on an in-depth assessment, interventions are often required to:

- target difficulties in parenting skills
- target aggressive and rejecting behaviour by the parents
- enable parents to use positive management strategies, improve communication and adopt stress management techniques.

Working with severe failure to thrive (Iwaniec *et al.* 2002)

- *Stage one*: Feeding is tackled in a highly structured and directive manner. The therapist assists, models, reassures, observes and prompts to create a calm, soothing, reassuring context.

- *Stage two*: To create positive interactions and reduce negative interactions, to desensitise the child's anxiety and fear of the mother's feeding and caregiving activities, to desensitise the mother's tension, anger and resentment, to promote more secure attachment behaviours. Considerable support is required to reinforce the programme.
- *Stage three*: A phase of deliberate, intensified mother/child interaction.
- *Stage four*: Some older children presenting require development of prosocial behaviour in other areas.
- *Stage five*: To broaden out the mother's social context. Structured parenting training, parent self-help groups resolve issues with wider family and history.

Treatment where illness has been fabricated or induced

Understandably a key focus in considering this unusual form of abuse and harm has been the identification and initial management of the abuse within a child protection framework. Forty-one children at Great Ormond Street Hospital for Children (Gray *et al.* 1995) in whom illness had been fabricated or induced were followed up. This sample included children who were failing to thrive as a result of the withholding of food or beliefs that the child had severe allergic states. A variety of symptoms were described and medical investigation demanded, and these children were made ill through the ingestion of substances such as salt or inappropriate medication. It was possible to identify the following outcomes:

- Whether the child's health and developmental milestones had progressed well.
- Whether there were further episodes of fabricated or induced illness.
- What intervention had taken place.

At follow-up a number of children (4) had died, indicating the potential seriousness of the condition. Of the remaining 37, 21 were found to have poor outcomes and 16 to have good outcomes. The question was, what were the factors and what form of intervention had led to success? The following were associated with a successful outcome:

1. The initial suspicion of abuse and its identification needs to be successfully managed. A parent who presented as deeply caring could also induce harm due to deeply ambivalent feelings about their children. A multidisciplinary/multi-agency approach to management brings together the child protection, the child mental health and child health teams.
2. A high standard of information needs to be obtained and an in-depth understanding of the family gained through effective teamwork.
3. The protection needs of the child had to be an essential focus. There was a poor outcome if intervention was short term, not adequately coordinated, and there was inadequate assessment and understanding of what needed to change in order for the child to be able to thrive within their family.
4. There was a better outcome if the assessment was comprehensive and well-coordinated, and the therapeutic intervention included individual and family factors occurring over a reasonable period of time within the context of a child protection plan.

The treatment of child sexual abuse

If physical abuse occurs as a result of perversion of punishment, then sexual abuse is a perversion of closeness and sexuality. There is an addictive compulsive element in the inappropriate sexual activities of the sex offender. Punitiveness is triggered by the defiance or perceived defiance of the child and the sexual abuser describes themselves as being helpless in the face of what they perceive as the sexualised signals and behaviour of the child. Sexuality with children is rationalised as psychological and physical boundaries are overcome. The child who is perceived as 'bad' and deserving punishment may also be perceived as deserving sexual action perpetrated against them.

Extensive grooming of the child and of the family context occurs, the protective parent's capacity to care is undermined, the child feels blamed and responsible for abuse perpetrated against them, and is therefore silenced and adapts to the role attributed to them – a 'corrupting process'. Professionals who are involved are perceived as misinformed and prejudiced against the family rather than seeing abusive reality for what it is.

The first stage of work – identification and protection from harm – is often prolonged and extensive, requiring collaboration between social work, police and specialist interviewers with children and with adults. Difficult decisions have to be taken about child protection action, about criminal action, the likelihood of success of such processes and the role of potential therapeutic work. In the Great Ormond Street research (Monck *et al.* 1996) fewer than 9% of abusers (both adults and older siblings) took responsibility for abuse. Children perceived only a third of their maternal carers as believing them, a third doubtful, and a third disbelieving. The state of the child (mental health indices, anxiety, depression, post-traumatic stress) is affected in part by the severity of abuse; a further key factor is whether the child perceives themselves to be supported. Adolescent girls are at risk of being disbelieved by a mother who puts her need for her partner above the protection of the child. Parents may come together in opposition to authorities who are accused of fabricating evidence. The young person is thus doubly rejected, being both abused and disbelieved. Over half (60%) of the children referred to the Great Ormond Street study were living apart from their original family at the time of referral, and had suffered separation not only from their parents, but also in many cases from their siblings. Mothers who had chosen to support their abused child frequently had to adjust to considerable changes: not only that abuse had occurred, but also to face the loss of a partner or another child.

Family work approaches to sexual abuse

Examination of a series of cases in the treatment outcome study (Monck *et al.* 1996) demonstrated that although treatment of the family was a focus of the therapeutic programme, family treatment sessions were far more often held with parts of the family (e.g. the mother and victim), reinforcing individual or group work approaches. When the offender had admitted responsibility for abuse, there were family sessions at a later stage.

All family members were seen during the evaluation period, but very young siblings were often not included in ongoing therapeutic sessions. Abused children were often reluctant to include younger siblings, fearing they would gossip about the abuse. It was important to work towards some inclusion of younger siblings in order to identify any help they might need in dealing with the sudden loss of a father or stepfather. Responsibility was seen as lying clearly with the individual abuser, but family attitudes (e.g. if the abused child had a different father) that might have contributed to the vulnerability of a particular child or children needed to be addressed.

A positive relationship between a mother and a female victim prior to the abuse being revealed might become undermined as a result of feelings of guilt, rivalry and responsibility, however misplaced. Relations following disclosure by a younger child could become complex if abuse was perpetrated by an older sibling, with parents becoming confused about how best to support each of the children. During the initial crisis the primary aims were to ensure appropriate protection for the victim(s) and any other children, supporting them and involving ourselves with court proceedings, both civil and criminal. Secondly, it was essential to prevent the family closing up and so refusing or becoming unavailable for treatment. Denial or minimisation of the seriousness leads to a refusal of professional help, insisting there was no risk of further abuse or harmful sequelae to the child or family.

During the crisis phase those offenders who accepted some responsibility almost invariably denied the possibility of their abusing again. Denial serves the purpose of protective self-interest or a need to minimise and deny even to themselves to avoid what could be suicidal guilt.

The different family contexts where treatment was offered include:

- those families where there was no change of membership because the abuser had left prior to disclosure, enabling the child to disclose abuse perpetrated against them
- families which hoped to reintegrate the offender or the victim if she had been moved out
- families where there was no intention to reunite with the offender.

Specific areas of work carried out at Great Ormond Street, London, are outlined below.

The process of clarification, taking appropriate responsibility and apology

- The process of clarifying exactly what abuse has occurred, to whom, how extensively and who is responsible needed to be a theme kept in mind throughout therapeutic work.
- Work with the abused child begins at the point of identification and needs to be extended both during the initial diagnostic phase and during the phase of exposure in the individual/group therapeutic phase.
- The notion of the development of a coherent narrative of the traumatic experience is essential to help the child or young person process the experience, to emerge as a 'survivor' and to understand that anxiety, fear and frozenness were protective strengths, not weaknesses, and can be 'let go'. A supportive parent can participate and reinforce the process (Cohen & Mannarino 2000).
- Perpetrators in treatment also need to acknowledge and share the extensiveness of their abusive action, using victim statements as a key to their work. Individual and group work with perpetrators, adult and adolescent, has now developed extensively as a key element in a 'multimodal' approach (Fisher & Beech 2002, Edwards *et al.* 2006).
- Both victims and perpetrators need to share with protective parents, and with victims acknowledging and attributing responsibility for abuse and failure to protect, and giving appropriate apologies.
- Acknowledging appropriate responsibility and apologising for harm caused to a victim can be a key moment in therapeutic work for the whole family, helping free the victim from responsibility.

Working on denial, minimisation and projection of blame

- A continuing process of family work is the constant revisiting of the issue of who is responsible for abusive action, resisting the desire to blame the victim and minimise the extent of abusive action and its impact.
- A helpful therapeutic approach is to constantly ask the questions:
  - What would happen if there was no denial, if there was no minimisation, if the victim was not blamed?
  - What would be the consequence for a mother if the abuser took full responsibility for their action?
  - Is a degree of denial essential for parents to maintain a relationship and function as parents?
  - If a mother were to acknowledge that she was aware, even peripherally, of abusive action, what would be the consequences? Would there be depressive, suicidal behaviour?
- An approach which positively connotes denial as a means of self-protection, or dissociation as a defence, makes it possible to work with denial, minimisation and blame.
- A denying parent or an older sibling may be asked what would be the consequences if they did recall that abuse had occurred. If they woke up one morning and became aware that the allegations made were true, and they realised they had indeed been responsible for abuse, what would their partner say/think, would they be able to live with themselves, might there be a risk of suicide? Could this sort of behaviour be treated adequately? Serious suicidal wishes could be positively connoted.
- Denial can be positively connoted because the court will protect the child; this could be the best outcome for the child.

Addressing abuse of power, powerlessness and empowerment

- Traumatic responses (e.g. flashbacks, visualisations) associated with a sense of powerlessness experienced by perpetrators, victims and other family members can trigger abusive behaviour.
- Another mechanism is 'identification with the aggressor' in the use of oppressive and violent strategies in relationships and parenting.
- Work with individuals and in family contexts needs to focus on developing appropriate non-coercive self-management, anger management, different ways of assertiveness and a contract of no violence, as in the treatment of physical abuse.
- Intergenerational patterns of abuse, coercive strategies and power-orientated approaches need to be explored through genograms and parents' own development, resolving earlier traumatic and stressful life events, as well as finding appropriate pathways to safe modes of relating.

Work with guilt and rivalry in the mother/child relationship

- Guilt was found to be one of the most prevailing feelings amongst both mothers and victims, particularly if they were female. Offenders contributed actively by shifting responsibility, avoiding blame and anger, and maintaining a sense of power and control. There is always a painful tension for mothers who wanted to support both their partner and child because of the conflict of need and wish.

- Children often felt let down and angry, yet because of their dependency it was difficult to show such feelings openly. There was anger on the mother's side that the child's needs could prohibit her meeting her own emotional needs, and feelings of jealousy that their daughter had been 'another woman' for their partners, despite rejecting the partner to support and protect the child. Adolescent daughters were particular sources of such jealousy.
- Sharing a full account of their abusive experiences – their 'trauma narrative' – often helped mothers understand the extensiveness of traumatic memories and anxieties triggered by thoughts of meeting or seeing the abuser.
- A mother faces a sense of push/pull between her feelings of having to be protective of a younger sibling and excluding an older. When a former partner has initiated abusive patterns the degree of pressure and anxiety on the parent was considerable. The mother needs to deal with her own sense of guilt and her inability to be able to meet her own needs and the needs of both her children adequately. Mothers can be helped to facilitate an apology session and reconciliation between siblings, which in turn helps her manage her own feelings.

Work on sexual feelings, beliefs and activities

- A major problem presented by victims of sexual abuse is sexualisation or anxieties and inhibitions about touching of any kind. Mothers needs to be actively helped to assist the child to overcome confusions and to learn appropriate boundaries for sexual behaviour.
- Learning appropriate touch, modesty and assertion skills can often be carried out in groups with peers; generalisation and reinforcement within the family context often consolidates what the child had learnt within group contexts. Societal norms and personal upbringing often inhibit the discussion of normality of masturbation and childhood erotic pleasure.
- Group work for parents focuses on approaches to sex education, giving explanations of sexual matters as an important training ground for family work. Books and drawings were helpful tools for mothers and older children, and young adolescents found such publications very helpful.
- Individual and group contexts, as well as work within the family, need to address the mother's difficulties in perceiving.

Focusing on blurred and confused role boundaries

- Blurred and confused role boundaries need to be addressed in family work; for example, the abusive father who creates a pseudo-partnership role with a child, putting the mother into a childlike rejected role. The relationship between the child and the mother is undermined, maintaining silencing, blame and guilt. The child is organised into an adult partnership role, becoming the object of emotional and physical closeness, an eroticised partnership – a form of 'traumatic bonding'.
- Individual work enables adults and children to take on appropriate roles and is an essential preliminary task before family work to reinforce appropriate boundaries. Sculpting techniques can help look at the pattern of relationships of family members whilst abuse was continuing, the process leading to a safe family context.
- A rehabilitation programme will include apology sessions when abusers take appropriate responsibility and describe the ways in which abuse has been

perpetrated, and the family manipulated and organised, allowing abusive behaviour to be maintained in secrecy.

■ In one family the father created the role as the authority, the controlling agent; mother and children were seen at a lower level. He belittled and diminished the mother's sense of herself through criticising her sexuality; the mother's silence about her own childhood abuse was rationalised on the basis that she must have enjoyed the sexual experiences. He set up a punitive organising approach and the daughter's ordinary desires for autonomy were labelled bad and rebellious. He then secretly groomed and abused his daughter, demanding silence and continuing secrecy. Following a period of individual and group therapeutic work, the mother began to assert her authority and the father moved down to a more appropriate level. The mother took a central role in the family, both protecting and negotiating the relationship between her children and her partner, the daughter processing her abusive experiences and 'resuming' her adolescent development.

Loss and bereavement

■ In many families there was no proposal to reunite with the offender, resulting in mothers becoming single-parent families without wishing to do so. In such situations therapeutic attention needs to be paid to issues of loss and bereavement.

■ It was important to try to involve all family members suffering loss. Non-abused siblings sometimes felt the loss very differently from the victims, and there needed to be an acceptance of difference.

■ Active involvement of the extended family may be supportive. Mothers were encouraged to share openly with extended family or friends in order to gain social support.

Meeting of individual needs

■ Understanding the impact of abuse on their children, regressed behaviour, aggression, dissociation, traumatic phenomena such as flashbacks, re-enactments, depressed affect, fears and phobias are an essential aspect of family work.

■ Promoting communication, seeking solutions, offering support and constantly linking the care professionals with the therapeutic needs of the family is an essential therapeutic task.

■ There is no one set of techniques that are useful in every context. Structural family therapy approaches help parents and children work through a problem to a solution. Problematic behaviour may need to be connoted positively as steps to healing.

■ Children need help to repair disrupted attachments, develop more satisfactory emotional dysregulation and reverse their negative sense of self. Abusive parents need help to face the nature of their abusive action, to understand its origins and the factors which maintain, and how to prevent relapse and recurrence. Protective parents need to understand how the addictive needs of a partner can distort and destroy family life. These are all important elements which need to be confronted to create a healthy family life for those who are willing to undertake the long journey to health.

- When considering work with abusive families, it is important to understand such families in the wider context of normal family processes. The family, through its functions and tasks, is an organisation which can inherently support and provide for the development and care of children and assist them to achieving maturity and resilience. Alternatively, the characteristics of family functioning – time spent together, intensity, competing activities and interests and proneness to stress from families of origin and currently – make it a context which can be vulnerable to conflict and violence.

- There are a variety of models to understand the nature of families where abuse occurs. Current theories, which stress the cumulative effects of genetic, biological, social, current and family historical factors and family situations, are most valuable to understand the complex processes associated with family violence.

- The introduction of the eco-systemic framework, which considers the way in which the needs of children can be met through the capacity of parents to provide for their needs and the influence of family and environmental factors, has proven a helpful approach. Evidence-based approaches to assessment are essential to ensure that a focused approach to the longer-term needs of children can be assessed.

- A number of factors can be brought together which can demonstrate a hopeful prognosis versus one where there is little prospect of rehabilitation because of the risk of repeated abuse. Situations which are doubtful require a period of continuing work to assess whether the situation is hopeful, or whether rehabilitation cannot be achieved within the child's timeframe.

- There are stages of therapeutic work from the phase of identification of abusive action, the assessment of individuals and the family context, to working in a context of protection, a rehabilitation programme or from children to have a new family. Initially, work is conducted with individuals or in group contexts to ensure that traumatic experiences are processed, protective parents' capacities are reinforced and abusive parents helped to develop safer ways of relating. Conjoint family work often takes place at a later stage when rehabilitation is being considered.

- A variety of approaches have now been demonstrated to be effective with physical and sexual abuse. These include cognitive–behavioural, dynamic and systemic approaches. Therapeutic work needs to be carried out in a context of close liaison between therapeutic, statutory and legal services so that the work is integrated and the protective needs of children are always kept central.

- Neglect remains a challenging and difficult area of work, and emotional abuse is being better understood; however, therapeutic work follows generic principles rather than specific approaches.

- When planning therapeutic work with families where abusive action has occurred, it is essential that a multidisciplinary approach is taken; no one professional can carry out the assessment of all family contexts as is required. A full understanding of the individuals in the family is necessary, as well as the impact of abusive action on children and young people, the parental family and environmental factors associated with abusive action, and an understanding of history, relationships, parenting and the response to the particular child.

- Approaches to assessment and therapeutic work need to be founded on evidence-based approaches to assessment and an awareness of developing knowledge about effective therapeutic approaches. Therapeutic work does not take place in isolation but must be provided in the service of protection authorities and statutory agencies that are responsible for the protection and well-being of children. Motivation for therapeutic work is often limited initially, the aim of maintaining a child within a family is an appropriate place to start; a true desire for change can grow by building on small successes.

■ It is essential to understand the stages of therapeutic work from the phase when abusive experiences are being identified, an understanding of the family context, the developing stages of therapeutic work with children and parents in a context of protection, to the stage where rehabilitation may be tested or a new family is going to be required.

■ There is no one approach that is more effective than another with children and parents in families where abuse has taken place. Approaches need to be multimodal, delivered with individuals, in groups and in family contexts. Work which is focused and addresses abusive and traumatic experiences directly is more effective than waiting for children and young people to take the lead. Work needs to be focused on a number of areas including parenting capacities, the management of boundaries between parents and children, ensuring protective functions are primary, protective parents are supported to care for children and children's traumatic experiences are resolved.

Annotated further reading

Bentovim A 1995 Trauma organised systems: physical and sexual abuse in families. Karnac, London

This text provides a systemic theoretical framework for understanding the impact of both physical and professional systems. In particular, sociological, social interactions and system perspectives, which describe how family systems become organised around the trauma of family violence, are described. A systemic account of trauma-organised systems associated with different forms of family violence is addressed. The need to break the denial process inherent in trauma-organised families is essential in planning therapeutic work. The book is illustrated with numerous case examples and provides child protection professionals with a valuable framework for understanding and assessing families in which child abuse has occurred.

Furniss T 1991 The multiprofessional handbook of child sexual abuse: integrated management, therapy and legal intervention. Routledge, London

This book makes a more direct link between child abuse and family therapy. It is a good resource for readers who wish to look in more depth at working with families where sexual abuse has taken place. Using a systems approach, Furniss considers child sexual abuse as a syndrome of addiction and secrecy which requires a multidisciplinary response. He presents an integrated approach to the management, therapeutic work and legal frameworks involved in the care and treatment of sexually abused children and their families, and shows how practical steps in therapy and management directly influence each other. The first part of the book outlines the principal ways and basic concepts used in dealing with child sexual abuse. The second part focuses on practical problems, ranging from the evaluation of suspicion, the management of disclosure and interprofessional problems through a wide range of treatment issues relating directly to working with abusing families. The theoretical and practice sections are cross-referenced, so that the reader can use the conceptual framework to inform their therapeutic work in a direct and specific way.

Jones D P H, Ramchandani P 1999 Child sexual abuse: informing practice from research. Radcliffe Medical Press, Oxford

A research/evidence-based review of many aspects of work with child sexual abuse. Brings together recently commissioned research by the Department of Health in an accessible, clear and well-argued way. Essential to assist in developing practice, and to clarify the family role in work with sexual abuse.

Browne K, Hanks H, Stratton P, Hamilton C 2002 Early prediction and prevention of child abuse: a handbook. Wiley, Chichester

This is an update of an earlier volume and provides a guide to the prediction of various forms of abuse including fatal child abuse and neglect, physical maltreatment, emotional child abuse and neglect and sexual abuse and neglect. It provides an account of primary and secondary prevention using an ecological analysis, focusing on positive parenting and prevention through prenatal and infancy home visiting. There is also an account of tertiary prevention, helping children and families affected by abuse by examining the impact of abusive experiences, a focus on intergenerational transmission, the role of family therapy, focusing on emotionally abused and neglected children, and working with offenders including my own chapter on preventing the victim-to-offender cycle. This text is written by leading American and UK authors. It provides an excellent view on a systemic approach by taking a broad updated view of the field.

Working with adult survivors of childhood sexual abuse: trauma, attachment and the search for meaning

Liz Hall and Siobhan Canavan

INTRODUCTION

This chapter examines a number of issues relating to working with adults who were sexually abused as children. We acknowledge that the impact of sexual abuse by a trusted adult has specific consequences in adulthood and that it is also important for practitioners to recognise that physical and emotional abuse and neglect may have many similar effects (Wilson & Ryan 2005). Adult survivors of sexual abuse are likely to have experienced other forms of abuse and/or neglect and it is often difficult to separate the impact of each of these types of abuse on an individual. Nor is it helpful to pursue the effects of one form of abuse or neglect over another. Recently there have been many developments in our understanding of therapeutic work with adults abused as children and there are a number of reasons for including this chapter in a book which deals primarily with child protection.

1. An understanding of the long-term effects of abuse into adulthood reminds us of the need to help children in similar situations to be protected and safe. The impact of sexual abuse on the developing child can continue well into adulthood (Browne & Finkelhor 1986, Russell 1986, Hall & Lloyd 1993, Kendall-Tackett *et al*. 1993). The long-term effects are significant and remind us that prevention and early identification of child abuse should be a high priority for all health and social services agencies.
2. Adult survivors of child abuse have provided professionals of all disciplines with significant knowledge about the nature of child abuse, the coping strategies of children subjected to abuse and the specific complexity surrounding child sexual abuse. Child sexual abuse affects every member of a family, but most of all the victims.
3. Our understanding of the impact of child sexual abuse on the development of attachments, which are so necessary for emotional development, has improved. The work of Schore (1994, 2003a, 2003b), Briere (1996), Siegel (1999), Levy and Orlans (1998) and Gerhardt (2004) has shown that the experience of sexual and other abuse disturbs and disrupts a child's ability to form secure attachments. As 80% of abused children are abused by people known to them, their ability to trust and attach to adults in general can become distorted and disrupted. This also has a serious effect both on the

developing brain and on subsequent emotional development (Schore 1994, 2003a, 2003b).

4. Where children grow up in a climate of abuse and neglect, they learn a model of parenting that leaves them poorly prepared to manage the needs of their own children. Many adult survivors manage very successfully to raise their children but there is a large number for whom parenting becomes a significant problem.

5. Recent neurobiological research conducted by van der Kolk (van der Kolk 1994, van der Kolk & Fisler 1995, van der Kolk *et al.* 1996a, 1996b), the work of Nijenhuis *et al.* (2001) and Schore (1994, 2003a) is beginning to clarify the exact nature of the impact of trauma on the brain with the advent and development of appropriate scanning technology.

6. Finally, whilst the body of literature on all aspects of therapeutic work with children and adults who have experienced sexual abuse has expanded in the last two decades, it is only more recently that the effects on helpers of doing this work have begun to be examined (Perlman & Saakvitne 1995).

For all of these reasons, it is timely to revisit key issues in working with adult survivors of abuse.

Attachment

Attachment in children is the most fundamental process that is essential for the child's development. It has been defined as:

the deep and enduring connection established between a child and caregiver in the first several years of life. It profoundly influences every component of the human condition – mind, body, emotions, relationships and values ... attachment is a physiological, emotional, cognitive, and social phenomenon.

(Levy & Orlans 1998)

It is created between caregiver and child through a process of attunement and mutual reciprocity. A secure attachment provides not only safety and protection for the vulnerable child, but is also vital for a number of other reasons:

■ Secure attachments shape brain development in the most optimal way and stimulate further brain development (Schore 1994, Siegel 1999)
■ To learn basic trust and reciprocity that acts as a template for future relationships
■ To explore the environment safely and securely which in turn facilitates both cognitive and social development
■ To develop the ability to self-regulate at an emotional level; this is vital for managing impulsive behaviour and emotional reactions
■ It establishes the basis for the formation of identity which includes a sense of self-worth, self-efficacy and a balance between dependency and autonomy
■ To establish conditions for the development of empathy, compassion and conscience
■ To generate a core belief system about oneself and others and about life in general
■ To provide a defence against trauma and stress. The literature demonstrates that resilience in children is associated with positive secure attachments (Schofield 2001).

Secure attachments develop where the caregiving relationship establishes safe and nurturing touch, appropriate eye contact, smile and positive emotional responses and a meeting of the child's needs. By meeting the child's needs consistently, the child's distress and arousal are reduced, and attachment is reinforced and developed.

Without a secure attachment, the child is at risk of serious problems throughout its development. There are a number of situations that can result in the disruption of attachment formation. They include:

- all forms of abuse (physical, emotional, sexual, verbal and psychological)
- neglect of all types
- alcoholism or drug abuse in the parent, especially the mother prenatally
- separation from the primary caregiver
- separation from other key family members, e.g. grandparents, siblings
- frequent moves in the looked-after system.

Gerhardt (2004) discusses the difficulties that result from these early experiences in terms of emotional regulation. She notes that there are considerable difficulties for the child in learning to manage the high physiological arousal of fear if the child's carers fail to manage this through the development of a positive attachment. Equally, difficulties are created when carers themselves behave in ways that heighten the child's physiological arousal beyond the capacity of the developing brain and connected systems. She discusses the negative effects of poor management of high physiological arousal on the developing brain of the child, and the consequences for the health and well-being of the child into adulthood.

Briere (1996) describes further difficulties for the traumatised child. These, combined with the attachment problems, underpin many of their later difficulties, particularly in relationships. The neglectful and/or abusive behaviour of the child's carers leads to the poor or impoverished development of key psychological processes that have considerable repercussions for the formation of stability, self-esteem and stable relationships. These core self-capacities are as follows:

- *A sense of identity*: Recognising the unique features that are personal to the individual. This incorporates values, beliefs and a sense of identity that comes from being part of a family/community/ethnic group
- *Boundaries*: These indicate where the individual begins and ends in relation to others, and includes acceptable interpersonal boundaries that reinforce positive relationships
- *Emotional tolerance*: This describes the ability to tolerate strong negative feelings without dissociation
- *Emotional modulation*: This describes the capacity to moderate strong feelings so that they become more manageable
- *Relatedness*: The capacity to form and maintain meaningful relationships. Deficits in this area lead to interpersonal conflicts and a tendency to be involved in chaotic and short-lived relationships. Additional problems include idealisation or disillusionment with people and concerns about abandonment.

Long-term consequences of sexual abuse

An understanding of the long-term effects has been known and accepted for a number of years (Browne & Finkelhor 1986, Russell 1986, Lew 1990, Hall & Lloyd 1993, Kendall-Tackett *et al.* 1993). Mullen and Fleming (1998) divide the long-term effects into primary issues and consequential secondary issues. They consider that difficulties with intimacy, trust, personal effectiveness, self-esteem and sexuality are the primary consequences of child sexual abuse; other issues, particularly those involving mental health, are second-order effects. However, it is also accepted that some of the consequences fall within a post-traumatic paradigm and include complex post-traumatic stress and complex dissociative processes.

Hall and Lloyd (1993) drew attention to some of the common parenting problems for adult survivors although it is important to note that a history of abuse does not *per se* lead to parenting problems. The importance of an individual's attachment history and reactions to the abuse is significant in this context. Common problems include:

- difficulties in meeting the emotional needs of a child, a consequence of having no internalised model of safe parenting from childhood, or because of dissociative and other emotional consequences of the abuse/neglect
- constant fears for the safety of the child, leading to damaging over-protection, hypervigilance, and providing a highly anxious environment for the child
- failures of protection of the child from risky or abusive adults, possibly because of a lack of awareness of the danger signs because of dissociative problems, or a lack of an internalised model of appropriate supervision and vigilance around children
- difficulties with touch, leading to a fear that they might abuse the child or be seen to do so, problems with showing physical affection and engaging in play that involves touch.

There still exists a cultural belief that suggests that an adult who was abused as a child will become an abuser of children. This is known as the victim–victimiser cycle of abuse. Glasser *et al.* (2001) noted that, in a sample of 747 males attending a specialist forensic psychotherapy centre (i.e. a clinical sample), 18% reported a history of child sexual abuse. Of these, 54% abused by males went on to offend against a child. This study showed that boys abused both at home by a family member and outside the home were more likely to become a perpetrator. The comparable figures for females in this study were that 43% reported a history of child abuse and 2% had, in adulthood, sexually abused a child. Two points need to be made about these statistics: firstly, from a forensic population we cannot generalise the findings to the general population; and secondly, although they do not provide an indication of the gender of the original perpetrator, the figures clearly illustrate a gender dimension to one of its consequences – insofar as women are more likely to experience sexual abuse than men but they are much less likely than males to go on to become abusers in adulthood.

Research into the long-term impact has included a link between a history of child abuse, particularly child sexual abuse, with a history of a variety of physical illnesses (Bachmann *et al.* 1988, Cunningham *et al.* 1988, Arnold *et al.* 1990, Felitti 1991). There is still much research to be done in this area.

The history of help for survivors

In the past 20 years, ways of helping adults abused as children have seen many changes. The voice of the survivor has been and continues to be a critical part of that history, informing professionals and the general population that the issue of child sexual abuse cannot be ignored. Survivors have also been crucial in informing professionals about what sort of therapeutic work is helpful, what is not and what the main issues in the work are likely to be. Here, as in no other area of therapeutic endeavour, the voice of the client is heard with consistency. In the UK this came through the advent of Rape Crisis Centres in the early 1980s and the development of ChildLine later in that decade. Initially, it was thought that telling the story about what had happened was an important and almost sufficient part of the healing process. The experience of the abuse is clearly critical but there is a risk of re-traumatising the individual by being exposed again to the details of the story. It is now accepted that telling the story in very small amounts, with the survivor in control of what is told, how and when, is the best way of preventing the individual from being re-traumatised.

Long-term therapy was offered by many agencies but long waiting lists have always been a problem. Some survivors sought help through hospital-based services; others accessed community and volunteer-based resources. Survivors set up their own groups and were involved in professionally led groups. Inevitably, demand outstripped resources, and agencies were continually reviewing the work offered to survivors in the light of best practice guidelines which have been established by most professional bodies, especially in the area of recovered memories.

New models incorporating the effect on the body of the traumatic material derive from the study of brain mechanisms involved in traumatic reactions (van der Kolk 1994, van der Kolk & Fisler 1995, van der Kolk *et al.* 1996a, 1996b) and the body-oriented psychotherapies such as sensorimotor psychotherapy (Ogden & Minton 2000). van der Kolk *et al.* (1996a) clearly indicate that 'the body keeps the score' of the trauma, both in terms of lack of control of physiological arousal and in terms of memory. The importance of the problems of emotional regulation at all levels is now firmly on the map.

Why now?

Many adults abused as children manage during some of their adult lives to cope with their difficult experiences from childhood. Memories and consequences of these experiences can erupt in adulthood, often triggered by current events and reactions. Having children, being involved in medical procedures, the survivor's children reaching the age when the abuse started and issues relating to the abuser (e.g. death, illness or even simply coming to visit) or a non-abusing caregiver are common triggers for the individual beginning to search for help.

Another situation that can bring a survivor for help is involvement in care proceedings relating to their own parenting. This may relate to the poor attachment history that they had as children, to the poor model of parenting they were exposed to or to negative reactions and problems relating to their own history of abuse, or becoming involved in abusive and violent relationships (Maltz 1991).

Problems in seeking help

There are a number of issues for an adult survivor of child abuse seeking help. Firstly, the search for help by adults abused as children leads them into a situation where many of their difficulties immediately come to the fore. Being in a room with one other individual where there is an expectation that the survivor will attempt to talk to a therapist or health professional can lead to significant physiological arousal, hypervigilance and generalised fear and anxiety. For many survivors who have experienced long-term abuse and neglect within their family of origin, forming an attachment to another individual is extremely difficult. Issues of relationship and trust may immediately arise.

Secondly, many survivors of abuse have limited recall of their past childhood experiences. Williams (1994) found that for the documented incidents of sexual abuse that had occurred 17 years earlier, one in three women did not report those abuse experiences. In a second study (Williams L 1995), it was found that one in 10 of the women who reported the abuse at the time of the study, reported that at some time in the past they had forgotten about the abuse. These findings are important because they were not based on a retrospective reporting of child abuse by adults. Thus, amnesia for the experiences of abuse is not uncommon, and any memories that emerge are often accompanied by a high level of anxiety and the desire to avoid them.

Thirdly, there is some anecdotal evidence that the development and increased use of short-term therapy which is offered now instead of longer-term psychotherapy has made it more difficult for adults abused as children to find the sustained support and help they need. This can increase a sense of isolation and difficulty for the individual in this situation.

Fourthly, child abuse involves not only specific acts of abuse and neglect but also involves the misuse of power and the loss of choice and control. These issues emerge throughout the search for help and within therapy itself. Finally, gender issues are also important because many survivors find they cannot work with a therapist who is the same gender as the person who abused them. Where there have been multiple abusers, this presents many problems in establishing a trusting therapeutic relationship. Simply being in a room with someone of the same gender as the abuser gives rise to the possibility that the survivor will be triggered into remembering the abuse, having flashbacks and high physiological reactions or to a collapse into a dissociative or hypo-aroused process, with numbing and switching off being key characteristics.

A framework for working with survivors of child abuse and neglect

Meaning of the abuse

To consider sexual abuse as a traumatic event or series of traumas offers a helpful conceptual framework for thinking about the long-term effects of such abuse and issues in working with survivors. Responses to traumatic events are highly idiosyncratic. Many factors, both internal and external, influence how the individual processes and internalises a traumatic event such as sexual abuse and how they manage this personal meaning in the aftermath of the trauma.

Trauma always involves loss. The losses may be actual losses, such as the loss of significant aspects of childhood, or they may be more psychological (e.g. the loss of identity, meaning or optimism). Often in the course of therapeutic work the traumatised person is faced with both and they can feel that they do not know who they now are in the world. There is considerable pain involved in working through and bearing these levels of loss. Levy and Lemma (2004) have argued that when an acknowledgement of the internal losses and mourning for these losses parallel 'an impoverishment in the person's social reality, the likelihood of a complicated post-traumatic reaction is significantly increased' (p. 7). They propose that an acknowledgement of both kinds of loss is vital and that the way in which a traumatised person processes an experience of loss is central to an understanding of the impact of trauma on the psyche. They establish a link between complex responses to trauma and a breakdown in the capacity to mourn which is distorted (they use the word perverted) as a way of managing the unbearable and unthinkable nature of the traumatic loss.

When an individual is traumatised by a sudden or unexplained event, the impact on mental functioning is considerable. There is an immediate period of shock and denial – but this does not always work, and the person's defences are shattered so that their capacity to trust in the predictability of the world creates a 'loss in the structure of meaning' (Marris 1974). This effect is much greater when the individual is a child and is not in an environment that allows the formation of secure attachment and capacity to trust. This can create a difficulty in processing information – the ability to represent events to oneself mentally in a way that enables them to be processed without being plunged again into feeling that it is happening in the present. This is represented in flashbacks. Garland (2002, 2004) notes that recent work in neuroscience connects this process with the work of the amygdala, now thought of as the brain's 'smoke detector', in which the work of the higher cortical centres, necessary for rational thought, are bypassed. The significance of this understanding for therapeutic work with survivors is that it helps us consider how therapeutic work might impact on the survivor, especially in relation to remembering aspects of the abuse or in the therapeutic relationship itself.

Warner (2000) argues that a development of the person-centred idea of 'process' offers a model for 'understanding extreme affective and relational sensitivity'. One aspect of the relational complexity is in a 'fragile' process, where clients have difficulty with emotional reactions, or understanding the points of view of other people without breaking contact with their own experience. This offers an understanding of survivors who, in the middle of a fragile process, experience very high levels of shame and self-criticism about their experience. A second type is in a 'dissociated process' in which aspects of the person's experience are separated into parts which may be totally unaware of each other's presence. Warner argues that these two styles of processing emerge when a child's earliest experience is not adequately accepted, protected or responded to by adult caregivers. They have experienced a high level of empathic failure in childhood so the presence and maintenance of empathy on the part of the therapist is of primary importance in the therapeutic relationship.

This framework fosters an understanding that links the survivor's experiences as a child with their difficulties, strengths and resources as an adult. The key aim of the approach is to create a relationship between the therapist and the survivor that acts as a partnership, using their collective resources to enable the survivor to come to terms with the past.

As an abused child grows into adulthood, issues of attachment and trust are obvious within the therapeutic relationship; feelings of powerlessness and lack of choice and control can continue, resulting in an expectation of betrayal by others. The framework for therapeutic work should therefore address the key issues of attachment and trust, power, choice, boundaries and understanding (Briere 1996). It is also vital to consider issues relating to the silence and secrecy surrounding the abuse.

Attachment and trust

Children who have been abused by an adult, particularly one known to them, have been betrayed by people who should have been protecting them from harm and danger. This fundamentally affects every other relationship for the child, and therefore prevents the establishment of or disrupts an existing attachment. As we have seen, attachment patterns underpin much of the child's later development. Where the abuse has occurred early in the child's life (before the age of 5 years) and has been perpetrated by one of the child's main caregivers, the effect on later development is the most significant. Schore (1994) notes that when a child is unable to develop a secure attachment in those early years, and if they live in fear on a regular basis, optimal brain development is not possible, with the negative consequences for emotional regulation, organisational skills, relationship skills and learning.

Attachment to the perpetrator is common and comprehensible in terms of the development of a trauma bond (James 1994). In spite of the abuse and neglect, adult survivors may retain a bond with the perpetrator and other family members who failed to protect them from the perpetrator. The bond is often one which is based on fear and not on the normal rules of attachment (Levy & Lemma 2004). Therapists and other helpers often find it difficult to understand how an individual could retain an attachment to someone who has hurt them. However, we have a salutary reminder of the way in which this process happens in the accounts of adults without a previous history of poor attachments forming attachments to those who have taken them hostage. This has become known as the Stockholm syndrome, following a bank raid in Stockholm where the captives actively resisted rescue at the end of their 6 days of captivity. They refused to testify against their captors, and raised money for their legal defence. If adults with no known history of attachment difficulties can form an attachment in 6 days to their captors, the power of this for children who are in a similarly captive and abusive situation is much greater.

It is perhaps surprising, therefore, that so many adult survivors of abuse and neglect manage to come for help at all since the therapeutic process immediately produces triggers to the very experiences that are most difficult. For example, the survivor may find that they become attached to the therapist, overdependent or avoidant of them. These experiences are likely to raise issues for the therapeutic alliance that can be both useful and inhibitory for the survivor, but need to be addressed by the therapist.

Many survivors come for help having had previous unsuccessful or unhelpful contacts with helping agencies. It is therefore important for the survivor to be given enough time to learn to trust the helper and not be pressurised to say more than they want to. Building trust takes time, and this process can easily be disrupted by situations that seem unimportant to the helper. For example, trust tends to be experienced as 'all or nothing' by survivors, so that even one error by a helper, such as failing to return a telephone call, may make it difficult for the survivor to trust them.

Power issues

Children have little or no power and are expected to obey the adult who is abusing them. In some situations it would be dangerous for the child to resist. The abuser, however, has misused their position of power and the responsibility they have over the child. At the outset the therapist is likely to be seen by the survivor as more knowledgeable, powerful, expert and important. This imbalance of power can reflect the survivor's view of authority figures and can also reinforce a lack of self-esteem. This is the reality of many therapeutic situations and, in order to redress this imbalance of power to some extent, the survivor's strengths, resources and courage should be acknowledged, valued and used within the therapeutic environment. Ultimately, the survivor is the best judge of how they feel, even if the therapist has to assist in finding the right words to describe reactions and interventions to help with this.

The therapeutic process can be very empowering because of the close attention that is paid to the survivor. This is often a new experience for the individual who may have experienced many disempowering experiences during childhood and into adulthood. However, there is also a downside to this therapeutic attention in that it could also be triggering and frightening for the survivor who is simply not used to having the spotlight turned on them except possibly during abusive experiences. The shift from feeling disempowered to being able to value oneself is a gradual process that comes partly through being valued within the therapeutic relationship. This process may be changing a lifelong pattern and therefore may impact on other relationships and situations outside the therapeutic process. Survivors often find that their relationships can change radically as they become aware of power imbalances and any abusive qualities within them. For the individual concerned, this may be a very uncomfortable and unsettling experience.

Choice and control

A child has little or no choice or control over what happens in an abusive situation, although the abuser may have led the child to believe that they did have a choice. The therapeutic framework can reverse this by providing choice over many aspects of the helping situation. The most important relates to disclosure of details of the abusive experiences. Survivors should have choice about when, how much and to whom they choose to tell about the abuse. They often report feeling forced to tell a helper what happened to them as children, with no consideration given to the consequences this might have in terms of continuing contact after the disclosure and their possible need for support. The gender of the therapist can be very important here, because many survivors find it difficult to work with someone of the same gender as the abuser. For women who were abused by men, the initial choice is often for a female worker, but a male worker can have beneficial effects in learning to trust a man.

Other areas where the survivor can have some choice relate to the location and timing of sessions with the therapist and other people available for support. The process of coming to terms with sexual abuse can be greatly facilitated if the survivor feels comfortable, unpressured and in control of aspects of the therapeutic process. Unfortunately, this is where the demand for longer-term work often outstrips the available resources, especially in agencies where brief therapy is the main therapy on offer. The therapist may also only have a limited range of options for timing and location which have to form part of the boundaries for the work.

Boundaries

Normal physical and emotional boundaries between adult and child are violated when an adult sexually abuses a child. This can leave a child and subsequently the adult survivor with problems in developing a clear sense of boundaries. Common problems with boundaries include the following:

- The individual develops poor boundaries and can be said to be under-boundaried (Fisher 2005). In this situation, the survivor is unable to say 'No', is over-compliant, and cannot identify their own feelings and reactions separately from those of others. They will often appear unguarded or over-relaxed physically, and may give too much in relationships because of the difficulty in distinguishing between self and others. The difficulty with this is that the individual is often flooded with too much information, obligation and activity, although they may also be able to develop good levels of empathy and insight which can be used to make changes.
- The individual develops an over-boundaried style of relating. This leads to being very guarded physically and emotionally. The individual is likely to have

problems with trust, intimacy and any experience of feeling vulnerable because they cannot let their guard down. As a result, they may feel isolated and unable to receive any positives from others. The first response is usually to say 'No', even when saying 'Yes' might be more appropriate or beneficial. The difficulties for this style of relating are that the individual has to live very rigidly and without spontaneity, and is often terrified of being overwhelmed by emotion. The task is to help the survivor to relax some of the control in small ways so that they can benefit from more flexible boundaries.

■   Other survivors develop a 'pendulum' boundary (Ogden *et al.* 2006) where they swing between the two styles described above.

It is also not uncommon to find that survivors have a different boundary in relation to their family of origin. Whereas the normal interpersonal boundary may be adequate in many circumstances, some survivors are either over- or under-boundaried in relation to their family of origin or the abuse experiences. This can create problems for therapeutic work where the individual may either become flooded by the physiological arousal associated with the triggers to the abuse experiences or maintain a rigid boundary round those experiences and refuse to discuss them at all. This variation can lead to considerable confusion and sense that at any time they might be overwhelmed, which in turn leads to increased rigidity in relating style.

An individual's boundary style may give the therapist clues about early family experiences, but may need to be actively worked with to establish predictable, non-abusive boundaries within the therapeutic work. These different styles give rise to differing reactions in the therapist which are useful pieces of information. The therapist may be invited to be a 'rescuer' by the individual, which would suggest an under-boundaried style in the client. The over-boundaried client often gives rise to increasing feelings of helplessness and frustration in the therapist. The client who swings between the various styles of relating can lead to more confusion and disappointment with and in the therapist.

It is essential that clear, safe boundaries are established, so that there is no danger of the survivor being victimised again by the therapeutic situation. Boundaries relating to confidentiality, the length and frequency of sessions, and the level of support available between sessions should be established early and may need regular review, especially at times of crisis or other difficulty. The issue of confidentiality should be discussed openly, with the survivor's wishes respected in this matter. Information about the agency's policy concerning confidentiality should be given so that the survivor knows what the guidelines are. It is also important to indicate how much of the content of sessions with the helper will be recorded and how much, when and with whom the survivor may be discussed by the therapist in supervision and support meetings, in meetings with other helpers or with members of the survivor's wider support network.

Problems relating to confidentiality may arise when a survivor is being seen by a number of different agencies or by several members of a multidisciplinary team. In these situations, it is important to inform the survivor of any policies regarding confidentiality, particularly about any information that may have to be passed to another worker. The therapist and other workers are responsible for drawing the boundaries clearly and for explaining them to the survivor.

It is also essential that boundaries relating to touch are agreed. Touch should be used with great caution and if at all, in a limited way, only with the survivor's permission. Issues of gender are very important in this respect. Regrettably, some survivors have been sexually abused by their helpers (Armsworth 1989, Rutter 1990, Russell 1993). Therapists need to be aware of any of their actions which might be felt by survivors to be in any way abusive. This clearly calls for a substantial degree of self-awareness on the part of the therapist.

The establishment of more appropriate boundaries comes through awareness, consistency of a safe and appropriate approach from the therapist, learning new ways of managing control of a situation and by learning positive levels of assertiveness. Clearly this is a process that develops over time. With the more severely abused and/or neglected survivor, establishment of secure and flexible interpersonal boundaries is difficult because the early trauma has taken away some of the necessary building blocks.

Understanding

An important aspect of the framework for helping adult survivors of child abuse is to facilitate an understanding of how the experience of being abused has affected them, both as a child and as an adult. This should include recognising the ways the child used to cope with and survive the trauma. Linking the abuse with adult difficulties enables survivors to recognise the relevance of the abuse to their development and facilitates the process of coming to terms with it. Helping the survivor regain a sense of their own resources can help with the process of building self-worth and feelings of self-efficacy. However, the issue of loss always emerges in this process.

Breaking the silence and secrecy

A child is often unable to tell anyone about the abuse. The abuser may have used threats of violence or threatened the family. The child may also be unable to tell because of a sense of guilt and shame, or because there was no one to tell who might have believed them. The child's coping mechanisms may complicate this further, as a child may deny, dissociate from, minimise or rationalise the abuse, so that telling someone becomes even more difficult. Finally, a young child does not have words and concepts to describe the abuse, thus making disclosure nearly impossible.

The burden of keeping the secret can cause many psychological and physical problems that can be resolved through talking about these experiences (Lister 1982). Disclosure requires sensitive handling and careful monitoring afterwards, as it can be both a liberating and a painful process. Through disclosure, however, the survivor can discover that the abuser was responsible, that a child has a right to have protection and care from an adult, and that the emotional energy used to maintain the silence can become available for more positive use in adult life. The legacy of sexual abuse and the burden of responsibility for the abuse can then be shifted to the abuser – where it unequivocally belongs.

Adult survival strengths

One of the main resources available in coming to terms with the abuse is those personal resources and strengths developed by the survivor in order to survive the abuse. Confirmation of the strength and courage involved in surviving into adulthood and in seeking help is important for empowering a survivor to value their own coping strategies, even those which might have been less productive for them. There is a continuum of coping strategies used by survivors ranging from alcohol and drug abuse, suicide attempts and other types of self-injury to those who channel all their energies into being high achievers in education or employment.

Some coping mechanisms develop into clear strengths, such as becoming self-sufficient or being steady in a crisis. Others can develop into self-destructive patterns of behaviour. There are also behaviours that have both healthy and destructive aspects – high achievement in academic matters may secure a college place or a good job, but it may lead the survivor into becoming more socially isolated from other people as their energy is channelled into the pursuit of academic success.

In recent years, the resourcefulness of survivors has been shown in the growth of published material written by survivors themselves in the form of poems, autobiographical accounts, songs, letters and self-help books (Evert & Bijkerk 1987, Spring 1987, Finney 1990, Malone *et al.* 1996). These have been crucial in breaking the silence about child sexual abuse and in educating professionals about the experience and effects of abuse in a very direct, accessible way. This literature has also played an important part in enabling survivors to see that they are not alone in their experience, that other survivors have struggled with similar difficulties and that recovery is possible.

Issues for therapists and other helpers

Working with survivors can be slow, exhausting, sad, angry, despairing and tense. It can also be exhilarating, exciting, energising and rewarding work. A survivor may have invested a great deal in undertaking therapeutic work but there may also be significant others in their life who are of equal importance as they work on coming to terms with their experiences. Working with sexual abuse significantly changes the therapist. We have experienced the process as 'a loss of innocence', as our view of the world – especially in relation to issues of child safety, appropriate adult/child boundaries and the experience of being a child – is challenged and changed forever. Working with survivors of sexual abuse can mean that helpers give up their familiar ways of being in the world.

One of the consequences of this is that they can experience the effects of vicarious traumatisation. This has been defined as 'the transformation of inner experience of the therapist that comes about as the result of empathic engagement with clients' traumatic experience' (Perlman & Saakvitne 1995). It is best understood as an occupational hazard in working with sexual abuse. Therapists may hear accounts of abusive experiences which are brutalising, cruel and persistently painful on many levels. In order to share with clients their journey towards a different reality, therapists need to be open. Yet their empathy can be a source of vulnerability to emotional pain and scarring. Since it is difficult to protect oneself from knowing the truth of what children and adults have endured, this can result in feelings of helplessness and of being a helpless witness to trauma, which in itself can be traumatising. Vicarious traumatisation is more of a process than an event; it is a normal reaction and response to intolerable experiences. Once it is acknowledged, the therapist can think about ways in which they can look after themselves in their work so that they continue to be available for their clients.

Vicarious traumatisation also carries a social cost. Many people come to work in a helping capacity because they are hopeful about humanity and the possibility for a better world. Unaddressed, vicarious traumatisation can lead to feelings of hopelessness, helplessness, cynicism and despair, and ultimately to burn-out and depression.

Therapeutic contexts

There are a variety of contexts where a survivor of abuse may find relevant help. Since we wrote the chapter for the first edition of this book, these have changed somewhat in that group facilities appear to be less available than previously, and there has been a growth in the private sector where therapists, psychologists and counsellors have established private practices, some of which offer a specific resource for survivors of sexual abuse. The following is a brief description of potential sources of help.

One-to-one settings

Most survivors choose a one-to-one therapeutic situation, preferring the confidentiality and sense of security it offers. Waiting times for an appointment can be a problem, however, and this can sometimes leave the survivor feeling abandoned after having made the courageous first step in seeking help.

There are a number of issues which can arise for both the survivor and helper in a one-to-one setting. It can establish a long-term trusting relationship with someone who believes the survivor, details of the abuse are confidential to one person and the therapeutic work can be done at the survivor's own pace. Survivors can sometimes fear the intensity of the work. They can also be concerned with burdening the helper with details of the abuse, and this can result in protecting the helper from their pain. For the helper, on the other hand, there may be concerns about over-involvement or dependency on the part of the survivor.

Survivors' groups

Groups can be open-ended or closed, and there are advantages and disadvantages to each. The former can provide immediate access when it is needed, and members at different stages can give each other encouragement and support. It is, however, difficult to build trust and to undertake planned work when group membership constantly changes. Variable attendance and issues relating to confidentiality are additional problems in open-ended groups. Closed groups have the advantage of a more easily established climate of trust and greater ease in establishing and maintaining a group culture. Members can also get to know each other over a period of time, and can move on together from one issue to another. One disadvantage is the difficulty of leaving if the group is not meeting the needs of the individual.

Working with partners

As more survivors seek help in dealing with issues from their past, a partner is often the first person a survivor tells about the abuse. This may be the result of feeling secure in a relationship, often for the first time; it can be the result of issues relating to pregnancy or children, or of difficulties which the couple experience in their relationship.

Partners themselves may need support during times of disclosure. There are three areas in which it can be helpful for partners to talk to someone:

- understanding the long-term effects of sexual abuse
- gaining an understanding of the process of recovery for the survivor
- consideration of the potential effects on the couple's relationship in the future.

At some point, a survivor and their partner may wish to deal with the effects of the abuse on their sexual relationship (Maltz 1991).

Assessment

The following issues are important to establish towards the beginning of any therapeutic work with an adult who has experienced any form of abuse as a child. There may be issues which are specific to adult survivors of sexual abuse and we would ask readers to bear this in mind when considering assessment for therapeutic work:

- *Boundaries*: The boundary style of the survivor is very useful information and may determine some of the problems in this area. The need for establishing the boundaries of the therapeutic contact, confidentiality, time and support is critical near the beginning although may have to be reiterated many times in a consistent and supportive way;
- *Psychological difficulties*: The level and type of these difficulties, and whether the problems have a long or more recent history. This will become clearer over time but an initial exploration does enable us to determine the likely course of therapy and whether additional professional supports are necessary.
- *Why now?*: It is useful to check what has triggered the request for help at this point.
- *The strengths of the survivor*: These include coping strategies, resilience and resourcefulness. They should also include capacities to regulate high physiological arousal (e.g. ability to relax, participation in physical activities, exercise, dissociation, self-harm).
- *The support network available to the individual*: This should include both professional and other sources of support such as friends, family and community-based supports.
- *Childhood history*: A thumbnail sketch of the individual's childhood history is advantageous so that the therapist has some knowledge of the family background. No pressure should be exerted for the individual to say more than they are comfortable with.
- *Previous help*: Any previous help received and the outcome of that help.
- *Expectations* of coming for help now.

Although this list is not exhaustive, these issues should be explored gently, always giving the choice and control to the individual about how much they discuss. The aim is to discover whether the survivor has the resources, stability and support to embark on a period of therapy, or whether these will need to be established first before looking more at the impact of the childhood experiences.

It is important for any therapist or worker in this field to be aware of and follow the good practice guidelines set by a number of organisations about memory work (British Psychological Society 1995). The survivor should have control over how much information is disclosed and there should not be any pressure on them to remember. Dissociating from the memories is common and protective, and should always be respected.

Conclusion

The partnership between survivors and their therapists has invoked a language to describe the child's experience in a way that has facilitated workers to suspend judgement and to dispel any remaining myths about sexual abuse. Throughout the last two decades, the voice of survivors heard in prose, poetry, song, letters and novels have provided a powerful testimony of painful childhood experiences. Despite advances in the use of appropriate methods for communicating with children when there is a suspicion of abuse, it has been and continues to be adult survivors who convey a fuller knowledge of the child's experience.

Acknowledging the strengths of survivors in seeking help and working on issues from their past means taking a perspective that genuinely empowers the survivor and confirms that workers acknowledge at the outset that the 'expert' view is that of the survivor, that survivors have power and control over the pace and depth of the work, and that their helpers are facilitators and enablers rather than experts who 'help victims'. Survivors have many strengths, not least their courage in breaking the silence about sexual abuse. Although there may be times when survivors feel overwhelmed by the experience of recalling events they thought were long-buried, the trauma of sexual abuse can be resolved, and survivors can begin to lead happier lives without being haunted by its legacy.

Coming to terms with the experience of childhood sexual abuse can be a long process. Many survivors are now embarking on that process, and they show great determination and courage in their ability to recover. Working with survivors is likely to challenge workers in a number of ways. Methods of working may need to be reassessed, and long-held assumptions about the nature of the family and the status of childhood may need to be questioned. Being creative in the work, ensuring that there is good support and supervision, evaluating the work in the light of progress, knowledge and experience, encouraging survivors to write about their experiences and always being aware of the magnitude for a survivor in disclosing details of the abuse are vital.

Key points and messages for practice

- A theoretical framework which recognises the significance of trauma, attachment and loss is helpful in understanding the impact of abuse on children and its implications in adulthood.

- The long-term effects of sexual abuse have specific implications for adults and these need to be taken into account in all aspects of therapeutic work.

- Therapeutic work with adult survivors of abuse can be supported within an attachment framework.

- Recent developments in neuroscience support work with survivors of abuse in a way that facilitates the work and recognises the importance of the therapeutic relationship.

- Helpers need to educate themselves about the long-term effects of abuse and to keep these in mind when working therapeutically with survivors.

- Assessment at the start of the work can be a collaborative venture which establishes trust and the possibility of good work.

- An acknowledgement of professional limitations in working with survivors of abuse keeps the work realistic, boundaried and safe for the client.

- Working with adult survivors of abuse can be hard work in which the helper needs to be aware of self-care; this has implications both personally and professionally.

27 Out-of-home care for the abused or neglected child: a review of the knowledge base for planning and practice

June Thoburn

INTRODUCTION

Developments in the provision of out-of-home care for children who have been abused or neglected mirror more general developments in child and family policy, law and practice. When the emphasis has been on the importance of the birth family, greater efforts have been made to provide residential placements and foster carers who will support the family at times of stress by providing good care for the children and facilitating positive contact with family members so that they can return home as soon as possible. At other times, an emphasis on rescue and a fresh start has led to more resources being available for the placement of children with permanent new families, preferably for adoption. This chapter starts from the premise that this either/or approach to child placement is detrimental to children whose protection or other needs require them to be placed away from home.

The Department of Health's *Introduction to the Children Act* (DoH 1989b, p. 5) states:

The Act seeks to protect children both from the harm which can arise from failures or abuse within the family and from the harm which can be caused by unwarranted intervention in their family life.

The Adoption and Children Act 2002 reinforced this direction of travel by bringing the principles underlying adoption work into line with 1989 Act principles and emphasising the role of the independent reviewing officer (IRO) as the 'guardian' of the child's care plan. The Children Act 2004 makes no changes to the main legislative provisions for looked-after children but the proposed structural changes should make multi-agency planning for and working with children for whom the state is the 'corporate parent' more effective. The Children (Leaving Care) Act 2000 strengthens the duties of the corporate state to continue to provide an individualised service when young people leave care.

Other chapters in this *Handbook* have referred to research findings on the impact of abuse and severe neglect on the long-term health and well-being of children. The research findings discussed here on the outcome of a range of substitute placements indicate that 'love is not enough', that a substantial minority of children placed with loving and dedicated new parents will still need additional services if they are to overcome the harmful effects of their early experiences, and that a proportion will not totally recover and will remain emotionally vulnerable. The children who we most want to rescue are most vulnerable to the sort of adversities that can happen once they leave home, most obviously renewed abuse, multiple placements and leaving care at the age of 18 without a secure base to provide the support they will need as young adults. (See Triseliotis 1983, Bowlby 1988, Thoburn 2000 and Schofield 2002a for detailed discussions of the concepts of 'a family for life' and a 'secure base'.)

In short, the early optimism of the 1970s and 1980s that, if restoration back home was not easily achievable, children could be placed successfully for adoption has been shown in many cases to have been wishful thinking rather than a realistic appraisal of the long-term problems and needs of abused and neglected children.

This chapter will review the research findings and place particular emphasis on what they tell us about how practice might be improved. It will highlight the crucially important tasks of assessment and making decisions about the type of placement and other services that are most likely to ensure that the short- and long-term needs of the child are met.

The literature on out-of-home placement

There is an extensive literature on the placement of children in residential care, foster care and with adoptive families. The Department of Health publications which accompanied the Children Act 1989 are still important sources, especially Guidance volumes 2 and 3 on family support and foster care placements, and volume 4 on residential care. *Principles and Practice in Regulations and Guidance* (DoH 1989c) summarises the principles that should underlie all family social work, including the placement of children away from their families of origin. These are given more concrete form in the *National Adoption Standards for England* (DoH 2001c) and the *National Minimum Standards for Fostering Services in England* (DoH 2002d) which were produced after extensive consultation with researchers and practitioners as part of the *Quality Protects* programme* (DoH 1998d). The Utting Report (Utting *et al.* 1997), the government's response (DoH 1998c) and the *Quality Protects* performance indicators (DoH 2002d, National Statistics/DfES 2005) provide the most recent guidance for policy and practice to safeguard the welfare of children looked after away from their families.

The British research that has been most influential is summarised in the series of DoH-sponsored research reviews that started with the 1985 *Social Work Decisions in Child Care* (DHSS 1985b, DoH 1991b, 1998c, 1999d, 2001c, Quinton 2004, Sinclair 2005). The studies involving larger numbers are those of Rowe *et al.* (1989) of the extent to which over 10 000 placements met the desired aims, Bullock *et al.* (1998a) of 875 children, most of whom returned home from care, Thoburn and Rowe of 1165 placements with permanent new families (in Fratter *et al.* 1991) and the most recent series of studies of Sinclair and colleagues (Sinclair *et al.* 2004, 2005a, 2005b) of 1528 foster carers and 596 foster children. These are complemented by a large number of smaller-scale studies which give a more detailed picture of child placement work in the UK. Other overviews considering research evidence and the practice literature are those of Sellick and Howell (2004), Sellick *et al.* (2004) and Wilson *et al.* (2004). Barth *et al.* (1994), Maluccio *et al.* (2000) and Whittaker and Maluccio (2002) review the North American and Australian

---

* Although references to policy documents and statistics are mainly to England, it is important to note that there are both similarities and differences for Northern Ireland, Scotland and Wales.

literature. Thoburn *et al.* (2005) provide an overview of mainly UK research findings on the placement of minority ethnic children. Triseliotis *et al.* (1997), Howe (1998), Thoburn (2000) and Rushton (2003) review the research and child development literature on the outcomes of adoption. Brophy *et al.* (2003b) describe the background and court processes concerning 183 children of minority ethnic heritage considered by the courts following allegations of maltreatment, most of whom were in out-of-home care at some stage in the proceedings.

However, professionals who make recommendations about plans for specific children are advised to use these overviews merely as a starting point in the search for research literature that is relevant to any particular child, since the range of options to meet individual needs is wide, and some studies are more relevant to some types of need and placements than others. Over-simplification of research findings can lead to avoidable mistakes, the price of which will be paid by the children. I shall therefore consider the importance of assessing the needs of individual children before considering the possible alternative placements that might be available to meet those needs.

Assessing the placement needs of children who cannot remain safely at home

The Children Act 1989 and guidance make it clear that out-of-home placement should be considered, not only as a 'last resort' but also as a support service available to families under stress, including in cases where there might be a need for protective services. Packman and Hall (1998) found that accommodation under voluntary arrangements for children about whom there were protection concerns increased following the implementation of the Act. Brandon *et al.* (1999) found that 65% of 105 children newly identified as suffering or likely to suffer significant harm were placed in out-of-home care at some point during the following 12 months. When plans are being made for the placement of a child who cannot remain safely at home, the following questions have to be considered:

- What sort of placement?
- For how long?
- What will be the appropriate legal status for the placement?
- What sort of contact with birth relatives and previous carers will be appropriate?
- What services, support or therapy will be needed by all those involved in the placement – the child, the carers and members of their own families, the original family members and relatives?
- What financial help and practical support will be needed to maintain the placement?

The answers to all these questions must come from a view about the long-term aims, which in turn have to be based on a painstaking and individually planned assessment process, leading to a detailed statement of the child's needs and the extent to which the adults who are currently a part of the child's life are willing and able to meet those needs.

Professionals who are considering long-term plans for a child must have a clear idea of what they consider to be a successful outcome. It is important to note that the Adoption and Children Act 2002 requires that the decisions made at the time that adoption is being considered take account of the lifetime impact on the child and other family members. It also reinforces the importance of continuing support after the making of an adoption order for adopted children and also for adopters and birth family members. As well as seeking to meet the needs common to all children, professionals should be conscious that the impact of separation and loss can be particularly injurious to long-term self-esteem. Research has indicated that self-esteem is most likely to be enhanced if children have a *sense of permanence* in their relationships with their primary carers, and a *sense of identity*, and that these two must be kept in balance (Thoburn 1994). Without a sense of permanence, the child will not feel secure enough to take the risks which go with new attachments, whether to new parents, siblings or friends. Without a sense of personal identity, which includes knowing about, and preferably being in contact with, members of the birth family and important people from the past, racial and cultural identity, and being valued as the individuals they *are*, there is a risk that children will grow up with a sense of 'incompleteness'. Howe and Feast (2000) provide detailed accounts of how some adopted adults seek to make sense of their identities, often through seeking more information or renewed contact with birth family members. Thoburn *et al.* (2000b, 2005) conclude from a longitudinal study of minority ethnic children in permanent placements and from a review of the research that, whilst adopters and foster carers can successfully parent a child of a different ethnic background, the differences in culture and appearance add an additional challenge to what is already a challenging form of family life. Some interview-based studies of adopted adults and young people leaving care find that some of those interviewed had been seriously harmed by the experience of growing up in a family visibly different from themselves and were not provided with strategies to confront racist behaviour (Ince 1998, Kirton *et al.* 2000).

It is essential therefore for practitioners making decisions about placement to list each of the child's needs and consider the 'job description' for the carers who are most likely to be able to meet the needs identified, and to do so in the light of research findings on outcomes for the different placement options. There is no point in identifying the perfect placement if research suggests that it is unlikely to be successful given the particular circumstances of this particular child. A solution that is likely to be successful in most respects may be preferable to an 'ideal' solution that carries a higher risk of either not being achieved or breaking down.

Information must be collected about the characteristics, personality, aptitudes and any particular disabilities – whether emotional, behavioural, learning or physical – of each child. The age of the child is another important dimension, since age at placement has been associated by several researchers with outcome. Children who are older when placed are more likely to experience placement breakdown and are therefore likely to need more skilled parenting and more extensive services (Wilson *et al.* 2004). The third dimension is the relationship of the child with significant others. This will involve a consideration of the child's attachments.

The assessment must also consider whether the people who are significant to the child wish the child to remain where they currently are, to return to them or to be placed elsewhere, and, if they have parental responsibility, whether they will consent to a particular form of placement but not to another form of placement. This occurs most obviously when a parent who acknowledges that the child cannot return home will consent to a placement with a view to a residence order or the more secure Special Guardianship Order introduced by the Adoption and Children Act 2002, but not to a placement for adoption. Human rights, children and adoption legislation require that the child, and all those who have parental responsibility, be consulted and due consideration given to their views, wishes and feelings and that all the alternatives are considered. Whilst the wishes of important people, including the children themselves, may sometimes have to be overruled, it is desirable to avoid this if accommodating their wishes will not clearly be detrimental to the child's long-term well-being.

Having formed a picture of the child's needs and relationships, and having consulted all those whose wishes and feelings must be given due consideration (ss.1 and 22 of the Children Act 1989 and s.1 of the Adoption and Children Act 2002), those considering the child's placement will be in a better position to answer the key placement questions listed above.

For how long?

Clarity is always needed about the approximate length of any placement, and this should be stated in the placement agreement. Where the situation is unclear, it is preferable to overestimate the time needed, and thus avoid an unnecessary change of placement. Data on children looked after provided on an annual basis by the Department for Education and Skills record the proportion of children in each authority who have had three or more placements. In 2003–4, 13% of all looked-after children had to cope with at least two changes of placement in the past year (Commission for Social Care Inspection 2004, National Statistics/DfES 2005). The Department of Health (now DfES) *Quality Protects* and *Choice Protects* programmes have sought to reduce the extent of placement change. If an older child has been harmed by earlier experiences, and assessment indicates that a permanent or long-term placement is needed, 18 months to 2 years is a realistic outer limit which allows for assessment followed by the search for the right placement and preparation for the move. However, for infants, court protocols and practice arrangements should seek to ensure that wherever possible the child returns home or joins a substitute family within 6 months of coming into care. Speeding up court processes and working intensively with birth families are important aspects of the 'concurrent planning' demonstration projects described by Monck *et al.* (2003). Another, more controversial aspect of these projects is the placement with foster carers who are also approved as adopters in the event of it being found that those children placed with them cannot safely be returned home. This has the advantage of avoiding another placement, but numbers in the evaluation are small and it is not clear which of the three main 'prongs' of this approach to infant placement made the greatest contribution to the generally positive outcomes reported. If the intention is that the placement should be until the child is an adult, this should be clearly stated and recorded in the agreement. Brandon *et al.* (1999) found that just over half of the 68 children in their significant harm study who left home at any point during the 12-month follow-up period were back home after 12 months. Nearly a quarter had been adopted or were placed with adoptive families. All except one of the youngest children were either at home or in a stable long-term placement. Stability was more difficult to achieve for those over 10 and still looked after.

The crucial role of 'emergency', 'assessment' or 'bridge' placements

When parents or older children request out-of-home care, or social workers consider a child's needs are not being adequately met and the child is suffering significant harm or likely to do so without an out-of-home placement, an early discussion of the sort of care that may be appropriate will alleviate the need for emergency placements and allow for better planning in more cases. Introductions can then be made, agreements about placement carefully negotiated and the trauma of the separation minimised. In some abuse cases, it is inevitable that emergency action is taken. However, even here it is possible to minimise the harm by providing care for the whole family, or perhaps 'crash pad' facilities in residential care or family centres, so that time can be taken for a more careful decision about the placement of the child, or indeed about whether an alleged abuser is willing to move out temporarily and can be offered help to find accommodation outside the home. In the 1950s and 1960s, many writers emphasised the value of short-term foster placements as an essential part of a family support service. However, increased concern about child abuse, which followed death and subsequent inquiries, together with a realisation that many children did not return to their families of origin and remained in unplanned care (Rowe & Lambert 1973), led to a greater emphasis on the placement of children in care with permanent new families, and to a concentration on the skills of permanent family placement to the exclusion of skills in recruiting, training and supporting short-term foster carers. The exception to this was the creative thinking and positive practice which went into the recruitment, training and support of carers for teenagers, no doubt because the concern about child abuse at that period was rivalled only by concern about troublesome teenagers (Shaw & Hipgrave 1983, Hazel & Fenyo 1993, Hill *et al.* 1993).

The attempt to have a permanence policy without a comprehensive and properly resourced foster care policy led to a new problem identified by the researchers whose work was reported in the Department of Health overviews. Drift, or lack of planning, ceased to be a significant problem, and was replaced by two equally serious problems: poor quality short-term foster care, which led to a succession of different placements while the child was awaiting a long-term placement; and poor and inflexible planning, which replaced a lack of planning. These two were interrelated, in that it is not possible adequately to assess the needs of children and undertake the work that is necessary with the parents, the child and the new family to prepare them for a permanent placement which is going to have a chance of succeeding, if the child is not in the interim period offered stable and skilled care by either residential workers or foster parents.

What legal status?

The first option (following the Children Act 1989 principle that orders should only be made if they are clearly necessary to safeguard and promote the child's welfare) is for voluntary arrangements (accommodation in the terminology of the 1989 Act). In these cases, parents retain full parental responsibility, but there may be the intention, if all are agreed, that the relatives or foster parents will make an application for a residence order once the child appears to be settled. In some cases where there is serious risk to the child, even though the plan might be to work towards rehabilitation, it may be appropriate for a residence order or an interim care order to be sought early on in the placement to give legal security. This might also be appropriate if a parent is impulsive or suffers from a mental illness or an addiction associated with impulsive behaviour, or there is evidence from the past that an agreement may not be adhered to. Where there is evidence that a child is suffering or is likely to suffer significant harm and an agreement cannot be reached to secure the child's immediate placement in accommodation, or for the child to remain in a placement until a residence, special guardianship or care order is sought, it may be necessary to apply for an emergency protection or care order to secure the placement. If a child looked after review considers that adoption is in the child's best interest, the local authority adoption panel will review the case and make a recommendation to the Director of Children's Services. An application for a placement order under the provisions of the Adoption and Children Act 2002 can be made at the same time as, or instead of, an application for a care order. Alternatively, the child may remain with the same family or be placed with another family as a 'long-term' or 'permanent' foster child, in which case it will be important to have a very clear agreement that this is intended to be a *permanent* foster placement, especially if the child is placed under voluntary arrangements (see Thoburn 1991 for a fuller discussion of the importance of ensuring that the child and the carers have a sense of permanence in such situations, and ways in which this sense of permanence can be facilitated).

The question of financial support should be considered separately from legal status. Financial support to substitute families can be available when appropriate through adoption or 'special guardianship' allowances, residence order allowances, foster care payments, grants made under s.17 of the Children Act, settling-in grants and one-off grants (e.g. if a child is particularly destructive). Financial support to birth family members, whether to facilitate contact or to maintain a child visiting in the family home, can be made either under the adoption support provisions if there is a plan for adoption, as part of s.34 contact arrangements or under s.17 of the Children Act 1989.

What sort of contact and with whom?

The work of Millham *et al.* (1986) played a major part in emphasising the importance of continued contact for children who are looked after by the local authority, not only with their parents but also with siblings if they are not placed together, and with relatives and friends. Research on 'open adoption' and the issues surrounding openness when children are placed with permanent new families is summarised by Fratter (1996), Grotevant and McRoy (1998), Neil *et al.* (2003), Wrobel *et al.* (2003) and Neil and Howe (2005). Cleaver (2000) describes contact arrangements for 185 children in long- or intermediate-term placements after the implementation of the Children Act 1989. She found that children who had contact with at least one parent did so more frequently and regularly than was reported in earlier studies, and that decisions to refuse contact with one or more birth relatives were usually taken for a good reason. There is not sufficient space here to cite all the research evidence on contact with members of the birth family but the cumulative findings can be summarised as follows.

- Continuing contact is associated with a greater likelihood that children will return home from care. The majority of children looked after or adopted from care when past infancy want to have continued contact with some if not all birth family members, and most want it to be more frequent or to be of longer duration (Thomas & Beckford 1999, Cleaver 2000, Thoburn *et al.* 2000b, Timms & Thoburn 2003, Beek & Schofield 2004, Neil & Howe 2005, Sinclair 2005b).
- No large-scale longitudinal study of children in long-term or permanent family placement has concluded that cessation of face-to-face contact is associated with lower rates of placement breakdown, and some have found associations between continuing contact and greater placement stability and other welfare benefits (Fanshel & Shinn 1978, Aldgate 1990, Fratter *et al.* 1991).
- Neil (2002) concludes from her study of contact arrangements for children placed for adoption from care when under the age of 4 years that, of itself, face-to-face contact with birth parents and other relatives does not impede the growth of attachments with the adoptive family.

Less easily measurable benefits of continued contact which have been pointed out by research studies of a more qualitative nature include the following:

- Members of the birth family can offer some continuity of relationships to those children who experience a series of different placements whilst in care.
- It may help in a crisis or with a contingency if a placement in care breaks down and no suitable placement is available. On occasion in such circumstances, a reassessment may lead to the conclusion that the child may safely return home. On other occasions, members of the family, perhaps grandparents or relatives, may provide a bridge placement until a new placement can be identified.
- Continued contact increases the chances of the child having 'a family for life'. If the placement works well, they may have the benefit as an adult of two 'families for life'. If the placement in care does not lead to a good long-term attachment and a secure base, family members who have not been able to meet their children's needs when young may be able to do so when they are young adults (Marsh & Peel 1999). The particular importance of siblings must not be forgotten, since the relationship between siblings is potentially even more long-lasting than is the parent–child relationship. This may apply to siblings born after the child left home, and there are many examples of siblings forming close friendships as adults, even if they never actually lived together as children.

However, studies also provide evidence that continuing birth family contact for some abused or neglected children with some birth family members may contribute, alongside other factors, to placement disruption and further harm, and that facilitating safe contact and keeping stress on all concerned to a minimum is a complex task. From their recent cross-sectional study of a large sample of children in foster care, Wilson and Sinclair (2004) and Sinclair *et al.* (2005b) found that, for children with a history of abuse prior to placement and no termination of contact with at least one family member, breakdown of their placement in foster care was three times more likely and the chance of re-abuse increased. Some smaller-scale studies have also pointed to problems resulting from specific factors such as inconsistency.

Several of the studies, especially those of Cleaver (2000), Schofield *et al.* (2000), Beek and Schofield (2004) and the authors contributing to Neil and Howe (2005), indicate how practice with birth and substitute parents and the children can reduce stress and improve the quality of contact. When there is a plan for reunification, contact will be an opportunity for the foster carers to 'model' appropriate responses, especially with adolescents or if the child's behaviour is challenging (Chamberlain & Reid 1998). Neil *et al.* (2003) looked at the differences between post-adoption and long-term foster care contact and provide guidance for practitioners. For both short-term and permanent placements, an early facilitated meeting between the prospective carers/new parents and the adult birth relatives and/or the carers of siblings who will be having contact greatly contributes to the success of both direct and indirect arrangements. Although supervision alongside facilitation by professionals may sometimes be essential, all studies indicate that contact arrangement works best when the carers play a major part in facilitating it. Researchers also comment on the importance of the review process, and reviews of post-adoption support services, and conclude that (unless this cannot be managed without risk to the carers or child) a facilitated meeting between the carers and those having contact should be arranged prior to the review. Support from the social worker to the carers and the child at this time (especially if contact is infrequent) will often be important. Where contact arouses painful feelings for birth relatives (as is usually the case) a support worker will often be essential to help them to manage their feelings before and after contact and assist them in ensuring that the meeting, phone calls or letters have benefits for the child, the carers and themselves.

Placement options

In the following sections, the range of short- and long-term placements which might be chosen in order to meet the assessed needs of abused and neglected children are considered.

Shared care, therapeutic care and respite

Sometimes parents will themselves request out-of-home care to tide them over particularly stressful periods in their lives, or residential therapy for a child whose behaviour is particularly difficult, or this may be an agreed part of a support package for the family of a child with a disability. In some cases, the family may be most appropriately supported by the provision of regular planned periods of respite care in the same foster home or residential placement. In other circumstances, the family may be linked with a foster carer or residential placement which will provide accommodation at times of stress, as when a parent suffers from a recurring mental illness such as schizophrenia or clinical depression. Stalker (1990) has reviewed the mainly positive outcomes of respite care for children with disabilities, and Aldgate and Bradley (1999) describe and evaluate the (generally positive) impact of respite care for children whose families are under stress for reasons other than disability. Howard (2000) provides a detailed account of the role of foster carers in providing a flexible range of support services to birth parents alongside periods of respite care. 'Task-centred' and 'shared care' arrangements are particularly relevant to the needs of older children, including those whose challenging behaviour results from earlier abuse or neglect. Accounts of specialist projects for teenagers date back to the 1980s. Shaw and Hipgrave (1983) report on evaluations of early UK projects and Walker *et al.* (2002) describe and evaluate a specialist project in Scotland to provide foster care for young people who would otherwise be in secure accommodation.

Evaluations of the work of the Oregon *Family Connections* foster care treatment programme for delinquent and otherwise troubled adolescents (Chamberlain & Reid 1998) indicate that parallel support and training for foster carers and the birth relatives to whom the children will return are centrally important aspects of the work.

If, following assessment either before or after a child leaves home, a decision is made that a child may not safely remain at or return home, at least for the present, the alternatives will be placement with relatives or friends, foster family care, adoption or placement in some form of group care which may be a children's home, boarding education or a small family-based children's home providing long-term care (Cairns 1984, 2004). A careful assessment should allow a decision to be made as to whether what is needed is a placement where the birth parent or parents will remain the 'psychological' parents, or whether substitute parents are needed. Dickens *et al.* (2005) and National Statistics/DfES (2005) show that around 70% of children entering care in a given year will have returned to the parents or relatives within 2 years. The majority of those returning home do so within the first 6 months. This 'leaving care curve' has been misinterpreted to imply that if a child is still away from home after 6 months, they are unlikely to return and should therefore be placed for adoption. The majority of the long stayers are not infants who will easily be placed with a new family, but are older children, many of whom have behaviour problems. Bullock *et al.* (1998a) found from their study of over 800 children entering care in the 1980s that around 90% eventually returned to parents or relatives. Even in the USA, where permanence policies require parental rights to be terminated after 6 months in care if reunification plans are not already well advanced, a recent large scale study by Courtney *et al.* (2001) found that a substantial number return to live with or be near to birth relatives.

If it appears that the child will not be able to return home in the near future, but that there is a strong and mainly positive relationship between parent and child, a placement is needed where the carers will *supplement* the care of the parent. The parent will remain the main attachment figure and the placement carers will need to be chosen for their skills in facilitating this. If such a placement is likely to last for a period of years, and especially if the child is quite young, it may be that the birth parents and the carers will *both* fulfil psychological parenting roles. (See Thoburn 1996 for a fuller discussion of the issues around 'dual' or 'multiple' psychological parenting.) This most often happens when a child remains with a relative such as a grandparent, but there are cases when 'dual psychological parenting' is appropriate for lengthy periods of time with children in foster or adoptive families.

Although, as noted above, the emphasis on permanence policies in the 1980s and 1990s led to reduced interest in foster care policy and research, the *Choice Protects* programme initiated in 2002 has led to renewed interest in its place in providing for children's needs in a range of circumstances. Rowe *et al.* (1989) identified the tasks of short-term or bridge carers as temporary care (including short periods of planned respite care to alleviate family stress); emergency placements – to offer a roof for a very limited period; preparation for long-term or permanent placement, whether back home or with a new family; assessment; treatment; and a bridge to independence. Utting (1992) identified similar tasks for residential care.

In the Rowe *et al.* (1989) study of nearly 6000 children and 10 000 placements, short-term placements had a lower breakdown rate than long-term placements, but the proportion breaking down – almost one in five in the Berridge and Cleaver (1987) study – is still alarming when one considers that they were only intended to last for up to 8 weeks. Few writers have measured outcomes other than placement breakdown for children who stay away from home for short periods. However, Packman (1986) found higher satisfaction rates amongst parents whose children were temporarily accommodated than amongst those whose request for temporary care was refused. One explanation for those who were reported in some studies as 'staying too long' in short-term foster care is that foster parents all too quickly come to see the children as 'theirs', and in subtle and unsubtle ways start to discourage contact between the parents and children, thus inhibiting the social worker's efforts to keep a space for child and parents in each other's practical and emotional lives. A key message from research for those selecting and training short-term foster carers is that they should be looking for those who can empathise with and facilitate positive contact with birth families and work positively with social workers and others to get children safely back home. However, they have also to be mindful to the fact that the best option for some children who cannot go home is for their short-term placement to be confirmed as a 'permanent' one, and thus to have an eye to the suitability of all short-term carers to take on a long-term parenting role.

Mention has already been made of the importance of clarity about who is intended to play the psychological parenting role for a child living away from home. It has also been suggested that on occasions birth and substitute parents will fulfil a 'psychological parenting' role. More often, however, the intention of using these options will be to maintain a strong attachment with the parents and other family members, including siblings. Longer-term shared care options are particularly appropriate when a parent and child are closely attached but there is danger to the child if they continue to live at home. It is often possible to arrange for visits home to be fully supervised, or for the adult believed to be a danger to the child to be out of the home when the child returns home for visits. If this is not possible, a comfortable environment is needed so that the parents and children can spend time together.

Long-term placement with relatives

The Children Act 1989 encourages placement with relatives as a preferred option if children cannot return home. Although these placements are often made when parents have severe problems, often involving mental ill-health, domestic violence or drugs or alcohol addictions, there are often elements of 'shared family care' even when kinship placements are made for the purposes of care and upbringing. Indeed, a major advantage of such placements, which generally result in higher rates of satisfaction amongst young people, is that they can stay in touch with their kinship networks, even when actual contact with birth parents may be difficult or impossible. Rowe *et al.* (1984) found that relatives were particularly good at keeping the child in touch with both sides of the family, as well as offering long-term stability and good parenting to the children in their care. Sinclair (2005) notes that in 2004 around 16% of all foster care placements were with kinship carers. This may be an underestimate of the numbers of maltreated children living with relatives, since many authorities prefer to use Children Act 1989 s.17 or residence order provisions to support these placements rather than formally 'looking after' the children.

It is important to note that Hunt (2001) concludes that the UK research on kinship care is mostly dated and inconclusive with respect to outcomes. A DfES-funded study by Farmer and Moyers (2002) is currently evaluating kinship care arrangements and there is some evidence on outcomes from other countries (especially New Zealand and the USA). Wulczyn *et al.* (2003) review the evidence on stability and well-being and report, from a longitudinal study of over 11 000 children entering care in New York City followed up for 3 years, that 'children first placed in relatives' homes move much less than children placed in other family settings' (p. 224). Only on the measure of leaving care through return to birth parents or through adoption are kin placements rated less positively than 'stranger' foster placements. Other USA studies (reviewed by Wilson *et al.* 2004) have less clear-cut findings. However, the context and legislation in those countries are very different. The Rowe *et al.* (1989) placement survey is still the largest UK empirical study comparing kinship placements with other placement options. This study, a smaller-scale early study by Berridge and Cleaver (1987) and contributors to the edited book by Broad (2001) suggest that such placements are less likely to break down. However, from their more recent study involving 70 relative carers and 25 children placed with relatives, Sinclair *et al.* (2004, 2005a, 2005b) concluded that 'outcomes were neither better nor worse for kinship care' (Sinclair 2005b, p. 42). It may be that differences in findings on placement stability reflect differences in the samples. In addition, caution is needed in interpreting earlier findings since the increased use of kinship foster care encouraged by the Children Act 1989 may have resulted in a less risk-averse attitude on the part of placement agencies.

All studies note that kinship carers tend to live in more disadvantaged circumstances and tend to be less well supported than 'stranger' foster carers. Contributors to Broad (2001) build on research and practice to suggest how outcomes could be improved by the provision of more practical as well as emotional support services and advocacy, particularly to ensure that educational needs are met.

Long-term group care placements

Long-term substitute care will normally be with adoptive or permanent foster parents, but some children may have been so hurt by early experiences within a family that a long-term group care placement will be appropriate. Some small children's homes are able to offer psychological parenting within a family-based group care environment where skilled and loving carers are sometimes able to help older children to develop trust and indeed form long-term relationships with them which may offer a secure base from which to launch out into adult life (Cairns 2002, 2004). In some cases, boarding education may be an appropriate way of maintaining the child's attachment to birth relatives. Some older children and their parents, stepparents or adopters are unable to live harmoniously together, but their fragile relationship can be maintained if they keep some distance between them, and may strengthen as the child becomes a young adult. Research on children in residential care reports mixed results. Rowe *et al.* (1989) found that, when age at placement was controlled for, placements in children's homes were least likely to break down and were as likely to achieve their aims as foster care placements. However, Colton (1989) compared the nature of caring in specialist foster homes and children's homes and concluded that, irrespective of the skills of the carers, those looking after young people in family environments are more able to be child-oriented than residential workers who can provide less individual attention. In their study of abused and abusing young people, Farmer and Pollock (1998) point out that there are differences between young people placed in foster care and those placed in residential care. Although breakdown rates are quite high, many adolescents speak well of their residential and foster carers, and it should be noted that adolescents are in any case a group of people 'on the move'. Berridge and Brodie (1998) and Sinclair and Gibbs (1998) report more negative results.

Longer-term care in foster families

In some cases, assessment will make it clear that the child needs substitute parents, either because there is no attachment or a very destructive or ambivalent attachment with the birth parents, or the child is young and it is not feasible for them to remain psychologically attached to two sets of parents. Longer-term foster care with families not previously known to the child (sometimes referred to as 'stranger' or 'matched' foster placements) is most often the placement of choice for older children who make it clear that they wish to maintain a relationship with birth relatives. In these cases, particular attention must be paid to ensuring that the birth parents and the foster parents get on well enough with each other to reach agreement about how contact might best be achieved and on other aspects of shared parental responsibility.

In some cases, the child will remain in accommodation on a voluntary basis, in which case the parents retain full parental responsibility. The placement agreement must spell out which responsibilities are delegated to the foster carers and the actions that all parties will take as contingencies if the arrangements break down. It is often small things such as a change in hairstyle or the choice of a birthday gift that can cause trouble between the two sets of parents, and creative social workers and skilled foster carers must think ahead to pre-empt such difficulties. Even when there is a care order, the Children Act 1989 requires that the parents are enabled to retain as much of their parental responsibility as possible, and that the authority only takes away that much of their parental responsibility as is necessary to secure the child's well-being.

The major British sources of information about the success of intermediate- or long-term foster placements are found in the work of Rowe *et al.* (1984, 1989), Millham *et al.* (1986), Berridge and Cleaver (1987), Aldgate (1990), Kelly and MacAuley (1995), Beek and Schofield (2004) and Sinclair *et al.* (2005a). Sellick and Connolly (2002) provide data on children placed with independent foster care agencies. Kufeldt and Allison (1990) and Courtney *et al.* (2001) report on studies in North America, Fernandez (1999) and Barber and Delfabbro (2004) report on young people in care in Australia, and Dumaret *et al.* (1997) and Andersson (2005) report on long-term outcomes for young adults brought up in foster care in France and Sweden, respectively. The voice of the children and young people is included in most of these studies, but the views of larger numbers are provided through the surveys conducted by Fletcher (1993), Shaw (1997), Timms and Thoburn (2003) and Sinclair *et al.* (2005a). Triseliotis *et al.* (2000) (with respect to Scotland) and Waterhouse (1997) and Sinclair *et al.* (2004) (with respect to England) provide information on the characteristics of foster carers and the foster care services.

Rowe *et al.* (1989) found that 27% of the 194 children placed in long-term foster care had experienced breakdown between 12 and 24 months later. However, Aldgate (1990) found that children in long-term foster placements were doing as well educationally, and in other aspects of their well-being, as were children who were on the social workers' preventative case loads but were not looked after by the local authority. They also note that increased well-being and satisfactory educational progress were associated with having a sense of stability and security within the foster home.

Reviewing the evidence on long-term foster care, Sinclair (2005) concludes that:

> foster care can provide long-term stable care in which children remain in contact with their foster family in adulthood. This is particularly so when the placement is intended to be permanent from the start. (p. 10)

He adds the important warning that more effort must be made to improve stability since research indicates that 'for most children the care system did not provide this long-term stable alternative to care at home'. Sinclair *et al.* (2004) found from their 'snapshot' sample of 596 children in (mainly long-term) foster placements that only a minority of the children who wanted to remain in those placements were still there 2 years later. The qualitative interviews reported in this study (Sinclair *et al.* 2005b), in Thoburn *et al.* (2000b) and in Schofield (2002b) provide important pointers to how more children brought up in foster family care might gain from the benefits of a sense of permanence and family membership whilst retaining links with their birth families. The longitudinal study reported by Schofield *et al.* (2000) and Beek and Schofield (2004) provides detailed descriptions of patterns of attachment with their birth and foster families of 58 children placed specifically with the aim of achieving family membership in long-term foster families. They review the important role played by long-term foster parents in meeting the needs of some of the most damaged children in care. This work on foster care is important since, even with the increasing use of adoption from care, given the ages, characteristics and wishes of children starting to be looked after, many more children will spend large periods of their childhoods in foster care than will leave care through adoption.

Most studies note that there is a higher breakdown rate of placements of teenagers, regardless of whether or not they are placed in specialist or professional foster schemes, in 'ordinary' foster homes, in lodgings or in residential care. Sallnas *et al.* (2004) summarise the international literature on teenage foster and residential care placements and provide data on the long-term outcomes of 776 teenagers who entered care in Sweden in 1991. They note that between 30 and 37% of placements broke down (depending on the definition of placement breakdown used). Kinship care and secure unit placements were less likely to break down than placements with 'stranger' foster families and residential care other than secure units.

UK studies tend to provide more detailed information but on smaller numbers. Berridge and Cleaver (1987) and Thoburn *et al.* (2000b) noted high breakdown rates amongst youngsters placed when aged 7–11 years as well as amongst those placed as teenagers. Farmer *et al.* (2004) provide a detailed account of the foster care placements of 68 adolescents and report that, 12 months after placement, 56% of placements had not disrupted but only 47% were rated as successful.

Most studies also consider whether placements of children of minority ethnic origin are any more or less successful than those of children whose parents are both white. Taken as a group, minority ethnic children are over-represented amongst children in out-of-home care. However, Rowe *et al.* (1989) and Thoburn *et al.* (2005) point out that over-simplification may lead to inappropriate placement planning. Children of south Asian heritage and those of east Asian heritage are under-represented, whilst children with one or both parents of African–Caribbean or African heritage are over-represented, particularly amongst those in short-term placements. Thoburn *et al.* (2000b) found that children both of whose parents were of minority ethnic origin were more likely than those of mixed heritage to be placed in permanent foster placements rather than for adoption, to have continuing contact with birth relatives, to be placed with siblings and to be in broadly ethnically matched placements.

To summarise this section on placement options, child protection and child placement studies, including studies that compare children who are looked after with similar children remaining with parents (Aldgate 1980, Packman 1986) indicate that the goalkeeping – 'care is bad for your health' or 'once they are in care, you can never get them back home' – attitudes and policies of the 1980s represented an over-simplification and must be adapted in the light of new knowledge. Well-resourced policies and knowledge-based practice to ensure that children can remain safely at home can prevent the need for some children to be placed in out-of-home care and can result in others returning home safely. But there is much evidence that short- and long-term foster care, alongside reunification and adoption, have important parts to play in child protection practice. There is much in the studies to indicate how practice can improve to reduce the incidence of poor outcomes, and to help identify the potential casualties, so that services (both when children are being looked after and when they leave) can be of a higher quality.

The fact that the majority of placements are reasonably successful should not, however, prevent us from recognising the extreme vulnerability of children who *do* become split off from their families of origin, and whose placements in care or for adoption are unsuccessful. Studies of care leavers, homeless young people and of young people in custody indicate that a substantial proportion of these were originally abused, placed in care for their own protection and re-abused, or felt so unprotected or alone in care that they ran away and preferred to trust to their own devices (Biehal *et al.* 1995, Wade *et al.* 1998, Courtney *et al.* 2001).

Adoption as a route out of care for maltreated infants and older children

It has already been noted that only a small proportion of the children entering out-of-home care will be placed for adoption, although more will spend long periods in foster family care and some will achieve the benefits of family membership and stability with foster families. Adoption as a route out of care is rarely used outside the USA, Canada and the UK, and most reports of adoption outcomes from other countries focus mainly on inter-country adoption. Particularly within the last 10 years or so, government policy in the UK has encouraged the use of adoption as a placement of choice (Performance and Innovations Unit 2000) and National Statistics/DfES (2005) data show that in 2004 6% of children in care were adopted. However, most children adopted from care enter care when under the age of 2 years and a much lower proportion of those adopted from care are in the older age groups than was the case in the 1980s (Thoburn 2003).

Over the past 25 years there have been many English language accounts of the adoption of children in care, both from practitioners and researchers. American studies are summarised by Barth and Berry (1988), Barth *et al.* (1994), Maluccio *et al.* (2000) and Festinger (2002); the British research studies are summarised by Triseliotis *et al.* (1997), Department of Health (1999d) and Sellick *et al.* (2004). There have also been many studies over the years of the placement of infants for adoption which are also relevant to this volume, since some children are placed for adoption at birth if it is believed they are likely to be significantly harmed in the light of the experience of siblings.

The psychology of adoption

Space precludes a full consideration of the subject, but readers are referred to the work of Brodzinsky and Schechter (1990), who have brought together their own writings and those of other researchers and practitioners on the psychology and outcomes of adoption. Although care must be exercised when applying their conclusions to children adopted when older, these writers do throw light on the problems adopted children and their new families may encounter. Their thesis is that the adoptive family faces additional challenges which result from the loss experienced by the child, and the loss for some adopters of the child by birth which they had hoped to have – the 'double jeopardy' theory. There may be additional challenges if the child carries the scars of earlier harm, and if the child is of a different skin colour or cultural background from the adoptive family (Thoburn *et al.* 2000b). These writers join Kirk (1964, 1981) in postulating that successful adopters are those who accept the special challenges of adoptive parenting which make it different from parenting a child born to them. They consider that an adoptive family is a dual identity family, in that it has to incorporate the original family of the child conceptually, even if there is no actual contact. Wrobel *et al.* (2003), reporting on post-adoption contact, refer to the 'adoptive kinship network' which links together the first and the adoptive family. Accordingly, these writers strongly support some form of contact between the birth family and the adoptive family, even if this is only by way of letters and photographs, partly because this reminds the adopters that they have extra parenting challenges to overcome, and partly because it avoids the risks of the child fantasising and idealising the first family, or the sense for the adopters of 'sitting on a time bomb' and wondering if and when the child will wish to seek out a birth relative and what they may find when they do so.

This adoption research gives clues about the characteristics of families who are likely to be most successful with a child who has been abused or neglected. Since they have to be comfortable with the child's first identity, it is especially important that they can empathise with the parent who was responsible for the abuse or neglect. A child whose parent is a known abuser is likely to need help in establishing a positive sense of self, and this will not be helped if the adopters or foster carers maintain a condemnatory attitude towards the first parents and can find nothing positive to say about them.

Adoption of children past infancy

Lowe *et al.* (1999) and the British Agencies for Adoption and Fostering (1998, 2000) give detailed information on adoption policy and practice, and the numbers and ages of children being placed for adoption in the UK. Lowe and Murch (2002) and Selwyn *et al.* (2003) compare the characteristics of children placed for adoption with those placed in long-term or permanent foster care.

Within the last few years, several outcome studies of permanent family placement of older children have been published, and their findings are generally similar. Some of these have included in the sample some children in permanent foster placements (Rushton *et al.* 1988, Thoburn 1990, Fratter *et al.* 1991, Quinton & Rushton 1998, Thoburn *et al.* 2000b). Some larger-scale surveys use placement breakdown within varying lengths of time since placement as the outcome measure. Other generally smaller-scale studies use standardised well-being measures, educational achievement or a range of more subjective measures, such as the satisfaction or otherwise of the parents, the child or other members of the family. Thomas and Beckford (1999) provide important insights into the lives and opinions of 41 children who were placed for adoption when over the age of 5.

Turning to outcomes of adoption, the percentage of placements that had broken down between 18 months and 6 years after placement in the large-scale survey of 1165 placements with new parents not previously known to the child was 22% (Fratter *et al.* 1991). However, it is not particularly helpful to have a global breakdown or success rate and indeed success rates vary in different studies because of the characteristics of the children in the sample. Some studies include children whose placement with a temporary foster family is confirmed as a permanent placement, whilst others only include new placements with parents who were previously unknown to the child. (Around 14% of English children adopted from care are adopted by their short-term foster carers. The proportions in the USA adopted by either relatives or foster carers with whom they were initially placed temporarily are even higher.) These foster care adoptions are less likely to break down, perhaps because the new parents and child have already got to know each other before deciding that this should be a permanent placement (Lahti 1982, Fein *et al.* 1983). Sinclair *et al.* (2005b) found that carer adoptions tended to do rather better than adoptions by strangers, a finding which replicates the American research. Other variables which may result in different 'success' rates in different studies are the ages of the children placed, the quality of the social work support and the agency policies. Older age at placement has been identified by all large-scale studies in Britain and America as associated with placement breakdown (Fratter *et al.* 1991, Selwyn *et al.* 2003). Young children who have disabilities might be hard to find families for, but once the family has been found these placements seem to be particularly successful. Around 22% of placements of 8-year-old children break down, and this rises to almost a half of the placements of 12 year olds. One factor identified by most researchers as being associated independently with breakdown is that the child has been abused or neglected prior to the placement (Fratter *et al.* 1991). Gibbons *et al.* (1995a), in a study of children who were physically abused or severely neglected when under the age of 5 years, found that 8 years later the well-being of those placed for adoption or in foster care was, on average, no higher than that of children who returned home, and lower than for a matched sample of children who had not been abused. Other factors associated with breakdown were the child being described as institutionalised, or behaviourally or emotionally disturbed. Several studies (Barth & Berry 1988, Borland *et al.* 1990, Fratter *et al.* 1991, Grotevant & McRoy 1998) found that placements where there was face-to-face contact with the birth parents after the placement were either less likely to break down or it made no difference. Neil (2000, Neil & Howe 2005) reports on the first two stages of a longitudinal study of 168 children placed from care for adoption before the age of 4, with a particular focus on arrangements for birth family contact. Even with this younger age group, those placed past infancy, and those who had suffered early trauma were doing less well 5 years after placement than the youngest children. She found that 'indirect' contact arrangement presented as many if not more challenges to all concerned as did face-to-face arrangements. Direct contact, although bringing with it some stress to older children and those with other problems, did not appear to have impeded the growth of attachments in the adoptive family.

Thoburn *et al.* (2000b) found that children with both parents of minority ethnic origin were no more likely to experience breakdown than children of two white parents, but those of mixed-race parentage were significantly more likely to experience placement breakdown. When variables such as age at placement were controlled for, there was no difference in placement breakdown rates between those placed in ethnically 'matched' families and those placed with white parents. These authors looked in more detail at the long-term outcomes of 297 children of minority ethnic origin. Outcome measures of 51 children included well-being, ethnic pride and self-esteem. On the basis of this detailed information provided by the adoptive parents and young people, the authors concluded that the requirements in the Children Act 1989 (re-stated in the Adoption and Children Act 2002) that children should be placed wherever possible with families of similar ethnic and cultural background is likely to be associated with more successful outcomes. However, if this is not possible, some families can successfully parent children of a different ethnicity and heritage from themselves if they are carefully selected, trained and supported.

In the full cohort of 1165 children, there was no difference in breakdown rate between those who were permanently fostered and those who were adopted. However, it should be noted that these children were all placed with the intention that the placement would be permanent, and the practice of the workers was aimed at giving them and the new parents a sense of permanence from the beginning of the placement. In that sense, they differed from long-term placements which, at least early on, were accompanied by uncertainty about the future. Gibbons *et al.* (1995a) found that more of the children maltreated when under the age of 5 were in the higher well-being groups when placed with foster parents than with adopters. However, other smaller-scale, qualitative studies have found that higher levels of satisfaction among the children and higher educational achievement were associated with placement for adoption rather than foster care (Triseliotis & Russell 1984, Hill *et al.* 1989). The conclusion to be drawn from these studies is that the decision about legal status should depend on the wishes, attitudes and temperament of all concerned, especially the child. The apparent cost advantage of adoption should not play a major part in this decision, since it is likely that a high proportion of maltreated children who are adopted will need support through adoption allowances, and the costs of long-term post-placement support are likely to be incurred whatever the legal status. In more complex cases in order to avoid unnecessary delay, there are advantages in seeking, concurrently, adoptive or permanent foster families, thus broadening the choice of families and making it more likely that the special needs of maltreated children will be met.

The task and skills of carers and those who support them

An overview of the social work task

There are several dimensions under which this work can be considered. Firstly, there are organisational decisions to be made about who will be primarily responsible for providing a social work service to the birth parents and their relatives, the child, the carers and possibly members of their family. In some cases, it may be appropriate for the same worker to provide all these services. More often, a specialist worker will be responsible for the recruitment and approval process, and will support the carers or new parents whilst the worker for the child remains principally concerned with the child's welfare. The English National Adoption Standards recognise that, particularly if there is a conflict of interest between the child and the birth family, or strong disagreement about the plans that have been made, it will be appropriate for support to be offered to the parents by another worker or even another agency.

It will be clear from the previous sections that the role of carers and, therefore, the skills and attributes needed are varied. Most obviously, carers fall into two groups: those who for a shorter or longer period or episodically will join with natural parents, social workers and therapists in caring for children in need; and those who will take on the prime parenting responsibility until the child becomes a young adult and beyond. The tasks of the social workers with these two groups are in many respects similar, but in other respects there are important differences. These tasks need to be considered in respect of the following stages:

- recruitment
- selection and preparation
- training
- matching the carers with the child
- preparing for the placement
- providing support and, when appropriate, therapy for the child, the carers and the birth parents when the child is in placement
- when appropriate, helping all those involved to ensure a smooth transfer back to the birth family or on to a new family.

On recruitment, research studies differ in their findings about the sort of people who can successfully provide long- or short-term care for children who have been abused or neglected. Some studies find that more experienced and older parents are more successful, but some (e.g. Wedge & Mantle 1991) have found that younger childless couples have been particularly successful with groups of siblings. Moving away from these more obvious characteristics, writers agree about the attitudes, personal characteristics and skills of successful carers, and these will be discussed in the next section. Foster and adoptive parents have a range of reasons for undertaking this task and research does not point to clear desirable or undesirable motivations.

Once approved, guidance and regulations requires that all foster families should be visited annually for the purposes of reviewing whether they are succeeding in undertaking the tasks they wish to undertake, with the sorts of children and families with whom they have skills and can empathise. The review is also an opportunity for them to discuss their training and support needs, and the adequacy of the support service they have received over the previous year. It is also an opportunity for the agency to monitor how effectively they have discharged their obligations to the children placed with them during the year.

All children who are away from home should be offered a reliable and empathic relationship with the social worker who is responsible for the child's care plan. This area of social work practice has now been well documented and a wide range of practice guidance is available. The term 'life story work' is most frequently used to describe some of the work undertaken with children away from home, but a classic article by Claire Winnicott (first published in 1966 and reprinted in 1986) is still the best statement of the principles and values that must underpin such work. Aldgate and Simmonds (1987), Redgrave (1987), Fahlberg (1991), Ryan and Wilson (2000a), Jones (2003), Rose and Philpot (2004) and Wilson and Ryan (2005) are all useful sources on working directly with children in placement about the circumstances of their lives.

Useful practice texts on social work practice in foster care are those on group work edited by Triseliotis (1988) and on the support of short-term foster parents by Sellick (1992) and Triseliotis *et al.* (1995). Hill and Shaw (1998) and Hill (1999a) have selected articles from the journal *Adoption and Fostering* – many of which provide 'signposts' for practitioners. Argent (2002) and Neil and Howe (2005) have drawn together research and practice guidance on the social work task in facilitating birth family contact. Fisher *et al.* (2000) report findings from their study concerning relationships between foster carers, family placement social workers and the children's social worker. Sellick and Howell (2004) review accounts of 'good practice in fostering'.

Task-centred, 'bridge' or 'therapeutic' carers

While some foster parents and most adopters will care for only one child or sibling group, the majority will look after many children, with a wide range of needs, during their foster care careers. Matching is therefore only possible in the broader sense of a particular age group, or children with particular characteristics or disabilities. Enjoying the company of children and feeling comfortable with them is an essential prerequisite, as are flexibility, negotiation skills and non-judgemental attitudes. Since some children will be placed before it becomes clear that they have been abused, all task-centred carers must be able to understand and empathise not only with the child who has been abused, but also (and more of a challenge) with the parent who was unable to protect the child or was the abuser. If these characteristics are present, it will be possible to provide training and support both before and during placements, so that the special needs of each child and family can be met. Batty (1991), Macaskill (1991), Downes (1992) and Farmer and Pollock (1998) write specifically about the foster care task and the support needs of carers of children who have been sexually abused.

Substitute parents

When children are placed with the intention that the new parents will become the psychological parents, many of the qualities required of them and the skills of the social workers are the same as for task-centred carers. There are, however, important differences, most notably that permanent carers will usually care for only one child or sibling group, and may be approved with specific children in mind. At the approval and matching stages a broad range of skills may be less important than the matching of their skills and needs with the needs and potential of the particular child to be placed.

The art of making permanent placements appears to be in learning what the new parents have to give, and what they will hope for in return, and matching these with what the child can give and needs and is willing and able to take from the new parent. It would thus be a mistake to place with a childless couple who want to love a child who will quickly return their love, a youngster who has been so hurt by earlier experiences that it is not at all obvious that the child will be able to become fully attached to them. Such a child will be more likely to settle with new parents who have already had the rewards of successfully parenting their own children, are motivated by a love of children and the desire to help a youngster in difficulties, and can accept that the youngster may never grow to love them in the same way that their own children have grown up loving them from their early months.

Assessing and matching, then, are the major social work tasks in permanent family placement on which can be built the later work of supporting the new family. Permanent placement work differs from work with task-centred carers in the sense that a family approved to take a child on a permanent basis should not have a child placed with them unless the match seems an appropriate one. For that reason, an even wider range of families may be approved. Indeed, many successful substitute parents have been turned down by foster care or more traditional adoption agencies as being unsuitable (Thoburn *et al.* 1986).

Another difference lies in the nature of social work practice. Once a child has been placed, most researchers have concluded that it is most appropriate for the long-term support of the placement to be undertaken by the specialist worker or agency who undertook the home study and approval work (Thoburn *et al.* 1986, Lowe *et al.* 1999). Beek and Schofield (2004) and Sinclair *et al.* (2005a) use detailed interviews with parents and young people on which to base recommendations about how social work practice might lead to greater placement stability. Cleaver (2000) and Neil *et al.* (2003) draw lessons from their research about the social worker role with birth parents, adopters and foster carers in order to facilitate birth family contact.

Allegations of abuse in adoptive and foster family care

Children who have been abused are vulnerable to renewed abuse by residential or family carers or by birth family members during contact or on return home. Some children who have been abused in the past may make reference to abuse they have already suffered which may be misinterpreted as having been inflicted by foster or adoptive parents and some young people with challenging behaviour use threats to 'expose' carer abuse when angry with their carers (Nixon 1997, Thoburn *et al.* 2000b). It has been noted by some practitioners and foster care support groups that the incidence of unsubstantiated suspicion and false allegation is higher when children are in foster care. Great sensitivity is especially needed when investigating allegations or suspicions of abuse when children are with adoptive or 'permanent' foster families. Procedures for investigating allegations must be followed, as when children are living with their original families, but children should not be removed without careful planning and consideration of their wishes and long-term needs unless this is absolutely necessary for their immediate protection.

Summary and conclusion

This chapter has emphasised that removal from home of a child who may be in need of protection may solve one set of problems but makes the child vulnerable to a new set of hazards. It has also referred to research findings which suggest that if temporary or permanent removal *does* become necessary, a course has to be steered between excess optimism and excess pessimism about the likely outcome for the child.

A succession of studies on short term and on permanent family placement and on the impact of abuse or severe neglect on children has indicated that it is the lucky or the temperamentally resilient minority who remain relatively unscathed. The majority will need more than replacement parent figures, no matter how much love they have to offer. Their fragile identities will require skill as well as love. If they cannot return safely home, their carers must work hard at understanding their past, and substitute parents must incorporate it into the life of the new family. Direct contact with members of the first family will usually be the best way of doing this, but a two-way exchange of letters and photographs may at times have to take the place of direct contact, sometimes for only temporary periods.

For those who help and support the children, their first families, their temporary carers or new families, the keys to success are good planning which adapts to the needs of each child and each situation, imaginative and sensitively negotiated agreements and an adequate supply of 'bridge' carers with choices between family and group care settings. Above all, children need carers and professional workers who will go on fighting on their behalf but who can live with uncertain outcomes and the lack of tidy solutions.

Key points and messages for practice

- Most children entering out-of-home care do so on a voluntary basis and return home fairly quickly. However, around a third need long-term care and the majority of these will have been maltreated before leaving home and/or have challenging behaviour.

- Despite adverse media publicity when things go wrong, the majority of children entering public out-of-home care benefit from the stability and good parenting it can provide. However, an important minority, whether returning home, being adopted or remaining in long-term care, are further harmed by multiple moves in care, adoption breakdowns and less frequently by maltreatment by carers.

- A minority leave care through adoption but most will have their needs for stability and family membership met through foster care, or will be exposed to further harm through instability in care. For children past infancy, once the characteristics of the child (or children in sibling groups) are considered, the research on outcomes indicates that there is no automatic advantage of adoption over long-term foster care, provided that steps are taken to ensure a sense of permanence for carers and child. Adoption works better for some; foster care (or guardianship) works better for others. For a small number of young people, group care is the best option.

- Unnecessary delay results in further harm for too many children. However, rushing a child into a placement that fails to meet important needs can be even more harmful. Failing to meet children's expressed wishes is to be avoided if at all possible. Doing so increases the likelihood of placement breakdown and impairs the development of self-esteem and self-efficacy.

- Child placement work is both 'science' and 'art' – there are no 'quick fixes' and no 'slide-rule' answers based on age or type of abuse. There is a great deal of research and practice literature to help the child placement worker, but the complexity of children's needs requires placement and practice decisions for each child to be made in the light of individual circumstances.

- The majority of children entering care will return home to parents or birth relatives and more resources should be put into, and skills developed in, respite care and facilitating and supporting reunited families.

- Central to effective decision making is getting a balance between the child's need for stability and family membership and their need for identity and continuity. Deciding about and facilitating contact can only be done by skilled and knowledgeable practitioners able to make empathic relationships with young people, parents and carers. More adopters and foster carers must be recruited who understand the value of nurturing a child's links with the past through facilitating appropriate contact and valuing prior relationships.

- Additional caring, empathic, well-trained and well-supported professionals working in partnership with each other, parents, children and carers are essential if good outcomes are to be achieved for a higher proportion of the maltreated children who need out-of-home care.

Annotated further reading

The literature has been reviewed in the body of the chapter, and there are no shortcuts when considering placement for a particular child. There is now no shortage of practice texts on working with children and families, most of which include references to practice with children living away from their parents. The ones listed below are those which specifically focus on children in out-of-home placement, an increasing proportion of whom have been abused or neglected.

Choice of placement and evidence-based practice

Department of Health (1989c, 1991c, 1999d), National Statistics/DfES (2005), Sellick *et al.* (2004), Sinclair (2005), Thoburn (1994), Thomas (2005), Wilson *et al.* (2004).

On short-term and task-centred placements

Aldgate & Bradley (1999), Cleaver (2000), Farmer & Pollock (1998), Howard (2000), Millham *et al.* (1986), Packman & Hall (1998), Rowe *et al.* (1989), Sellick (1992), Thoburn (1994). Triseliotis *et al.* (1995), Wheal (2005).

On residential care

Department of Health (1998b), Grimshaw & Berridge (1994), Sinclair & Gibbs (1998), Utting (1992).

On placement with relatives

Berridge & Cleaver (1987), Broad (2001), Farmer & Moyers (2002), Hunt (2001), Rowe *et al.* (1989).

On permanent placement with substitute parents

Beek & Schofield (2004), Brodzinsky & Schechter (1990), Howe (1998), Neil & Howe (2005), Quinton & Rushton (1998), Sinclair (2005), Sinclair *et al.* (2005a), Thoburn (2002), Thoburn *et al.* (2000), Triseliotis *et al.* (1997).

On work with birth relatives and facilitating contact

Argent (2002), Cleaver (2000), Fahlberg (1991), Morgan (2005), Neil *et al.* (2003), Neil & Howe (2005), Wrobel *et al.* (2003).

On social work practice with children in out-of-home care

Batty (1991), Beek & Schofield (2004), Bell (2002), Cairns (2002), Downes (1992), Fahlberg (1990), Jones (2003), Rose & Philpot (2004), Ryan & Wilson (2000a), Schofield (2002a),Wilson & Ryan (2005).

Useful websites

British Association of Adoption and Fostering: www.baaf.org.uk

The Fostering Network – this website has links to sister organisations in Northern Ireland, Scotland and Wales: www.thefostering.net

Commission for Social Care Inspection Children's Rights Office reports: www.csci.org.uk/child/childrens_rights_director.aspx

Department for Education and Skills Choice Protects: www.dfes.gov.uk/choiceprotects

DfES statistics on children looked after: www.dfes.gov.uk/rsgateway/DB/VOL/v000569/vweb01-2005_2.pdf

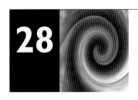

28 Safeguarding children: the manager's perspective

Martin C. Calder

INTRODUCTION

We are currently operating in a time of enormous managerial as well as structural change across the child care field, with many areas of overlap. The government shift towards performance management is a part of their drive for efficiency and accountability and there are enormous implications for all tiers of management. Senior managers are involved in major restructuring tasks such as the merger of education and social services, links with primary care trusts (PCTs) through the Children's Trust initiative, and they have to prioritise performance management, linked directly to the performance management framework (Commission for Social Care Inspection 2005c), which introduces the financially and status-driven council star-rating systems. Departments stand or fall according to their overall social service and council ratings, which in turn impact directly on staff morale and practice.

First-line managers are the first tier of management and they are expected to deliver quality frontline services through the staff they manage, as well as ensuring that the delivery of services is performance compliant. This is difficult in a context of poor staffing levels across key professional agencies (Cooper 2005b). They also have to act as a shock absorber between central government and local initiatives, as well as between social workers and families and, occasionally, other professionals. These are the latest tasks they face in a long list of delicate balancing acts and this chapter focuses on their role in the current and incoming system of child protection.

The role of the social services first-line manager

The role of the social services first-line manager is pivotal to effective multidisciplinary child protection practice. First-line managers must attempt to create and sustain a working environment in which professionals and families can work together. In addition, they supervise and manage the key worker, occasionally intervene to resolve conflict between professionals and between agencies, and tackle any dangerous practice, as well as ensuring that all planning is clear, and outcome as well as output focused.

First-line managers undertake a number of delicate balancing acts in this area of practice. Firstly, they are responsible for ensuring that children are protected by the social workers they manage, through the implementation of departmental procedures and ensuring that statutory responsibilities are met. Currently, this is undertaken in a climate of continuous change and diminishing resources, in which they and social workers are pilloried by the media and the general public if they fail to protect children (e.g. Victoria Climbié) or are perceived as being too interventionist (e.g. Cleveland, the Sally Clarke case). Secondly, they must manage a balance between preventive, investigative and post-registration work.

These varied and multiple roles and responsibilities need to be located in the ever-changing external landscape that has seen the demise of a professional vocabulary relating to child protection (see Munro & Calder 2005). I will not attempt to replace the excellent chapter in the previous edition by Paul Dyson (2002), but rather aim to build on the theoretical, historical and operational foundations he set down. This chapter therefore echoes his view that the child is at the core of the manager's role and that it is the joint task of employers, managers and practitioners to ensure that the child's welfare is paramount. It also accepts that it is too easy for children's needs to be lost in the pressures that are faced in running large, complex and ever-changing health and social care agencies.

This chapter is based on English law for reasons of space and the avoidance of confusion. The Scottish system operates under its own legal system and system of guidance, while in Northern Ireland the Health and Social Services Boards comprise a very different organisational context for child protection work. The devolved national assemblies in Scotland and Wales further add to this diversity.

Review of recent literature and research

What is the child protection system?

The child protection system is a formal system established by central government (through guidance and legislation). It encourages professionals to unite to work collaboratively in the pursuit of protecting children, embracing the family, in order to produce plans designed to prevent or reduce the likelihood of repeat harm to children in the family. Little attention is focused on reparation from harm experienced or treatment options/interventions because of the time they take to achieve, the cost of these and because the government requires short-term fixes to secure acclaim and political security (Calder 2003a).

There have been a number of shifts in the focus of public concern about child abuse over the years that have resulted in changing government guidance (see Parton, Chapter 1, in this volume). This has seen the landscape of child protection change from a focus on sexual and physical abuse to one concerned with emotional abuse and neglect, with therefore less emphasis on immediate risk and harm and more on cumulative concerns and early preventative intervention. Emerging evidence suggests, however, that universal service provision and early intervention lead to the identification of a greater volume of child protection work and thus specific skills and frameworks are needed for both, even when subsumed under a safeguarding umbrella (Jones & O'Loughlin 2003).

The Victoria Climbié Inquiry was not the only factor precipitating change. A further shift was caused by the Bichard Inquiry Report (2004) which examined the circumstances in which Ian Huntley was able to gain employment in a school setting and how he was able to have sexual relationships with a large number of under-age girls without criminal sanction, culminating in the murder of Holly Wells and Jessica Chapman. The Report recommended the introduction of a register of those who wish to work with children or vulnerable adults – perhaps evidenced by a licence or card. The inclusion of an individual on this register would reassure employers that nothing was known by any of the relevant agencies about that individual that would disqualify them from working with children or vulnerable adults. This is currently being explored by central government but is unlikely to be introduced as suggested.

The allegations that medics have over-stepped their mark in the child protection field has also appeared many times in a variety of contexts in recent years. One prominent example is that of Professor Roy Meadow, who was accused of presenting misleading and flawed evidence to a number of high-profile criminal courts relating to sudden unexplained death in infancy (SUDI). Sally Clarke and Angela Cannings were both convicted and imprisoned for killing their children but were subsequently acquitted on appeal. Whilst these events have induced intense and inquisitorial media attention, there has been an immense and potentially grave backlash from such critical attention. Many doctors have relinquished their designated child protection responsibilities and many more are more reticent about providing clear diagnoses. This can impact on the manager who is concerned that a child is being harmed but cannot substantiate it or act in the absence of a medical opinion.

Child protection at the crossroads

As has recently been argued (Calder 2004b), child protection is at a critical crossroads in its evolutionary journey. There is rightly a debate about the need for early identification of and intervention in problems that will hopefully reduce the number of child abuse tragedies; there is rightly an emphasis on joined-up professional thinking, planning and intervention packages in order to reduce potential conflict and pool limited resources; and there is also rightly a need to examine how we can maximise the efficiency of a bureaucratic child protection system. However, there are a great many areas of concern arising from this debate, not least the over-emphasis on professional output measurement (performance indicators) rather than on child-orientated outcomes (Calder 2005b).

There are some particular barriers to working together which have an enormous influence on the functionality of the child protection system. These are summarised elsewhere (Calder 1999b) but several relating specifically to the manager's role are worth detailing here.

Thresholds for the provision of a social work service

Identified need outstrips fiscal resources by a ratio of 3:1 (Bullock *et al.* 1998b) and thus there is a need to restrict the provision of scarce resources to the most deserving cases. This is transparent but creates additional tensions when potential child protection cases are left to deteriorate to the point of crisis, often resulting in harm to the child before they are acted on by social services. This generates professional division and resentment that can also generate new problems for managers to resolve.

Information sharing confusion

Currently, there is a very strong emphasis on building systems that promote information exchange at an earlier point in the intervention process, but this has to be balanced against a sense of professional paralysis about what information can and cannot be shared. What seems essential to communicate for one may seem a breach of confidentiality or peripheral to another. Professionals from different fields are used to working within their own particular culture and organisational structure, with their own rules on issues such as confidentiality.

In addition, however, at a time when agencies need to work together more closely to prevent abuse and protect children, there is a concern that to do so requires parental consent. This is problematic when so many child protection clients are involuntary and, in neglect cases, often passive and unmotivated to effect the required change. For professionals, the increasing focus on neglect and emotional abuse has revealed very clear divisions concerning the point at which, and with what characteristics, a case becomes abusive. This changing face of child protection requires clarity of thought, consistency and commonality of language across professions. Without this, managers will be distracted by disputes between professionals who will continue to disagree on whether a particular concern requires a child protection or a child in need approach, or by having to deal with the consequences of non-identification if a child is seriously harmed.

To compound this confusion further, there are a number of information exchange systems currently being promoted and developed by different departments in government, which work against each other rather than clarifying the professional task. The number of databases that could warn of dangers to children is mushrooming and at present includes the following.

- Care records service: An NHS system of health and social care records accessed by a national 'data spine'
- Citizen Information Project (CIP): A national database of UK residents proposed by the Office for National Statistics
- Common Assessment Framework (CAF): A strategy for assessing the needs of children across different agencies, proposed by the Green Paper, *Every Child Matters* (DfES 2003b).
- Framework for Multi-agency Environments (FAME): A national project funded by the Office of the Deputy Prime Minister's local e-government programme
- Information referral and tracking (IRT): A local authority-based IT system for sharing information about children between agencies
- Information sharing and assessment (ISA): The current programme is sponsored by the Department for Education and Skills for information-sharing between agencies; it includes the work on IRT
- Reducing Youth Offending Generic National Solution (Ryogens): A system for sharing data about children and young people at risk of falling into crime, developed under the Office of the Deputy Prime Minister's local e-government programme.

But whether and how these will all fit together is still unclear and, as Cross (2004) has argued, local authorities have waited years for decent IT to alert them when children are in danger and now several systems are coming all at once. The problem is that from a relative clarity of approach in child protection, a shift in government policy has seen the publication of materials which generate and sustain chaos and which create a huge operational dilemma for managers in terms of understanding and explaining these to their staff, and applying, operationalising and coordinating them in practice.

Changing roles and responsibilities

The issue of role clarity is important, particularly when the blurring of roles can serve to relieve staff of knowing who is doing what and why, and who should be held accountable in the event of failure. The last 10 years has seen the role of the front-line social services manager both change and expand. Not only are they responsible for the supervision of team members, essential in light of the findings of Lord Laming (Laming Report 2003), but the destructuring and delayering that has occurred in many social services departments has meant that they are also now responsible for significant budgets and for the management of additional staff.

This has had an impact on supervision. Marsh and Triseleotis (1996) noted that 25% of staff in social services reported that they had received no supervision within their first year of practice and for many others it was unplanned and erratic. Horwath (1997) commented that the pressures placed on front-line managers meant that decisions were made 'on the hoof' as they rushed from one meeting to another. She also noted that many managers found they did not have the time to read case files in detail and were increasingly dependent on social workers to give them verbal details, which could lead to subjective assessments.

Managers are also operating in a climate of changing philosophies, where the emerging paradigm is one that requires a wider, more holistic view of the needs of vulnerable children and their families. Burton (1996) reported the findings of a study which highlighted the impact of this changing philosophy: front-line managers reported a number of concerns that centred on anxiety over the ability to balance support for staff and the protection of children, fear regarding the management of risk, low professional esteem, lack of emphasis on enhancing the professional knowledge of managers and budgets structured in favour of intervention.

Performance targets

Dyson (2002) noted that the performance culture has evolved a framework for monitoring the public sector through national performance indicators. This encourages individual agencies to look inwardly in order to meet their own targets and to look outwardly only if there is any remaining time, energy and inclination. This rarely happens, which impacts significantly on working together and consequently on the manager's role. Caulkin (2001) usefully explored the issue of management being tied to set goals, concluding that it could be meaningless and counterproductive, as well as potentially leading to disaster. It systematically lowers quality, raises costs and wrecks systems, making them less stable and therefore harder to improve. When people are given targets and their careers become dependent on delivering them, they will strive to meet the targets – even if they subvert or destroy the enterprise to do it.

Rather, the current high-profile nature of the performance management systems that regulate and prioritise the activities of many agencies needs to give way to child-outcome orientated thinking and practice. The balance for managers is to achieve outputs in a way that does not impact negatively on the provision of a quality front-line social work service, since failure to meet targets can have consequences for the department in terms of star ratings, status and self-esteem of staff and, as such, cannot be ignored by managers trying to recruit and retain a dwindling professional workforce.

Organisational restructuring

The variety of structures and systems within different agencies creates difficulties and makes coordination difficult: different agencies hold different powers and duties and some do not have coterminous geographical boundaries. Morrison (1998) notes that the organisational context has become less predictable, less stable and more conflict-ridden in the short term, as the competition for resources has become even more acute. Whilst the emphasis on contractual, accountable and targeted services may, in the longer term, result in strategic inter-agency partnerships for the planning, commissioning and evaluating of child protection services, in the short term at least, 'partnerships' across agencies are under severe strain.

The combination of market forces and government restructuring of funding impacts on the role of the manager directly: they have to steer their staff through changes in structure and philosophy and motivate them to work with change; they also have to work indirectly, through an expanding public relations role, with other agencies concerned about the elevated threshold for the provision of a social work service, as well as being distracted from their ever-expanding frontline roles.

An analysis of policy issues

The Victoria Climbié Inquiry (Laming Report 2003) clearly reveals how the failure to identify accurately a child in need of protection can have disastrous consequences. This has resulted in a full-frontal attack on the child protection system when what is needed is a strengthening of the preventative, legal and therapeutic options to support, rather than challenge or replace, the child protection function. Child protection as we know it is no longer an accepted term in central government guidance and the ensuing Children Act 2004 and *Working Together* guidance* has resulted in:

- no place for the established view of child protection
- the language of 'safeguarding' predominating
- 'risk' being deleted from the social work vocabulary
- no clear assessment structure existing to integrate the multiple structures in existence
- the number of new initiatives continuing in the absence of integration, evaluation or review (e.g. the Integrated Children's System was introduced even before the Assessment Framework upon which it was built had been evaluated; similarly, the concept of Children's Trusts was heralded post-Laming without any evaluation of the pilot projects).

The following analysis of the current structural initiatives from central government is not designed to offer a detailed résumé of each but a flavour of the specific issues within each that relate to the managerial role, as well as identifying the compounding effect of fragmented, even contradictory, initiatives.

Universal and standardised services

The government's aim was for the *Framework for the Assessment of Children in Need and their Families* to be adopted universally by all professionals and used with all children, in order to create a common language and structure (DoH 2000). Unfortunately, only social services were included in the consultation process and other government departments (cited below) issued parallel mandatory frameworks for the assessment of children, such as ASSET (and now ONSET) by the Youth Justice Board, APIR (Assessment, Planning, Intervention and Review) (Connexions Service National Unit 2001), OASYs (Offender Assessment Systems) (HM Prison Service/National Probation Service 2001) and Matrix 2000 by the police. This clearly illustrates the enduring incapacity within government for different departments of state

---

* The most up-to-date version of this document was published by HM Government in 2006. For a full discussion of this, see Chapter 11.

to liaise and to unify their individual responsibilities within a collective framework of response.

The problem for managers trying to make sense of this situation is compounded further when one considers the different basis upon which some of the tools have been developed. For example, the world of criminal justice (police, probation, prisons) is evolving actuarial, statistically derived tools that deny the use of professional judgement and which focus on the risk of offending over a lifetime within a group or category of offenders. This may be useful when examining policies relating to supervision and predicting reconviction rates but it does not inform the issue of child protection when workers have to consider the specific risk of offending by an individual perpetrator resident in a particular family.

To compound this, there has been a refinement and extension of risk tools within the sexual abuse arena at a time when, it has been argued, 'risk' is no longer acceptable in the vocabulary of social work (see Calder 2003b for a detailed discussion of this point). Managers and workers who wish to assess risks in cases need to be aware, however, that importing refined risk tools from elsewhere can be problematic if these were designed in different contexts to measure different outcomes (Calder 2000).

The lack of fit between parallel government publications addressing child protection

For managers, it is alarming that there are inconsistencies between the child protection guidance (DoH *et al.* 1999) and the Assessment Framework (DoH 2000), given they are the two essential documents in their toolkit. For example, whilst there is an expectation that we move towards a 'children in need' perspective, it is confusing and contradictory that the criteria for adding a child's name to the child protection register appear to have been broadened to include children exposed to or involved in internet sexual abuse, female genital mutilation, domestic violence and prostitution and, in more recent times, managing licensing applications.

Risk deletion

The concept of risk has been abolished within government guidance involving child protection, since 'risk' is equated with the idea of child protection (s.47 Children Act 1989) that the government is seeking to redefine. Instead, it has been replaced with concepts of 'weaknesses' and 'strengths' in order to reinforce the preferred notion of children in need. This suggests that there has been a misunderstanding about the meaning of risk in government circles, since need clearly must be balanced with risk when weighing up the options in the light of all the available information (Calder 2003b). Had this more balanced view of risk been embraced, it would have been consistent with holistic assessments and provided an opportunity to debate a more contemporary view of risk located within the change agenda.

The relegation of risk from the framework also creates huge operational problems. Frontline staff undertaking primarily child protection work cannot talk about 'risk' and therefore struggle to incorporate risk into their assessment practice. For managers this means that they have the task of furnishing frontline staff with circumstance-specific risk assessment frameworks to overcome the generic, strengths-loaded assessment framework and this is challenging since managers will struggle to have the necessary range and depth of evidence-based and up-to-date knowledge.

Evidence-based practice

There is now an expectation that social workers should operate within an evidence base and there is little disagreement with the view that good practice ought to derive from research evidence about the nature, causes or typical pathways of social problems, and about the success of methods for dealing with those problems (Hill 1999b). The demands of evidence-based practice therefore require practitioners to seek out and critically assess relevant research literature and findings. Evidence-based practitioners should themselves collect data systematically, specify outcomes in measurable terms, and systematically monitor and evaluate their interventions (Hill 1999b). There are, however, some potential problems with evidence-based practice, including whether research should be the sole basis for developing or sustaining services, whether things as complex as human interactions can be measured, and whether paying attention to the efficacy of interventions diverts attention away from the root of problems.

Whilst the definition of evidence-based practice adopted within the Assessment Framework allows for the use of practice wisdom to offset the limitations of any research, this is problematic since it is the lowest acceptable form of evidence on the evidence-base continuum (Ramchandani *et al.* 2001) and workers often lack the opportunity for reflective practice or time to read and digest the emerging materials.

The evidence-based movement also fails to address issues raised by the skill deficit currently facing providers of frontline health and social services. The latter have taken to importing workers from abroad to try to deal with the situation; for managers, this can mean having to train and supervise newly qualified staff from a different country who are unfamiliar with British culture or current legal and operational guidance and systems.

The emergence of the Advanced Child Care Award (PQ2-6) is also to be welcomed in that it provides the opportunity for staff to be released to learn about the necessary evidence base, whilst also promoting a greater emphasis on the use of professional judgement alongside research by building in reflective opportunities lacking in frontline practice. Releasing social workers for such training creates problems of staff replacement, however, and it has also catapulted managers into an assessor role, which is time consuming and takes them into the territory of being academic markers in addition to their operational responsibilities.

The consequences of rigid timescales

The promulgation of tight timescales for conducting the required assessments also detracts from frontline work because they form a central plank of performance management and the associated stars and status for departments. The unfortunate result of these is that managers are pressured to become output-focused rather than child-outcome compliant and the child is forced to work at the professional's pace rather than vice versa. An example of this is interviewing children under the timescales recommended by the *Achieving Best Evidence* guidelines (Home Office *et al.* 2002) and the Assessment Framework, regardless of a child's readiness and willingness to disclose sensitive information in this context – practice which completely undermines the emphasis on partnership and consumer participation.

The decline of sexual abuse

In the early 1980s there was an explosion of sexual abuse work and the focus of much child protection work, and many publications were on this area. Since that time we have seen a significant decrease in the number of cases of sexual abuse falling within the child protection system, despite the problems of internet sexual offending, children and young people with sexual behaviour problems, children involved in prostitution, child trafficking and female genital mutilation that should arguably have seen a continued increase in such cases.

For managers, this raises a number of issues. At a fundamental level, they have to examine strategically whether there is simply a failure to recognise sexual abuse, exposing potential victims to terrible harm: many offenders do not differ from other fathers/partners apart from their offending, which renders detection very difficult. Once sexual abuse has been identified, staff and managers need to understand just how different this type of abuse can be and that there are specific rather than general assessment frameworks to ensure a focus on the risks/harm rather than simply the strengths. Indeed, focusing only on strengths arguably colludes with such behaviour. The Assessment Framework is not applicable to sexual abuse cases, however: it only allows the worker to conduct a general and not a specific assessment, which is problematic given the unique causal factors and, more importantly, the variance across the ever-expanding range of sexual abuse scenarios (Calder 2000).

Information storage and retrieval systems

Integrated Children's System (ICS): the manager's dream?

The ICS has been developed to help workers and managers in social services improve the outcomes of their work with children and families. It was originally designed to achieve two objectives: to unify the two major frameworks used within children's services (the Assessment Framework and the Looked After Children materials) and to do some reparatory work across professional boundaries and between agencies by creating a truly universal framework for assessment. However, the government agenda has forced some significant changes, consolidating and possibly deepening, rather than resolving, the existing chaos (Calder 2004b).

One example of this relates to the question of which agency will utilise the ICS. From the outset, social services retained lead responsibility for coordinating the implementation of the ICS, although the intention was for it to be issued beyond social services to embrace Connexions, Children's Fund, Sure Start and Youth Offending Teams. This was in recognition of the fact that all providers of services for children and families would benefit from a common approach to assessment, intervention and review, and from being able to share relevant information with each other. This seems to mirror the situation that existed with the Assessment Framework and assumes that there is a common language and assessment tool.

This has now been changed, however, with the ICS becoming the exclusive property of social services and other organisations having been given a separate assessment tool (the CAF), although the two are intended to dovetail with each other to provide a seamless service. Both the ICS and the CAF are systems without any detailed operational assessment tools, however, these having been left for managers to develop and implement locally. One further challenge to managers is to operationalise a system designed principally as a performance tool, but furnishing frontline staff with it as an exemplar for their practice is contentious as well as generating many new IT challenges for managers and workers alike. The ICS exemplars, which provide standardised templates for different tasks such as initial and core assessments, or pathway planning, form the basis for designing the necessary IT software to run the templates and assist social workers in collecting, organising, retrieving and analysing information about cases. They will also constitute the e-social record required by government by 2005.

Information sharing and assessment (ISA)

ISA is the government's response to Lord Laming's call for better joint working practices and data sharing between all agencies involved in the care of vulnerable children. Hunter (2004) examined some of the problems associated with development of effective information sharing and assessment and blames difficulties on central government. He argued that insufficient resources, poor communication and a lack of guidance from central government were severely hampering the drive to identify children at risk of social exclusion, refer them to services and monitor them through information sharing between agencies. In particular, the conflicting guidance on information sharing from the Department of Constitutional Affairs and from the DfES (2004h) has hindered progress and it is ironic to note that the government's drive to encourage working together is again being hampered by different departments of state working completely independently of each other.

As identified earlier, there is a multitude of information-sharing initiatives being introduced within a variety of different agencies, apparently without thought as to how and when they might be integrated. In simple terms, there is still no clarity about what the full ISA framework will look like and no coherent guidance that clarifies how it will operate or integrate with other data-sharing initiatives, such as the CAF and the ICS. This renders effective implementation impossible and leaves managers with a very difficult task in terms of having to work with internal procedures, families and other agencies without any blueprint for application. Managers again have a key role in progressing this – that of troubleshooting central guidance and developing possible local solutions.

Common Assessment Framework

The *Every Child Matters* Green Paper (DfES 2003b) proposed the introduction of a Common Assessment Framework (CAF) as a central element of the strategy for helping children, young people and their families. Most agencies and practitioners undertake some form of needs assessment to determine what services should be offered in each case but, because each agency has its own approach to assessment, there is a lack of coordination and consistency between them. In some cases this leads to important needs not being picked up early enough, if at all, and in other cases, to agencies asking families for similar information time and time again. Some practitioners routinely refer children and young people to other agencies, most notably to social services, with only a very minimal needs assessment, with the consequence that sometimes the child/young person is found not to qualify for any support.

The government intends that a common assessment would be undertaken at the first sign of difficulty, most likely outside of the particular context of social services, in order to enable early intervention and thus prevent a child's needs becoming more serious. Common assessment is therefore particularly aimed at 'vulnerable children' and the challenge for managers is to ensure that, when developed locally, it feeds the ICS. In this sense it can best be construed as a template for an inter-agency referral form into social services. Figure 28.1 illustrates how the current initiatives may sit

Figure 28.1
A visual contextualisation of current systems (adapted with permission from Calder 2004b).

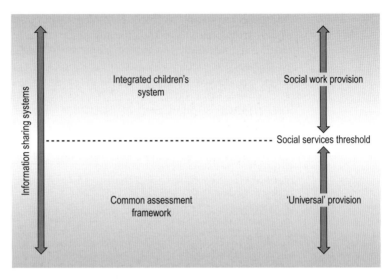

together, although it does not capture the detailed planning that will be required in relation to each initiative and to apply them in a meaningful and integrative way.

Additional structural additions

Children's Trusts

The government's view of Children's Trusts is premised on a belief that there is a case for structural change in order to effect better coordination of children's services. They are considered to be a means of achieving better outcomes for children, a means of commissioning services and as an entity that must include PCTs and social services, and hopefully education. In so doing, they will unify at local level the various agencies involved in providing services to children, enabling local partners to jointly plan, commission, finance and deliver services and cut through inter-agency boundaries. There is significant discretion as to how broadly or narrowly the Children's Trust concept is interpreted and applied locally, however, so, once again, this draws managers into a significant volume of strategic local negotiation to colour in the picture outlined by central government – but without the evaluation of the pilot projects to provide an embryonic evidence base from which to draw.

Local Safeguarding Children's Boards

LSCBs were advocated by Lord Laming to replace the toothless Area Child Protection Committees. There are a number of managerial challenges arising from this important change.

■   Broader definition of safeguarding. We have already seen what this may look like with the enactment of the Licensing Act on April 1 2005, which confers the responsibility for child protection on the ACPC, although managers have no history of vetting such applications and there has been little training or additional resources. There is also a very real need to look at where domestic violence fora will be located within the safeguarding agenda, since a significant percentage of the current child protection population come from families where there has been such a problem.

■ Building structures and services that are best placed to deliver on the agenda.
■ Establishing clear relationships, including scrutiny and commissioning arrangements, across the various strategic planning fora.
■ Developing work across agencies, including establishing LSCBs, shared performance indicators, planning, screening and auditing arrangements.
■ Involvement of communities and users.
■ Equipping the workforce – managing structural and cultural change, training requirements, thresholds, CAF, accountabilities, etc.

Education Act 2002

S.175 of the 2002 Act, which came into force on 1 June 2004, places a duty on local education authorities, and on the governing bodies of schools and further education institutions, to make arrangements for carrying out their functions with a view to safeguarding and promoting the welfare of children. It expands the traditional child protection responsibilities to include the prevention of bullying, dealing with attendance issues, making provision for children who are excluded from school, meeting the needs of sick children and for school security. Subsequent guidance has addressed how allegations of abuse by teaching staff should be managed, proposing the introduction of an allegations manager. These developments impact on managers through an expansion and adjustment of their role in a changing context.

Associated educational developments

For the government, education holds the key to personal fulfilment, social inclusion, cohesion and economic competitiveness. It plays a critical role in the vision for and delivery of children's services as a 'universal service' and 'children at risk'. Schools are 'at the heart' of their local communities although they need encouragement to play their part in a vision for improving children's services. The Education Act gives schools powers to procure community-based services and education is at the heart of growing partnerships which are developing preventative services, including Sure Start, Early Years and Childcare Partnerships, Children's Fund and Connexions.

Extended schools

The concept of establishing schools as the hub of children's services, within which wrap-around care of pupils takes place from 8 a.m. until 6 p.m., is a further development in the configuration of service structures that have implications for safeguarding children and young people. Many schools already provide additional services and activities centred on their premises such as counselling, attached social workers, after-school homework and sport. In addition, a new role is being prescribed for school nurses by the Chief Nursing Officer whereby they will be much more actively involved in child protection, health promotion and parent support.

Many child care organisations have pointed out, however, that a significant number of children and young people are not engaged in schools and do not naturally regard them as a positive resource. Pupils who are excluded, receiving home tuition, attending specialist pupil referral units or involved in regular truanting will need to be reached in other more creative ways if their needs are not to be neglected: they are arguably more in need than those already participating in school life and will be at higher risk of abuse and/or tempted into antisocial behaviour.

Children's centres

It is envisaged that about 2500 children's centres will be established by the year 2008 as part of the current government plan to provide universal access to affordable, flexible childcare. They are another example of integrated strategic thinking where provision for under-5s, early education, full day-care, parental outreach, family support and health services can be offered. Children's centres are also expected to have a role in identifying and providing for children with special educational needs, providing a base for child minders, acting as a service hub for other childcare providers, and offering management and workforce training.

These new centres are set to develop in different ways according to local need and local authority priorities. The concept includes full-scale centres in areas of high need and one-stop advice centres in areas where little more than information and signposting is required. Criticisms of the children's centre plan include the concern that they are replacing Sure Start programmes, in which there was an ethos of flexibility and innovation built around parental expectations. In addition, the role of the independent and voluntary sectors seems to have been minimised in the strategic planning, which does not bode well for partnership practice and integrated services.

With the merger of education and social services post-Climbié, there is a tremendous responsibility on managers to try to translate rhetoric into reality, extending their remit to prevention as well as protection and providing social work services across new boundaries, with partners who may be simultaneously struggling with this expanding role on a shoestring budget and with only skeletal guidance. Achieving this is important since it is not the only bridge they will have to cross: the separation of adult and children's services creates major challenges for managers to grapple with simply in order to maintain the status quo, such as ensuring that protocol agreements reached with adult mental health and drug and alcohol services are transferred and hopefully consolidated and extended. This is important because the identification of parental problems is central to safeguarding and the separation of services is likely to make understanding of their respective roles, responsibilities and procedures less likely. A further demand on managers' time is to advise the newly appointed Directors of Children's Services: since most of these have no history of social work operations, they are reliant on managers who have to guide them into their new roles.

Implications for practice

A conceptual model has been developed (Calder 1999b; see Fig. 28.2) to help local authorities, ACPCs/LSCBs and individual practitioners cope with both the contradictions and lack of detail that is evident in most central government guidance: the role of managers is critical in this respect.

This model has been used by managers to develop an effective response to specific presenting concerns, such as prostitution (Calder 2001b) or domestic violence (Calder *et al.* 2004), or to negotiate across agencies about what is needed and what the respective roles and responsibilities should be, or to consider how best to implement changes such as those contained in the Children Act 2004. The implications of the current agenda for practice include managing change in systems as well as operational practice. This must be done with a diminished and confused workforce, who are being denied the vocabulary, specific procedures and assessment frameworks for an ever-increasing range of child protection situations and yet who are

Figure 28.2
A framework for local responses (reproduced with permission from Calder 1999b).

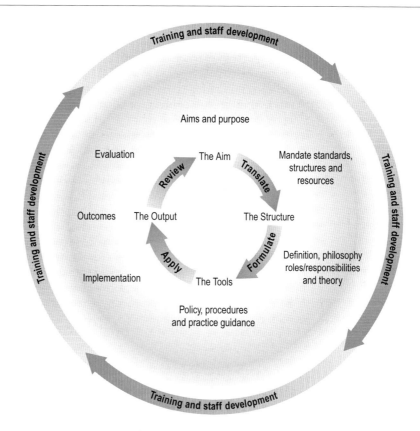

expected to deploy their skills to develop individualised evidence-based frameworks that will be critically examined by courts and others and where they are left culpable for mistakes.

This seems ironic when it is the system itself that is creating the problems and when the consultation document (DfES 2005a*) is adding to the confusion by amalgamating enquiries under s.47 of the Children Act 1989 with core assessments, ostensibly as a means of ensuring performance compliance for departments. The most crucial need for managers is time in which to work with the workforce to help them to understand and incorporate the change agenda into their practice in a manageable way, as well as working with others to furnish them with practice guidance that moves beyond general processes to offer guidance on the 'how'. It is therefore perhaps unsurprising that problems of recruitment and retention are no longer restricted to frontline social workers but now extend to first-line managers.

Conclusion

The pace of change for the child care and protection field is accelerating at the same time that it is also becoming less prescriptive, creating immense operational and strategic challenges for managers locally to resolve. This is to be welcomed if it

---

* The most up-to-date version of this document was published by HM Government in 2006. For a full discussion of this, see Chapter 11.

allows for creativity but the performance culture tends to stifle this. The manager has the difficult task of responding to the required changes, whilst continuing to support staff and manage their work, as well as motivating them to accept and contribute to the change agenda. Managers thus act as a shock absorber and a juggler, as well as representing the lynchpin for successful multi-agency working.

It is in this difficult context that first-line managers need to ensure that the focus remains firmly on the child; that the risks to the child are monitored, reviewed and reassessed; and that the work with the child and the family is planned. This chapter has highlighted the complex and demanding role of the first-line manager in both the management of their social workers as well as the multidisciplinary network. Managers also need opportunities to develop their own skills, however, as a prerequisite for their being able to manage the multiple demands made of them. Organisational change and restructuring can increase these demands, however, as resources and support become more limited and managers are forced to fight to protect shrinking resources, whether material or human. This chapter has also identified the operational considerations for managers, which are coupled with management expectations and responsibilities that are also changing with the growing influence of market forces and performance management. This is a challenging time to be a first-line manager, especially when one considers the difficulties in staff recruitment, retention and morale.

Key points and messages for practice

- Managers need to consider the effects of pursuing a performance-driven agenda for frontline social work practice and child outcomes. This has the potential to alienate staff and families.

- The Laming Inquiry re-emphasised the centrality of effective supervision to the attainment of safe outcomes for children and workers.

- Managers need to consider how to develop an evidence-based knowledge base within the teams they manage so that there is a reservoir of specific rather than general assessment frameworks available to their staff.

- Change is an inevitable feature of current practice and managers need to ensure that appropriate time and focus are given to keeping staff informed, whilst also channelling their views upwards so that they influence the systems and structures being developed. Ownership often stems from influence.

Annotated further reading

Calder M C 2004 The integrated children's system: out of the frying pan and into the fire? Child Care in Practice 10(3):225–240
A critical analysis of the system and the predecessors upon which it is based.

Adair J 2005 How to grow leaders. Kogan Page, London
Looks at the nature of leadership and how it can be encouraged and developed. Topics discussed include the manager as leader, how people become leaders, training team leaders and learning to be a top strategic leader.

Walker S, Thurston C 2005 Safeguarding children and young people: a guide to integrated work. Russell House, Lyme Regis
Examines in a simple accessible way the influences behind the incoming safeguarding agenda as well as a guide to the relevant legislation and how they sit together.

Buckley H 2003 Child protection work: beyond the rhetoric. Jessica Kingsley, London
Examines what professionals actually do in the child protection field. Looking beyond procedural guidance, the book explores practice frameworks in a number of forums, including the conference.

Smith D (ed) 2004 Social work and evidence-based practice. Jessica Kingsley, London
This excellent text explores evidence-based practice – what it might mean, how it can be achieved – and examines these issues in a range of contexts from child abuse and domestic violence to looked-after children and disability.

Useful websites

Bichard Inquiry Report: www.bichardinquiry.org.uk/report
Calder Social Work Training and Consultancy: www.caldertrainingandconsultancy.co.uk
Child Welfare Information Gateway (formerly the National Clearinghouse on Child Abuse and Neglect Information and the National Adoption Information Clearinghouse): www.childwelfare.gov
Department for Education and Skills: www.dfes.gov.uk
Minnesota Center Against Violence and Abuse: www.mincava.umn.edu
Victoria Climbié Inquiry: www.victoria-climbie-inquiry.org.uk

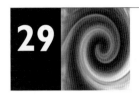

29

Where are we now? Themes and future directions

Olive Stevenson

INTRODUCTION

It is 5 years since the second edition of the *Child Protection Handbook* was published. That there is a need for a revised third edition is evident from the substantial modifications and additions to this volume. Indeed, when one reflects upon trends and events in relation to 'protecting' and 'safeguarding' children during the first years of the millennium, they are quite bewildering in their extent and diversity. In consequence, the range of responses they elicit, political and professional, are equally extensive and diverse. Because these are dynamic processes, set in a wider social context, there cannot be a simple linear reaction from a trend or event to a response. Rather, issues get swept up in the high winds of social and political controversy. Arguments about safeguarding children are bound up with the deepest feelings and the strongest opinions about child welfare, the rights of parents and family life generally. Of course, it was ever thus. But there are some factors which pose particular challenges at the present time in the United Kingdom. These may be categorised as follows:

- Dealing with the widening and changing understanding of child maltreatment and of the circumstances in which it occurs
- Coming to terms with the cultural issues raised for child protection practice in multicultural Britain
- The widening of professional and community involvement in protecting children from maltreatment
- Working together – inter-agency and inter-professional activity
- Managing the tensions between political and professional worlds
- Critical issues for practice, education and professional development.

These matters are all extremely complex: some are profound, touching as they do some basic values in our society. This analysis will show how hard, and in how many ways, those involved are struggling with the implications of 'protecting' children.

The discussion which follows has to be set in the context of developments in government policy, following the Victoria Climbié Inquiry (Laming Report 2003), the succeeding Green Paper *Every Child Matters* (DfES 2003a) and the Children Act 2004. The draft guidance (DfES 2005a) on *Working Together** marks a move away from earlier comparable documents, in that it places issues of child protection within a wider framework of 'safeguarding' children; this in turn is within the framework of 'supporting children and families'. The five desired outcomes

---

* The most up-to-date version of this document was published by HM Government in 2006. For a full discussion of this, see Chapter 11.

identified in *Every Child Matters* 'that are key to children and young people's well-being' (DfES 2003a) are:

- Being healthy
- Staying safe
- Enjoying and achieving
- Making a positive contribution
- Achieving economic well-being.

This is a hugely ambitious agenda, albeit one to which we can all subscribe in theory. Parton (Chapter 1) and Luckock (Chapter 14), both in this volume, together provide a comprehensive description and analysis of the history behind the present situation and of its implications for us today. Both authors express fundamental doubts about the viability of the proposals and concern about their effect on the child protection agenda. Parton argues that the impact of the changes 'will be to fundamentally reconfigure the relationship between the state, professionals, parents and children' and that 'new and wide-ranging systems of surveillance are being introduced'. However, he suggests that 'because the systems are so extensive, the definitions of concern so broad and the fact that the professionals who have responsibilities for children are held so … accountable', there is a danger of the focus on the real needs and rights of children and young people being diluted or dispersed by the excessive organisational 'busyness'. He fears a preoccupation with boundaries and roles. Luckock considers in detail the effects, already present or emerging, of the drive towards service integration, matters to which I shall return later in this chapter.

In this, the final chapter of the *Handbook*, I can only point to the uncertainties raised by these current trends. However, one thing is sure: there will be a continuing need and cry for better services to protect children from maltreatment by adults or their peers. The substitution of the word 'safeguarding' for 'protection' in government discourse may widen the scope for prevention and intervention but it should not lessen vigilance and focus on that group of children and young people whose tragic experiences have darkened the last 40 years of child welfare. This chapter will focus on the challenge of protecting children from serious maltreatment whilst acknowledging that the reframing of policy and practice in line with the changed focus of current trends will have a substantial impact on the work of many professionals in health and social care.

Dealing with widening and changing understandings of child maltreatment and of the circumstances in which it occurs

Since the 1960s, we have continuously expanded our understanding and definitions of child abuse. Whilst the conventional categories of physical, sexual, emotional abuse and neglect have been familiar for many years, the emphasis on, and interpretation of, them constantly changes or evolves. In the last decade, we have seen increased emphasis on neglect and emotional abuse.

These two forms of maltreatment have been defined as distinct categories in relation to the 'at risk register' (DoH *et al.* 1999). However, as we understand better the interaction of body, mind and feelings in the development of a child, it has become clearer that the two categories of 'emotional abuse' and 'neglect' overlap, to the point when their separation may not be logically sustainable. Thus, for example, a child who is physically neglected may suffer both emotional and cognitive harm; a child who is emotionally abused, for example, by isolation or scapegoating, is in fact being emotionally neglected, even if their physical care is adequate. It may be that, for the time being, the distinction between the terms has its uses; however, it is important to recognise that 'significant harm' to a child cannot be compartmentalised. The official definitions of emotional abuse and neglect, as they stand at present are as follows:

- *Emotional abuse* – the persistent emotional ill-treatment of a child such as to cause severe and persistent adverse effects on the child's emotional development. It may involve conveying to children that they are worthless or unloved, inadequate or valued only insofar as they meet the needs of another person, age or developmentally inappropriate expectations being imposed on children, causing children frequently to feel frightened, or the exploitation or corruption of children.
- *Neglect* – the persistent failure to meet a child's basic physical and/or psychological needs, likely to result in the serious impairment of the child's health or development, such as failing to provide adequate food, shelter and clothing, or neglect of, or unresponsiveness to, a child's basic emotional needs (DoH *et al.* 1999). (It should be noted that the definition of neglect does not include cognitive neglect, which is of particular importance in infancy because of its long-lasting effects on the development of the brain.)

Table 29.1 shows the significance of the two categories for the years 2000–2004. 'Neglect' has been significantly higher than other categories during these years.

The emergence of the two categories as a current cause of particular concern suggests that we are becoming more sophisticated in our understanding of what may cause 'significant harm' to children's development. Emotional abuse emerges as a concept underpinning all aspects of child maltreatment. However, it takes us into more contested territory than many aspects of physical and sexual abuse. Whilst few would deny that emotional abuse is a component of physical and sexual abuse, the concept itself rests on basic assumptions about children's needs or rights which include, for example, the development of their sense of identity and of self-esteem. Once we begin to unpick the underlying values and associated theories of child development, it becomes clear that there will on occasion be tensions, if not clashes, between the prevailing orthodoxy in our society and those of other groups or societies. Probably the clearest example is in the matter of gender. Any society or social group which values girls less than boys, or which requires women to be subservient to men, is bound to have a different understanding of what may contribute emotional abuse of girls. 'Forced marriages' are a current example of such controversy; it is interesting that the issue merits two paragraphs in the draft government guidance on 'safeguarding children' (DfES 2005a, para. 7.100/101).

Sometimes these value clashes are seen in sharp focus through comparisons between countries. For example, my own recent experience as a supervisor of a South Korean doctoral student raised some theoretical questions about the concept of emotional abuse. It is well known that South Korean parents are amongst the most ambitious in the world for their children's educational attainment. Yet this has led to criticism by the United Nations Children's Rights Council which found that the rights of Korean children had been violated because of this excessive emphasis (as it is perceived) (Ministry of Health and Welfare 2003). To this end, many sacrifices are made by parents and children, to the point that it may be argued to result in emotional abuse. Yet these parents believe that their love for their children

Table 29.1
Numbers and percentages of children suffering from abuse and neglect in England, 2000–2004[1]

Categories of abuse	Numbers					Percentages				
	2000	**2001**	**2002**	**2003**	**2004**	**2000**	**2001**	**2002**	**2003**	**2004**
Neglect	12900	12400	10800	11700	12600	44	46	39	39	41
Physical abuse[2]	9500	8000	5300	5700	5700	32	30	19	19	19
Sexual abuse[2]	5100	4300	2800	3000	2800	17	16	10	10	9
Emotional abuse[2]	4800	4600	4700	5400	5600	17	17	17	18	18
Categories not recommended by *Working Together*[3]	310	420	–	–	–	1	2	–	–	–
No category available (transfer pending conferencing)[3]	320	180	–	–	–	1	1	–	–	–
Mixed/not recommended by *Working Together*[4]	–	–	4100	4400	4300	–	–	15	15	14

[1] Where a child was registered more than once in the year, each registration has been counted. Registrations include unborn children.
[2] These three main categories also featured in the 'mixed' categories from 1998 to 2001 only. This table incorporates these 'mixed' categories with the main categories in order to show the total number of children for whom each category of abuse was cited on the register. The total of the percentages will exceed 100 for these years because the children in the 'mixed' categories are counted more than once.
[3] These categories were discontinued from 1 April 2001.
[4] This category was introduced from 1 April 2001.
(Reproduced with permission from DfES 2005)

requires them to bring the maximum pressure to bear on them about their education. Furthermore, they may not accept that such pressure causes 'significant harm' to a child's development. Rather, they see educational achievement as a passport to success and a good life; the stresses of study are a price worth paying (Yang 2005).

Putting this example in such bald terms and without illustration, it is easy to see the parallels with our own contemporary society. Indeed, there is concern within the UK about the strains placed increasingly on children by our own educational system. Thus, the debate turns on matters of degree, not on absolute difference in values. However, it is crucially affected by the frames of reference used to understand child development; for example, the effect on children of reward or punishment, of praise or criticism. Behind those lie fundamental questions about the goals of socialisation, in which education plays such a vital part. In particular, the extent to which conformity, with its associated repression of argument, is a goal has a crucial bearing on the ways in which adults interact with children.

In short, the generally accepted maxim that child abuse is a socially constructed concept raises particularly contentious questions in relation to emotional abuse. We enter the debate about cultural relativity and the extent to which we modify our definitions in relation to a given society or social group. Difficulties arise across all aspects of child abuse but the starker aspects of it, such as physical or sexual harm, do not usually pose the same dilemmas in making moral judgements (although there may be dreadful professional dilemmas) as those when the primary concern is that of emotional abuse. It is easier to 'come off the fence' of cultural relativity when children are physically damaged.

The increased emphasis on neglect raises issues similar to those of emotional abuse regarding the underpinning assumptions about the conditions necessary for healthy development and, in particular, the effects of 'omission' of care. Perversely, the focus of British social services has been on the grosser forms of neglect, especially physical, on which there are fewer grounds for dispute. The vast majority of cases registered as 'neglect' under child protection procedures display a range of parental behaviours and serious ill-effects on children which would be recognised across cultures as unquestionably harmful. However, when 'neglect' is considered at the less serious end of a continuum, more controversy may arise. Examples include leaving children alone or in the care of young teenagers (Thoburn *et al.* 2000a; see also Korbin, Chapter 7).

Thus it can be seen that a major challenge for workers in child protection today lies in the understanding and definition of some aspects of child abuse. Its cultural and social implications are matters to which I shall return later.

A second challenge for today's workers is a result of the widening expectations of their responsibilities to safeguard children and young people. Although in theory, all children and young people were to be offered protection where appropriate, in practice there have been strange blind spots so that certain groups were largely invisible to the eyes of the relevant authorities. In the 1970s and 1980s, before the period we are considering, a significant number of children and young people in residential care (public and voluntary) were subjected to appalling abuse (see Butler, Chapter 10). Systems which were developed quickly in order to protect children in their own homes were not adequately applied to the most vulnerable. The inquiries in the 1990s exposed this and shone a light into some very dark places (Utting *et al.* 1997). There are also a number of similar 'black holes' that have taken longer to recognise, illustrated by the following four examples:

1. The area of private fostering is generally conceded to have been a grossly neglected area of policy, in which the legal framework has proved quite inadequate to protect children. The latest legislation (Children Act 2004) should begin to rectify this.
2. We have been slow to include child prostitutes within the category of 'the sexually abused'. (Does this say something about confused moral judgements?)
3. Another example, well illustrated by Kitson and Clawson (Chapter 9), concerns disabled children. The authors show what a long road we have to travel in affording adequate protection to such children. Their reference to residential schools is of particular concern.
4. Lastly, and most recently, concerns are mounting about some migrant children, unaccompanied or 'trafficked', and about the position of some children in families housed in detention centres. Phillips (Chapter 8) stresses this last point in her *Key Points and Messages for Practice*, pointing to the dangers of a preoccupation with gatekeeping resources and establishing legal entitlement.

Thus, there is a need for constant vigilance as social changes alter the pattern of relationships between adults and children and the circumstances of particular groups.

Summary

Those who seek to safeguard children are faced with the need constantly to review their responsibilities, both in terms of the types of abuse to which children and young people are subjected and the settings or situations in which it may occur. This onerous duty is made more complex by the shift of emphasis in government policy, which has placed 'protection' within an overall context of 'safeguarding'.

Coming to terms with cultural implications of child protection in the UK

Cultural conflict and tension in relation to the upbringing of children arise not only from ethnic or religious diversity, but also from social class variations, although in recent years this has not been the focus of much debate in professional circles. It seems likely that, in the next few decades, the extent and diversity of ethnic and religious groups within the UK population will raise serious and urgent matters related to family values, concerning the upbringing of children, when these appear to conflict with the majority view of the general population. Unfortunately, the sensitivity of these issues may be heightened by the increased social unease about relations between different religious and ethnic groups. Phillips (Chapter 8) points out the dangers for practitioners in accepting or perpetuating cultural 'myths' (or stereotypes) as a basis for assessment. She stresses the importance of basing child protection work on well-founded evidence on the effect of certain patterns of child rearing. Yet it has to be said that we are a long way from having a solid body of knowledge about these matters (see Korbin, Chapter 7).

It is my contention that many workers and teachers in child welfare have turned away from the responsibility to achieve what has been described as 'cultural competence'. Korbin (Chapter 7) discusses this. The case has been well argued by Korbin and Spilsbury (1999) in *Cultural Competence and Child Neglect*. They argue that 'the foundation of cultural competence ... is the development of skills and knowledge that allow one to take multiple perspectives' (p. 69) and that 'cultural competence avoids both unmoderated ethnocentrism and unmoderated relativism' (p. 71). Such statements, however valuable, leave safeguarding agencies in the UK in the twenty-first century with a huge task.

Indeed, as I have argued elsewhere, there is a kind of inverted racism in the extreme reluctance to examine the matter of cultural variations, presumably because of fear of being perceived as racist (Stevenson 1998a). It can be argued that the 'anti-oppression' era of social work in the 1980s suppressed this debate. Yet it is of the utmost importance to build reasonably strong foundations of cultural knowledge upon which to build practice. It involves workers in a scrutiny of their own assumptions as to what is good, bad or unimportant in child rearing and putting them to the test of available evidence. Although evidence, rather than preconceptions, is essential, so are values, drawn from basic philosophical or religious tenets, which underlie some of the agonising decisions that workers have to make.

Of particular difficulty are those situations when there appears to be a basic difference in the ways that boys and girls are valued and how girls are expected to behave. A worker involved in a situation like this will be well aware that the actions taken by authority may have grave consequences for the long-term relationships of a girl within her own family. Recent reports in the press that the government is considering whether new legislation on 'forced marriages' is necessary pinpoint this kind of dilemma.

There has been an understandable reluctance to place too much emphasis on aspects of maltreatment which shock many of our citizens and which may cause antagonism and racist responses, inflaming already difficult situations. When the Victoria Climbié report was published (Laming Report 2003), concerns were expressed that so little attention had been paid to the role of a particular church in that tragedy and its influence in suggesting that Victoria was demonically possessed. Four years later we read more in the media of concern about that phenomenon and about missing African children. Police have spoken on these matters but there has been little comment from the social services. Another issue which has been recently raised more starkly is that of female genital mutilation. The latest 'Safeguarding' draft* states: 'Female genital mutilation is much more common than most people realise, both worldwide and in the UK. ... There are substantial populations where female genital mutilation is endemic in London, Liverpool, Birmingham, Sheffield and Cardiff, but it is likely that communities in which female genital mutilation is practised reside throughout the UK' (DfES 2005a, p. 154, para. 7.96).

These two examples – the idea of demonic possession in children and of female genital mutilation – will be morally abhorrent to the vast majority of professionals in child welfare and to our ethnic minorities. They cannot be sidestepped although they pose exceedingly difficult problems in terms of action and intervention. Such stark issues, however, should not dominate debate. They form only a very small part of the careful, sensitive work needed to understand better the values and assumptions underlying parenting behaviours which do not carry such dramatic overtones. The task – and it is an onerous one – is twofold. First, we must learn as much as possible about the beliefs and values which underpin child care in particular ethnic groups, some of which should change and inform our own assumptions; secondly, we must face with honesty and openness whether those beliefs and values differ so much from those of the prevailing majority that they cannot be accepted. This requires a readiness to examine our own preconceptions, both personal and cultural. Nor can we approach these issues from an assumption of an established consensus within traditional British society and set this against a range of ethnic variations. On the contrary, one can see some deep tensions in contemporary society, often expressed in political arguments about 'the best ways' of correcting delinquent young people. Arguments about corporal punishment have revealed how uncertain we are.

The new Local Safeguarding Children Boards will have to translate the general imperative for 'cultural competence' into strategies and policies which foster better understanding of the different approaches to child rearing and identify those issues which may have implications for children's well-being. This requires a degree of openness and humility about some established and 'taken for granted' practices in the majority population as well as genuine 'cultural curiosity'. As a first step, local surveys to determine the nature and extent of the diversity may well be required.

Summary

The reality of our large and growing cultural diversity demands that all professionals in child welfare make a substantial effort to inform themselves about parenting

---

*A number of parts of the 2005 draft have been omitted from the final version in favour of references to specific documents such as those on *Forced Marriage* and *Female Genital Mutilation*, which are now referred to in detail in the Annotated Further Reading to Chapter 11 by Professor C M Lyon.

practices and child rearing in different groups. This must go alongside work to combat racism, both institutional and personal – the latter being often oblique rather than overt. When we are better informed, judgements have to be made concerning particular practices and behaviours based on explicit values and the best available evidence of children's needs for healthy development.

The widening of professional and community involvement in protecting children from maltreatment

Earlier in this chapter, reference was made to the need to place protection against maltreatment within a wider context of safeguarding and supporting children. To see child welfare as a continuum from provision for universal need via preventative services to protection from abuse is clearly desirable. For example, Lord Laming pointed to the perverse consequences of the (then) current system whereby social services used 'registration' as a decision which could unlock resources (Laming Report 2003). However, it is not yet obvious how the wide range of agencies involved in child welfare generally will define and develop their role in relation specifically to child abuse (see Parton, Chapter 1, and Luckock, Chapter 14).

Recent years have seen a significant enlargement of the circle of those who are expected to play a part in protecting children and young people from maltreatment. Within some of the broad groupings are large and diverse populations and organisations; for example, 'sport, culture and leisure organisations' and 'the voluntary and private sectors'. Some of these categories have come to public attention because of scandals. For example, certain cases concerning the relationship of young people to their sports instructors or coaches have drawn attention to their vulnerability to maltreatment. It is likely that the stimulation given to sports activities by the successful Olympic bid will result in increased anxiety about risk in that area, some increase in investigations and more criminal prosecutions. Religious organisations, such as the Catholic and Anglican churches, have been active in recent years in developing child protection procedures; this has been given powerful impetus by the disturbing examples of widespread sexual and physical abuse found in such settings. It is therefore somewhat surprising that there is no specific reference to religious organisations in the list given in the draft guidance (DfES 2005a) of those who should be involved. (The paragraphs on 'the voluntary and private sectors make no reference to religious bodies.) It seems likely that these issues will arise, uncomfortably, in relation to some religious groups and may in some cases be related to basic assumptions in certain religious communities, such as those of 'demonic possession' referred to earlier.

It is also important to note that 'child care services', both statutory and private, which have long formed a core part of the protective network, have expanded exponentially in the wake of government support for a range of day care facilities from nurseries to child minders. This has already led to some unease, seen in changes in the Office for Standards in Education (OFSTED) regulations policy to include unannounced inspections.

Agencies which have long been identified as critical in the protection of children are also subject to new scrutiny, as we become aware of specific issues affecting their performance. As Taylor and Corlett (Chapter 16) point out, the range of health professionals who have a role at least in raising awareness of risk is extensive. This will be of increasing importance in relation to growing numbers of children where the concerns are focused upon neglect. Thus, for example, the observations of midwives can be of critical importance when involved in the birth of a child where families are neglectful. I have commented elsewhere (Stevenson 2005b) that there are major problems of communication *between* health professionals in such families, especially when there are large numbers of children.

A further example of new challenges in agencies accepted from many years as critical to child protection lies in the educational sphere (see Baginsky and Green, Chapter 17). As schools have established their independence from local education authorities, their involvement in routine child protection activities (e.g. case conferences) has become more problematic. Current policies to maximise the number of disabled children attending mainstream schools may bring with them some dangers that their vulnerability to abuse may be overlooked.

The growing expectation that such a wide range of agencies, with diverse personnel, should take responsibility for protecting children has, of course, resulted in a huge increase in the number of individuals whose criminal records are checked before they are allowed to enter occupations in which contact with children is required. There are also centrally held lists of individuals who are thought to pose a risk to children, including those who have no criminal record. The recent political tension and media excitement concerning the decision not to put a teacher on 'List 99' held by the DfES who had been cautioned over a sexual offence illustrates one aspect of this issue.

These matters are part of a wider trend in our society in which the avoidance of risk has assumed greater significance. 'Risk assessments' are now required procedures in many different situations, of which child maltreatment is only one, albeit an important one. There is a considerable degree of social tension and ambivalence about the detailed operation of these policies and procedures in practice. This can arise when a particular situation is felt to be 'heavy handed'; the required behaviour can seem to create a different kind of problem, even if it is designed simply to protect the individual (be it a child or adult). Relevant examples are when a foster child is not allowed 'sleepovers' at a friend's house without police checks of the family concerned, or when the reading of bedtime stories in the bedroom by the foster father is thought to be too 'risky' lest sexual allegations are made by children damaged by past experience. Behind this, of course, lies the fear of those responsible that they would be held accountable 'if something happened'.

On the other hand, amongst experienced professionals (see Calder, Chapter 28), there has been much anxiety that, despite broader social trends which emphasise 'risk assessment', the concept has been played down in some recent government publications concerning child welfare, notably in *Working Together to Safeguard Children* (DoH *et al.* 1999).

It is not yet clear whether those who are now being drawn into the network will find themselves under similar constraints as those described in the fostering situations (which do raise some specific and special concerns). What, for example, are sports instructors or the clergy being told they can or cannot do when they engage with children or young people? The sadness of this phase in our society's reaction to children's maltreatment is that there is a sense of a grievous betrayal of children's trust in adults. We now know much more about the extent of abuse to which generations of children have been subjected and about the sickening ways some adults behave. We should not be surprised that, in a surge of reaction against this, policies are framed in order to protect vulnerable children better. But, as Lyth (1988) argued, the classic institutional response to anxiety about risk is to attempt to proceduralise behaviour along fairly rigid lines. To an extent, this is necessary. The question is – when does it become disproportionate and so create a different kind of problem, possibly even become abusive. These are matters too far reaching to be developed here. They bear on the crucial issue of social trust between those who serve and those who are served, which O'Neill explored in the BBC Reith lectures (O'Neill 2002).

Closer to our topic, however, are key questions of professional competence in the assessment of people, not simply of 'risk'. The making of judgements about people's reliability, as well as the formulation of policies, lie at the heart of effective child protection. The implications of widening the network of those supposed to keep children safe are far reaching and extremely complex. Of course, the occupations and organisations involved vary greatly in the extent and nature of their involvement. For many, the raising of awareness of the problem and understanding of where to go with their worries is enough. That being said, thousands across the country need such information and advice and the process is ongoing as staff come and go in various occupations. (A recent example, shown on television, was of 'dinner ladies' in a particular school who were the subject of an NSPCC project to include them in the protective network.)

Summary

The last decade has seen a significant increase in the number of agencies and professionals expected to participate in the protection of children from maltreatment and in the roles they are expected to play in the process. The implications of this are both far reaching and profound, above all because of the expectations that they will 'work together' to these ends, an issue to which I now turn.

Working together: inter-agency and inter-professional activity

Since the report of the Maria Colwell Inquiry in 1974 (DHSS 1974b), successive governments have placed great emphasis on the importance of communication and cooperation between agencies and individuals in the protection of children. In fact, the issue was raised well before the Maria Colwell Inquiry, although it was given greater impetus thereafter (see Home Office 1950). Thus, recent developments and trends can be seen as part of an ongoing process in which central government has sought to achieve more effective 'working together' at local levels.

Luckock (Chapter 14) has comprehensively explored the current position and the changes now being implemented. In essence, they represent a huge effort by the present government to improve structures and systems for the safeguarding of children. There are five key factors in this:

- to put in place a database on which causes of concern about children are noted and made available to the range of professionals who work for them
- to rationalise the processes of assessment so that they do not duplicate or overlap
- to ensure that there are 'lead professionals' to oversee processes of assessment and intervention
- to ensure greater agency accountability by the creation of new coordinating structures – Local Safeguarding Children Boards (LSCBs)
- to create structures designed to facilitate integrated services, Children's Trusts and Children's Centres being two examples at different levels of organisation.

Much effort has already been devoted at local level to developing these arrangements, some of which involve sophisticated information technology. In particular, the Children Act 2004 authorises the setting up of a database, known as information sharing and assessment (ISA). It is intended that about eleven million children in England and Wales will be entered on this database, and 'a flag of concern' (not just about abuse) will note potential or actual problems. The resource implications in terms of staff time and equipment are great. Munro (2005c) has argued trenchantly that this emphasis is misplaced. She suggests that the primary thrust should have been in finding the way to help professionals with their main problems in sharing information – 'in collecting information … in understanding what it means … and in communicating it effectively to other professionals' (p. 375). She claims that the concentration on the database will do little to help professionals and that, indeed 'it may do more harm than good' (p. 375). She argues, *inter alia*, that the proliferation of data in all aspects of children's health and development may actually obscure the victims of abuse.

It was predictable that administrative and professional energy would be heavily invested in the myriad details such changes require. It is too early to see whether the new arrangements will stand up when exposed to the rough and tumble of practice. However, whatever their merits, it remains a source of great concern that so little emphasis has been placed on the need to understand better the underlying dynamics, especially those at an interpersonal level, which so often impede or distort the quality of working relationships. Luckock (Chapter 14) argues that policy makers have neglected 'the psychosocial research literature on the dynamics of intervention and decision making in child protection'. There are various dimensions of these theoretical perspectives. Some relate to role; how professionals perceive and understand their own role, and those of others, affects critically their interaction with others (Stevenson O 1999). Some relate to the psychodynamic forces which lie beneath professional interaction (Cooper 2005a, Rustin 2005). Over some years the work of Reder and colleagues (Reder *et al.* 1993, Reder & Duncan 1999, 2004b) has been much appreciated by practitioners. They have also explored psychodynamic and social psychological factors in professional reactions to child abuse.

The work referred to above is rooted in evidence, especially from a wide range of inquiries into the deaths of children. Experienced practitioners recognise its salience and readily accept this approach as throwing light on the subtler aspects of 'working together'. Of particular importance are the difficulties that have arisen in achieving satisfactory 'working together' between certain key adult and children's services. This has been acknowledged by government in cautious words in the draft guidance:

> The Local Safeguarding Children Boards (LSCB) should make appropriate arrangements to involve … some organisations or individuals which are in theory represented by statutory board partners but in which need extra effort to engage them (drug and alcohol abuse are given as examples).
>
> (DfES 2005a, paras 5.18 and 5.20)

There is substantial research evidence (see Stevenson 2005c) which suggests that the reasons for this lie in part in the workers' identification with particular clients within a family, which develops as a result of the ascribed role but which also may reflect the emotions of the professionals. These problems may be compounded by reference to the issue of confidentiality. Whatever the underlying explanations, there is no doubt that there have been major barriers to, and failures in, communication and cooperation for the protection of children between these services.

Where are we now? Themes and future directions   543

It is unfortunate that there has been relatively little recognition of the importance of these elements in inter-professional work in official guidance. They have important implications for the supervision of workers and for the development of education and training. Changes in systems and structures, however desirable, will not alone achieve the desired improvements unless the interpersonal factors are given adequate attention. Furthermore, the problems arising from frequent changes in personnel complicate these processes.

The new LSCBs, which replace the Area Child Protection Committees (ACPCs), are pivotal if the widening and strengthening of the network is to become an effective reality and not a kind of bureaucratic fantasy – which would be most dangerous. There are formidable implications for LSCBs in this drive to increase the number and range of those who have defined roles in relation to the prevention of abuse, and to improve the understanding of its importance amongst others who have been reluctant to 'work together'. It is disappointing that the very considerable resource implications are not identified with any precision in the draft guidance (DfES 2005a), in which no specific financial requirements are placed on the constituent agencies of the LSCBs or on the various agencies included in the networks. In the past, the constituent agencies of the ACPCs have varied greatly between one locality and another in the resources made available for this work. So far, there is no indication that this will become more standardised.

LSCBs will have to develop plans to meet the challenge to widen and to consolidate the protective network. Some of these plans concern general strategies for inclusion which are proactive – 'reaching out' to many agencies and individuals hitherto little involved in the work. One of its most crucial functions will be in the development and oversight of programmes of training and staff development. Some ACPCs have laid good foundations for future work; for example, in the development of models in which likely numbers, timescales and different levels required have been formulated. These will require constant revision. To base these soundly, the LSCBs will need to keep abreast of relevant developments in research, social trends and policy. They will need to ensure that agencies develop 'in-house' training at basic level and audit the process. A second role is to provide direct multidisciplinary training for many who need to learn together. All this represents a huge task. At local level, thousands of people each year will potentially be involved in various forms of training to raise awareness, taking account of staff mobility and new knowledge. Many hundreds will need more detailed help.

Summary

We do not know whether the radical changes proposed by government in the working together arrangements will work out as planned and whether there will be unintended negative consequences. The new LSCBs will have a pivotal role in carrying out the changes. It is to be hoped that they will be innovative in pursuing the subtle, but crucial, aspects of communication and cooperation upon which effective working together at practitioner level is founded.

Managing the tensions between political and professional worlds

The years since the death of Maria Colwell in 1973 have been marked by increasing control and scrutiny by central government of those considered crucial to the protection of children from harm. These trends are seen in legislation concerning children's welfare (Children Act 1975, 1989, 2004), in more specific guidance – above all, in succeeding versions of *Working Together* (e.g. DHSS 1974a, DoH 1988b, Home Office *et al.* 1991, DoH *et al.* 1999, HM Government 2006a) – and in inspections, which became more precise and rigorous during this period. In common with many other areas of public welfare, we have seen the emergence of 'targets' and 'goals' as key elements in the management of social services. All this, together with an insistence on evidence-based research and on evidence of outcomes in evaluation have created new forms of stress for workers and what may be described as 'anxious environments' in which practice takes place. In relation to the safeguarding children agenda, although social workers are central, there are also certain key workers in other services who are increasingly aware of this scrutiny – notably police, paediatricians and health visitors, especially those who act as 'designated' officers for child protection. Such workers are subject to similar stresses in other spheres of their work.

It seems clear that action of this kind was required to raise standards and to ensure greater equity of provision across the country. The depressing, repetitive findings of dozens of inquiries into the deaths of children between that of Maria Colwell in 1974 (DHSS 1974a) and of Victoria Climbié in 2003 (Laming Report 2003) showed beyond doubt that, in too many instances, standards of practice within and between agencies were unacceptable. Furthermore, the general criteria used and the targets set for the development of good practice were in general sound and not incompatible with professional values of good practice (Stevenson 2003). Yet the widening and tightening of government control has had certain worrying effects.

The overall impact of repeated inquiries and repeated policy directives, often requiring substantial effort and resources to implement, has created a deep fatigue in many workers, often summed up by references to 'more forms and paperwork'. Furthermore, this fatigue results not only from the amount of work required, but also from the nature of activity required. There is a strong, if somewhat imprecise, feeling amongst many workers that these requirements are too mechanical and procedurally driven and that this will result in the essence of good practice being lost. This is particularly evident in responses to the guidance designed to improve the assessment of child and family (DoH *et al.* 2000). The initial 'assessment framework' was generally welcomed by social workers but the subsequent advice, examples and timescales gave rise to anger and dismay amongst practitioners (see Calder, Chapter 28). There was also considerable resentment that its launch did not involve the many professionals and agencies outside social services, whose expertise was crucial to effective assessment.

Furthermore, there is the well-known phenomenon of perverse incentives to good practice, arising as the 'unintended consequences' of certain requirements. Of particular relevance to this discussion are issues surrounding the performance assessment framework and the child protection register (although the register itself is now being reconsidered). For example, one important measure of good performance for some social services departments is a reduction in numbers on the register and of re-registrations over a given period. These are not in themselves undesirable but workers worry whether they may be pressurised to take decisions to achieve policy objectives rather than on the merits of particular circumstances in each case. This is especially pertinent to cases of long-term neglect in which children may be at risk of significant harm but in which there are no immediate precipitating events.

Overall, the effect of scrutiny and control within social services can lead to serious tensions between the managerial layers of the hierarchy and the workers at field level. Team leaders and middle managers, in particular, maybe trapped between the organisational goals set by senior managers in response to government requirements and the responses and attitudes of field workers to them. Calder (Chapter 28) comments in detail on these issues.

In any case, government policy does not evolve systematically. The proliferation of different initiatives which bear on the development of better safeguarding arrangements have complex consequences which may not always be foreseen. One major example in recent years has been the emergence of the Sure Start programmes and their location outside the mainstream social services departments not usually staffed by social workers. These important programmes (which are now intended to be universal but which initially focused on the support of the more vulnerable children and families) must be adequately connected to those social services which have responsibility for the most worrying cases. The ideal of a continuum of services from 'children in need' to 'children in need of protection' cannot be translated into effective reality without close connections between the agencies at field level. Sure Start is only one of a range of initiatives which have implications for direct services to families whose children are at risk from significant harm.

There is also the problem of change, uncertainty or inconsistency, which may be perceived in government policy as it emerges. This is obvious at times of political change. Thus, initiatives such as Sure Start were launched after 1997 when the new government in power was willing to intervene in family problems at an earlier stage. There were ideological differences at the root of that shift in emphasis. However, policy shifts are often more subtle than that and may occur within the framework of the political party in power. This is seen most clearly in the discourse surrounding juvenile crime and delinquency and the emergence of new forms of correction or punishment, such as Anti-Social Behaviour Orders. Because new structures (Youth Justice Boards) and new roles have been created for workers in relation to delinquency, child protection workers are not formally involved in the care and supervision of such offenders. But labels and boxes disguise the reality – that there are many children and young people who are both delinquent and abused or neglected in a range of ways. Workers involved in such families cannot be unaffected by the roles ascribed to them by government. This issue was (crudely) described in the 1970s as the difference between 'the depraved and the deprived'. The terms may change but the underlying tension is unresolved; furthermore, views of 'the causes of crime' have a powerful effect on the choice of intervention. We do not know how far social workers in child protection are consciously aware, or affected by, these underlying conflicts or inconsistencies. For example, how do they view their colleagues in the Youth Justice Boards when both are involved in certain families? Is there agreement or conflict about objectives and methods of working? Is there any consensus, in practice, to disregard or circumvent some of the punitive views and measures emerging from central government?

Summary

I have argued that, because of the degree of central government control over child protection services, there are considerable tensions and difficulties between government and the relevant professions. This is particularly so for social workers. This is not to deny that there was a strong case for better leadership from government. However, the ways in which this control has been exercised have led to a pervasive sense of anxiety, discomfort and fatigue, especially amongst field workers.

Critical issues for the improvement of practice

This section focuses on two aspects of practice which may at first sight appear to be particularly relevant to social workers. However, in my opinion, improvements in these matters are crucial to overall standards of 'working together'. They are the necessary foundations on which to build inter-professional work.

The first concerns assessment, a topic which consumes a great deal of energy and time – perhaps disproportionately so – for reasons explored in this volume by Horwath (Chapter 13) and Calder (Chapter 28).

It is my opinion that the considerable value of the basic assessment framework (see Fig. 3.4, p. 62) has been undermined by a failure to relate it adequately to the theories on which it is based. It is unclear whether this springs from government concern to be seen as neutral in theoretical areas that may seem contentious (albeit that much of this theory is now well founded). Although there may be an implicit assumption that the theoretical base for the framework is the business of the educators, it is doubtful whether educational programmes have systematically addressed theoretical issues in such a way as to illuminate guidance on assessment. The effect has been to weaken the credibility of the analysis – the underlying meaning and significance of the detailed information gathered is not adequately conceptualised. Often, there is too much undigested description.

There is no simple way to correct this. It has to be a part of a wider programme to raise the quality of education and supervision. This is not achieved by a breathless tour round a variety of theories. Rather, it is about drawing attention to the significance of certain theories to specific aspects of the process. A topical example is that of attachment theory, on which there is substantial literature (e.g. Howe 2005). This important knowledge may, however, be used loosely and uncritically by social workers. In cases of neglect, for example, there are sometimes complex patterns of distorted attachment that are not adequately described by statements such as 'she is very attached to her children'. In working with other professionals, social workers need to understand something about the theoretical perspectives of their colleagues and have some ability to draw various theories together to form a picture of the family functioning.

A further crucial issue for effective assessment relates to the roles and skills involved in the process. Local authority social workers often voice anger and disappointment that their contribution to the process is not sufficiently valued, especially in the courts. In the courts, children's guardians (see Head, Chapter 19), themselves social workers, and others, 'the experts', such as psychologists, are seen to hold the status and the influence. These issues need to be addressed in different ways, including more respect from members of the legal profession, including lawyers in local authority practice (Dickens 2005), for the social worker's contribution. However, the recognition which social workers understandably crave must be won in part by improvement in their own competence and presentation. Social workers have different roles in relation to the assessment process. They must draw together the information and evidence from a variety of sources. Some of this is from other official and professional sources; it is important to know at local level the skills and interests which particular professionals have, as well as a good working knowledge of their roles in general. A major source of information is, of course, from the family and this requires different skills and techniques. A first principle of this is to recognise that assessment is not a neutral, detached process. It is interactive and the feelings aroused on both sides in those interviews are often intense.

Future relationships with social services will be much affected by these initial relationships.

There are two specific areas in which social work expertise in assessment is critical. The first concerns the bottom line of the 'assessment triangle', which focuses on material, environmental and extended family matters (see Fig. 13.1). No other contributors to the assessment process will put this crucial information into the process – it is integral to the social work task. The second concerns the feelings and perception of the children. Social workers have been much criticised for failure to communicate effectively with the children they are required to safeguard. Yet, as remarked earlier, they also feel strongly that their skills are often disregarded, when 'experts' are called in to assess children coming before the courts (sometimes very briefly and outside the home). Whilst this may be necessary for the assessment of particular aspects of a child's functioning, social workers who have visited the home a number of times, made appropriate observations and established good communication with children, have a key role in evaluating the child's development in relation to the risks of 'significant harm'. Unfortunately, it seems that the quality of such work has been very variable.

In short, social workers must work to establish their credibility but the attitudes of other professionals towards them, especially in the judicial system, is also critical. Greater confidence and clarity about the theoretical basis for their judgements is important but it needs to run parallel with work at managerial levels to increase understanding of their proper role.

Throughout the process of the work in this field, there are crucial issues for social workers in child protection concerning the nature of their relationship with children's caregivers. At the assessment stage, progress in completing this task is critically affected by the willingness or unwillingness of the adults to cooperate. This is particularly difficult – and vital – in cases of neglect, where fundamental non-compliance may be overt or covert and may thus impede decisions regarding the future of these children (see Horwath, Chapter 13).

It is sometimes suggested that the local authority workers who have carried out the assessment process, inevitably painful for parents, cannot hope to forge a positive relationship with those they have assessed and, by definition, 'found wanting' in some aspects of their parental capabilities (see Petrie, Chapter 21). If parents are effectively under supervision or being monitored in order to protect the children, can the worker responsible gain the trust of parents so that they believe that the worker cares for them as well? Should not the functions of 'care and control', as it has long been described, be split between workers and perhaps agencies (e.g. between the local authority and the voluntary sector)?

The issue has been painfully illustrated by inquiries into the deaths of children in which social workers have been accused of naivety or gullibility and/or of fear of parents (e.g. Jasmine Beckford, London Borough of Brent 1985). There are also difficulties when workers become over-identified with needy parents so that they lose sight of the primary duty to protect the child (e.g. Lucie Gates, London Borough of Bexley 1982). Such cases are most likely when a parent (or parents) has learning disabilities and in which neglect is the primary cause of concern. Certainly, managing the tension and the ambivalence which the role creates requires a high level of professional awareness.

However, to assume that a division between workers is often necessary or helpful for effective protection of the child is unsound and may be dangerous. There need to be judgements made about particular cases that examine the extent to which parents have acknowledged some deficits in their own parenting about which they are willing to work in partnership with professionals. Farmer and Owen

(1995) discuss the complex factors at play in such cases. The skilful and self-aware professional can manage the 'care and control' balance, provided they are adequately supported and supervised, especially when the parent in question is vulnerable and dependent. However, there are cases in which there is no genuine acceptance by parents of the need to change and the implications of this for constructive work have not been faced. It may sometimes be that, despite this lack of compliance, evidence sufficient to take the child to court is missing. Alternatively, the problem may arise from undue caution or confusion in the minds of workers, or the negative impact of changes in parental circumstances, such as a new partner, may not be taken on board by the workers.

On occasion, there will be the need for fairly heavy 'surveillance', in which a range of workers from different disciplines is necessary to keep children safe. The social worker alone is neither fitted nor competent in their role to do this alone. Indeed, examination of some cases after tragedies has shown that there had been a progressive 'shut down' by parents on visiting professionals. In such cases, earlier involvement of police, under their powers to gain entrance at a stage when anxiety mounts, may sometimes be essential. In this sense, social workers have a key 'warning' role, but one in which a range of others, perhaps especially the police, must provide a network of safety for the children.

Thus, effective working with parents in these circumstances is critically dependent on the judgements made at the beginning, and throughout the process, about the genuineness of parental participation and their capacity to change. This is highly skilled, difficult work and requires effective supervision and consultation of a higher quality than is usually available at present. It may also be that, on occasion, 'two heads are better than one' in appraising the situation at particular times. Furthermore, one must be alert to the dangers of working on false premises, assuming a degree of compliance where it does not exist.

The forging of a meaningful relationship with a parent must rest on the capacity of the worker to understand and to work with the negative as well as the positive feelings that are aroused in such a process (see Petrie, Chapter 21). To be afraid of failing as a parent is a most distressing experience, and a flight from thinking about that possibility may lead to all manner of psychic defences, played out with the worker involved. These have to be held within the relationship.

Summary

This section has addressed specific aspects of current practice which are pivotal to more effective intervention. Although the focus has been primarily on social workers, whose role in child protection remains crucial, there are significant implications for other professionals; for example, in the development of adequately grounded assessment and in the appreciation of the intense and conflicting emotions aroused at every stage in the work with families.

Conclusion

This chapter has sought to show some of the ways in which the task of protecting children has changed and become more complex in recent years. The push and pull of diverse social trends and political influences, discussed here, reminds us that the concept of child maltreatment as socially constructed must be at the core of our understanding. At various times, there are major shifts in the way the issue is perceived and it may be that time will show that in the last decade such a shift was, in fact, taking place. We are not yet in a position to make such a judgement, but the debate, national and international, about Human Rights and, within that, children's rights, has introduced powerful new elements into the way the safeguarding and protection of children is viewed. It is perhaps significant that the year 2000 saw a special issue on children's rights and child protection in *Child Abuse Review*. Hallett, in her editorial, and Cleave (2000) draw attention to the tensions between 'liberationist' and 'protectionist' policies regarding child protection. However this plays out, the last 5 years have seen increasing recognition of children's rights to be heard and increasing acceptance of their rights to play a part in decisions about their lives. It remains to be seen whether a theoretical emphasis on social justice and the associated concept of 'rights' results in the improvements in practice that are so urgently needed.

Further reading

Cooper A 2005 Surface and depth in the Victoria Climbié Inquiry Report. Child and Family Social Work 10(1):1–9

Dickens J 2005 Being 'the epitome of reason': the challenge for lawyers and social workers in child care proceedings. International Journal of Law, Policy and the Family 19:73–101

Home Office, Department of Health, Department of Education and Science, Welsh Office 1991 Working together under the Children Act 1989: a guide to arrangements for inter-agency cooperation for the protection of children from abuse. HMSO, London

Korbin J E, Spilsbury J 1999 Cultural competence and child neglect. In: Dubowitz H (ed) Neglected children: research, practice and policy. Sage, Newbury Park, CA, pp. 69–88

Munro E 2005 What tools do we need to improve identification of child abuse? Child Abuse Review 14:374–388

Reder P, Duncan S 2004 From Colwell to Climbié: inquiry into fatal child abuse. In: Stanley N, Manthorpe J (eds) The age of the inquiry. Brunner-Routledge, London, pp. 92–115

Stevenson O (ed) 2005 Special issue: interdisciplinary working in child welfare. Child and Family Social Work 10(3)

References

In 2005, the government issued a number of draft consultation papers on *Working Together to Safeguard Children*, through the auspices of the Department for Education and Skills and HM Government. These culminated in the publication, in April 2006, of the definitive document *Working Together to Safeguard Children* (HM Government 2006a; see also Lyon, Chapter 11, in this volume).

Abel G, Rouleau J 1990 The nature and extent of sexual assault. In: Marshall W, Laws D R, Barbaree H (eds) Handbook of sexual assault. Plenum, New York

Abel G, Becker J, Cunningham-Rathner J, Mettleman M, Rouleau J 1988 Multiple paraphilic diagnoses among sex offenders. Bulletin of the Academy of Psychiatry and the Law 16:153

Abney V 1996 Cultural competence in the field of child maltreatment. In: Briere J, Berliner L, Bulkley J, Jenny C, Reid T (eds) The APSAC handbook on child maltreatment. Sage, Thousand Oaks, CA, p 409–491

Adams N 1981 Lambeth Directorate of Social Services. London Borough of Lambeth, London

Adcock M 2001 The core assessment – how to synthesise information and make judgements. In: Horwath J (ed) The child's world: assessing children in need. Jessica Kingsley, London

Adcock M, White R (eds) 1998 Significant harm: its management and outcome. Significant Publications, London

Ahmed S, Cheetham J, Small J (eds) 1986 Social work with black children and their families. Batsford/BAAF, London

Ainsworth M D S, Blehar M C, Waters E, Wall S 1978 Patterns of attachment: a psychological study of the strange situation. Erlbaum, Hillsdale, NJ

Aldgate J 1980 Identification of factors which influence length of stay in care. In: Triseliotis J P (ed) New developments in foster care and adoption. Routledge and Kegan Paul, London

Aldgate J 1990 Foster children at school: success or failure. Adoption and Fostering 7(2):38–45

Aldgate J, Bradley M 1999 Supporting families through short-term fostering. TSO, London

Aldgate J, Simmonds J (eds) 1987 Direct work with children. Batsford, London

Aldgate J, Statham J 2001 The Children Act now: messages from research. TSO, London

Aldgate J, Tunstill J, McBeath G 1992 National monitoring of the Children Act: Part III, Section 7 – the first year. Oxford University/NCVCCO, Oxford

Aldgate J, McBeath G, Ozolins R, Tunstill J 1994 Implementing Section 17 of the Children Act – the first 18 months. Leicester University School of Social Work, Leicester

Aldridge M 1994 Making social work news. Routledge, London

Allan J 1988 Inscapes of the child's world: Jungian counselling in schools and clinics. Spring Publications, Dallas, TX

Allanson S 2002 Jeffrey the dog: a search for shared meaning. In: Cattanach A (ed) The story so far: play therapy narratives. Jessica Kingsley, London, p 59–81

Andersson G 2005 Family relations, adjustment and well-being in a longitudinal study of children in care. Child and Family Social Work 10:43–56

Appleton J V 1994 The role of the health visitor in identifying and working with vulnerable families in relation to child protection: a review of the literature. Journal of Advanced Nursing 20:167–175

APSAC (American Professional Society on the Abuse of Children) 1995 Guidelines for the psycho-social evaluation of suspected psychological maltreatment in children and adolescents. APSAC, Charleston, SC

Archard D 1993 Children: rights and childhood. Routledge, London

Archer J 2000 Sex differences in aggression between heterosexual partners: a meta-analytic review. Psychological Bulletin 126:651–680

Archer J 2002 Sex differences in physically aggressive acts between heterosexual partners: a meta-analytic review. Aggression and Violent Behavior 7:313–351

Argent H (ed) 2002 Staying connected: managing contact arrangements in adoption. BAAF, London

Armstrong H (ed) 1991, 1997 Taking care: a response to children, adults and abuse for churches and other faith communities. National Children's Bureau, London

Armstrong H 1997 Refocusing children services conferences. DoH, London

Armsworth M W 1989 Therapy of incest survivors: abuse or support? Child Abuse and Neglect 13:549–562

Arnold E, Cloke C 1988 Society keeps abuse hidden – the biggest cause of all: the case for child friendly communities. Child Abuse Review 7:302–314

Arnold R P, Rogers D, Cook D A G 1990 Medical problems of adults who were sexually abused in childhood. British Medical Journal 300:705–708

Arnstein S 1969 A ladder of citizen participation. American Institute of Planners Journal 35:216–224

Asen G E, Piper R, Stevens A 1989 A systems approach to child abuse. Child Abuse and Neglect 13:45–58

Association of Directors of Education and Children's Services, Association of Directors of Social Services, Confederation of Education and Children's Services Managers and Local Government Association 2005 Omitting schools from consultation means vulnerable children might suffer [press notice, 17 June]. Online. Available: www.adss.org.uk/pres/2005/omitting.shtml

Association of Directors of Social Services (ADSS) 1987 Child abuse: incidence of registrations for child abuse between 1985 and 1986 [press release]. Berkshire Social Services Department, Slough

Audit Commission 1994 Seen but not heard: coordinating child health and social services for children in need. Detailed evidence and guidelines for managers and practitioners. HMSO, London

Audit Commission 2002 Integrated services for older people: building a whole system approach. Audit Commission, London

Australian Institute of Health and Welfare (AIHW) 2004 Child Protection Australia 2003–04. AIHW cat. No. CWS24. AIHW (Child Welfare Series no. 36), Canberra

Axford N, Bullock R 2005 Child death and significant case reviews: international approaches. Report to the Scottish Executive. Scottish Executive Education Department, Edinburgh

Axford N, Little M 2004 Refocusing children's services towards prevention: lessons from the literature. Research Report RR 510. Darlington Social Research Unit, Darlington

Axline V 1947 Play therapy: the inner dynamics of childhood. Houghton Mifflin, Boston

Axline V 1971 Dibbs: in search of self. Penguin, Harmondsworth

Axline V 1987 Play therapy, revised edn. Ballantine Books, New York

Ayre P 1998 Significant harm: making professional judgements. Child Abuse Review 7(5):330–342

Ayre P 2001 Child protection and the media: lessons from the last three decades. British Journal of Social Work 31(6):887–891

Ayres M 1989 Sexual abuse in institutional care. Sexual Abuse Newsletter 6(1):7

Azar S T 1997 A cognitive–behavioural approach to understanding and treating parents who physically abuse their children. In: Wolfe D A, McMahon R J, Peters R D (eds) Child abuse: new directions in prevention and treatment across the lifespan. Sage, Thousand Oaks, CA

Bachmann G A, Moeller T P, Benett J 1988 Childhood sexual abuse and the consequences in adult women. Obstetrics and Gynecology 71(4):631–642

Badgley R F, Allard H A, McCormick N et al 1984 Sexual offences against children, Vol. 1. Report of the Committee on Sexual Offences Against Children and Youths. Minister of Supply and Services, Ottawa, Canada

Baginsky M 2000a Child protection and education. NSPCC, London

Baginsky M 2000b Report on the evaluation of the piloting of Child Protection in Initial Teacher Training, 1999–2000. NSPCC, London

Baginsky M 2003a Newly qualified teachers and child protection. A survey of their views, training and experiences. Child Abuse Review 12:119–127

Baginsky M 2003b Responsibility without power? LEAs and child protection. NSPCC, London

Baginsky M (forthcoming) Schools, social services and safeguarding children: past practice and future challenges. NSPCC, London

Bagley C 1992 Characteristics of 60 children with a history of sexual assault against others: evidence from a comparative study. Journal of Forensic Psychiatry 3:299–309

Bailey R, Boswell G 2002 Sexually abusive adolescent males: a literature review. De Montfort University, Leicester, Monograph 4

Bainham A 1993 Care after 1991: a reply. Journal of Child Law 99:103

Bairstow K, Hetherington R 1998 Parents' experience of child welfare interventions: an Anglo-French comparison. Children and Society 12:113–124

Baker A W, Duncan S P 1985 Child sexual abuse: a study of prevalence in Great Britain. Child Abuse and Neglect 9:453–467

Baldwin N, Spencer N 1993 Deprivation and child abuse: implications for strategic planning in children's services. Children and Society 7(4):357–375

Baldwin N, Spencer N J 2005 Economic, cultural and social contexts of neglect. In: Taylor J, Daniel B (eds) Child neglect: practice issues for health and social care. Jessica Kingsley, London

Bandura A 1973 Aggression: a social learning analysis. Prentice Hall, Englewood Cliffs, NJ

Bannister A 1989 Healing action – action methods with children who have been sexually abused. In: Wattam C, Blagg H, Hughes J A (eds) Child sexual abuse: listening, hearing and validating the experiences of childhood. Longman/NSPCC, Harlow, p 78–94

Bannister A (ed) 1998 From hearing to healing: working with the aftermath of child sexual abuse, 2nd edn. Wiley/NSPCC, Chichester

Bannon M J, Carter Y H, Barwell F, Hicks C 1999a Perceptions held by general practitioners in England regarding their training needs in child abuse and neglect. Child Abuse Review 8:276–283

Bannon M J, Carter Y H, Ross L 1999b Perceived barriers to full participation by general practitioners in the child protection process: preliminary conclusions from focus group discussions in West Midlands, UK. Journal of Interprofessional Care 13:239–248

Bannon M J, Carter Y H, Jackson N R, Pace M, Thorne W 2001 Meeting the training needs of GP registrars in child abuse and neglect. Child Abuse Review 10:254–261

Barbaree H, Marshall W, McCormick J 1998 The development of deviant sexual behaviours among adolescents and its implications for prevention and treatment. Irish Journal of Psychology 19:1–31

Barber J G, Delfabbro P H 2004 Children in foster care. Routledge, London

Barford R 1993 Childrens' views of child protection social work. University of East Anglia Monograph, Norwich

Barlow J 1999 What works in parent education programmes? In: Lloyd E (ed) Parenting matters: what works in parenting education? Barnardo's, Barkingside, Ilford

Barlow J, Stewart Brown S 2005 Individual and group-based parenting programmes for the prevention of child abuse and neglect. Wiley, London

Barn R 1990 Black children in local authority care: admission patterns. New Community 16(2):229–246

Barn R 1993 Black children in the public care system. Batsford/BAAF, London

Barn R, Sinclair R, Ferdinand D 1997 Acting on principle: an examination of race and ethnicity in social services provision for children and families. BAAF, London

Barnett D, Manly J T, Cicchetti D 1993 Defining child maltreatment: the interface between policy and research. In: Cicchetti D, Toth S (eds) Child abuse, child development, and social policy. Ablex, Norwood, NJ

Barter C 2003 Abuse of children in residential care. NSPCC Information Briefing October 2003. Online. Available: www.nspcc.org.uk/inform

Barth R, Berry M 1988 Adoption and disruption: rates, risk and responses. Aldine de Gruyter, New York

Barth R P, Courtney M, Berrick J D, Albert V 1994 From child abuse to permanency planning: child welfare services pathways and placements. Aldine de Gruyter, New York

Bartholomew K, Henderson A J Z, Dutton D G 2001 Insecure attachment and partner abuse. In: Clulow C C (ed) Attachment and couple work: applying the secure base concept in research and practice. Routledge, London

Batchelor J, Kerslake A 1990 Failure to find failure to thrive: the case for improving screening, prevention and treatment in primary care. Whiting and Birch, London

Bates P 1999 New legislation: the Youth Justice and Criminal Evidence Act – the evidence of children and vulnerable adults. Child and Family Law Quarterly 11(8):289–303

Batta I D, McCulloch J W, Smith N J 1979 Colour as a variable in Children's Sections of Local Authority Social Services Departments. New Community 7:78–84

Batty D (ed) 1991 Sexually abused children – making their placements work. BAAF, London

Batty D 2006 Paedophile monitoring systems need more resources. Guardian Unlimited 18 January

BBC 1986 Childwatch – overview of results from 2530 self-completion questionnaires. BBC Broadcasting Research, London (unpublished)

BBC 1987 Childwatch – national survey on child abuse. BBC Press Briefing, 9 July

BBC News 2004 Wider cot deaths review considered. 20 January. Online. Available: http://news.bbc.co.uk/2/hi/uk_news/3412307.stm

Bebbington A, Beecham J 2003 Children in need 2001: ethnicity and service use. University of Kent, Canterbury

Bebbington A, Miles J 1989 The background of children who enter local authority care. British Journal of Social Work 19(5):349–368

Bedingfield D 1998 The child in need: children, the state and the law. Family Law, Bristol

Beek M, Schofield G 2004 Providing a secure base in long-term foster care. BAAF, London

Bell M 1999 Child protection: families and the conference process. Ashgate, Andover

Bell M 2000a Social work responses to domestic violence within the context of child protection. In: McCluskey U, Hooper C A (eds) Psycho-dynamic perspectives on abuse: the cost of fear. Jessica Kingsley, London

Bell M 2000b Children speak out: the views of children and young people in York on their experience of a child protection investigation. University of York, York

Bell M 2002 Promoting children's rights through the use of relationship. Child and Family Social Work 7(1):1–11

Bell M 2003 Working with families where there is domestic violence. In: Bell M, Wilson K (eds) The practitioner's guide to working with families. Palgrave, London, p 188–208

Bell M 2005 Community based parenting programmes: an exploration of the interplay between environmental and organizational factors in a Webster Stratton project. British Journal of Social Work 35:1–18

Bell M, Wilson K 2006 Children's views on their participation in family group conferences. British Journal of Social Work (forthcoming[AU2])

Belsky J 1980 Child maltreatment: an ecological integration. American Psychologist 35:320–335

Belsky J, Stratton P 2002 An ecological analysis of the etiology of child maltreatment. In: Browne K, Hanks H, Stratton P, Hamilton C (eds) Early prediction and prevention of child abuse: a handbook, 2nd edn. Wiley, Chichester, ch 6

Benedict M I, Zuravin S, Brandt D, Abbey H 1994 Types and frequency of child maltreatment by family foster care providers in an urban population. Child Abuse and Neglect 18(7):577–585

Benn M 1998 Madonna and child: towards a new politics of motherhood. Jonathan Cape, London

Bennett F 2005 Promoting the health and well-being of children: evidence of need in the UK. In: Scott J, Ward H (eds) Safeguarding and promoting the well-being of children, families and communities. Jessica Kingsley, London

Bennett N, Blundell J, Malpass L, Lavender T 2001 Midwives' views on redefining midwifery 2: public health. British Journal of Midwifery 9:743–746

Bentovim A 1992 Trauma organised systems: physical and sexual abuse in families. Karnac, London

Bentovim A 1995 Trauma organised systems: physical and sexual abuse in families (revised edition). Karnac, London

Bentovim A 1998 Significant harm in context. In: Adcock M, White R (eds) Significant harm, its management and outcome. Significant Publications, Croyden

Bentovim A 2002 Preventing the victim to offender cycle: risk and protection factors, and the implication for therapeutic intervention. In: Browne K, Davies C, Stratton P (eds) Early prediction and prevention of child abuse: a handbook, 2nd edn. Wiley, Chichester, p 289–290

Bentovim A, Bingley Miller L 2001 The family assessment. Assessment of family competence, strengths and difficulties. Pavilion, Brighton

Bentovim A, Elton A, Tranter M 1987 Prognosis for rehabilitation after abuse. Adoption and Fostering 34:821–826

Bentovim A, Elton A, Hildebrand J et al (eds) 1988 Child sexual abuse within the family. Wright, London

Berger A M, Knutsen J F, Mehm J G, Perkins K A 1988 The self-report of punitive childhood experiences of young adults and adolescents. Child Abuse and Neglect 12(2):251–262

Bergner R M, Delgado L K, Graybill D 1994 Finkelhor's risk factor checklist: a cross validation study. Child Abuse and Neglect 18(4):331–340

Berkowitz L 1989 Laboratory experiments in the study of aggression. In: Archer J, Browne K (eds) Human aggression: naturalistic approaches. Routledge, London, p 42–61

Berlin L J, Ziv Y, Amaya-Jackson L, Greenberg M T 2005 Enhancing early attachments: theory, research, intervention and policy. Guilford Press, London

Berliner L 2002 The traumatic impact of abuse experiences: treatment issues. In: Browne K, Davies C, Stratton P (eds) Early prediction and prevention of child abuse: a handbook, 2nd edn. Wiley, Chichester

Berridge D 1996 Foster care – a research review. HMSO, London

Berridge D, Brodie I 1996 Residential child care in England and Wales – the inquiries and after. In: Hill M, Aldgate J (eds) Child welfare services – developments in law, policy, practice and research. Jessica Kingsley, London

Berridge D, Brodie I 1998 Children's homes revisited. In: DOH Caring for children away from home: messages from research. Wiley, Chichester

Berridge D, Cleaver H 1987 Foster home breakdown. Basil Blackwell, Oxford

Bettelheim B 1976 The uses of enchantment: the meaning and importance of fairy tales. Thames and Hudson, London

Bibby P C 1996a Organised abuse: the current debate. Arena, Aldershot

Bibby P C (ed) 1996b Definitions and recent history. In: Organised abuse – the current debate. Arena, Aldershot

Bichard Inquiry Report 2004 A public inquiry report on child protection procedures in Humberside Police and Cambridge Constabulary, particularly the effectiveness of relevant intelligence-based recording, vetting practices since 1995 and information sharing with other agencies. HC 653. TSO, London. Online. Available: www.bichardinquiry.org.uk

Biehal N, Clayden J, Stein M, Wade J 1995 Moving on: young people and leaving care schemes. HMSO, London

Birchall E, Hallett C 1995 Working together in child protection. HMSO, London

Birminghan Women and Social Work Group 1985 Women and social work in Birmingham. In: Brook E, Davis A (eds) Women, the family and social work. Tavistock, London

Blair M E, Pullan C R, Rands C E, Crown N 2000 Community paediatrics moves on – an analysis of changing work patterns 1994–97. Public Health 114:61–64

Blair T 1999 Beveridge revisited: welfare state for the 21st century. In: Walker R (ed) Ending child poverty: popular welfare. Policy Press, Bristol

Blatt E R I 1992 Factors associated with child abuse and neglect in residential care settings. Child and Youth Services Review 15:493–517

Blatt E, Brown S 1986 Environmental influences on incidents of alleged child abuse and neglect in New York State psychiatric facilities: towards an ecology of institutional child maltreatment. Child Abuse and Neglect 10:171–180

Bloom R B 1992 When staff members sexually abuse children in residential care. Child Welfare LXXI(2):131–145

Blues A, Moffat C, Telford P 1999 Working with adolescent females who sexually abuse. In: Erooga M, Masson H (eds) Children and young people who sexually abuse others: challenges and responses. Routledge, London

Boateng P 1999 The government's role in early intervention. In: Bayley R (ed) Transforming children's lives: the importance of early intervention. Family Policy Studies Centre, London

Boddy J, Skuse D 1994 Annotation: the process of parenting in failure to thrive. Journal of Child Psychology and Psychiatry 35(3):401–424

Bograd M 1988 Power, gender and the family: feminist perspectives on family systems therapy. In: Dutton-Douglas M A, Walker L A (eds) Feminist psychotherapies: integration of therapeutic and feminist systems. Ablex, Norwood, NJ

Bolen R 2001 Child sexual abuse: its scope, our failure. Kluwer Academic/Plenum, New York

Booth Dame M E 1996 Avoiding delay in Children Act cases. Lord Chancellor's Department, London

Borkowski A 1995 Police protection and s46 CA 1989. Family Law, p 204–206

Borland M, Triseliotis J, O'Hara G 1990 Permanency planning for children in Lothian region. University of Edinburgh, Edinburgh

Bowlby J 1951 Maternal care and mental health. World Health Organization, Geneva

Bowlby J 1969 Attachment and loss, Vol. 1: Attachment. Hogarth Press, London

Bowlby J 1980 Attachment and loss, Vol. 3: Loss, sadness, and depression. Hogarth Press, London

Bowlby J 1984 Violence in the family as a disorder of attachment and caregiving systems. American Journal of Psychoanalysis 44(1):9–31

Bowlby J 1988 A secure base: clinical applications of attachment theory. Routledge, London

Boyle S 1997 Introduction. In: Bray M (ed) Sexual abuse: the child's voice: poppies on the rubbish heap, 2nd edn. Jessica Kingsley, London, p vii–xiii

Bradshaw J 2002 Comparisons of child poverty and deprivation internationally. In: Bradshaw J (ed) The well-being of children in the UK. University of York/Save the Children, York

Brandon M, Dodsworth J, Rumball D 2005 Serious case reviews: learning to use expertise. Child Abuse Review 14:160–176

Brandon M, Lewis A, Thoburn J, Way A 1999 Safeguarding children with the Children Act 1989. TSO, London.

Brandwein R (ed) 1999 Battered women, children and welfare reform. Sage, Thousand Oaks, CA

Brannen J, Heptinstall E, Bhopal K 2000 Connecting children: care and family life in later childhood. Routledge/Farmer, London

Brassard M R, Hardy D B 1997 Psychological maltreatment. In: Helfer M E, Kempe R S, Krugman R D (eds) The battered child. University of Chicago Press, Chicago

Bratton S, Ray D, Rhine T, Jones L 2005 The efficacy of play therapy with children: a meta-analytic review of treatment outcomes. Professional Psychology: Research and Practice 36(4):376–390

Braun D, Schonveld A 1994 Training teachers in child protection: INSET. In: David T (ed) Protecting children from abuse: multi-professionalism and the Children Act 1989. Trentham, Stoke-on-Trent

Bray M (ed) 1997 Sexual abuse: the child's voice: poppies on the rubbish heap, 2nd edn. Jessica Kingsley, London

Bridge Child Care Consultancy Service 1991 Sukina – an evaluation report of the circumstances leading to her death. Bridge Child Care Consultancy Service, London

Briere J N 1992 Child abuse trauma. Sage, Newbury Park, CA

Briere J 1996 A self-trauma model for treating adult survivors of severe abuse. In: Briere J, Berliner L, Bulkley J A et al (eds) The ASPAC handbook on child maltreatment. Sage, Walnut Creek, CA

Briggs F, Broadhurst D, Hawkins R 2004 Violence, threats and intimidation in the lives of professionals whose work involves children, Criminology Research Council, Australia

British Agencies for Adoption and Fostering 1989 After abuse: papers on caring and planning for a child who has been sexually abused. BAAF, London

British Agencies for Adoption and Fostering 1998, 2000 Working with children. BAAF, London

British Psychological Society 1995 Recovered memories. The report of the working party of the BPS. British Psychological Society, London

Broad B (ed) 2001 Kinship care: the placement choice for children and young people. Russell House, Lyme Regis

Brodzinsky D, Schechter M (eds) 1990 The psychology of adoption. Oxford University Press, Oxford

Bronfenbrenner U 1979 The ecology of human development. Harvard University Press, Cambridge, MA

Brophy J 2000 Race and ethnicity in public law proceedings. Family Law 30:740–743

Brophy J 2003 Diversity and child protection. Family Law 33:674–678

Brophy J, Jhutti-Johal J, Owen C 2003a Assessing and documenting child ill treatment in ethnic minority households. Family Law 33:756–764

Brophy J, Jhutti-Johal J, Owen C 2003b Significant harm: child protection litigation in a multi-cultural society. Lord Chancellor's Research Programme, Research Series 1/2003. Department of Constitutional Affairs, London

Brophy J, Jhutti-Johal Y, McDonald E 2005 Minority ethnic parents, their solicitors and child protection litigation. DCA Research Series 5/05. DCA, London. Online. Available: www.dca.gov.uk/research/2005/5_2005_1.pdf

Brown C 1984 Child abuse parents speaking: parents' impressions of social workers and the social work process. School of Advanced Urban Studies, University of Bristol, Bristol

Brown E, Bullock R, Hobson C, Little M 1998 Making residential care work – structure and culture in children's homes. In: DOH Caring for children away from home: messages from research. Wiley, Chichester

Brown J, Cohen P, Johnson J G, Salzinger S 1998 A longitudinal analysis of risk factors for child maltreatment: findings of a 17-year prospective study of officially recorded and self-reported child abuse and neglect. Child Abuse and Neglect 22:1065–1078

Brown L 2003 Mainstream or margin? The current use of family group conferences in child welfare practice in the UK. Child and Family Social Work 8:331–340

Brown S 2005 Treating sex offenders. Willan, Cullompton

Browne A, Finkelhor D 1986 Initial and long-term effects. A review of the research. In: Finkelhor D (ed) A sourcebook of child sexual abuse. Sage, Beverley Hills, CA

Browne K D 1986 Methods and approaches to the study of parenting. In: Sluckin W, Herbert M (eds) Parental behaviour. Blackwell, Oxford, p 344–373

Browne K D 1988 The nature of child abuse and neglect. In: Browne K D, Davies C, Stratton P (eds) Early prediction and prevention of child abuse: a handbook. Wiley, Chichester, p 15–30

Browne K D 1989 The naturalistic context of family violence and child abuse. In: Archer J, Browne K D (eds) Human aggression: naturalistic approaches. Routledge, London, p 182–216

Browne K D 1993 Violence in the family and its links to child abuse. In: Hobbs C J, Wynne J M (eds) Clinical paediatrics: international practice and research. Baillière Tindall, London, p 149–164

Browne K D 1995a Preventing child maltreatment through community nursing. Journal of Advanced Nursing 2:57–63

Browne K D 1995b The prediction of child maltreatment. In: Reder P, Lucey C (eds) The assessment of parenting. Routledge, London, p 118–135

Browne K D 2002 Child protection. In: Rutter M, Taylor E (eds) Child and adolescent psychiatry, 4th edn. Routledge, London, p 1158–1174

Browne K D, Hamilton C 1999 Police recognition of links between spouse abuse and child abuse. Child Maltreatment 4:136–147

Browne K D, Hamilton-Giachritsis C E 2003 Prevention: current and future trends. In: Bannon M J, Carter Y H (eds) Protecting children from abuse and neglect in primary care. Oxford University Press, Oxford, p 233–247

Browne K D, Hamilton-Giachritsis C 2005 The influence of violent media on children and adolescents: a public health approach. Lancet 365:702–710

Browne K D, Herbert M 1997 Preventing family violence. Wiley, Chichester

Browne K D, Howells K 1996 Violent offenders. In: Hollin C R (ed) Working with offenders. Wiley, Chichester, p 188–210

Browne K D, Lynch M 1995 The nature and extent of child homicide and fatal abuse. Child Abuse Review 4(5):309–316

Browne K D, Saqi S 1987 Parent–child interaction in abusing families: possible causes and consequences. In: Maher P (ed) Child abuse: an educational perspective. Blackwell, Oxford, p 77–104

Browne K D, Saqi S 1988a Approaches to screening families at high risk for child abuse. In: Browne K D, Davies C, Stratton P (eds) Early prediction and prevention of child abuse: a handbook. Wiley, Chichester, p 57–85

Browne K D, Saqi S 1988b Mother–infant interactions and attachment in physically abusing families. Journal of Reproductive and Infant Psychology 6(3):163–282

Browne K D, Davies C, Stratton P 1988 Early prediction and prevention of child abuse: a handbook. Wiley, Chichester

Browne K D, Hamilton C, Hegarty J, Blissett J 2000 Identifying need and protecting children through community nurse home visits. Representing Children 13:111–123

Browne K D, Hanks H, Stratton P, Hamilton C (eds) 2002a Early prediction and prevention of child abuse: a handbook, 2nd edn. Wiley, Chichester

Browne K D, Falshaw L, Dixon L 2002b Treating domestic violence offenders. In: Browne K D, Hanks H, Stratton P, Hamilton C E (eds) Early prediction and prevention of child abuse: a handbook, 2nd edn. Wiley, Chichester, p 317–336

Browne K D, Douglas J, Hamilton-Giachritsis C E, Hegarty J 2006 A community health approach to the assessment of infants and their parents: the CARE programme. Wiley, Chichester

Brunk M, Henggeler S W, Whelan J P 1987 Comparison of multisystemic therapy and parent training in the brief treatment of child abuse and neglect. Journal of Consulting and Clinical Psychology 55:171–178

Bryans A N 2004 Examining health visiting expertise: combining simulation, interview and observation. Journal of Advanced Nursing 47:623–630

Bryson V 2002 Feminist debates: issues of theory and political practice. Palgrave Macmillan, Basingstoke

Buckley H 2003 Child protection work. Beyond the rhetoric. Jessica Kingsley, London

Buckley H, Horwath J, Whelan S, Health Service Executive 2005 A framework for assessing vulnerable children and their families. Unpublished report. Trinity College Dublin and University of Sheffield

Bullock R, Little M, Millham S 1993 Residential care for children – a review of the research. HMSO, London

Bullock R, Gooch D, Little M 1998a Children going home: the reunification of families. Dartmouth, Aldershot

Bullock R, Gooch D, Little M, Mount K 1998b Research into practice: experiments in development and information design. Ashgate, Aldershot

Bulmer M 1996 The ethnic group question in the 1991 Census of Population. In: Coleman D, Salt J (eds). HMSO, London

Burgess C 2005 Interim report of evaluation of Aberlour National Parenting Development Project (unpublished). Stirling University, Stirling

Burton M 1996 Child protection issues in general practice: an action research project to improve inter-professional practice. Essex Child Protection Committee, Chelmsford

Busfield J 1996 Men, women and madness: understanding gender and mental disorder. Macmillan, Basingstoke

Butler I 1996 Safe? Involving children in child protection. In: Butler I, Shaw I (eds) A case of neglect? Children's experiences and the sociology of childhood. Avebury, Aldershot

Butler I 1997 Used and abused? Engaging the child in child protection. In: Pithouse A, Williamson H (eds) Engaging the user. Venture Press, Birmingham

Butler I, Drakeford M 2005a Scandal, social policy and social welfare, 2nd edn. BASW/Policy Press, Bristol

Butler I, Drakeford M 2005b Trusting in social work. British Journal of Social Work 35:639–653

Butler I, Williamson H 1994 Children speak: children, trauma and social work. Longman, London

Butler-Sloss Lady Justice E 1988 The report of the inquiry into child abuse in Cleveland 1987. Cmnd 412. HMSO, London

Butt J, Box L 1998 Family centred: a study of the use of family centres by black families. REU, London

CAFCASS 2003 Service principles and standards. CAFCASS, London

CAFCASS 2004 Business Plan 2004–05. CAFCASS, London. Online. Available: www.cafcass.gov.uk/english/Publications/reports/Business%20Plan%202004.pdf

Cairns B 1984 The children's family trust: a unique approach to substitute family care? British Journal of Social Work 14:457–473

Cairns B 2004 Fostering attachments: long-term outcomes in family group care. BAAF, London

Cairns K 2002 Attachment, trauma and resilience: therapeutic caring for children. BAAF, London

Calam R, Cox A, Glasgow D, Jimmieson P, Groth Larsen S 2005 In my shoes: a computer assisted interview for children and vulnerable adults. Child and Family Training, Department for Education and Skills, London

Calder M C 1999a Assessing risk in adult males who sexually abuse children: a practitioner's guide. Russell House, Lyme Regis

Calder M C (ed) 1999b A conceptual framework for managing young people who sexually abuse: towards a consortium approach. In: Working with young people who sexually abuse: new pieces of the jigsaw puzzle. Russell House, Lyme Regis, p 109–150

Calder M C 2000 A complete guide to sexual abuse assessments. Russell House, Lyme Regis

Calder M C 2001a Juveniles and children who sexually abuse: frameworks for assessment, 2nd edn. Russell House, Lyme Regis

Calder M C 2001b Child prostitution: developing effective protocols. Child Care in Practice 7(2):98–115

Calder M C 2003a The assessment framework: a critique and reformulation. In: Calder M C, Hackett S (eds) Assessment in child care: using and developing frameworks for practice. Russell House, Lyme Regis, p 3–60

Calder M C 2003b Risk and child protection. CareKnowledge Briefing Number 9. OLM CareKnowledge, London

Calder M C (ed) 2004a Child sexual abuse and the internet: tackling the new frontier. Russell House, Lyme Regis

Calder M C 2004b Child protection: current context, central contradictions and collective challenges. Representing Children 17(1):56–73

Calder M C (ed) 2005a Children and young people who sexually abuse: new theory, research and practice developments. Russell House, Lyme Regis

Calder M C 2005b From system-orientated outputs to child-orientated outcomes. OLM Briefing Paper. OLM CareKnowledge, London

Calder M, Horwath J 1999 Working for children on the child protection register. Ashgate, Aldershot

Calder M C, Goulding S, Hanks H et al 2001 The complete guide to sexual abuse assessments. Russell House, Lyme Regis

Calder M C, Harold G T, Howarth E L 2004 Children living with domestic violence: towards a framework for assessment and intervention. Russell House, Lyme Regis

Caldwell B M, Bradley R H 2001 Home observation for measurement of the environment: administration manual, 3rd edn. University of Arkansas, Little Rock, Arkansas

Cameron A, Lart R 2003 Factors promoting and obstacles hindering joint working: a systematic review of the research evidence. Journal of Integrated Care 11:9–17

Campbell-Smith M 1983 The school – liberator or censurer? Child Abuse and Neglect 7:329–337

Cann J, Falshaw L, Friendship C 2004 Sexual offenders discharged from prison in England and Wales: a twenty-one year reconviction study. Legal and Criminological Psychology 9(1):1

Cantwell H B 1997 The neglect of child neglect. In: Helfer M E, Kempe R S, Krugman R D (eds) The battered child. University of Chicago Press, Chicago

Carbino R 1991 Advocacy for foster families in the United States facing child abuse allegations: how social agencies and foster parents are responding to the problem. Child Welfare LXX(2):131–149

Carbino R 1992 Policy and practice for response to foster families when child abuse or neglect is reported. Child Welfare LXXI(6):497–509

Carich M, Calder C 2003 Contemporary treatment of adult male sex offenders. Russell House, Lyme Regis

Carlson V, Cicchetti D, Barnett D, Braunwald K 1989 Disorganised/disorientated attachment relationships in maltreated infants. Developmental Psychology 25:525–531

Carpenter J, Griffin M, Brown S 2005 The impact of Sure Start on social services. Durham Centre for Applied Social Research. University of Durham. Sure Start Evidence and Research. SSU/2005/FR/015. DfES Publications, Nottingham

Carroll J 1994 The protection of children exposed to marital violence. Child Abuse Review 3(1):6–14

Carter Y H, Bannon M J 2002 The role of primary care in the protection of children from abuse and neglect: a position paper for the Royal College of General Practitioners with endorsement from the Royal College of Paediatrics and Child Health, the National Society for the Prevention of Cruelty to Children, the British Association of Medical Managers and the NHS Confederation. RCGP, London

Cashmore J, Bussey K 1996 Judicial perceptions of child witness competence. Law and Human Behaviour 20(3):313–334

Cassidy J, Shaver P R 1999 Handbook of attachment: theory, research and clinical applications. Guilford Press, New York

Cassidy J, Woodhouse S S, Cooper G et al 2005 Examination of the precursors of infant attachment security: implications for early intervention and intervention research. In: Berlin L J, Ziv Y, Amaya-Jackson L, Greenberg M T (eds) Enhancing early attachments: theory, research, intervention and policy. Guilford Press, London, p 34–60

Cattanach A 2001 The story so far: play therapy narratives. Jessica Kingsley, London

Caudill W, Plath D 1966 Who sleeps by whom? Parent–child involvement in urban Japanese families. Psychiatry 29:344–366

Caulkin S 2001 On target for destruction. The Observer, 5 August

Cawson P, Wattam C, Brooker S, Kelly G 2000 Child maltreatment in the United Kingdom: a study of the prevalence of child abuse and neglect. NSPCC, London

CCETSW 1991 The teaching of child care in the Diploma in Social Work: guidance notes for programme planners: improving social work education and training, No. 6. CCETSW, London

Central Advisory Council for Education 1967 Children and their primary schools (Plowden Report). HMSO, London

Central Statistical Office 1993 Social Trends 23, 1993 edn. HMSO, London

Centre for Community Child Health 2004 Literature review: parenting information project. Royal Children's Hospital, Melbourne

Chaffin M 2004 Is it time to rethink Healthy Start/Healthy Families? Child Abuse and Neglect 28:589–595

Chalmers K I 1992 Working with men: an analysis of health visiting practice in families with young children. International Journal of Nursing Studies 29:3–16

Chamberlain P, Reid J 1998 Comparison of two community alternatives to incarceration for chronic juvenile offenders. Journal of Consulting and Clinical Psychology 66(4):624–633

Chand A 2000 The over-representation of black children in the child protection system: possible causes, consequences and solutions. Child and Family Social Work 5(1):66–67

Chapman T 2002 Safeguarding the welfare of children: 1. British Journal of Midwifery 10:569–572

Chesson R, Chisholm D 1995 Issues relating to child residential psychiatric units. In: Chesson R, Chisholm D (eds) Child psychiatric units: at the crossroads. Jessica Kingsley, London, p 234–247

Chief Secretary to the Treasury 2003 Every child matters. Cmnd 5860. TSO, London

ChildLine 1997 Children living away from home. ChildLine, London

Children Act Advisory Committee Report 1997 Lord Chancellor's Department, London

Children's Rights Alliance for England 2004 State of children's rights in England 2004: annual review of UK government action on 2002 concluding observations of the United Nations Committee on the Rights of the Child. Children's Rights Alliance for England, London

Cicchetti D, Lynch M 1993 Toward an ecological/transactional model of community violence and child maltreatment: consequences for children's development. Psychiatry 56:96–118

Cicchetti D, Toth S I 1995 A developmental psychopathology perspective on child abuse and neglect. Journal of the American Academy of Child and Adolescent Psychiatry 34:541–565

Cigno K, Ryan V 1998 Making therapy work for children using non-directive play therapy and cognitive–behavioural therapy. Paper presented at the 28th Congress of the European Association for Behavioural and Cognitive Psychotherapists, University of Cork, Ireland

Clarke S, Popay J 1998 'I'm just a bloke who's had kids.' Men and women on parenthood. In: Popay J, Hearn J, Edwards J (eds) Men, gender divisions and welfare. Routledge, London, p 196–230

Claussen A, Crittenden P 1991 Physical and psychological maltreatment: relations among types of maltreatment. Child Abuse and Neglect 15:5–18

Cleave G 2000 The Human Rights Act 1998 – how will it affect child law in England and Wales. Child Abuse Review 9(6):394–402

Cleaver H 2000 Fostering family contact. TSO, London

Cleaver H, Freeman P 1995 Parental perspectives in cases of suspected child abuse: studies in child protection. HMSO, London

Cleaver H, Nicholson D 2005 The development and use of a local prototype common referral, information and assessment record in Cumbria. Cumbria Children's Fund, Cladbeck, Cumbria

Cleaver H, Walker S 2004 From policy to practice: the implementation of a new framework for social work assessments of children and families. Child and Family Social Work 9(1):81–90

Cleaver H, Wattam C, Cawson P 1998 Assessing risk in child protection. NSPCC, London

Cleaver H, Unell I, Aldgate J 1999 Children's needs – parenting capacity: the impact of parental mental illness, problem alcohol and drug abuse, and domestic violence on children's development. TSO, London

Cleaver H, Barnes J, Bliss D, Cleaver D 2004a Developing information sharing and assessment systems. Research Report RR597 for DfES, University of London

Cleaver H, Walker S, Meadows P 2004b Assessing children's needs and circumstances: the impact of the assessment framework. Jessica Kingsley, London

Cleaver H, Cleaver D, Cleaver C, Woodhead V 2004c Information sharing and assessment. The progress of 'non-trailblazing' local authorities. Research Report 566. DfES Publications, London

Cloke C, Davies M (eds) 1995 Participation and empowerment in child protection. Pitman, London

Clothier C 1994 The Allitt Inquiry. Independent inquiry relating to deaths and injuries on the children's ward at Grantham and Kesteven General Hospital during the period February to April 1991. HMSO, London

Cohen J A, Mannarino A 2000 Predictors of treatment outcome in sexually abused children. Child Abuse and Neglect 24:983–994

Cohen J A, Mannarino A P, Berliner L, Deblinger E 2000 Trauma-focussed cognitive–behavioural therapy for children and adolescents: an empirical update. Journal of Interpersonal Violence 15:1202–1223

Cohen J, Deblinger E, Mannarino A, de Arellano M 2001 The importance of culture in treating abused and neglected children: an empirical review. Child Maltreatment 6:148–175

Colton M 1989 Dimensions of substitute care. Avebury, Aldershot

Colton M 2002 Factors associated with abuse in residential child care institutions. Children and Society 16:33–44

Colton M, Vanstone M 1996 Betrayal of trust: sexual abuse by men who work with children ... in their own words. Free Association Books, London

Colton M, Drury C, Williams M 1995 Children in need: family support under the Children Act 1989. Avebury, Aldershot

Commission for Racial Equality 2003 Statistics: Education. CRE, London. Online. Available: www.cre.gov.uk/research/statistics_education.html

Commission for Social Care Inspection 2004 Performance assessment framework 2003–4. CSCI, London

Commission for Social Care Inspection 2005a Safeguarding children. The second joint Chief Inspectors' Report on arrangements to safeguard children. CSCI, London. Online. Available: www.safeguardingchildren.org.uk

Commission for Social Care Inspection 2005b Making every child matter. Messages from inspections of children's social services. CSCI, London

Commission for Social Care Inspection 2005c Performance indicators for 2005–6. CSCI, London

Commission to Inquire into Child Abuse 2005 www.childabusecommission.ie

Committee of Ministers 2005 Reply by the Committee of Ministers of the Council of Europe adopted 20 April 2005 at the 924th meeting of the Ministers' deputies to Recommendation 1666 (2004) of the Parliamentary Assembly that there should be a 'Europe wide ban on corporal punishment of children'. Council of Europe, Strasbourg

Committee on Local Authority and Allied Personal Social Services 1968 Report of the Committee on Local Authority and Allied Personal Social Services (Seebohm Report). Cmnd 3703. HMSO, London

CommunityCare.co.uk 2005 What did we learn? www.communitycare.co.uk/Articles/2005/11/24/51912/What+did+we+learn.html

Connell S, Sanders M R, Markie-Dadds C 1997 Self-directed behavioral family intervention for parents of oppositional children in rural and remote areas. Behavior Modification 21(4):379–408

Connexions Service National Unit 2001 The Connexions framework for assessment, planning, implementation and review. Connexions Service National Unit, Sheffield

Connolly M 1994 An act of empowerment: the Children, Young Persons and their Families Act 1989. British Journal of Social Work 24:87–100

Connolly M 2006 Fifteen years of family group conferencing: coordinators talk about their experiences in Aotearoa, New Zealand. British Journal of Social Work 36:523–540

Coohey C 2001 The relationship between familism and child maltreatment in Latino and Anglo families. Child Maltreatment 6:130–142

Cooke P 2000 Final report on disabled children and abuse – research project funded by Children-in-Need October 1996–December 1999. Ann Craft Trust, Centre for Social Work, Nottingham University, Nottingham

Cooke P 2004 AC Ting to support parents with learning disabilities. Ann Craft Trust, Centre for Social Work, Nottingham University, Nottingham

Cooper A 2005a Surface and depth in the Victoria Climbié Inquiry Report. Child and Family Social Work 10(1):1–9

Cooper A 2005b The children's workforce in England: a review of the evidence. DfES, London

Cooper A, Lousada J 2005 Borderline welfare. Feeling and fear of feeling in modern welfare. The Tavistock Clinic Series. Karnac, London

Cooper A, Hetherington R, Bairstow K, Pitts J, Spriggs A 1995 Positive child protection: a view from abroad. Russell House, Lyme Regis

Cooper A, Hetherington R, Katz I 2003 The risk factor. Making the child protection system work for children. Demos, London

Cooper D 2005 Pigot unfulfilled: video recorded cross examination under Section 28 of the Youth Justice and Criminal Evidence Act 1999. Criminal Law Review 456 at p 458

Corby B 1987 Working with child abuse. Open University Press, Milton Keynes

Corby B 2000 Child abuse: towards a knowledge base, 2nd edn. Open University Press, Buckingham

Corby B, Millar M 1997 Parents' view of partnership. In: Bates J, Pugh R, Thompson N (eds) Protecting children: challenges and change. Avebury, Aldershot

Corby B, Miller M, Young L 1996 Parental participation in child protection work: rethinking the rhetoric. British Journal of Social Work 26(4):475–492

Corby B, Doig A, Roberts V 2001 Public inquiries into abuse of children in residential care. Jessica Kingsley, London

Corden J, Somerton J 2004 The trans-theoretical model of change: a reliable blueprint for assessment in work with children and families? British Journal of Social Work 34:1025–1044

Corlett J, Twycross A 2006 Negotiation of parental roles within family-centred care: a review of the research. Journal of Clinical Nursing 15:1308–1316

Courtney M, Piliavin I, Grogan-Kaylor A, Nesmith A 2001 Foster youth transitions to adulthood: a longitudinal view of youth leaving care. Child Welfare 80(6):685–717

Cox A, Bentovim A 2000 Framework for the assessment of children in need and their families. The family pack of questionnaires and scales. TSO, London

Cox A, Walker S 2001 Home observation for measurement of the environment. UK version. Pavilion, Brighton

Cox A, Walker S 2002 The HOME inventory: a training approach for the UK. Pavilion, Brighton

Coyle C 1987 The practitioner's view of the role and tasks of guardians ad litem and reporting officers. Barnardo's Research and Development Section, London

Craft A 2005 The National Service Framework for children. Archives of Disease in Childhood 90:665–666

Creighton S J 1992 Child abuse trends in England and Wales 1988–1990 and an overview from 1973–1990. NSPCC, London

Creighton S J, Noyes P 1989 Child abuse trends in England and Wales 1983–1987. NSPCC, London

Creighton S J, Russell N 1995 Voices from childhood. A survey of childhood experiences and attitudes to child rearing among adults in the United Kingdom. NSPCC, London

Crisp B R, Lister P G 2004 Child protection and public health: nurses' responsibilities. Journal of Advanced Nursing 47:656–663

Crittenden P M 1985 Maltreated infants: vulnerability and resilience. Journal of Child Psychology and Psychiatry 26(1):85–96

Crittenden P M 1988 Family and dyadic patterns of functioning in maltreating families. In: Browne K D, Davies C, Stratton P (eds) Early prediction and prevention of child abuse: a handbook. Wiley, Chichester, p 161–189

Crittenden P M 2002 If I knew then what I know now: integrity and fragmentation in the treatment of child abuse and neglect. In: Browne K, Hanks H, Stratton P, Hamilton C (eds) Early prediction and prevention of child abuse: a handbook, 2nd edn. Wiley, Chichester

Crittenden P, Ainsworth M 1989 Child maltreatment and attachment theory. In: Cicchetti D, Carlson V (eds) Child maltreatment: theory and research on the causes and consequences of child abuse and neglect. Cambridge University Press, Cambridge

Crittenden P, Claussen A (eds) 2003 The organization of attachment relationships: maturation, culture and context. Cambridge University Press, Cambridge

Crompton M 1980 Respecting children: social work with young people. Edward Arnold, London

Crompton M 1990 Attending to children: direct work in social and health care. Edward Arnold, Dunton Green

Crompton M 1991 Invasion by Russian dolls: on privacy and intrusion. Adoption and Fostering 15:31–33

Crompton M 1992 Children and counselling. Edward Arnold, Dunton Green

Crompton M 1998 Children, spirituality, religion and social work. Ashgate, Aldershot

Crompton M 2001 Who am I? Promoting children's spiritual well-being in everyday life: a guide for all who care for children. Barnardo's, Barkingside, Ilford

Crompton M, Jackson R 2004 Spiritual well-being of adults with Down syndrome. Down Syndrome Educational Trust, Southsea

Cross M 2004 All systems go for child protection. The Guardian, 22 September

Cross T, Bazron B J, Dennis K W, Isaacs M R 1989 Towards a culturally competent system of care. CASSP Technical Assistance Center, Georgetown University, Washington, DC

Crosse S B, Kaye E, Ratnofsky A C 1993 A report on the maltreatment of children with disabilities. National Centre on Child Abuse and Neglect, Washington DC

Crouch J L, Milner J S, Thomsen C 2001 Childhood physical abuse, early social support, and risk for maltreatment: current social support as a mediator of risk for child physical abuse. Child Abuse and Neglect 25:93–107

Culp R E, Little V, Letts D, Lawrence H 1991 Maltreated children's self-concept effects of a comprehensive treatment. American Journal of Orthopsychiatry 61:114–121

Cummings C, Dyson A, Papps I et al 2005 Evaluation of the full service extended schools project: end of first year report. School of Education, Language and Communication Sciences, University of Newcastle, Education in Urban Contexts Group, School of Education, University of Manchester, Tecis Ltd. Research Report RR680. DfES Publications, Nottingham

Cunningham J, Pearce T, Pearce P 1988 Childhood sexual abuse and medical complaints in adult women. Journal of Interpersonal Violence 3:131–134

Curtis M 1946 Report of the Care of Children Committee. Cmnd 6922. HMSO, London

CYPU (Children and Young People's Unit) 2002 Local preventative strategy: interim guidance for local authorities and other local agencies (statutory and non-statutory) providing services to children and young people. Online. Available: www.cypu.gov.uk/corporate/services/preventative.cfm

Dale P 2004 'Like a fish in a bowl': parents' perceptions of child protection services. Child Abuse Review 13:137–157

Dale P, Davies M, Morrison T, Waters J 1986a Dangerous families: assessment and treatment of child abuse. Tavistock, London

Dale P, Waters J, Davies M et al 1986b The towers of silence: creative and destructive issues for therapeutic teams dealing with sexual abuse. Journal of Family Therapy 8:1–25

Dale P, Green R, Fellows R 2005 Child protection assessment following serious injuries to infants. Fine judgements. Wiley, Chichester

Dalgleish L 2003 Risk, needs and consequences. In: Calder M C, Hackett S (eds) Assessment in child care. Using and developing frameworks for practice. Russell House, Lyme Regis, p 86–99

Dallos R, Draper R 2005 An introduction to family therapy: systemic theory and practice. Open University Press, London

Daniel B, Taylor J 2001 Engaging with fathers: practice issues for health and social care. Jessica Kingsley, London

Daniel B, Taylor J 2005 Do they care? The role of fathers in cases of child neglect. In: Taylor J, Daniel B (eds) Child neglect: practice issues for health and social care. Jessica Kingsley, London

Daniel B, Wassell S 2002 The early years: assessing and promoting resilience in vulnerable children I. Jessica Kingsley, London

Daniel B, Featherstone B, Hooper C-A, Scourfield J 2005 Why gender matters for Every Child Matters. British Journal of Social Work 10:207–216

Daro D 1996 Current trends in child abuse reporting and fatalities: NCPA's 1995 annual fifty-state survey. APSAC Advisor 9(2):21–24

Daro D 2002 Educating and changing parents. In: Browne K D, Hanks H, Stratton P, Hamilton C (eds) Early prediction and prevention of child abuse: a handbook, 2nd edn. Wiley, Chichester p 127–144

Daro D, Mitchel L 1990 Current trends in child abuse reporting and fatalities: the results of the 1989 annual fifty-state survey. Working Paper No. 808. National Center on Child Abuse Prevention Research, Chicago

Daro D, Migely G, Wiese D, Salmon-Cox S 1996 World perspectives on child abuse: the second international resource book. National Committee to Prevent Child Abuse, Chicago

Data Protection Act 1998 Information Commissioner, London

David T 1993 Child protection and early years teachers: coping with child abuse. Open University Press, Buckingham

David T (ed) 1994 Protecting children from abuse: multi-professionalism and the Children Act 1989. Trentham, Stoke-on-Trent

Davis L V, Carlson B E 1987 Observation of spouse abuse: what happens to the children? Journal of Interpersonal Violence 2(3):320–345

Davies L, Krane J 2006 Collaborate with caution: protecting children, helping mothers. Critical Social Policy 26:412–425

Dawson S 2004 Representation of children in proceedings under Rule 9(5) of the Family Proceedings Rules 1991: a balance of rights and welfare? Seen and Heard 14(1):40

De Wolff M S, van Ijzendoorn M H 1997 Sensitivity and attachment: a meta-analysis on parental antecedents of infant attachment. Child Development 68:571–591

Deblinger E, Hope Heflin A 1996 Treating sexually abused children and their nonoffending parents. Sage, Newbury Park, CA

Department for Constitutional Affairs 1999 Human Rights Act. Core guidance for public authorities: a new era of rights and responsibilities. DCA, London

Department for Education and Skills 2003a Every Child Matters: change for children. A consultation document. Home Office, London

Department for Education and Skills 2003b Every child matters. Cmnd 5860. TSO, London

Department for Education and Skills 2004a Every child matters: next steps. DfES Publications, Nottingham

Department for Education and Skills 2004b Every child matters: change for children (DfES/1081/2004). TSO, London

Department for Education and Skills 2004c Every child matters: change for children in social care (DfES/1090/2004). TSO, London

Department for Education and Skills 2004d Get it sorted. Guidance on providing effective advocacy services for children and young people making a complaint under the Children Act 1989. Online. Available: www.dfes.gov.uk/childrensadvocacy/docs/GetitSorted.pdf

Department for Education and Skills 2004e Common assessment framework. Introduction and practitioners' guide. DfES, London. Online. Available: www.dfes.gov.uk/consultations

Department for Education and Skills 2004f Safeguarding children in education. DfES, London. Online. Available: www.teachernet.gov.uk/childprotection/guidance.htm

Department for Education and Skills 2004g Five year strategy for children and learners. TSO, London

Department for Education and Skills 2004h Information sharing and assessment: the progress of 'non-trailblazer' local authorities. DfES, London. Online. Available: www.dfes.gov.uk/research

Department for Education and Skills 2005a Working together to safeguard children: a guide for inter-agency working to safeguard and promote the welfare of the child. Draft guide for consultation. DfES, London

Department for Education and Skills 2005b Referrals, assessments and children and young people on child protection registers. Year ending 31 March 2004. TSO, London

Department for Education and Skills 2005c Working together to safeguard children and Local Safeguarding Children Board Regulations. Consultation draft. DfES, London. Online. Available: www.dfes.gov.uk/consultations

Department for Education and Skills 2005d Outcome indicators for looked after children: twelve months to 30th September 2004, England. DfES, London

Department for Education and Skills 2005e Common assessment framework: introduction and practitioners guide. Draft consultation document. DfES, London

Department for Education and Skills 2005f Cross-government guidance on sharing information on children and young people. DfES, London

Department for Education and Skills 2005g Lead professional good practice. Guidance for children with additional needs. Every child matters: change for children. July. Online. Available: www. everychildmatters.gov.uk

Department for Education and Skills 2005h Multi-agency working. Fact sheet. Online. Available: www.everychildmatters.gov.uk/multiagencyworking

Department for Education and Skills 2005i Extended schools: access to opportunities and services for all. A prospectus. Every child matters: change for children. DfES Publications, Nottingham

Department for Education and Skills 2005j Safeguarding children: safer recruitment and selection in education settings. TSO, London

Department for Education and Skills 2005k Safeguarding children in education: dealing with allegations of abuse made against teachers and other staff. DfES, London. Online. Available: www. teachernet.gov.uk/_doc/9350/this%20one.doc

Department for Education and Skills 2005l National statistics of education. DfES, London

Department for Education and Skills 2006 Children and young people on child protection registers year ending 31st March 2005, England (Personal Social Services and Local Authority Statistics). Government Statistical Service, London

Department for Education and Skills, Department of Health 2004a Change for children – every child matters. Executive summary. TSO, London

Department for Education and Skills, Department of Health 2004b Change for children – every child matters: disabled children and young people and those with complex health needs. TSO, London

Department for Education and Skills, Department of Health, Home Office 2003 Keeping children safe: the government's response to the Victoria Climbié Inquiry Report and the Joint Inspectors Report Safeguarding Children. Cmnd 5861. TSO, London

Department for Work and Pensions 2000/2001 Households below average income family resources survey. DWP, London

Department of Education and Employment 1995 Protecting children from abuse: the role of the Educational Service (Circular 10/95). DfEE, London

Department of Education and Science 1988 Working together for the protection of children from abuse: procedures within the Education Service (Circular 4/88). DES, London

Department of Health 1988a Protecting children: a guide for social workers undertaking a comprehensive assessment. HMSO, London

Department of Health 1988b Working together: a guide to arrangements for interagency cooperation for the protection of children from abuse. HMSO, London

Department of Health 1989a The care of children: principles and practice in regulations and guidance. HMSO, London

Department of Health 1989b Introduction to the Children Act 1989. HMSO, London

Department of Health 1989c Principles and practice in regulations and guidance. HMSO, London

Department of Health 1991a Child abuse: a study of inquiry reports 1980–1989. HMSO, London

Department of Health 1991b The Children Act 1989: guidance and regulations. HMSO, London

Department of Health 1991c Patterns and outcomes in child placement: messages from current research. HMSO, London

Department of Health 1991d Guidance and regulations, Children Act 1989. Vol. II, Family support, day-care and educational provision for young children. HMSO, London

Department of Health 1991e Guidance and regulations, Children Act 1989. Vol. I, Court orders. HMSO, London

Department of Health 1991f Working together under the Children Act 1989: a guide to arrangements for inter-agency cooperation for the protection of children against abuse. HMSO, London

Department of Health 1992a Choosing with care – the report of the committee of inquiry into the selection, development and management of staff in children's homes. HMSO, London

Department of Health 1992b Manual of practice guidance for guardians ad litem and reporting officers. HMSO, London

Department of Health 1994a Children Act Report 1993. HMSO, London

Department of Health 1994b The extent and nature of organised and ritual abuse: research findings. HMSO, London

Department of Health 1994c Convention on the rights of the child: first report to the UN Committee on the rights of the child by the United Kingdom. DoH, London

Department of Health 1995a Child protection: messages from research. HMSO, London

Department of Health 1995b The challenge of partnership in child protection: practice guide. HMSO, London

Department of Health 1997 Utting Report: safety of children in the public care. TSO, London

Department of Health 1998a Modernising social services: promoting independence, improving protection, raising standards. Cmnd 4169. TSO, London

Department of Health 1998b Caring for children away from home: messages from research. Wiley, Chichester

Department of Health 1998c The government's response to the children's safeguards review. TSO, London

Department of Health 1998d Quality protects. Objectives for social services objectives for children. DoH, London

Department of Health 1999a The government's objectives for children's social services. TSO, London

Department of Health 1999b Care plans and care proceedings under the Children Act 1989. Local Authority Circular (99)29. DoH, London

Department of Health 1999c Convention on the rights of the child: second report to the UN Committee on the rights of the child by the United Kingdom. TSO, London

Department of Health 1999d Adoption now: messages from research. Wiley, Chichester

Department of Health 2000a Protecting children, supporting parents: a consultation document on the physical punishment of children. DoH, London

Department of Health 2000b Working together to safeguard children involved in prostitution. TSO, London

Department of Health 2000c Assessing children in need and their families: practice guidance. TSO, London

Department of Health 2000d Working together to safeguard and promote the welfare of children. TSO, London

Department of Health 2001a The Children Act now: messages from research. TSO, London

Department of Health 2001b Studies informing the framework for the assessment of children in need and their families. TSO, London

Department of Health 2001c National adoption standards for England. TSO, London

Department of Health 2002a Safeguarding children: a Joint Chief Inspectors report on arrangements to safeguard children. DoH, London

Department of Health 2002b Working together to safeguard children in whom illness is fabricated or induced. TSO, London

Department of Health 2002c Improvement, expansion and reform: the next three years. TSO, London

Department of Health 2002d National minimum standards for fostering services in England. TSO, London

Department of Health 2003a Children Act Report 2003. TSO, London

Department of Health 2003b What to do if you're worried a child is being abused. DoH, London. Online. Available: www.safeguardingchildren.co.uk/managed/files/dfes-what-to-do.pdf

Department of Health 2004 The Children Act 2004. TSO, London

Department of Health, Department for Education and Skills 2004 National Service Framework for children, young people and maternity services. TSO, London. Online. Available: www.dh.gov.uk/PublicationsAndStatistics/Publications/PublicationsPolicyAndGuidance/PublicationsPolicyAndGuidanceArticle/fs/en?CONTENT_ID 5 4089100&chk 5 Egpznc

Department of Health, Department for Education and Skills 2004 Children's and maternity services information strategy. Supporting the children's, young people and maternity services National Service Framework. DoH, London. Online. Available: www.dh.gov.uk/assetRoot/04/08/92/35/04089235.pdf

Department of Health, Home Office, Department of Education and Science, Welsh Office 1991 Working together under the Children Act 1989. A guide to arrangements for inter-agency cooperation for the protection of children from abuse. HMSO, London

Department of Health, Department for Education and Employment, Home Office 1999 Working together to safeguard children – a guide to inter-agency working to safeguard and promote the welfare of children. TSO, London

Department of Health, Department for Education and Employment, Home Office 2000 Framework for the assessment of children in need and their families. TSO, London

Department of Health, Department for Education and Employment, Home Office 2000e Framework for the assessment of children in need and their families. DoH, London

Department of Health, Department for Education and Skills, Home Office 2003 Keeping children safe: the government's response to the Victoria Climbié Inquiry Report and Joint Chief Inspectors' Report, Safeguarding Children. TSO, London

Department of Health and Social Security 1971 Better services for the mentally handicapped. Cmnd 4683. HMSO, London

Department of Health and Social Security 1974a Non-accidental injury to children. Local Authority Social Services Letter (74) (13)

Department of Health and Social Security 1974b Report of the Committee of Inquiry into the care and supervision provided in relation to Maria Colwell. HMSO, London

Department of Health and Social Security 1974c Memorandum on non-accidental injury to children. DHSS, London

Department of Health and Social Security 1976 Non-accidental injury to children: the police and case conferences. Local Authority Social Services Letter (76) (2)

Department of Health and Social Security 1982 Child abuse: a study of inquiry reports 1973–1981. HMSO, London

Department of Health and Social Security 1985a Review of child care law: report to ministers of an interdepartmental working party. HMSO, London

Department of Health and Social Security 1985b Social work decisions in child care: recent research findings and their implications. HMSO, London

Department of Health and Social Security 1986 Child abuse – working together. A guide to arrangements for inter-agency cooperation for the protection of children. HMSO, London

Department of Health and Social Security, Welsh Office 1988 Working together: a guide to arrangements for inter-agency cooperation for the protection of children from abuse. HMSO, London

Department of the Environment, Transport and the Regions (DETR) 2000 Indices of deprivation 2000. Regeneration Research Summary No. 31. DETR, London

Dickens J 2005 Being 'the epitome of reason': the challenge for lawyers and social workers in child care proceedings. International Journal of Law, Policy and the Family 19:73–101

Dickens J, Thoburn J, Howell D, Schofield G 2005 Children starting to be looked after by local authorities in England: an analysis of inter-authority variation and case-centred decision-making. British Journal of Social Work. Online. Available: http://bjsw.oxfordjournals.org/cgi/reprint/bch276v1.pdf

Digby A 1996 Contexts and perspectives. In: Wright D, Digby A (eds) From idiocy to mental deficiency. Routledge, London

Dingwall R 1986 The Jasmine Beckford affair. Modern Law Review 49:489–507

Dingwall R 1989 Some problems about predicting child abuse and neglect. In: Stevenson O (ed) Child abuse: public policy and professional practice. Harvester Wheatsheaf, Hemel Hempstead, ch 2

Dingwall R, Eekelaar J, Murray T 1983 The protection of children: state intervention and family life. Blackwell, Oxford

Dixon L, Browne K D, Hamilton-Giachritsis C 2005a Risk factors of parents abused as children: a mediational analysis of the intergenerational continuity of child maltreatment (Part I). Journal of Child Psychology and Psychiatry 46(1):47–57

Dixon L, Hamilton-Giachritsis C, Browne K D 2005b Risk factors and behavioural measures of parents abused as children: a mediational analysis of the intergenerational continuity of child maltreatment (Part II). Journal of Child Psychology and Psychiatry 46(1):58–68

Dobash R P, Dobash R E 2004 Women's violence to men in intimate relationships: working on a puzzle. British Journal of Criminology 44:324–349

Dolan M, Holloway J, Bailey S, Kroll L 1996 The psychosocial characteristics of juvenile sexual offenders referred to an adolescent forensic service in the UK. Medical Science and Law 36:343–352

Donald T, Jureidini J 2004 Parenting capacity. Child Abuse Review 13:5–17

Donzelot J 1988 The promotion of the social. Economy and Society 17(3):395–427

Doran C, Brannan C 1996 Institutional abuse. In: Bibby P C (ed) Organised abuse – the current debate. Arena/Ashgate, Aldershot

Dorfman E 1951 Play therapy. In: Rogers C R (ed) Client-centred therapy: its current practice, implications and theory. Constable, London, p 235–277

Downes C 1992 Separation revisited: adolescents in foster family care. Ashgate, Aldershot

Doyle C 1990 Working with abused children. Macmillan Education, Basingstoke

Drewe A, Carey L J, Schaefer C E (eds) 2001 School-based play therapy. Wiley, New York

Drewett R 2005 The importance of slow weight gain in the first 2 months in identifying children who fail to thrive. Journal of Reproductive and Infant Psychology 23(4):309–317

Dubanoski R 1981 Child maltreatment in European– and Hawaiian–Americans. Child Abuse and Neglect 5(4):457–466

Dubanoski R, Snyder K 1980 Patterns of child abuse in Japanese– and Samoan–Americans. Child Abuse and Neglect 4(4):217–225

Dubowitz H, DePanfilis D (eds) 2000 Handbook for child protection. Sage, Thousand Oaks, CA

Dumaret A, Coppel-Batsch M, Couraud S 1997 Adult outcome of children reared for long-term periods in foster families. Child Abuse and Neglect 21(10):911–927

Duncan S, Edwards R 1999 Lone mothers, paid work and gendered moral rationalities. Macmillan, Basingstoke

Dunn A, Jareg E, Webb D 2003 A last resort: the growing concern about children in residential care. Save the Children, London

Dunn J 1988 The beginnings of social understanding. Basil Blackwell, Oxford

Durkin R 1982 No one will thank you – first thoughts on reporting institutional abuse. Child and Youth Services Review IV(1–2):109–113

Dutt R, Phillips M 1996 Race, culture and the prevention of child abuse. Report of the National Commission of Inquiry into the Prevention of Child Abuse, Vol. 2: Background papers. TSO, London

Dutt R, Phillips M 2000 Assessing the needs of black children and their families. In: The framework for the assessment of children in need and their families: practice guidance. TSO, London

Dyer O 2005 Doctors reluctant to work on child protection committees, survey shows. British Medical Journal 328:327

Dyson P 2002 Child protection: the manager's perspective. In: Wilson K, James A (eds) The child protection handbook, 2nd edn. Baillière Tindall, Edinburgh, p 538–551

Eckenrode J, Munsch J, Powers J, Doris J 1988 The nature and substantiation of official sexual abuse reports. Child Abuse and Neglect 12(3):311–319

Edgerton R 1992 Sick societies: challenging the myth of primitive harmony. Free Press, New York

Edleson J L 1999 The overlap between child maltreatment and woman battering. Violence Against Women 5(2):134–154

Edleson J L, Mbilinyi L F, Beeman S K, Hagemeister A K 2003 How children are involved in adult domestic violence: results from a four-city telephone survey. Journal of Interpersonal Violence 18:18–32

Edwards H, Richardson K 2003 The child protection system and disabled children. In: It doesn't happen to disabled children. NSPCC, London

Edwards R, Dunn J, Bentovim A 2006 A multi-modal approach to treating sexually abusive young people and their families. In: Calder M (ed) Treating sexually abusive young people. Russell House, Lyme Regis

Egeland B, Jacobvitz D, Sroufe A 1988 Breaking the cycle of abuse. Child Development 59:1080–1088

Egeland B, Bosquet M, Chung A L 2002 Continuities and discontinuities in the intergenerational transmission of child maltreatment: implications for breaking the cycle of abuse. In: Browne K D, Hanks H, Stratton P, Hamilton C E (eds) Early prediction and prevention of child abuse: a handbook, 2nd edn. Wiley, Chichester, p 217–232

Eldridge H 1998 Therapist guide for maintaining change: relapse prevention for adult male perpetrators of child sexual abuse. Sage, Thousand Oaks, CA

Eldridge H 2000 Patterns of sex offending and strategies for effective assessment and intervention. In: Itzin C (ed) Home truths about child sex abuse. Routledge, London

Eldridge H, Still J 1998 Building networks: phase 1. In: Eldridge H (ed) Therapist guide for maintaining change: relapse prevention for adult male perpetrators of child sexual abuse. Sage, Thousand Oaks, CA

Elliott M (ed) 1993 Female sexual abuse of children. Longman, Harlow

Ellis L, Lasson I, Solomon R 1998 Keeping children in mind. A model of child observation practice. CCETSW, London

Ellison L 2003 The adversarial process and the vulnerable witness. Oxford University Press, Oxford

Engel B 1998 Living with the legacy of abuse: how to make your relationship work when your partner is a survivor of childhood sexual abuse. Camden, London

English D J 1999 Evaluation and risk assessment of child neglect in public child protection services. In: Dubowitz H (ed) Neglected children. Research, practice and policy. Sage, Thousand Oaks, CA, p 191–210

English D J (ed) 2005 Longitudinal studies of child abuse and neglect. Child Abuse and Neglect (Special Issue) 29(5):441–619

Erikson E H 1963 Childhood and society. Norton, New York

Erikson M, Egeland B, Pianta R 1989 The effects of maltreatment on the development of young children. In: Cicchetti D, Carlson V (eds) Child maltreatment: theory and research on the causes and consequences of child abuse and neglect. Cambridge University Press, Cambridge

Esping-Andersen G (ed) 2002 Why we need a new welfare state. Oxford University Press, Oxford

Eth S, Pynoos R S (eds) 1985 Post traumatic stress disorder in children. American Psychiatric Association, Los Angeles, CA

European Network of Ombudspersons for Children (ENOC) 2005 Online. Available: www.ombudsnet.org

Evert K, Bijkerk I 1987 When you're ready. Walnut Press, Walnut Creek, CA

Fagan D 1998 Child abuse and neglect: The knowledge base of the A&E nurse. Accident and Emergency Nursing 6:30–35

Fahlberg V 1990 Residential treatment: a tapestry of many therapies. Perspectives Press, New York

Fahlberg V 1991 A child's journey through placement. Perspectives Press, Indianapolis

Falkov A 1996 Study of Working Together 'Part 8' reports. Fatal child abuse and parental psychiatric disorder. An analysis of 100 area child protection committee case reviews conducted under the terms of Part 8 of Working Together under the Children Act 1989, Department of Health. In: Reder P, Duncan S 1999 Lost innocents: a follow up of fatal child abuse. Routledge, London, p 41–61

Falkov A (ed) 1998 Crossing bridges: training resources for working with mentally ill parents and their children. DoH, London

Faller K 1990 Sexual abuse by paternal caretakers. In: Horton A, Johnson B, Roundy L, Williams D (eds) The incest perpetrator: a family member no one wants to treat. Sage, Newbury Park, CA

Falshaw L, Friendship C, Bates A 2003 Sexual offenders – measuring reconviction, reoffending and recidivism. Home Office, London

Fanshel D, Shinn E B 1978 Children in foster care: a longitudinal study. Columbia University Press, New York

Farmer E 1999 Holes in the safety net: the strengths and weaknesses of child protection procedures. Child and Family Social Work 4(4):293–302

Farmer E, Moyers S 2002 Children placed with relatives or family. University of Bristol, Bristol

Farmer E, Owen M 1995 Child protection practice: private risks and public remedies – decision making, intervention and outcome in child protection work. HMSO, London

Farmer E, Pollock S 1998 Sexually abused and abusing children in substitute care. Wiley, Chichester

Farmer E, Moyers S, Lipscombe J 2004 Fostering adolescents. Jessica Kingsley, London

Fawcett B, Featherstone B, Goddard J 2004 Contemporary child care policy and practice. Palgrave Macmillan, Basingstoke

Featherstone B 1997 I wouldn't do your job: women, social and child abuse. In: Hollway W, Featherstone B (eds) Mothering and ambivalence. Routledge, London

Featherstone B 2003 Taking fathers seriously. British Journal of Social Work 33:239–254

Featherstone B 2004a Family life and family support: a feminist analysis. Palgrave Macmillan, Basingstoke

Featherstone B 2004b Feminist social work: past, present and future. In: Hick S, Fook J, Pozutto R (eds) Social work: the critical turn. Thompson Educational Press, Scarborough, ON

Featherstone B 2005 From Sure Start to Children's Centres: charting the journey. Social Policy Association Annual Conference, University of Bath, 27–29 June

Featherstone B 2006 Why gender matters in child welfare and protection. Critical Social Policy 26(2):294–314

Featherstone B, Evans H 2004 Children experiencing maltreatment: who do they turn to? NSPCC, London

Featherstone B, Lancaster E 1997 Contemplating the unthinkable: men who sexually abuse. Critical Social Policy 17(4):51–73

Featherstone B, Peckover S Where have all the violent fathers gone? Critical Social Policy (forthcoming)

Featherstone B, Trinder L 1997 Familiar subjects? Domestic violence and child welfare. Child and Family Social Work 2:147–159

Fein E, Maluccio A N, Hamilton V J, Ward D E 1983 After foster care: permanency planning for children. Child Welfare 62(6):483–558

Feldman W, Feldman E, Goodman J T et al 1991 Is childhood sexual abuse really increasing in prevalence? An analysis of the evidence. Pediatrics 88(1):29–33

Felitti V J 1991 Long-term medical consequences of incest, rape and molestation. Southern Medical Journal 84:328–331

Fenwick H 2004 Clashing rights: the welfare of the child and the Human Rights Act. Modern Law Review 67(6):889–927

Ferenczy S 1949 Confusion of tongues between the adult and the child. International Journal of Psycho-Analysis 30:225–230

Ferguson H 1990 Rethinking child protection practices: a case for history. In: The Violence Against Children Study Group (eds) Taking child abuse seriously: contemporary issues in child protection theory and practice. Unwin Hyman, London

Ferguson H 1996 The protection of children in time. Child and Family Social Work 1(4):205–218

Ferguson H 1997 Protecting children in new times: child protection and the risk society. Child and Family Social Work 2(4):221–234

Ferguson H 2004 Protecting children in time: child abuse, child protection and the consequences of modernity. Palgrave Macmillan, Basingstoke

Fergusson D, Flemming J, O'Neil D 1972 Child abuse in New Zealand. Government Press, Wellington

Fergusson D M, Horwood L J, Lynskey M T 1996 Childhood sexual abuse and psychiatric disorders in young adulthood. Part II. Psychiatric outcomes of sexual abuse. Journal of the American Academy of Child and Adolescent Psychiatry 35:1365–1374

Fernandez E 1999 Pathways in substitute care. Children and Youth Services Review 21:177–216

Festinger T 2002 After adoption: dissolution or permanence? Child Welfare 81(3):515–533

Figley C (ed) 1990 Treating stress in families. Brunner Mazel, New York

Finch J 1989 Family obligations and social change. Polity Press, Cambridge

Finkelhor D 1979 Sexually victimized children. Free Press, New York

Finkelhor D 1980 Risk factors in the sexual victimization of children. Child Abuse and Neglect 4:265–273

Finkelhor D 1984 Child sexual abuse: new theory and research. Free Press, New York

Finkelhor D 1986 A sourcebook on child sexual abuse. Sage, Beverley Hills, CA

Finkelhor D 1988 Initial and long-term effects of child sexual abuse. Paper at SRIP Conference, Leeds

Finkelhor D 1992 Child sexual abuse: recent developments in research. Paper presented at Surviving Childhood Adversity Conference, Trinity College, Dublin

Finkelhor D, Baron L 1986 Risk factors for child sexual abuse. Journal of Interpersonal Violence 1(1):43–71

Finkelhor D, Dziuba-Leatherman J 1994a Children as victims of violence: a national survey. Pediatrics 94:413–420

Finkelhor D, Dziuba-Leatherman J 1994b Victimisation of children. American Psychologist 49(3):173–183

Finkelhor D, Korbin J 1988 Child abuse as an international issue. Child Abuse and Neglect 12(1):3–23

Finkelhor D, Russell D 1984 Women as perpetrators: review of the evidence. In: Finkelhor D (ed) Child sexual abuse: new theory and research. Free Press, New York

Finney L D 1990 Reach for the rainbow. Changes Publishing, Park City, Malibu

Fisher D, Beech A 2002 Treating adult sexual offenders. In: Browne K D, Hanks H, Stratton P (eds) Early prediction and prevention of child abuse. Wiley, Chichester

Fisher D, Beech A 2004 Adult male sex offenders. In: Kemshall H, McIvor G (eds) Managing sex offender risk. Jessica Kingsley, London

Fisher J, Wilson K, Gibbs I, Sinclair I 2000 Sharing the care: what foster carers want from social workers. Child and Family Social Work 5(3):225–233

Fisher J J 2005 Trauma training in Lincoln UK. Sensorimotor Psychotherapy Institute, Boulder, CO

Fisher M, Marsh P, Phillips D, Sainsbury E 1986 In and out of care: the experiences of children, parents and social workers. Batsford, London

Flax J 1990 Postmodernism and gender relations in feminist theory. In: Nicholson L (ed) Feminism/postmodernism. Routledge, London

Fletcher J 1993 Not just a name: the views of young people in foster and residential care. National Consumer Council, London

Flin R, Spencer J R 1990 The evidence of children: the law and psychology. Blackstone Press, Oxford

Fontes L 2001 Introduction: those who do not look ahead, stay behind. Child Maltreatment 6:83–88

Fontes L 2005 Child abuse and culture: working with diverse families. Guilford Press, New York

Ford H 2006 Women who sexually abuse children. Wiley, Chichester

Fortin J 2003 Children's rights and the developing law, 2nd edn. Cambridge University Press, Cambridge

Foster V 2005 Success stories? A participatory arts-based research project at Sure Start. Unpublished document

Fox Harding L 1991 Perspectives in child care policy. Longman, Harlow

Fox Harding L 1997 Family, the state and social policy. Macmillan, Basingstoke

Frank D, Zeisel S 1988 Failure to thrive. Paediatric Clinics of North America 35:1187–1206

Franklin B (ed) 1986 The rights of children. Basil Blackwell, London

Franklin B (ed) 2002 The new handbook of children's rights: comparative policy and practice. Routledge, London

Franklin B, Parton N (eds) 1991 Social work, the media and public relations. Routledge, London

Franks S 1999 Having none of it: women, men and the future of work. Granta, London

Fraser D 1984 The evolution of the British welfare state, 2nd edn. Macmillan, Basingstoke

Fratter J 1996 Adoption and contact: implications for policy and practice. BAAF, London

Fratter J, Rowe J, Sapsford D, Thoburn J 1991 Permanent family placement: a decade of experience. BAAF, London

Freeman M D A 1983 The rights and wrongs of children. Francis Pinter, London

Freeman M D A (ed) 1997 Children's rights and cultural pluralisms. In: The moral status of children. Martinus Nijhoff, Dordrecht, The Netherlands

Freidrich W 1998 Behavioural manifestations of child sexual abuse. Child Abuse and Neglect 22:523–531

Freud S 1964 New introductory lectures on psychoanalysis (1932–36). Hogarth Press, London

Freyd J, Putnam F, Lyon T et al 2005 The science of child sexual abuse. Science 308:501

Friedrich W N, Boroskin J A 1976 The role of the child in abuse: a review of the literature. American Journal of Orthopsychiatry 46(4):580–590

Friendship C, Thornton D 2002 Risk assessment of offenders. In: Browne K, Hanks H, Stratton P, Hamilton C (eds) Early prediction and prevention of child abuse: a handbook, 2nd edn. Wiley, Chichester

Frosh S 2002 Characteristics of sexual abusers. In: Wilson K, James A (eds) The child protection handbook, 2nd edn. Baillière Tindall, Edinburgh

Frosh S, Phoenix A, Pattman R 2001 Young masculinities. Palgrave, Basingstoke

Frost N, Stein M 1989 The politics of child welfare: inequality, power and change? Harvester Wheatsheaf, New York

Frude N 1980 Child abuse as aggression. In: Frude N (ed) Psychological approaches to child abuse. Batsford, London, p 136–150

Frude N 1989 The physical abuse of children. In: Howells K, Hollin C (eds) Clinical approaches to violence. Wiley, Chichester, p 155–181

Frude N 1991 Understanding family problems: a psychological approach. Wiley, Chichester

Frude N 2003 A framework for assessing the physical abuse of children. In: Calder M, Hackett S (eds) Assessment in child care: using and developing frameworks for practice. Russell House, Lyme Regis

Fuller R, Hallett C, Murray C, Punch S 2000 Young people and welfare: negotiating pathways. Summary of research results. Report to the Economic and Social Research Council. University of Stirling, Stirling. Online. Available: www.data-archive.ac.uk/doc/4586/mrdoc/pdf/a4586uab.pdf

Furniss T 1991 The multiprofessional handbook of child sexual abuse: integrated management, therapy and legal intervention. Routledge, London

Fyson R 2005 Young people with learning disabilities who show sexually inappropriate or abusive behaviours. Ann Craft Trust, Nottingham

Fyson R, Eadie T, Cooke P 2003 Adolescents with learning disabilities who show sexually inappropriate or abusive behaviours. Child Abuse Review 12:305–314

Gallagher B 1998 Grappling with smoke: investigating and managing organised sexual abuse – a good practice guide. NSPCC, London

Gallagher B 2000 The extent and nature of known cases of institutional child sexual abuse. British Journal of Social Work 30:795–817

Gallimore R, Boggs J W, Jordan C 1974 Culture, behaviour and education: a study of Hawaiian Americans. Sage, Beverly Hills, CA

Gallo-Lopez L, Schaefer C E (eds) 2005 Play therapy with adolescents. Jason Aronson, New York

Gambrill E, Shlonsky A 2000 Risk assessment in context. Children and Youth Services Review 22(11–12):813–837

Garbarino J 1977 The human ecology of child maltreatment. Journal of Marriage and the Family 39(4):721–735

Garbarino J, Guttmann E, Wilson Seeley J 1986 The psychologically battered child. Jossey-Bass, San Francisco

Gardner R 1987 Who says? Choice and control in care. National Children's Bureau, London

Garland C 2002 Understanding trauma: a psychoanalytical approach. Karnac, London

Garland C 2004 Traumatic events and their impact on symbolic functioning. In: Levy S, Lemma A (eds) The perversion of loss: psychoanalytic perspectives on trauma. Whurr, London

Geach H, Szwed E (eds) 1983 Providing civil justice for children. Arnold, London

Gelles R J 1973 Child abuse as psychopathology: a sociological critique and reformulation. American Journal of Orthopsychiatry 43:611–621

Gelles R J 1983 An exchange/social control theory. In: Finkelhor D, Gelles R, Straus M, Hotaling G (eds) The dark side of the family: current family violence research. Sage, Beverly Hills, CA, p 151–165

Gelles R J 1987 Family violence, 2nd edn. Library of Social Research No. 84. Sage, Beverly Hills, CA

Gelles R J, Cornell C P 1997 Intimate violence in families, 3rd edn. Sage, Beverly Hills, CA

Gelles R J, Straus M A 1987 Is violence toward children increasing? A comparison of 1975 and 1985 national survey rates. Journal of Interpersonal Violence 2:212–222

General Social Care Council 2002 Code of practice for social care workers. GSCC, London

Gerhardt S 2004 Why love matters: how affection shapes a baby's brain. Routledge, London

Gershater-Molko R M, Lutzker J R, Sherman J A 2003 Assessing child neglect. Aggression and Violent Behaviour 8:563–585

Ghate D, Hazel N 2002 Parenting in poor environments. Jessica Kingsley, London

Ghate D, Spencer L 1995 The prevalence of child sexual abuse in Britain. HMSO, London

Ghate D, Hazel N, Creighton S J, Finch S, Field J 2003 The national study of parents, children and discipline in Britain. Summary of findings. Policy Research Bureau, London. Online. Available: www.prb.org.uk/publications/Parents%20Children%20and%20Discipline%20Summary%20final.pdf

Gibbons J, Gallagher B, Bell C, Gordon D 1995a Development after physical abuse in early childhood: a follow-up study of children on protection registers. HMSO, London

Gibbons J, Conroy S, Bell C 1995b Operating the child protection system. A study of child protection practices in English local authorities. HMSO, London

Gil D 1970 Violence against children. Harvard University Press, Cambridge, MA

Gil D 1978 Societal violence in families. In: Eekelaar J M, Katz S N (eds) Family violence. Butterworths, Toronto, p 14–33

Gil E 1982 Institutional abuse of children in out-of-home care. In: Hanson R (ed) Institutional abuse of children and youth. Haworth Press, New York

Gilbert P 1994 Male violence: towards an integration. In: Archer J (ed) Male violence. Routledge, London, p 352–389

Giller H 1993 Children in need: definition, management and monitoring: a report for the Department of Health. Social Information Systems, Manchester

Giller H, Gormley C, Williams P 1992 The effectiveness of child protection procedures. An evaluation of child protection procedures in four ACPC areas. Social Information Systems, Manchester

Gilligan R 2001 Promoting resilience: a resource guide on working with children in the care system. BAAF, London

Ginott H 1961 Group psychotherapy with children: the theory and practice of play therapy. McGraw-Hill, New York

Gladstone D 1996 The changing dynamic of institutional care. In: Wright D, Digby A (eds) From idiocy to mental deficiency. Routledge, London

Glaser D 1991 Therapeutic work with children. In: Wilson K (ed) Child protection: helping or harming? Papers in Social Policy and Professional Studies No. 15. University of Hull, Hull

Glaser D 1993 Emotional abuse. In: Hobbs C, Wynne J (eds) Baillière's clinical paediatrics. Baillière Tindall, London

Glaser D 2000 Child abuse and neglect and the brain: a review. Journal of Child Psychology and Psychiatry 41(8):1076

Glaser D 2002 Emotional abuse and neglect (psychological maltreatment): a conceptual framework. Child Abuse and Neglect 67:697–714

Glaser D 2005 Neurobiological effects of child maltreatment. Abstract Xth ISPCAN European Regional Conference on Child Abuse and Neglect, Berlin, Germany

Glaser D, Frosh S 1988 Child sexual abuse. Macmillan, Houndmills

Glaser D, Prior V 2002 Predicting emotional child abuse and neglect. In: Browne K, Hanks H, Stratton P, Hamilton C (eds) Early prediction and prevention of child abuse: a handbook, 2nd edn. Wiley, Chichester

Glasgow D, Horne L, Calam R, Cox A 1994 Evidence, incidence, gender and age in sexual abuse of children perpetrated by children: towards a developmental analysis of child sexual abuse. Child Abuse Review 3:196–210

Glass N 1999 Sure Start: the development of an early intervention programme for young people in the United Kingdom. Children and Society 13(4):257–264

Glass N 2000 Sure Start history: origins of the Sure Start Programme. Sure Start Unit, London

Glass N 2001 What works for children: the political issues. Children and Society 15:14–20

Glasser M, Kolvin I, Cambell D, Glasser A, Leitch I, Farrelly S 2001 Cycle of child sexual abuse: links between being a victim and becoming a perpetrator. British Journal of Psychiatry 179:482–494

Glennie S 2003 Safeguarding children together: addressing the inter-professional agenda. In: Leathard A (ed) Interprofessional collaboration. From policy to practice in health and social care. Brunner-Routledge, Hove

Glisson C, Hemmelgarn A 1998 The effects of organizational climate and inter-organizational coordination on the quality and outcomes of children's service systems. Child Abuse and Neglect 22(5):401–421

Goddard C 2005 The truth is longer than a lie: children speak of their experiences of abuse and protective intervention. Abstract and Presentation Xth ISPCAN European Regional Conference on Child Abuse and Neglect, Berlin, Germany

Goddard C, Hiller P 1993 Child sexual abuse: assault in a violent context. Australian Journal of Social Issues 28(1):20–33

Golden M H, Samuels M P, Southall D P 2003 How to distinguish between neglect and deprivational abuse. Archives of Disease in Childhood 88(20):105–107

Goldson B 2002 Vulnerable inside: children in secure and penal settings. The Children's Society, London

Goldstein J H 1986 Aggression and crimes of violence, 2nd edn. Oxford University Press, Oxford

Goldstein J, Freud A, Solnit A 1973 Beyond the best interests of the child. Free Press, New York

Goodey C 1996 The psychopolitics of learning and disability in seventeenth-century thought. In: Wright D, Digby A (eds) From idiocy to mental deficiency. Routledge, London

Goodman G S, Tobey A E, Batterman-Faunce J M et al 1998 Face to face confrontation: effects of closed-circuit technology on children's eyewitness testimony and jurors' decisions. Law and Human Behaviour 22:165–203

Goodyear R 1994 Training teachers in child protection: initial teacher education. In: David T (ed) Protecting children from abuse: multi-professionalism and the Children Act 1989. Trentham, Stoke-on-Trent

Gordon L 1986 Feminism and social control. In: Mitchell J, Oakley A (eds) What is feminism? Basil Blackwell, Oxford

Gordon L 1989 Heroes of their own lives: the politics and history of family violence. Virago, London

Gray J, Bentovim A, Miller P 1995 The treatment of children and families where illness induction has been identified. In: Horwath J, Lawson B (eds) Trust betrayed. National Children's Bureau, London

Green J W 1978 The role of cultural anthropology in the education of social service personnel. Journal of Sociology and Social Welfare 5(2):214–229

Green J W 1982 Cultural awareness in the human services. Prentice-Hall, Englewood Cliffs, NJ

Greenfields M, Statham J 2004 The use of child protection registers. Thomas Corum Research Unit, London

Griffiths R 1988 Community care: agenda for action. HMSO, London

Grimshaw R, Berridge D 1994 Educating disruptive children. National Children's Bureau, London

Grimshaw R, McGuire C 1998 Evaluating parenting programmes: a study of stakeholders' views. National Children's Bureau, London

Grotevant H D, McRoy R G 1998 Openness in adoption: exploring family connections. Sage, New York

Grubin D H 1991 Unfit to plead in England and Wales 1976–88: a survey. British Journal of Psychiatry 158:540–548

Grubin D 1998 Sex offending against children: understanding the risk. Home Office, London

Grubin D 2004 The risk assessment of sex offenders: In: Kemshall H, McIvor G (eds) Managing sex offender risk. Jessica Kingsley, London

Guerney L F 1984 Client-centred (non-directive) play therapy. In: Schaefer C, O'Conner K (eds) Handbook of play therapy. Wiley, New York

Gully K J, Dengerink H A 1983 The dyadic interaction of persons with violent and non-violent histories. Aggressive Behaviour 9(1):13–20

Guterman N B 1999 Enrolment strategies in early home visitation to prevent physical child abuse and neglect and the 'universal versus targeted' debate: a meta-analysis of population-based and screening-based programs. Child Abuse and Neglect 23(9):863–890

Hackett S 2004 What works for children and young people with harmful sexual behaviours? Barnardo's, Barkingside, Ilford

Hackett S, Telford P, Slack K 2002 Groupwork with parents of children who sexually harm. In: Calder M (ed) Children and young people who sexually abuse: new theory, research and practice developments. Russell House, Lyme Regis

Hacking I 1988 The sociology of knowledge about child abuse. Nous 2:53–63

Hacking I 1991 The making and moulding of child abuse. Critical Inquiry 17(Winter):253–288

Hacking I 1992 World-making by kind-making: child abuse for example. In: Douglas M, Hull D (eds) How classification works: Nelson Goodman among the social sciences. Edinburgh University Press, Edinburgh

Haeri A 1998 Overcoming abuse: an Islamic approach. In: Patel N, Naik D, Humphries B (eds) Visions of reality: religion and ethnicity in social work. Central Council for Education and Training in Social Work, London, p 97–101 (first published in Open Mind 1994, 69, June/July)

Hagell A 1998 Dangerous care. Reviewing the risks to children from their carers. Policy Studies Institute, London

Hagood M M 2001 The use of art in counselling child and adult survivors of sexual abuse. Jessica Kingsley, London

Hahn R, Mercy J, Bilukha O, Briss P A 2005 Assessing home visiting programs to prevent child abuse: taking silver and bronze along with gold. Child Abuse and Neglect 29:215–218

Haj-Yahia M M, Tamish S 2001 The rates of child sexual abuse and its psychological consequences as revealed by a study among Palestinian university students. Child Abuse and Neglect 25:1303–1327

Hall D, Elliman D (eds) 2003 Health for all children, 4th edn. Oxford University Press, Oxford

Hall L, Lloyd S 1993 Surviving child sexual abuse: a handbook for helping women challenge their past, 2nd edn. Falmer Press, London

Hallett C 1995 Interagency coordination in child protection. HMSO, London

Hallett C 2000 Children's rights [editorial]. Child Abuse Review 9(6):389–393

Hallett C, Birchall E 1992 Coordination and child protection: a review of the literature. HMSO, London

Hallett C, Stevenson O 1980 Child abuse: aspects of inter-professional cooperation. Allen and Unwin, London

Hallstrom I, Runeson I, Elander G 2002 An observational study of the level at which parents participate in decisions during their child's hospitalization. Nursing Ethics 9:202–214

Halperin D S, Bouvier P, Jaffe P D et al 1996 Prevalence of child sexual abuse among adolescents in Geneva: results of a cross-sectional survey. British Medical Journal 312:1326–1329

Hamilton C E 2002 Editor's introduction: Section IV. Daro D (2002) Educating and changing parents. In: Browne K D, Hanks H, Stratton P, Hamilton C (eds) Early prediction and prevention of child abuse: a handbook, 2nd edn. Wiley, Chichester, p 279–282

Hamilton C E, Browne K D 1998 The repeat victimisation of children: should the concept be revised? Aggression and Violent Behavior 3(1):47–60

Hamilton C E, Browne K D 1999 Recurrent maltreatment during childhood: a survey of referrals to police child protection units in England. Child Maltreatment 4(4):275–286

Hamilton C E, Browne K D 2002 Predicting physical maltreatment. In: Browne K D, Hanks H, Stratton P, Hamilton C (eds) Early prediction and prevention of child abuse: a handbook, 2nd edn. Wiley, Chichester, p 41–56

Hamilton-Giachritsis C E, Browne K D 2005 A retrospective study of risk to siblings in abusing families. Journal of Family Psychology 19(4):619–624

Hampton R L 1999 Family violence: prevention and treatment. Sage, London

Hampton R L, Senatore V, Gullotta T P 1998 Substance abuse, family violence and child welfare: bridging perspectives. Sage, London

Hanks H 1993 Failure to thrive: a model for treatment. In: Hobbs C, Wynne J (eds) Baillière's clinical paediatrics. Baillière Tindall, London

Hanks H, Hobbs C 1993 Failure to thrive: a model for treatment. In: Hobbs C, Wynne J (eds) Baillière's clinical paediatrics. Baillière Tindall, London

Hanks H, Saradjian J 1991 Women who abuse children sexually. Human Systems: The Journal of Systemic Consultation and Management 2:247–262

Hanks H, Wynne J 2001 Females who sexually abuse: an approach to assessment. In: Calder M C (ed) Juveniles and children who abuse, 2nd edn. Russell House, Lyme Regis

Hansard 1988 House of Lords Debates, Vol. 502, col. 488, 6 January. HMSO, London

Hansard 1989 House of Lords Debates, Vol. 503, cols 354 and 355. HMSO, London

Hansard 2004 House of Lords Debates, cols 563–564, 5 July. TSO, London

Hanson R K, Bussiere M 1998 Predicting relapse: a meta-analysis of sexual offender recidivism studies. Journal of Consulting and Clinical Psychology 66(2):348

Hanson R K, Gordon A, Harris A, Marques J, Murphy W, Quinsey V 2002 First report of the collaborative outcome data project on the effectiveness of psychological treatment for sex offenders. Sexual Abuse: A Journal of Research and Treatment 14(2):169–194

Harder M, Pringle K (eds) 1997 Protecting children in Europe: towards a new millennium. Aarlborg University Press, Aarlborg

Harlow H F 1959 Love in infant monkeys. Scientific American 200(6):68–74

Harris P L 1989 Children and emotion. Basil Blackwell, Oxford

Hart S, Laws D R, Kropp P R 2003 The promise and the peril of sex offender risk assessment. In: Ward T, Laws D R, Hudson S (eds) Sexual deviance – issues and controversies. Sage, Thousand Oaks, CA

Hartley C C 2002 The co-occurrence of child maltreatment and domestic violence: examining both neglect and child physical abuse. Child Maltreatment 7:349–358

Hawley D R, DeHaan L 1996 Toward a definition of family resilience: integrating life-span and family perspectives. Family Process 35:283–298

Hayes S 1991 Sex offenders. Australia and New Zealand Journal of Developmental Disabilities 17:220–227

Hazel M, Fenyo A 1993 Free to be myself: the development of teenage fostering. Human Service Associates, London

Head A 1998 The child's voice in child and family social work decision making: the perspective of a guardian ad litem. Child and Family Social Work 3(2):189–196

Heard D, Lake B 1997 The challenge of attachment for caregiving. Routledge, London

Heider F 1958 The psychology of interpersonal relations. Wiley, New York

Helfer M E, Kempe R S, Krugman R D 1997 The battered child. University of Chicago Press, Chicago

Helfer R 1990 The neglect of our children in child abuse. Paediatric Clinics of North America 37(4):923–942

Heller S S, Larrieu J A, D'Imperio R, Boris N W 1999 Research on resilience to child maltreatment: empirical considerations. Child Abuse and Neglect 23:321–338

Hendrick H 1994 Child welfare in England 1872–1989. Routledge, London

Hendrick H 2003 Child welfare: historical dimensions, contemporary debates. Policy Press, Bristol

Hendry E 1997 Engaging general practitioners in child protection training. Child Abuse Review 6:60–64

Her Majesty's Court Service 2004 Practice directions. President's direction on representation of children in family proceedings. HMCS, London. Online. Available: www.hmcourts-service.gov.uk/cms/949.htm

Herbert M, Harper-Dorton K V 2002 Working with children, adolescents and their families. BPS/Blackwell, Oxford

Herman J 1992 Trauma and recovery: from domestic violence to political terror. Harper Collins, New York

Hershell A D, McNeil C B 2005 Parent–child interaction therapy for children experiencing externalizing behavior problems. In: Reddy L A, Files-Hall T M, Schaefer C E (eds) Empirically based play interventions for children. American Psychological Association, Washington, DC, p 169–190

Hetherington R, Cooper A, Smith P, Wilford G 1997 Protecting children: messages from Europe. Russell House, Lyme Regis

Hetherton J, Beardsall L 1998 Decisions and attitudes concerning child sexual abuse: does the gender of the perpetrator make a difference to child protection professionals? Child Abuse and Neglect 22:1265–1283

Heywood J S 1969 Childhood and society 100 years ago. National Children's Home, London

Heywood J S 1978 Children in care: the development of the service for the deprived child, 3rd edn. Routledge and Kegan Paul, London

Hildebrand J 1988 The use of group work in treating child sexual abuse. In: Bentovim A, Elton A, Hildebrand J et al (eds) Child sexual abuse within the family. Wright, London

Hill M (ed) 1999a Signposts in fostering. BAAF, London

Hill M (ed) 1999b Effective ways of working with children and their families. Jessica Kingsley, London

Hill M, Hupe P 2002 Implementing public policy: governance in theory and in practice. Sage, London

Hill M, Shaw M (eds) 1998 Signposts in adoption. BAAF, London

Hill M, Lambert L, Triseliotis J 1989 Achieving adoption with love and money. National Children's Bureau, London

Hill M, Nutter R, Giltinan D et al 1993 A comparative survey of specialist fostering in the UK and North America. Adoption and Fostering 17(2):17–22

Hill S 2005 Partners for protection: a future direction for child protection. Child Abuse Review 14:347–364

HM Government 2005a Working together to safeguard children – a guide to inter-agency working to safeguard and promote the welfare of children. Draft for public consultation. Online. Available: www.dfes.gov.uk/consultations/downloadableDocs/Working%20together%20to%20safeguard%20children%20-%20July%2027th%20-%20final%20to%20pdf.pdf

HM Government 2005b Statutory guidance on inter-agency co-operation to improve the well-being of children: children's trusts. Every child matters: change for children. Statutory guidance. DfES Publications, Nottingham

HM Government 2005c Children's workforce strategy. A strategy to build a world-class workforce for children and young people. Consultation. DfES Publications, Nottingham

HM Government 2005d Common core of skills and knowledge for the children's workforce. Every child matters: change for children. Non-statutory guidance. DfES Publications, Nottingham

HM Government 2005e Higher standards, better schools for all. More choice for parents and pupils. Cmnd 6677. TSO, London

HM Government 2006a Working together to safeguard children – a guide to inter-agency working to safeguard and promote the welfare of children. TSO, London. Online. Available: www.everychild-matters.gov.uk/workingtogether

HM Government 2006b Making safeguarding everyone's business – response to the second joint Chief Inspectors' report on safeguarding children. TSO, London. Online. Available: www.everychildmatters.gov.uk/socialcare/safeguarding

HM Prison Service/National Probation Service 2001 OASYs (Offender Assessment Systems). Home Office, London

HM Treasury 2002 The 2002 spending review: opportunity and security for all. Investing in an enterprising society: new public spending plans 2003–2006. TSO, London

HMSO 1991 Patterns and outcomes in child placement. HMSO, London

HMSO 1995 Criminal statistics, England and Wales 1994. Cmnd 3010. HMSO, London

HMSO 2003 Ethnic group statistics. A guide for the collection and classification of ethnicity data. HMSO, London

Ho H 1999 A theory of hearsay. Oxford Journal of Legal Studies 19(3):403–420

Hobbs C 2005 The prevalence of child maltreatment in the United Kingdom. Child Abuse and Neglect 29(9):949–951

Hobbs C J, Wynne J M 1993 The evaluation of child sexual abuse. In: Hobbs C, Wynne J (eds) Baillière's clinical paediatrics. Baillière Tindall, London

Hobbs C, Hanks H, Wynne J 1993 Child abuse and neglect: a clinician's handbook. Churchill Livingstone, London

Hobbs C J, Hanks H G I, Wynne J M 1999 Child abuse and neglect: a clinician's handbook, 2nd edn. Churchill Livingstone, London

Hobbs C J, Wynne J M, Hanks H G I 2003 Child abuse and social aspects of pediatrics. In: McIntosh N, Helms P J, Smyth R L (eds) Forfar and Arneil's textbook of paediatrics, 6th edn. Churchill Livingstone, Edinburgh

Hogan C, Murphy D 2002 Outcomes: reframing responsibility for well-being. Annie Casey Foundation, Baltimore

Hoghughi M 1997 Sexual abuse by adolescents. In: Hoghughi M, Bhate S, Graham S (eds) Working with sexually abusive adolescents. Sage, London

Holgate E 1972 Communicating with children. Longman, London

Holland S 2004 Child and family assessment in social work practice. Sage, London

Holland S, Scourfield J 2004 Liberty and respect in child protection. British Journal of Social Work 34:21–36

Hollin C 1993 Contemporary psychological research into violence: an overview. In: Taylor P J (ed) Violence in society. Royal College of Physicians, London, p 55–68

Hollows A 2003 Making professional judgements in the framework for the assessment of children in need and their families. In: Calder M C, Hackett S (eds) Assessment in child care: using and developing frameworks for practice. Russell House, Lyme Regis, p 61–74

Holman B 1988 Putting families first: prevention and childcare? Macmillan Education, Basingstoke

Holman R 1996 Fifty years ago: the Curtis and Clyde reports. Children and Society 9(3):197–209

Holtzworth-Munroe A, Bates L, Smutzler N, Sandin E 1997 A brief review of the research on husband violence. Part I: Maritally violent versus nonviolent men. Aggression and Violent Behavior 2:65–99

Holtzworth-Munroe A, Meehan C, Herron K, Rehman U, Stuart G L 2000 Testing the Holtzworth-Munroe and Stuart (1994) batterer typology. Journal of Consulting and Clinical Psychology 68:1000–1019

Home Office 1945 Report by Sir Walter Monckton on the circumstances that led to the boarding-out of Dennis and Terence O'Neill at Bank Farm, Minsterley and the steps taken to supervise their welfare. Cmnd 6636. HMSO, London

Home Office 1950 Joint circular with Ministry of Health and Ministry of Education: children neglected or ill-treated in their own homes. HMSO, London

Home Office 1998 Speaking up for justice. Report of the Interdepartmental Working Group on the treatment of vulnerable or intimidated witnesses in the criminal justice system. Home Office, London

Home Office 2001 Criminal statistics, England and Wales 2000. Cmnd 5312. Home Office, London

Home Office 2003a MAPPA guidance. Home Office, London

Home Office 2003b Hidden harm: responding to the needs of children of problem drug users. Advisory Council on the Misuse of Drugs, London

Home Office 2004 Crime in England and Wales 2003/2004. Statistical Bulletin 10/04. National Statistics, London

Home Office 2005a Crime in England and Wales 2003/2004. Supplementary Volume 1: Homicide and Gun Crime 02/05. National Statistics, London

Home Office 2005b Criminal statistics 2004, England and Wales. Home Office Statistical Bulletin, London

Home Office 2005c The implementation of 'Speaking up for Justice': special measures. Provisions from the Youth Justice and Criminal Evidence Act 1999: Part Ii (Circular 39/2005). Home Office, London

Home Office, Department of Health, Department of Education and Science, Welsh Office 1991 Working together under the Children Act 1989: a guide to arrangements for inter-agency cooperation for the protection of children from abuse. HMSO, London

Home Office, Department of Health and Crown Prosecution Service 2001 Provision of therapy for child witnesses prior to a criminal trial: practice guidance. CPS Communications Branch, Bolton. Online. Available: www.dfes.gov.uk/qualityprotects/pdfs/therapy.pdf

Home Office, Lord Chancellor, Crown Prosecution Service, Department of Health, The National Assembly for Wales 2002 Achieving best evidence in criminal proceedings: guidance for vulnerable or intimidated witnesses, including children. Home Office Communications, London

Hong G K, Hong L K 1991 Comparative perspectives on child abuse and neglect: Chinese vs. Hispanics and Whites. Child Welfare 70(4):463–475

Hooper C-A 1992 Mothers surviving child sexual abuse. Routledge, London

Hooper C-A, Humphreys C 1997 What's in a name? Reflections on the term non-abusing parent. Child Abuse Review 6:298–303

Horwath J 1997 Child protection messages from research: issues for inter-agency practice in the late 1990s. Child Care in Practice 3(4):2–17

Horwath J (ed) 2001 Assessing the world of the child in need. In: The child's world: assessing children in need. Jessica Kingsley, London, p 23–34

Horwath J 2002 Maintaining a focus on the child? First impressions of the Framework for the Assessment of Children in Need and their Families in cases of child neglect. Child Abuse Review 11:195–213

Horwath J 2005a Identifying and assessing cases of child neglect: learning from the Irish experience. Child and Family Social Work 10:99–110

Horwath J 2005b The influences of differences in perceptions of child neglect in social work practice. In: Taylor J, Daniel B (eds) Child neglect. Practice issues for health and social care. Jessica Kingsley, London

Horwath J 2007 Child neglect: Identification & Assessment. Palgrave, London

Horwath J, Morrison T 2000 Identifying and implementing pathways for organisational change: using the framework for the assessment of children in need and their families as a case example. Child and Family Social Work 5:245–254

Horwath J, Morrison T 2001 Assessment of parental motivation to change. In: Horwath J (ed) The child's world: assessing children in need. Jessica Kingsley, London

House of Commons 1984 Children in care. Second report from the Social Services Committee, Session 1983–1984, Vol. 1. HMSO, London

House of Commons 2003 CAFCASS/Social Services Inspectorate Report 1990 House of Commons Committee on the Lord Chancellor's Department, Vol. 1, para. 62. TSO, London

House of Commons Education and Skills Committee 2005 Every child matters: Ninth Report of Session 2004–05, HC 40-1. TSO, London

Houston S 2001 Beyond social constructionism: critical realism and social work. British Journal of Social Work 31:845–861

Howard J 2000 Support care: a new role for foster carers. In: Wheal A (ed) Working with parents. Russell House, Lyme Regis

Howard League 1995 Banged up, beaten up, cutting up. Howard League, London

Howard League 1996 Lessons for policy and practice on 15-year-olds in prison. Troubleshooter Project Report. Howard League, London

Howe D 1992 Child abuse and the bureaucratisation of social work. Sociological Review 40(3):491–508

Howe D 1995 Attachment theory for social work practice. Macmillan, Houndmills

Howe D (ed) 1996 Attachment and loss in child and family social work. Avebury, Aldershot

Howe D 1998 Patterns of adoption. Blackwell Science, Oxford

Howe D 1999 Attachment theory for social work practice. Macmillan, Basingstoke

Howe D 2005 Child abuse and neglect: attachment, development and intervention. Palgrave Macmillan, Houndmills

Howe D, Brandon M, Hinings D, Schofield G 1999 Attachment theory, child maltreatment and family support. Macmillan, Basingstoke

Howe D, Feast J, Coster D 2000 Adoption search and reunion: the long term experience of adopted adults. Children's Society, London

Hoyano L 2000 Variations on a theme by Pigot: special measures directions for child witnesses. Criminal Law Review 250–273

Hudson B 2004 Whole systems working: a discussion paper for the Integrated Care Network. Online. Available: www.integratedcarenetwork.gov.uk

Hudson B 2005 Partnership working and the children's services agenda: is it feasible? Journal of Integrated Care 13(2):7–12

Hughes H M, Fantuzzo J W 1994 Family violence. In: Hersen M, Ammerman R T, Sisson L A (eds) Handbook of aggressive and destructive behavior in psychiatric patients. Plenum Press, New York, p 491–507

Human Rights Act 1998 TSO, London

Humphreys C 1999 Avoidance and confrontation: social work practice in relation to domestic violence and child abuse. Child and Family Social Work 4:77–87

Humphreys C, Atkar S, Baldwin N 1999 Discrimination in child protection work: recurring themes in work with Asian families. Child and Family Social Work 4(4):283–291

Hunt G (ed) 1998 Whistleblowing in the social services: public accountability and professional practice. Arnold, Aldershot

Hunt J 2001 Family and friends carers: a scoping paper prepared for the Department of Health. Online. Available: www.dfes.gov.uk/qualityprotects/pdfs/friends-family-paper.pdf

Hunt J, Lawson J 1999 Crossing the boundaries: the views of practitioners with experience of family court welfare and guardian ad litem work on the proposal to create a unified court welfare service. National Council for Family Proceedings, London

Hunt J, Macleod A, Thomas C, Freeman P 1999 The last resort: child protection, the courts and the 1989 Children Act. TSO, London

Hunt J, Drucker N, Gill B 2002 Understanding variation in the hours guardians take to complete care cases. Working Paper Series. Oxford Centre for Family Law and Policy, Oxford

Hunt J, Head A, Drucker N 2003 Capturing guardian practice prior to CAFCASS. Oxford Centre for Family Law and Policy, Oxford

Hunter M 1987 Julia: a 'frozen' child. Adoption and Fostering 11(3):26–30

Hunter M 2004 Councils demand coherent guidance. Community Care 9–15 September:18–19

Hutton D 2004 Filial therapy: shifting the balance. Clinical Child Psychology and Psychiatry 9(2):261–270

Hyde C, Bentovim A, Monck E 1996 Treatment outcome study of sexually abused children. Child Abuse and Neglect 19:1387–1397

Hyman C A, Mitchell R 1975 A psychological study of child battering. Health Visitor 48:294–296

Hyman C A, Parr R, Browne K D 1979 An observation study of mother–infant interaction in abusing families. Child Abuse and Neglect 3:241–246

Illingworth R S 1983 Weight and height. In: Hobbs C, Hanks H G I, Wynne J (eds) The normal child, some problems of the early years and their treatment. Churchill Livingstone, Edinburgh

Ima K, Hohm C F 1991 Child maltreatment among Asian and Pacific Islander refugees and immigrants: the San Diego case. Journal of Interpersonal Violence 6(3):267–285

Ince L 1998 Making it alone: a study of the care experiences of young black people. BAAF, London

Independent Representation for Children in Need (IRCHIN) 1985a Representing children. IRCHIN, Heswall, Wirral

Independent Representation for Children in Need (IRCHIN) 1985b Training notes for guardians ad litem. IRCHIN, Heswall, Wirral

Ironside V 1999 The huge bag of worries, 2nd edn. Macdonald, London

Island D, Letellier P 1991 Men who beat the men who love them: battered gay men and domestic violence. Harrington Park Press, New York

Itzin C (ed) 2000 Child protection and child sexual abuse prevention. In: Home truths about child sexual abuse. Routledge, London

Iwaniec D 1996 The emotionally abused and neglected child. Wiley, Chichester

Iwaniec D 2004 Children who fail to thrive. Wiley, Chichester

Iwaniec D 2006 The emotionally abused and neglected child: identification, assessment and intervention – a practice handbook. Wiley, Chichester

Iwaniec D, Herbert M, McNeish A 1985 Social work with failure to thrive children and their families. British Journal of Social Work 15:243–259

Iwaniec D, Herbert M, Sluckin A 2002 Helping emotionally abused and neglected children and abusive carers. In: Browne K D, Hanks H, Stratton P, Hamilton C (eds) Early prediction and prevention of child abuse: a handbook, 2nd edn. Wiley, Chichester

Iwaniec D, Donaldson T, Allweis M 2004 The plight of neglected children – social work and judicial decision making and the management of neglect cases. Child and Family Law Quarterly 16(4):423–436

Jack G 2001 Ecological perspectives in assessing children and families. In Horwath J (ed) The child's world: assessing children in need. Jessica Kingsley, London

Jack G, Owen G 2003 The missing side of the triangle: assessing the importance of family and environmental factors in the lives of children. Barnardo's, Ilford

Jaffe P, Wolfe D, Wilson S, Zak L 1986 Similarities in behaviour and social maladjustment among child victims and witnesses to family violence. American Journal of Orthopsychiatry 56:142–146

Jaffe P G, Wolfe D A, Wilson S K 1990 Children of battered women. Sage, Beverly Hills, CA

Jaffe P, Crooks C, Wolfe D 2003 Legal and policy responses to children exposed to domestic violence: the need to evaluate intended and unintended consequences. Clinical Child and Family Psychology Review 6(3):205–213

James A, James A 2001 Tightening the net: children, communities and control. British Journal of Sociology 52(2):211–228

James A, Neil P 1996 Juvenile sexual offending: one-year period prevalence study within Oxfordshire. Child Abuse and Neglect 20:477–485

James A, Prout A (eds) 1991 A new paradigm for the sociology of childhood? Provenance, promise and problems. In: Constructing and reconstructing childhood: contemporary issues in the sociological study of childhood. Falmer Press, London

James A, Wilson K (eds) 1988 Social work in family proceedings. A practice guide. Routledge, London

James A L, James A, McNamee S 2004 Can children's voices be heard in family proceedings? Family law and the construction of childhood in England and Wales. Representing Children 16(3):168–178

James B 1994 Handbook for treatment of attachment-trauma problems in children. Lexington Books, New York

Jay P 1979 Report of the Committee of Enquiry into Mental Handicap Nursing and Care. Cmnd 7468. HMSO, London

Jeffery L 2003 New Labour, new initiatives: Sure Start and the Children's Fund. In: Frost N, Lloyd A, Jeffery L (eds) The RHP companion to family support. Russell House, Lyme Regis

Jenson J, Saint-Martin D 2001 Changing citizenship regimes: social policy strategies in the investment state. Workshop on Fostering Social Cohesion: A Comparison of New Policy Strategies. Université de Montreal, 21–22 June

Johnson G, Kent G, Leather J 2005 Strengthening the parent–child relationship: a review of family interventions and their use in medical settings. Child: Care, Health and Development 31:25

Johnson S, Petrie S 2004 Child protection and risk-management: the death of Victoria Climbié. Journal of Social Policy 33(2):179–202

Johnson T C 1999 Understanding your child's sexual behaviour: what's natural and healthy. New Harbinger, Oakland, CA

Johnson T C, Doonan R 2005 Children with sexual behaviour problems: what have we learned in the past two decades? In: Calder M (ed) Children and young people who sexually abuse: new theory, research and practice developments. Russell House, Lyme Regis

Jones C 2001 Voices from the front line: state social workers and New Labour. British Journal of Social Work 31:547–562

Jones C, Novak T 1999 Poverty, welfare and the disciplinary state. Routledge, London

Jones D P H 1992 Interviewing the sexually abused child: investigation of suspected abuse. Gaskell/Royal College of Psychiatrists, London

Jones D P H 2003 Communicating with vulnerable children: a guide for practitioners. Gaskell, London

Jones J 1994 Towards an understanding of power relationships in institutional abuse. Early Childhood Development 100:69–76

Jones L, O'Loughlin T 2003 A child concern model to embrace the framework. In: Calder M C, Hackett S (eds) Assessment in childcare: using and developing frameworks for practice. Russell House, Lyme Regis, p 141–155

Jonker F, Jonker-Bakker I 1997 Effects of ritual abuse: the results of three surveys in the Netherlands. Child Abuse and Neglect 21:541–556

Jordan B 1988 What price partnership? Costs and benefits. In: James A, Scott D (eds) Partnership in probation, education and training. Central Council for Education and Training in Social Work, London

Jordan B 1998 The new politics of welfare. Sage, London

Jordan B, Jordan C 2000 Social work and the third way. Sage, London

Joseph R 1999 The neurology of traumatic 'dissociative' amnesia: commentary and literature review. Child Abuse and Neglect 23:715–727

Joseph Rowntree Foundation 2005 The role of family centres in encouraging learning and understanding within families. JRF, York

Kagan J, Kearsley R B, Zelazo P R 1978 Infancy: its place in human development. Harvard University Press, Cambridge, MA

Kaplan M J, Becker J V, Tenke C E 1991 Influence of abuse history on male adolescent self-reported comfort with interviewer gender. Journal of Interpersonal Violence 6(1):3–11

Kastell J 1962 Casework in child care. Routledge and Kegan Paul, London

Katz I 1997 Current issues in comprehensive assessment. NSPCC, London

Kaufman J, Zigler E 1987 Do abused children become abusive parents? American Journal of Orthopsychiatry 57:186–192

Kaufman J, Zigler E 1992 The prevention of child maltreatment. Programming, research and policy. In: Holden E W, Rosenberg M (eds) Prevention of child maltreatment: developmental and ecological perspectives. Wiley, New York, p 269–295

Kazdin A E, Bass D, Ayas W A, Rodgers A 1990 Empirical and clinical focus of child and adolescent psychotherapy research. Journal of Consulting and Clinical Psychology 58(6):729–740

Kellogg N D, Menard S W 2003 Violence among family members of children and adolescents evaluated for sexual abuse. Child Abuse and Neglect 27:1367–1376

Kelly G, MacAuley C 1995 Foster care in Northern Ireland. BAAF, London

Kelly L 1988 Surviving sexual violence. Polity Press, Cambridge

Kelly L 1992 The connection between disability and child abuse: a review of the research evidence. Child Abuse Review 1(3):157–167

Kelly L, Regan L, Burton S 1991 An exploratory study of the prevalence of sexual abuse in a sample of 16–21 year olds. Polytechnic of North London, Child Abuse Studies Unit, London

Kelly L, Regan L, Burton S 2000 Sexual exploitation. In: Itzin C (ed) Home truths about child sexual abuse. Routledge, London

Kempe R, Goldbloom B 1987 Malnutrition and growth retardation in the context of child abuse and neglect. In: Helfer R, Kempe R (eds) The battered child. University of Chicago Press, Chicago

Kempe S, Kempe C 1984 Sexual abuse of children and adolescents. W H Freeman, New York

Kempe C H, Silverman F N, Steel B F, Droegemueller W, Silver H K 1962 The battered child syndrome. Journal of the American Medical Association 181:17–24

Kemshall H 2001 Risk assessment and management of known sexual and violent offenders: a review of current issues. Home Office, London

Kemshall H, McIvor G (eds) 2004 Managing sex offender risk. Jessica Kingsley, London

Kendall L, Harker L (eds) 2002 From welfare to wellbeing: the future of social care. Institute of Public Policy Research, London

Kendall-Tackett K A, Williams L M, Finkelhor D 1993 Impact of sexual abuse on children: a review and synthesis of recent empirical studies. Psychological Bulletin 113(1):164–180

Kendrick A, Taylor J 2000 Hidden on the ward: the abuse of children in hospitals. Journal of Advanced Nursing 31:565–573

Kendrick D, Elkan R, Hewitt M 2000 Does home visiting improve parenting and the quality of the home environment? A systematic review and meta-analysis. Archives of Disease in Childhood 82:443–451

Kennedy I 2001 The report of the public inquiry into children's heart surgery at the Bristol Royal Infirmary, 1984–1995 (Kennedy Report). Cmnd 5207. TSO, London

Kennedy R 2001 Assessment and treatment in family law – a valid distinction. Family Law 31:676–681

Kenny G 2002 Children's nursing and interprofessional collaboration: challenges and opportunities. Journal of Clinical Nursing 11:306–313

Kent A, Waller G 1998 The impact of childhood emotional abuse: an extension on the child abuse and trauma scale. Child Abuse and Neglect 22(5):393–399

Kenward H 1989 Helping children who have been abused. In: British Agencies for Adoption and Fostering (ed) After abuse: papers on caring and planning for a child who has been sexually abused. BAAF, London

King M, Trowell J 1992 Children's welfare and the law: the limits of legal intervention. Sage, London

Kinsey A C, Pomeroy W B, Martin C E, Gebhard P H 1953 Sexual behaviour in the human female. W B Saunders, Philadelphia

Kirk H D 1964 Shared fate. Collier-Macmillan, London

Kirk H D 1981 Adoptive kinship: a modern institution in need of reform. Butterworths, Vancouver

Kirkwood A 1993 The Leicestershire inquiry 1992. Leicestershire County Council, Leicester

Kirton D, Feast J, Howe D 2000 Searching, reunion and transracial adoption. Adoption and Fostering 24(3):6–18

Kitchen S, Elliott R 2001 Key findings from the Vulnerable Witness Survey, Home Office Research. Findings No. 147. Home Office, London

Kmietowicz Z 2004 Complaints about doctors in child protection work have increased fivefold. British Medical Journal 328:601

Knopp F H, Stevenson W F 1990 Nationwide survey of juvenile and adult sex offender treatment programs and models. Safer Society Press, New York

Kolko D J 1996 Individual cognitive behavioural treatment and family therapy for physically abused children and their offending parents: the comparison of clinical outcomes. Journal of Child Maltreatment 1(4):322–342

Kolko D J, Swenson C C 2002 Assessing and treating physically abused children and their families: a cognitive–behavioural approach. Sage, Thousand Oaks, CA

Korbin J (ed) 1981 Child abuse and neglect: cross-cultural perspectives. University of California Press, Berkeley, CA

Korbin J 1987a Child abuse and neglect: the cultural context. In: Helfer R, Kempe R (eds) The battered child, 4th edn. University of Chicago Press, Chicago, p 23–41

Korbin J 1987b Child maltreatment in cross-cultural perspective. Vulnerable children and circumstances. In: Gelles R, Lancaster J (eds) Child abuse and neglect: biosocial dimensions. Aldine, Chicago, p 31–55

Korbin J 1990 Hana'ino: child maltreatment in a Hawai'ian–American community. Pacific Studies 13:6–22

Korbin J E 1994 Sociocultural factors in child maltreatment: a neighborhood approach. In: Melton G, Barry F (eds) Protecting children from abuse and neglect. Guilford Press, New York, p 182–223

Korbin J E 1997 Culture and child maltreatment. In: Helfer M E, Kempe R, Krugman R (eds) The battered child, 5th edn. University of Chicago Press, Chicago, p 29–48

Korbin J E 1998 'Good mothers', 'babykillers', and fatal child maltreatment. In: Scheper-Hughes N, Sargent C (eds) Small wars: the cultural politics of childhood. University of California Press, Berkeley, CA, p 253–276

Korbin J E, Spilsbury J 1999 Cultural competence and child neglect. In: Dubowitz H (ed) Neglected children: research, practice and policy. Sage, Newbury Park, CA, p 69–88

Korbin J E, Coulton C, Chard S, Platt-Houston C, Su M 1998 Impoverishment and child maltreatment in African–American and European–American neighborhoods. Development and Psychopathology 10:215–233

Krugman R D 1986 The relationship between unemployment and physical abuse of children. Child Abuse and Neglect 10(3):415–418

Kufeldt K, Allison J 1990 Fostering children fostering families. Community alternatives. International Journal of Family Care 2:1–17

La Fontaine J 1994 The extent and nature of organised ritual abuse. HMSO, London

Ladwa-Thomas U, Sanders R 1999 Juvenile sex abusers: perceptions of social work practitioners. Child Abuse Review 8:55–62

Lahti J 1982 A follow-up study of foster children in permanent placements. Social Service Review. University of Chicago, Chicago

Lamb M E, Lewis C 2004 The development and significance of father–child relationships in two-parent families. In: Lamb M E (ed) The role of the father in child development, 4th edn. Wiley, Chichester

Laming Report 2003 The Victoria Climbié Inquiry: report of an inquiry by Lord Laming. Cmnd 5730. TSO, London. Online. Available: www.victoria-climbie-inquiry.org.uk/finreport/finreport.htm

Land H 1999 New Labour, new families. In: Dean H, Woods R (eds) Social policy review II. Social Policy Association, Luton

Landreth G L 2002 Play therapy: the art of the relationship, 2nd edn. Brunner-Routledge, London

Langness L L 1981 Child abuse and cultural values. The case of New Guinea. In: Korbin J (ed) Child abuse and neglect: cross-cultural perspectives. University of California Press, Los Angeles, CA, p 13–34

Lanyon R 1991 Theories of sex offending. In: Hollin C, Howells K (eds) Clinical approaches to sex offenders and their victims. Wiley, Chichester

Lau A 1997 Cultural and ethnic perspectives on significant harm: its assessment and treatment. In: Adcock M, White R, Hollows A (eds) Significant harm. Significant Publications, Croydon

Laws D R (ed) 1989 Relapse prevention with sex offenders. Guilford Press, New York

Leathard S 2003 Models for interprofessional collaboration In: Leathard A (ed) Interprofessional collaboration: from policy to practice in health and social care. Brunner-Routledge, London

LeBlanc M, Ritchie M 2001 A meta-analysis of play therapy outcomes. Counselling Psychology Quarterly 14:149–163

Levine E M 1986 Sociocultural causes of family violence: a theoretical comment. Journal of Family Violence 1(1):3–12

Levitas R (ed) 1986 The ideology of the new right. Polity Press, Cambridge

Levy A, Kahan B 1991 The Pindown experience and the protection of children. Staffordshire County Council, Stafford

Levy S, Lemma A 2004 The perversion of loss. Psychoanalytic perspectives on trauma. Whurr, London

Levy T M, Orlans M 1998 Attachment, trauma, and healing: understanding and treating attachment disorder in children and families. CWLA Press, Washington, DC

Lew M 1990 Victims no longer. Harper and Row, New York

Lewis A, Shemmings D, Thoburn J 1992 Participation in practice: a reader. University of East Anglia, Norwich

Lewis C S 1950 The lion, the witch and the wardrobe. Penguin, Harmondsworth

Lewis J 2001 The end of marriage? Individualism and intimate relations. Edward Elgar, Cheltenham

Liebling A, Krarup H 1994 Suicide attempts in prison. Home Office Research Bulletin No. 36. Home Office, London

Lifton B 1989 The king of children. Pan, London

Lindsay M 1997 The tip of the iceberg: sexual abuse in the context of residential care. Centre for Residential Care, University of Strathclyde, Glasgow

Lister E D 1982 Forced silence: a neglected dimension of trauma. American Journal of Psychiatry 139:872–876

Lister R 1997 Citizenship: feminist perspectives. Macmillan, Basingstoke

Lister R 2003a Citizenship: feminist perspectives, 2nd edn. Palgrave Macmillan, Basingstoke

Lister R 2003b Investing in citizen-workers of the future: transformations in citizenship and the state under New Labour. Social Policy and Administration 37(5):427–443

Little M 1997 The re-focusing of children's services. In: Parton N (ed) Child protection and family support. Routledge, London

Little M, Mount K 1999 Prevention and early intervention with children in need. Ashgate, Aldershot

Local Safeguarding Children Boards Regulations 2006 Statutory Instrument 2006 No. 90. Online. Available: www.opsi.gov.uk/si/si2006/20060090.htm

London Borough of Bexley 1982 Report of the panel of inquiry into the death of Lucie Gates. London Borough of Bexley, London

London Borough of Brent 1985 A child in trust. The report of the panel of inquiry investigating the circumstances surrounding the death of Jasmine Beckford. London Borough of Brent, London

London Borough of Greenwich 1987 A child in mind: protection of children in a responsible society. Report of the Commission of Inquiry into the circumstances surrounding the death of Kimberley Carlile. London Borough of Greenwich, London

London Borough of Lambeth 1987 Whose child? The report of the Panel appointed to inquire into the death of Tyra Henry. London Borough of Lambeth, London

London Borough of Lambeth, Inner London Education Authority and Lambeth, Southwark and Lewisham Area Health Authority (Teaching) 1982 Report into the inquiry into the death of Richard Fraser. London Borough of Lambeth, London

Long A, Smyth A 1998 The role of mental health nursing in the prevention of child sexual abuse and the therapeutic care of survivors. Journal of Psychiatric and Mental Health Nursing 5:129–136

Long T 1992 'To protect the public and ensure that justice is done': an examination of the Philip Donnelly case. Journal of Advanced Nursing 17:5–9

Longo R, Calder M 2005 The use of sex offender registration with young people who sexually abuse. In: Calder M (ed) Children and young people who sexually abuse: new theory, research and practice developments. Russell House, Lyme Regis

Longo R, Groth N 1982 Juvenile sexual offences in the histories of adult rapists and child molesters. International Journal of Offender Therapy, Comparative Criminology 27:150–155

Longstaff D 1998 Partnership: a social work perspective on preparing children and families for the initial child protection conference. MSW Thesis, University of York, York

Lord Chancellor's Department 2002 Scoping study on delay in Children Act cases. Lord Chancellor's Department, London

Lorenz K 1965 Evolution and modification of behavior. University of Chicago Press, Chicago

Lorenz K 1966 On aggression. Harcourt, Brace and World, New York

Love A, Cooke P, Taylor P 2003 The criminal justice system and disabled children. In: It doesn't happen to disabled children. NSPCC, London

Lovell E 2002 'I think I might need some more help with this problem…' Responding to children and young people who display sexually harmful behaviour. NSPCC, London

Lowe M, Murch M 2002 The plan for the child: adoption and long-term fostering. BAAF, London

Lowe M, Murch M, Borkowski M et al 1999 Supporting adoption. BAAF, London

Loxley A 1997 Collaboration in health and welfare. Working with difference. Jessica Kingsley, London

Lupton C, North N, Khan P 2001 Working together or pulling apart? The National Health Service and child protection networks. Policy Press, Bristol

Luthar S S, Zelazo L B 2003 Resilience and vulnerability: adaptation in the context of childhood adversities. In: Luthar S (ed) Resilience and vulnerability. Cambridge University Press, New York

Lymbery M E F 2003 Negotiating the contradictions between competence and creativity in social work education. Journal of Social Work 3(1):99–118

Lynch M, Roberts J 1977 Predicting child abuse. Child Abuse and Neglect 1:491–492

Lyon C M 1994 Whatever happened to the child's right to refuse? Journal of Child Law 84:346

Lyon C M 2000 Loving smack – lawful assault. A contradiction in human rights and law. Institute of Public Policy Research, London

Lyon C M 2003 Child abuse, 3rd edn. Family Law, Bristol

Lyon C M 2004 Light taps and loving smacks. New Law Journal 1069

Lyon C M 2005 Toothless tigers and dogs breakfasts: enhancing or minimising the rights of children to better protection of their interests. Part I. Representing Children 17(4):226–238

Lyon C M 2006a Toothless tigers and dogs breakfasts: enhancing or minimising the rights of children to better protection of their interests. Part II. Representing Children 18(1):38–53

Lyon C M 2006b Toothless tigers and dogs breakfasts: enhancing or minimising the rights of children to better protection of their interests. Part III. Representing Children 18(2):128–143

Lyth I M 1998 Containing anxiety in institutions. Free Association Books, London

Macaskill C 1991 Adopting or fostering a sexually abused child. BAAF, London

Maccoby E E 1980 Social development: psychology growth and the parent–child relationship. Harcourt Brace Jovanovich, New York

Macdonald G, Roberts H 1995 What works in the early years? Barnardo's, Barkingside, Ilford

MacKay, Lord Chancellor 1990 The Joseph Jackson Memorial Lecture, 139 NLJ 505 at 508.

Macleod M 1999 The abuse of children in institutional settings: children's perspectives. In: Stanley M, Manthorpe J, Penhale J (eds) Institutional abuse – perspectives across the lifecourse. Routledge, London

Madu S N, Peltzer K 2000 Risk factors and child sexual abuse among secondary school students in the northern province (South Africa). Child Abuse and Neglect 24:259–268

Maher P (ed) 1987 Child abuse: the educational perspective. Blackwell, London

Main M, Solomon J 1986 Discovery of a new, insecure-disorganized/disoriented attachment pattern. In: Yogman M, Brazelton T B (eds) Affective development in infancy. Ablex, Norwood, NJ, p 95–124

Main M, Solomon J 1990 Procedures for identifying infants as disorganised/disoriented during the Ainsworth Strange Situation. In: Greenberg M, Cicchetti D, Cummings E (eds) Attachment in the preschool years. University of Chicago Press, Chicago, p 121–160

Mallon B 2002 Dream time with children: learning to dream, dreaming to learn. Jessica Kingsley, London

Malone C, Farthing L, Marce L (eds) 1996 The memory bird: survivors of sexual abuse. Virago, London

Maltz W 1991 The sexual healing journey: a guide for survivors of sexual abuse. Harper Collins, New York

Maluccio A N, Ainsworth F, Thoburn J 2000 Child welfare outcome research in the United States, the United Kingdom, and Australia. Child Welfare League of America, Washington, DC

Mandeville-Norden R, Beech A 2004 Community-based treatment of sex offenders. Journal of Sexual Aggression 10(2):193

Mann R E 2004 Innovations in sex offender treatment. Journal of Sexual Aggression 10(2):141–152

Manocha K, Mezey G 1998 British adolescents who sexually abuse: a descriptive study. Journal of Forensic Psychiatry 3:588–608

Marchant R, Jones M 2000 Assessing the needs of disabled children and their families. In: Assessing children in need and their families: practice guidance. DoH, London

Marchant R, Page M 2003 Child protection practice with disabled children. In: It doesn't happen to disabled children. NSPCC, London

Marchant S, Davidson L, Garcia J, Parsons J 2001 Addressing domestic violence through maternity services: policy and practice. Midwifery 17:164–170

Markie-Dadds C, Sanders M R 2006 A controlled evaluation of an enhanced self-directed behavioural family intervention for parents of children with conduct problems in rural and remote areas. Behaviour Change 23(1):55–72

Markowe H L J 1988 The frequency of childhood sexual abuse in the UK. Health Trends 20(1):2–6

Markowe H L J 1991 Epidemiological assessment of studies of child abuse. Paper given at BASPCAN conference Turning Research into Practice, Leicester

Marrett M 1991 Raw deal for black children in care. Community Care (Inside) 28 February:vii–viii

Marris P 1974 Loss and change. Routledge, London

Mars M 1989 Child sexual abuse and race issues. In: British Agencies for Adoption and Fostering (ed) After abuse papers: papers on caring and planning for a child who has been sexually abused. BAAF, London

Marsh D (ed) 1998 Comparing policy networks. Open University Press, Buckingham

Marsh D, Rhodes R A W 1992 Policy networks in British government. Clarendon Press, Oxford

Marsh M, Peel M 1999 Leaving care in partnership. TSO, London

Marsh P, Crow G 1998 Family group conferences in child welfare: working together for children, young people and their families. Blackwell, Oxford

Marsh P, Triseliotis J 1996 Ready to practice? Social workers and probation officers: their training and first year of work. Avebury, Aldershot

Marshall K 1997 Children's rights in the balance. TSO, Edinburgh

Marshall W L, Barbaree H E 1988 The long term evaluation of a behavioral treatment program. Behavior, Research and Therapy 26:499–511

Marshall W, Barbaree H 1990 An integrated theory of the etiology of sex offending. In: Marshall W, Laws D R, Barbaree H (eds) Handbook of sexual assault. Plenum, New York

Marshall W, Anderson D, Fernandez Y 1999 Cognitive–behavioural treatment of sex offenders. Wiley, Chichester

Martin H P, Rodeheffer M 1976 Learning and intelligence. In: Martin H P (ed) The abused child: a multidisciplinary approach to developmental issues and treatment. Ballinger, Cambridge, MA

Mason C, Regan S, Thorpe D, May-Chahal C 2004 Report on children and families referrals to Oldham Borough Council Social Services Department for the month of April 2003. Department of Applied Social Science, Lancaster University, Lancaster

Mason C, May-Chahal C, Regan S, Thorpe D 2004 Report on children and families referrals to Oldham Borough Council Social Services for the month of April 2003. Department of Applied Social Science, Lancaster University

Masson H 1995 Children and adolescents who sexually abuse other children: responses to an emerging problem. Journal of Social Welfare and Family Law 17:325–336

Masson H, Hackett S 2003 A decade on from the NCH Report 1992: adolescent sexual aggression policy, practice and service delivery across the UK and Republic of Ireland. Journal of Sexual Aggression 9:109–124

Masson J 2005 Emergency intervention to protect children using and avoiding legal controls. Child and Family Law Quarterly 17(1):75–96

Masson J, Winn Oakley M 1999 Out of hearing: representing children in care proceedings. Wiley, Chichester

Masson J, Winn Oakley M 2004 After dark – the use of police powers of protection. Online.

Mathews R, Matthews J, Speltz K 1989 Female sexual offenders. Safer Society Press, Orwell

May M 1973 Innocence and experience: the evolution of the concept of juvenile delinquency in the mid-nineteenth-century. Victorian Studies 181:7–29

May-Chahal C, CAPCAE 2006 Child maltreatment in the family: a European perspective. European Journal of Social Work 9(1):3–20

May-Chahal C, Cawson P 2005 Measuring child maltreatment in the United Kingdom: a study of the prevalence of child abuse and neglect. Child Abuse and Neglect 29(9):969–984

May-Chahal C, Coleman S 2003 Safeguarding children and young people. Routledge, London

Mayer J E, Timms N 1970 The client speaks. Routledge, London

McCann J, Stein A, Fairburn C, Dunger D 1994 Eating habits and attitudes of mothers of children with non-organic failure to thrive. Archives of Diseases in Childhood 70:234–236

McCarlie C, Brady M 2005 The extra dimension: developing a risk management framework. In: Calder M (ed) Children and young people who sexually abuse: new theory, research and practice developments. Russell House, Lyme Regis

McCurdy K, Daro D 1993 Current trends in child abuse reporting and fatalities: the results of the 1992 annual fifty-state survey. National Center on Child Abuse Research, Working Paper No. 808. National Committee to Prevent Child Abuse, Chicago

McDonald G 2001 Effective interventions for child abuse and neglect. Wiley, Chichester

McEwan J 1999 In defence of vulnerable witnesses: the Youth Justice and Criminal Evidence Act 1999. International Journal of Evidence and Proof 4:1–30

McGee H, Garavan R, de Barra M, Byrne J, Conroy R 2003 The SAVI report: sexual abuse and violence in Ireland. Dublin Rape Crisis Centre and the Liffey Press, Dublin

McGoldrick M, Giordano J, Pearce J (eds) 1996 Ethnicity and family therapy, 2nd edn. Guilford Press, New York

McIntyre C, Collinson M 1997 Failure to thrive: a prevalence audit to monitoring. Health Visitor 70:254–256

McKeigue B, Beckett C 2004 Care proceedings under the 1989 Children Act: rhetoric and reality. British Journal of Social Work 34:831–849

McKenna J, Mosko S, Dungy C, McAninch J 1990 Sleep and arousal patterns of co-sleeping human mother/infant pairs: a preliminary physiological study with implications for the study of Sudden Infant Death Syndrome (SIDS). American Journal of Physical Anthropology 83:331–347

McMillan H L, Fleming J E, Trocme N et al 1997 Prevalence of child physical and sexual abuse in the community. Journal of the American Medical Association 278(2):131–135

Meadow S 1993 ABC of child abuse, 2nd edn. BMJ Publishing, London

Mearns D, Thorne B 1988 Person-centred counselling in action. Sage, London

Melhuish E C 2004 A literature review of the impact of early years provision on young children, with emphasis given to children from disadvantaged backgrounds. Prepared for the Audit Office. National Audit Office, London

Melhuish E, Belsky J, Tunstill J, Meadows P 2005 National evaluation of Sure Start. University of London, London

Merkel-Holguin L, Nixon P, Burford G 2003 Learning with families: a synopsis of FGDM research and evaluation in child welfare. Protecting Children 18(1–2):2–11

Middleton L 1992 Children first: working with children and disability. Venture Press, Birmingham

Mihalopoulos C, Sanders M R, Turner K M T, Murphy-Brennan M, Carter R (in submission[AU10]) Does the Triple P – Positive Parenting Program provide value for money?

Miller D 2003 Disabled children and abuse. In: It doesn't happen to disabled children. NSPCC, London

Miller J, Ridge T 2002 Parents, children, families and new labour: developing family policy. In: Powell M (ed) Evaluating New Labour's welfare reforms. Policy Press, Bristol

Miller-Perrin C L, Perrin R D 1999 Child maltreatment: an introduction. Sage, Thousand Oaks, CA

Millham S, Bullock R, Hosie K, Haak M 1986 Lost in care: the family contacts of children in care. Gower, Aldershot

Milner J 1996 Men's resistance to social workers. In: Fawcett B, Featherstone B, Hearn J, Toft C (eds) Violence and gender relations: theories and interventions. Sage, London

Milner J, O'Byrne P 2002 Assessment in social work, 2nd edn. Palgrave, London

Milner P, Carolin B 1999 Time to listen to children: personal and professional communication. Routledge, London

Ministry of Health and Welfare (South Korea) 2003 Committee on the Rights of the Child. Ministry of Health and Welfare, Seoul

Minuchin S 1974 Families and family therapy. Harvard University Press, Cambridge, MA

Monck E, Bentovim A, Goodall G et al 1996 Child sexual abuse: a descriptive and treatment study. Studies in child protection. HMSO, London

Monck E, Reynolds J, Wigfall V 2003 Permanent placement for young children: the role of concurrent planning. BAAF, London

Moore J 1992 The ABC of child protection. Ashgate, Aldershot

Moran P, Ghate D, van de Merwe A 2004 What works in parenting support? A review of the international evidence. Policy Research Bureau. Research Report 574. DfES Publications, Nottingham

Morgan D 1996 Family connections: an introduction to family studies. Polity Press, Cambridge

Morgan R 2005 A national survey of the views of foster children, foster carers and birth parents about foster care. CSCI, London

Morris A, Giller H, Szwed E, Geach H 1980 Justice for children. Macmillan, London

Morris J 1998 Still missing? Vol 2: Disabled children and the Children Act. The Who Cares? Trust, London

Morris J 1999 Disabled children, child protection systems and the Children Act. Child Abuse Review 8:91–108

Morris J 2002 A lot to say! A guide for social workers, personal advisors and others working with disabled children and young people with communication disorders. Scope, London

Morrison T 1998 Partnership, collaboration and change under the Children Act. In: Adcock M, White R (eds) Significant harm: its management and outcome, 2nd edn. Significant Publications, Croydon, p 121–147

Morrison T 2000 Working together to safeguard children: challenges and changes for interagency co-ordination in child protection. Journal of Interprofessional Care 14(4):363–373

Morton N, Browne K D 1998 Theory and observation of attachment and its relation to child maltreatment: a review. Child Abuse and Neglect 22(11):1093–1104

Moss M 1990 Abuse in the child care system – a pilot study by the National Association of Young People in Care. NAYPIC, London

Moustakas C 1953 Children in play therapy. McGraw-Hill, New York

Moustakas C 1959 Psychotherapy with children: the living relationship. Harper and Row, New York

Mudaly N, Goddard C 2006 The truth is longer than a lie: children's experiences of abuse and professional interventions. Jessica Kingsley, London

Mullen P E, Fleming J 1998 Long-term effects of child sexual abuse. Issues in Child Abuse and Prevention 9. Australian Institute of Family Studies, Melbourne

Mullender A, Morley B (eds) 1994 Putting the abuse of women on the child care agenda. Whiting and Birch, London

Munby J 2004 Making sure the child is heard. Representing Children 17(1):10–25

Munro E 1997 Letter about judgement teaching. Cited in Hollows A 2003 Making professional judgements in the framework for the assessment of children in need and their families. In: Calder M C, Hackett S (eds) Assessment in child care: using and developing frameworks for practice. Russell House, Lyme Regis, p 61–74

Munro E 1998 Improving social workers' knowledge base in child protection work. British Journal of Social Work 28:89–105

Munro E 1999 Common errors of reasoning in child protection work. Child Abuse and Neglect 23(8):745–758

Munro E 2000 Effective child protection. Sage, London

Munro E 2004 State regulation of parenting. Political Quarterly 75(2):180–184

Munro E 2005a Snooper squad. Guardian 31 May

Munro E 2005b A system's approach to investigating child abuse deaths. British Journal of Social Work 35(4):531–546

Munro E 2005c What tools do we need to improve identification of child abuse? Child Abuse Review 14:374–388

Munro E, Calder M C 2005 Where has child protection gone? Political Quarterly 76(3):439–445

Munro M 2002 Effective child protection. Sage, London

Murch M, Bader K 1984 Separate representation for parents and children: an examination of the initial phase. Family Law, Bristol

Murch M, Hooper D 1992 The family justice system. Family Law, Bristol

Murphy-Berman V 1994 A conceptual framework for thinking about risk assessment and case management in child protective services. Child Abuse and Neglect 18(2):193–201

Murray C J L, Gakidou E E, Frenk J 1999 Health inequalities and social group differences: what should we measure? Bulletin of the World Health Organization 77(7):537–552

Murray K 1995 Live television link: evaluation of its use by child witnesses in Scottish criminal trials. Scottish Law Commission, Edinburgh

Myers J, Bays J, Becker J, Berliner L, Corwin D, Saywitz K 1989 Expert testimony in child sexual abuse litigation. Nebraska Law Review 68(1/2):1–145

Myers J E B, Berliner L, Briere J et al (eds) 2002 The APSAC handbook on child maltreatment. Sage, Thousand Oaks, CA

National Assembly for Wales, Home Office 2001 Framework for the assessment of children in need and their families. National Assembly for Wales, Cardiff. Online. Available: www.wales.gov.uk/subichildren/content/childrenfirst.htm

National Commission of Inquiry into the Prevention of Child Abuse 1996 Childhood matters. TSO, London

National Research Council 1993 Understanding child abuse and neglect. National Academy Press, Washington, DC

National Society for the Prevention of Cruelty to Children 1995 So who are we supposed to trust now? Responding to abuse in care: the experiences of young people. NSPCC/Safe and Sound Partnership, London

National Society for the Prevention of Cruelty to Children 2003 It doesn't happen to disabled children. Report of the National Working Group on Child Protection and Disability. NSPCC, London

National Society for the Prevention of Cruelty to Children/Council for Disabled Children 2004 Safeguarding disabled children in residential special schools. NSPCC, London

National Statistics 2005 Statistics of education: children looked after by local authorities, year ending 31st March 2004. Vol 1: Commentary and Tables. TSO, London

National Statistics, Department for Education and Skills 2005 Children looked after by local authorities, year ending 31 March 2004. DfES, London

National Statistics, Department of Health 2003 Children looked after by local authorities, year ending 31 March 2002, England. DoH, London

National Statistics Online 2005 www.statistics.gov.uk

NCH Action for Children 1996 Children still in need. Refocusing child protection in the context of children in need. ADSS and NCH, London

Neil E 2000 The reasons why young children are placed for adoption: findings from a recently-placed sample. Child and Family Social Work 5(4):303–316

Neil E 2002 Managing face-to-face contact for young adopted children. In: Argent H (ed) Staying connected: managing contact arrangements in adoption. BAAF, London

Neil E, Howe D 2005 Contact in adoption and permanent foster care. BAAF, London

Neil E, Beek M, Schofield G 2003 Thinking about and managing contact in permanent placements: the differences and similarities between adoptive parents and foster carers. Clinical Child Psychology and Psychiatry 8(3):401–418

Nelson S, Baldwin N 2005 The Craigmillar project: neighbourhood mapping to improve children's safety from sexual crime. Child Abuse Review 13:415–425

New York State Commission on Quality of Care 1992 Child abuse and neglect in New York State Office of Mental Health and Office of Mental Retardation and Developmental Disabilities Residential Programs. NYS Commission on Quality of Care, Schenectady, New York

Newcomb M D, Locke T F 2001 Intergenerational cycle of maltreatment: a popular concept obscured by methodological limitations. Child Abuse and Neglect 25:1219–1240

Nijenhuis E R S, Van Engen A, Kusters I, Van der Hart O 2001 Peritraumatic somatoform and psychological dissociation in relation to recall of childhood sexual abuse. Journal of Trauma and Dissociation 2(3):49–68

Nixon S 1997 The limits of support in foster care. British Journal of Social Work 27:913–930

Nobes G, Smith M 2000 The relative extent of physical punishment and abuse by mothers and fathers. Trauma, Violence and Abuse 1(1):47–66

Norfolk Health Authority 2002 Summary report of the independent health review. Norfolk Health Authority, Cambridge. Online. Available: www.nscha.nhs.uk/4856/5327/Report%20of%20the%20Independent%20Health%20Review%20-%20Lauren%20Wright.pdf

Novaco R W 1978 Anger and coping with stress. In: Forey J P, Rathjen D P, Rathjen D P (eds) Cognitive–behaviour therapy. Plenum, New York

Nunno M 1992 The abuse of children in out-of-home care. Paper given at the Conference on Institutional Abuse. NSPCC, London

O'Callaghan D 1999 Young abusers with learning disabilities: towards better understanding and positive interventions. In: Calder M (ed) Working with young people who sexually abuse: new pieces of the jigsaw puzzle. Russell House, Lyme Regis

O'Hagan K 1989 Working with child sexual abuse. Open University Press, Milton Keynes

O'Neill T 2001 Children in secure accommodation: a gendered exploration of locked institutional care for children in trouble. Jessica Kingsley, London

O'Neill O 2002 A question of trust. BBC Reith Lectures. Cambridge University Press, Cambridge

O'Toole R, Turbett P, Nalepka C 1983 Theories, professional knowledge and diagnosis of child abuse. In: Finkelhor D, Gelles R J, Hotaling G T, Straus MA (eds) The dark side of families. Sage, Beverly Hills, CA, ch 22

Oaklander V 1978 Windows to our children: a gestalt approach to children and adolescents. The Center for Gestalt Development, New York (first published in 1969 by Real People Press, Moab, Utah)

Office for Children, Victorian Government 2005 Protecting children: the next steps. State of Victoria, Department of Human Services, Melbourne

Office of the Children's Rights Director for England 2005 Getting the best from complaints – the children's view. Online. Available: www.rights4me.org.uk

Office of the High Commissioner for Human Rights 1989 Convention on the rights of the child. Office of the United Nations High Commissioner for Human Rights, Geneva. Online. Available: www.unhchr.ch/html/menu3/b/k2crc.htm

Ogden P, Minton K 2000 Sensorimotor psychotherapy: one method for processing traumatic memory. Traumatology 6(3):1–20

Ogden P, Minton K, Pain C 2006 Trauma and the body: a sensorimotor approach to psychotherapy. W W Norton, New York

Oldfield A 1999 Listening: the first step toward communicating through music. In: Milner P, Carolin B (eds) Time to listen to children: personal and professional communication. Routledge, London, p 188–199

Olds D L, Henderson C R, Phelps C et al 1993 Effect of prenatal and infancy nurse home visitation on Government spending. Medical Care 31(2):155–174

Olds D, Henderson C J, Kitzman H, Cole R 1995 Effects of prenatal and infancy home visitation on surveillance of child maltreatment. Pediatrics 95:365–372

Olds D, Eckenrode J, Henderson C R et al 1997 Long term effects of home visitation on maternal life course and child abuse and neglect: 15 year follow up of a randomised controlled trial. Journal of the American Medical Association 278(8):637–643

Olds D, Henderson C, Eckenrode J 2002 Preventing child abuse and neglect with parental and infancy home visiting by nurses. In: Browne K D, Hanks H, Stratton P, Hamilton C (eds) Early prediction and prevention of child abuse: a handbook, 2nd edn. Wiley, Chichester, p 165–182

Olds D, Robinson J, Pettitt L et al 2005 Effects of home visits by paraprofessionals and by nurses: age 4 follow-up results of a randomized trial. Child: Care, Health and Development 32:245–247

Otway O 1996 Social work with children and families: from child welfare to child protection. In: Parton N (ed) Social theory, social change and social work. Routledge, London

Owen M, Farmer E 1996 Child protection in a multi-racial context. Policy and Politics 24(3):299–313

Packman J 1981 The child's generation, 2nd edn. Basil Blackwell/Martin Robertson, Oxford

Packman J 1986 Who needs care? Social work decisions about children. Blackwell, Oxford

Packman J, Hall C 1998 From care to accommodation: support, protection and care in child care services. TSO, London

PAIN, NISW, NSPCC 1997 Enquiries into alleged child abuse: promoting partnership with families. A policy and practice guide for elected members, senior managers, first line managers and practitioners. NSPCC, London

Parenting Education and Support Forum 2004 National occupation standards – work with parents. Draft Version 3, Consultation Document. Parenting Education and Support Forum, London

Parker J, Bradley G 2003 Social work practice: assessment, planning, intervention and review. Learning Matters, Exeter

Parker R (ed) 1980 Caring for separated children: plans, procedures and priorities. A report by a Working Party established by the National Children's Bureau. Macmillan, London

Parker R 1995 A brief history of child protection. In: Farmer E, Owen M (eds) Child protection practice: private risks and public remedies. HMSO, London

Parker R, Ward H, Jackson S et al 1991 Assessing outcomes in child care. HMSO, London

Parliamentary Assembly Debate 23 June 2004. 21st Sitting-Doc.10199

Parton C, Parton N 1989a Child protection: the law and dangerousness. In: Stevenson O (ed) Child abuse: public policy and professional practice. Harvester Wheatsheaf, Hemel Hempstead, ch 3

Parton C, Parton N 1989b Women, the family and child protection. Critical Social Policy 24:38–49

Parton N 1979 The natural history of child abuse: a study in social problem definition. British Journal of Social Work 9:431

Parton N 1985 The politics of child abuse. Macmillan, Basingstoke

Parton N 1990 Taking child abuse seriously. In: The Violence Against Children Study Group (eds) Taking child abuse seriously: contemporary issues in child protection theory and practice. Unwin Hyman, London

Parton N 1991 Governing the family: child care, child protection and the state. Macmillan, Houndmills, Basingstoke

Parton N 1995 Neglect as child protection: the political context and the practical outcomes. Children and Society 9(1):67–89

Parton N 1996 Child protection, family support and social work: a critical appraisal of the Department of Health research studies in child protection. Child and Family Social Work 1(1):3–11

Parton N (ed) 1997 Child protection and family support: current debates and future prospects. In: Child protection and family support: tensions, contradictions and possibilities. Routledge, London, p 1–24

Parton N 1998 Risk, advanced liberalism and child welfare: the need to rediscover uncertainty and ambiguity. British Journal of Social Work 28(1):5–27

Parton N 1999 Ideology, politics and policy. In: Stevenson O (ed) Child welfare in the UK, 1948–1998. Blackwell Science, Oxford

Parton N 2002 Protecting children: a socio-historical analysis. In: Wilson K, James A (eds) The child protection handbook, 2nd edn. Baillière Tindall, Edinburgh

Parton N 2004 From Maria Colwell to Victoria Climbié: reflections on public inquiries into child abuse a generation apart. Child Abuse Review 13(2): 80–94

Parton N 2006 Safeguarding childhood: early intervention and surveillance in a late modern society. Palgrave Macmillan, Basingstoke

Parton N, Thorpe D, Wattam C 1997 Child protection: risk and the moral order. Macmillan, London

Patel N, Naik D, Humphries B (eds) 1998 Visions of reality: religion and ethnicity in social work. CCETSW, London

Patterson G R 1982 Coercive family process. Castalia, Eugene, OR

Patterson G R 1986 Maternal rejection. Determinant or product for deviant child behaviour? In: Hartup W W, Rubin Z (eds) Relationships and development. Lawrence Erlbaum, Hillsdale, NJ

Paul A, Cawson P 2002 Safeguarding disabled children in residential settings. Child Abuse Review 11:262–281

Paul A, Cawson P, Paton J 2004 Safeguarding disabled children in residential special schools. NSPCC, London

Peckover S 2003 'I could have just done with a little more help': an analysis of women's help-seeking from health visitors in the context of domestic violence. Health and Social Care in the Community 11:275

Peel M, Ward H 2000 North Lincolnshire parenting project: report to the Area Child Protection Committee. Loughborough University, Loughborough

Penna S 2005 The Children Act 2004: child protection and social surveillance. Journal of Social Welfare and Family Law 27(2):143–157

Performance and Innovations Unit 2000 Review of adoption: issues for consultation. Cabinet Office, London

Perlman L A, Saakvitne K W 1995 Trauma and the therapist. Countertransference and vicarious traumatisation in psychotherapy with incest survivors. W W Norton, London

Pernanen K 1991 Alcohol in human violence. Guilford Press, London

Petrie S, Wilson K 1999 Towards the disintegration of child welfare services. Journal of Social Policy and Administration 33(2):181–197

Petticrew M, Roberts H 2004 Child public health and social welfare: lessons from the evidence. Child: Care, Health and Development 30:667–669

Pfohl S J 1977 The 'discovery' of child abuse. Social Problems 24:310–323

Pieterse J J, Van Urk H 1989 Maltreatment of children in the Netherlands: an update after ten years. Child Abuse and Neglect 13:263–269

Pigot T 1989 The report of the Advisory Group on Video Evidence. Home Office, London

Pinchbeck I, Hewitt M 1973 Children in English society. Routledge and Kegan Paul, London

Pincock S 2004 Poor communication lies at heart of NHS complaints, says ombudsman. British Medical Journal 328:10–11

Pithers W 1990 Relapse prevention with sexual aggressors. In: Marshall W, Laws D R, Barbaree H (eds) Handbook of sexual assault. Plenum, New York

Platt D 2001 Refocusing children's services: evaluation of an initial assessment process. Child and Family Social Work 6(2):139–148

Platt D 2004 The Children Bill and what it means for children's services. The unresolved issues of the Bill: emerging themes and unresolved issues. Inter-Agency Group Conference, London, July 15

Platt D 2005 Investigation or initial assessment of child concerns? The impact of the refocusing initiative on social work practice. British Journal of Social Work 36(2):267–281

Plotnikoff J, Woolfson R (eds) 1996 Reporting to court under the Children Act 1989. HMSO, London

Polnay J 2000 General practitioners and child protection conference participation: reasons for non-attendance and proposals for a way forward. Child Abuse Review 9:108–123

Powell C 1997 Protecting children in the Accident and Emergency department. Accident and Emergency Nursing 5:76–80

Powers J L, Mooney A, Nunno M 1990 Institutional abuse – a review of the literature. Journal of Child and Youth Care 4:81–95

Pratt J, Gordon P, Plamping D 1999 Working whole systems: putting theory into practice in organisations. King's Fund, London

PricewaterhouseCoopers 2004 Scoping the market for children's services. Report for the Department for Education and Skills. Final Report October 2004. PricewaterhouseCoopers LLC, London

Prime Minister's Review of Adoption 2000 Performance and Innovation Unit. TSO, London

Pringle K 1998 Children and social welfare in Europe. Open University Press, Buckingham

Pritchard C 2004 The child abusers: research and controversy. Open University Press, Maidenhead

Prosser J 1992 Child abuse investigations: the families' perspective. Evaluation Unit, Westminster College, Oxford

Puckering C 2005 Does it matter if my mum is depressed? Paper presented at the Child Psychology Matters, BPS Faculty for Children and Young People 7th Annual Conference, 15–16 September, Edinburgh

Pugh G, Parton N (eds) 2003 New Labour policy and its outcomes for children. Children and Society (Special Issue) 17(3)

Pugh R 1992 Schools and child abuse: training for teachers. Social Work Education 11(1):47–53

Putallaz M, Costanzo P R, Grimes C L, Sherman D M 1998 Intergenerational continuities and their influences on children's social development. Social Development 7: 389–427

Pynoos R, Eth S 1984 The child as witness to homicide. Journal of Social Issues 40:87–108

Pynoos R, Eth S 1986 Witness to violence: the child interview. Journal of the American Academy of Child Psychiatry 25(3):306–319

Quayle E, Erooga M, Wright L, Taylor N, Harbinson D 2006 Only pictures? Therapeutic work with internet sex offenders. Russell House, Lyme Regis

Quinton D 2004 Supporting parents: messages from research. Jessica Kingsley, London

Quinton D, Rushton A 1998 Joining new families: adoption and fostering in middle childhood. Wiley, Chichester

Radnor H, Ball S 1996 Local education authorities; accountability and control. Trentham, Stoke-on-Trent

Rae M, Murphy M, Collins C 1997 Breaking the chains. Nursing Times 93(6):26–28

Ramchandani P, McConachie H 2005 Mothers, fathers and their children's health. Child: Care, Health and Development 31:5–6

Ramchandani P, Joughin C, Zwi M 2001 Evidence-based child and adolescent mental health services: oxymoron or brave new dawn? Child Psychology and Psychiatry Review 6(2):59–64

Randall J, Henggeller S W 1999 Multisystemic therapy. In: Russ S W, Ollendick T H (eds) Handbook of psychotherapies with children and families. Kluwer/Plenum, New York

Raynes B 2005 When words aren't enough. Paper presented at: From Area Child Protection Committee to Local Safeguarding Children Board, 21 September 2005, Plymouth

Read J 1998 Child abuse and severity of disturbance among adult psychiatric inpatients. Child Abuse and Neglect 22:359–368

Reading R 2004 Impact of a general practice based group parenting programme: quantitative and qualitative results from a controlled trial at 12 months. Child: Care, Health and Development 30:550–561

Reddy L A, Files-Hall T M, Schaefer C E (eds) 2005 Empirically based play interventions for children. American Psychological Association, Washington, DC

Reder P, Duncan S 1995 The meaning of the child. In: Reder P, Lucey C (eds) Assessment of parenting: psychiatric and psychological contributions. Routledge, London

Reder P, Duncan S 1999 Lost innocents: a follow-up study of fatal child abuse. Routledge, London

Reder P, Duncan S 2002 Predicting fatal child abuse and neglect. In: Browne K D, Hanks H, Stratton P, Hamilton C (eds) Early prediction and prevention of child abuse: a handbook, 2nd edn. Wiley, Chichester

Reder P, Duncan S 2003 Understanding communication in child protection networks. Child Abuse Review 12:82–100

Reder P, Duncan S 2004a Making the most of the Victoria Climbié Inquiry report. Child Abuse Review 13(2):95–114

Reder P, Duncan S 2004b From Colwell to Climbié: inquiry into fatal child abuse. In: Stanley N, Manthorpe J (eds) The age of the inquiry. Brunner-Routledge, London, p 92–115

Reder P, Lucey C (eds) 1995 Significant issues in the assessment of parenting. In: Assessment of parenting: psychiatric and psychological contributions. Routledge, London, p 3–17

Reder P, Duncan S, Gray M 1993 Beyond blame: child abuse tragedies revisited. Routledge, London

Redgrave K 1987 Child's play: direct work with the deprived child. Boys and Girls Welfare Society, Cheadle

Reece R M, Ludwig S 2001 Child abuse: medical diagnosis and management. Lippincott, Williams and Wilkins, Philadelphia

Rees S 1978 Social work face to face. Edward Arnold, London

Rees S, Wallace A 1982 Verdicts on social work. Edward Arnold, London

Reid B, Long A 2002 Suspected child abuse: communicating with a child and her mother. Journal of Pediatric Nursing 17:229–235

Renzetti C M 1992 Violent betrayal: partner abuse in lesbian relationships. Sage, London

Rindfleisch N, Rabb J 1984 How much of a problem is resident mistreatment in child welfare institutions? Child Abuse and Neglect 15:249–260

Ritchie C 2005 Looked after children: time for change? British Journal of Social Work 35:761–767

Ritchie J, Ritchie J 1981 Child rearing and child abuse: the Polynesian context. In: Korbin J (ed) Child abuse and neglect: cross-cultural perspectives. University of California Press, Berkeley, CA, p 186–294

Roberts A R 1987 Psycho-social characteristics of batterers: a study of 234 men charged with domestic violence offences. Journal of Family Violence 2:81–94

Roberts J 1993 The importance of self-esteem to children and young people separated from their families. Adoption and Fostering 17(2):48–50

Roberts M 2001 Childcare policy. In: Foley P, Roche J, Tucker S (eds) Children in society: contemporary theory, policy and practice. Palgrave/Open University, Basingstoke

Rodwell S 2005 Responding to children who witness domestic violence: an exploration of the views and experiences of community nurses and midwives. Third Annual Postgraduate Conference, University of Dundee

Rogers C R (ed) 1951 Client-centred therapy: its current practice, implications and theory. Constable, London

Rose N, Miller P 1992 Political power beyond the state: problematics of government. British Journal of Sociology 43(25):173–205

Rose R, Philpot T 2004 The child's own story: life story work with traumatised children. Jessica Kingsley, London

Rose W 2001 Assessing children in need and their families: an overview of the framework. In: Horwath J (ed) The child's world: assessing children in need. Jessica Kingsley, London

Rosenbaum A, Hog S K, Adelman S A, Warnken W J, Fletcher K E, Kane R L 1994 Head injury in partner-abusive men. Journal of Consulting and Clinical Psychology 62:1187–1193

Rosenberg M S, Repucci N D 1983 Abusive mothers: perceptions of their own and their children's behaviour. Journal of Consulting and Clinical Psychology 51(5):674–682

Rosenman S, Rodgers B 2004 Childhood adversity in an Australian population. Social Psychiatry and Psychiatric Epidemiology 39(9):695–702

Rosenthal J, Motz J, Edmonson D, Groze V 1991 A descriptive study of abuse and neglect in out of home placement. Child Abuse and Neglect 15:249–260

Ross C 1997 Something to draw on: activities and interventions using an art therapy approach. Jessica Kingsley, London

Rouf K 1989 Journey through darkness: the path from victim to survivor. In: Lindsay G, Peake A (eds) Child sexual abuse: educational and child psychology, Vol. 6(1). The British Psychological Society, Disley, p 6–10

Rouse S 2002 Protecting children: the role of the health visitor. In: Wilson K, James A (eds) The child protection handbook, 2nd edn. Baillière Tindall, Edinburgh, p 305–318

Rowe J, Lambert L 1973 Children who wait. Association of British Adoption Agencies, London

Rowe J, Cain H, Hundleby M, Keane A 1984 Long-term foster care. Batsford, London

Rowe J, Hundleby M, Garnett L 1989 Child care now: a survey of placement patterns. BAAF Research Series 6. British Agencies for Adoption and Fostering, London

Roy M 1982 The abusive partner. Van Nostrand Reinhold, New York

Ruegger M (ed) 2000 Children's experiences of the guardian ad litem service and public law proceedings. In: Hearing the voice of the child: the representation of children's interests in public law proceedings. Russell House, Lyme Regis, S.33–43

Rushton A 2003 The adoption of looked after children: a scoping review of research. SCIE, London

Rushton A, Treseder J, Quinton D 1988 New parents for older children. BAAF, London

Russell D E 1983 The incidence and prevalence of intrafamilial and extrafamilial sexual abuse of female children. Child Abuse and Neglect 7:133–146

Russell D E H 1986 The secret trauma: incest in the lives of girls and women. Basic Books, New York

Russell J 1993 Out of bounds. Sage, London

Russell M, Lazenbatt A, Freeman R, Marcenes W 2004 Child physical abuse: health professionals' perceptions, diagnosis and response. British Journal of Community Nursing 9:332–338

Rustin M 2005 Conceptual analysis of critical moments in Victoria Climbié's life. Child and Family Social Work 10:11–19

Rutter M 1985 Aggression and the family. Acta Paedopsychiatrica 6:11–25

Rutter M P 1990 Sex in the forbidden zone. Collins, London

Rutter M 1999 Resilience concepts and findings: implications for family therapy. Journal of Family Therapy 21:119–144

Ruxton S 2002 Men, masculinities and poverty in the UK. Oxfam, Oxford

Ryan J, Thomas F 1987 The politics of mental handicap (revised edition). Free Association Books, London

Ryan M 2000 Working with fathers. Radcliffe Medical Press, Abingdon

Ryan S, Wiles D, Cash S, Siebert C 2005 Risk assessments: empirically supported or values driven? Children Youth Services Review 27:213–225

Ryan V 1999 Building attachments: how play therapists help children develop loving relationships. Keynote address, British Association for Play Therapists 7th Annual Conference, Leicester

Ryan V 2004 Adapting non-directive play therapy interventions for children with attachment disorders. Clinical Child Psychology and Psychiatry 9(1):75–87

Ryan V Filial therapy: helping children and new carers to form secure attachment relationships. British Journal of Social Work (forthcoming)

Ryan V, Wilson K 1995a Child therapy and evidence in court proceedings: tensions and some solutions. British Journal of Social Work 25:157–172

Ryan V, Wilson K 1995b Non-directive play therapy as a means of recreating optimal infant socialisation patterns. Early Development and Parenting 4(1):29–38

Ryan V, Wilson K 2000a Case studies in non-directive play therapy. Jessica Kingsley, London

Ryan V, Wilson K 2000b Conducting child assessments for court proceedings: the use of non-directive play therapy. Clinical Child Psychology and Psychiatry 5(2):267–279

Ryan V, Wilson K, Fisher T 1995 Partnerships in therapeutic work with children. Journal of Social Work Practice 9(2):131–140

Ryburn M 1992 Contested adoptions. BAAF Adoption and Fostering Journal 16(4):29–38

Sainsbury E 1975 Social work with families. Routledge and Kegan Paul, London

Sainsbury E, Nixon S, Phillips D 1982 Social work in focus: clients and social workers' perceptions in long-term social work. Routledge and Kegan Paul, London

Saleeby D (ed) 1992 The strengths perspective in social work practice. Longman, New York

Sallnas M, Vinnerljung B, Westermark P K 2004 Breakdown of teenage placements in Swedish foster and residential care. Child and Family Social Work 9:141–152

Salter A 1988 Treating child sex offenders and victims? Assessment and treatment of child sex offenders. Sage, Beverley Hills, CA

Salter A 1995 Transforming trauma. Sage, Thousand Oaks, CA

Samra-Tibbetts C, Raynes B 1999 Assessment and planning. In: Calder M C, Horwath J (eds) Working for children on the child protection register. Ashgate, Aldershot, p 81–118

Sanders B, Becker-Lausen E 1995 The measurement of psychological maltreatment: early data on the child abuse and trauma scale. Child Abuse and Neglect 19:315–323

Sanders M 1999 The triple-P positive parenting program: towards an empirically validated multilevel parenting and family support strategy for the prevention of behaviour and emotional problems in children. Clinical Child and Family Psychology Review 2:71–90

Sanders M, Cann W 2002 Promoting positive parenting as an abuse prevention strategy. In: Browne K D, Hanks H, Stratton P, Hamilton C (eds) Early prediction and prevention of child abuse: a handbook, 2nd edn. Wiley, Chichester, p 145–164

Sanders R, Colton M, Roberts S 1999 Child abuse fatalities and cases of extreme concern: lessons from reviews. Child Abuse and Neglect 23(3):257–268

Sanders M, Cann W, Markie-Dadds C 2003 Why a universal population-level approach to the prevention of child abuse is essential. Child Abuse Review 12:145–154

Saradjian J (in association with Hawks H) 1996 Women who sexually abuse children. Wiley, Chichester

Sariola H, Uutela A 1994 The prevalence of child sexual abuse in Finland. Child Abuse and Neglect 18(10):827–835

Schaffer H R 1998 Making decisions about children, 2nd edn. Blackwell, Oxford

Schene P 1987 Is child abuse decreasing? Commentary on Gelles and Straus paper. Journal of Interpersonal Violence 2:225–227

Schofield G 2001 Resilience and family placement: a lifespan perspective. Adoption and Fostering 25(3):6–19

Schofield G 2002a The significance of a secure base: a psychosocial model of long-term foster care. Child and Family Social Work 7(4):259–272

Schofield G 2002b Part of the family. BAAF, London

Schofield G, Beek M, Sargent K 2000 Growing up in foster care. BAAF, London

Schore A N 1994 Affect regulation and the origin of the self. Lawrence Erlbaum, Hillsdale, NJ

Schore A N 2003a Affect regulation and the repair of the self. W W Norton, London

Schore A N 2003b Affect regulation and disorders of the self. W W Norton, London

Schultz L G 1960 The wife assaulter. Journal of Social Therapy 6:103–112

Schweinhart L J, Montie J, Xiang Z, Barnett W S, Belfield C R, Nores M 2004 Lifetime effects: the High/Scope Perry Preschool Study through age 40. High/Scope Press, Ypsilanti

Scottish Executive 2000 Report of the Joint Futures Group. Scottish Executive, Edinburgh

Scottish Executive 2002 It's everyone's job to make sure I'm alright: report of the Child Protection Audit and Review. Scottish Executive, Edinburgh

Scottish Executive 2005 Getting it right for every child: proposals for action. Scottish Executive, Edinburgh

Scourfield J 2003 Gender and child protection. Palgrave, Basingstoke

Scourfield J, Campling J 2002 Gender and child protection. Palgrave Macmillan, Basingstoke

Scutt N 1998 Child advocacy. In: Cloke C, Davis M (eds) Participation and empowerment in child protection. Pitman, London

Seaman S, Turner K, Hill M, Stafford A, Walker M 2005 Parenting and children's resilience in disadvantaged communities. Joseph Rowntree Foundation, York

Sebre S, Sprugevica I, Novotni A et al 2004 Cross-cultural comparisons of child-reported emotional and physical abuse: rates, risk factors and psychosocial symptoms. Child Abuse and Neglect 28:113–127

Secretary of State for Social Services 1974 Report of the inquiry into the care and supervision provided in relation to Maria Colwell. HMSO, London

Secretary of State for Social Services 1988 Report of the inquiry into child abuse in Cleveland. Cmnd 412. HMSO, London

Sedlak A J 1990 Technical amendment to the study findings: national incidence and prevalence of child abuse and neglect: 1988. Westat, Rockville, MD

Seebohm Report 1968 Report of the Committee on Local Authority and Allied Personal Social Services. Cmnd 3703. HMSO, London

Segal L 1987 Is the future female? Troubled thoughts on contemporary feminism. Virago, London

Segal L 1997 Slow motion: changing men, changing masculinities, 2nd edn. Virago, London

Seligman M E P, Peterson C 1986 A learned helplessness perspective on childhood depression: theory and research. In: Rutter M, Tizard C, Reads R (eds) Depression and young people: developmental and clinical perspectives. Guilford Press, New York

Sellick C 1992 Supporting short-term foster carers. Avebury, Aldershot

Sellick C, Connolly J 2002 National survey of independent fostering agencies. UEA Centre for Research on the Child and Family, Norwich

Sellick C, Howell D 2004 Innovative, tried and tested: a review of good practice in fostering. SCIE, London

Sellick C, Thoburn J, Philpot T 2004 What works in adoption and foster care? Barnardo's, Barkingside, Ilford

Selwyn J, Sturgess W, Quinton D, Baxter C 2003 Costs and outcomes of non-infant adoptions: report to the Department for Education and Skills. DfES, London

Senn C Y 1988 Vulnerable: sexual abuse and people with an intellectual handicap. Roecher Institute, Ontario

Sennett R 2003 Respect: the formation of character in an age of inequality. Penguin, London

Shapiro L 1984 The new short-term therapies for children: a guide for helping professionals and parents. Prentice-Hall, Englewood Cliffs, NJ

Shaughnessy M F 1984 Institutional child abuse. Children and Youth Services Review 6:311–318

Shaw C 1997 Remember my messages. The Who Cares? Trust, London

Shaw M, Hipgrave T 1983 Specialist fostering. Batsford, London

Sheinberg M 1992 Navigating treatment impasses at the disclosure of incest: combining ideas from family and social construction and family process. Family Process 31:201–216

Sheinberg M, True F, Frankel P 1994 Treating the sexually abused child: a recursive multi-model programme. Family Process 33:263–276

Shemmings D 2000 Professional attitudes to children's participation in decision-making: dichotomous accounts and doctrinal contests. Child and Family Social Work 5:235–243

Shemmings D, Shemmings Y 1996 Building trust with families when making enquiries. In: Platt D, Shemmings D (eds) Making enquiries into alleged child abuse and neglect: partnership with families. Pavilion, Brighton

Shemmings Y, Shemmings D 2001 Empowering children and family members to participate in the assessment process. In: Horwath J (ed) The child's world: assessing children in need. Jessica Kingsley, London, p 114–128

Shepherd A M 1994 Ensuring children's voices are heard in the child protection process and child care decision making: strategies for improving policy and practice. Advanced Practice Dissertation, University of East Anglia, Norwich

Shonkoff J, Phillips D (eds) 2000 National Research Council and Institute of Medicine. Neurons to neighborhoods: the science of early childhood development. National Academy Press, Washington, DC

Sidebotham P 2001 An ecological approach to child abuse: A creative use of scientific models in research and practice. Child Abuse Review 10(2):311–320

Sidebotham P 2003 Red skies, risk factors and early indicators. Child Abuse Review 12:41–45

Sidebotham P, ALSPAC Study Team 2001 Culture, stress and the parent–child relationship: a qualitative study of parents' perceptions of parenting. Child: Care, Health and Development 27:469–485

Siegal J M, Sorenson S B, Golding J M et al 1987 The prevalence of childhood sexual assault: the Los Angeles epidemiologic catchment area project. American Journal of Epidemiology 126:1141–1153

Siegel D J 1999 The developing mind: toward a neurobiology of interpersonal experience. Guilford Press, New York

Simmonds J 2004 Primitive forces in society: holding the unaccompanied asylum-seeking child in mind. Adoption and Fostering 28(2):68–75

Simpson C M, Simpson R J, Power K G, Salter A, Williams G-J 1994 GPs' and health visitors' participation in child protection case conferences. Child Abuse Review 3:211–230

Sinclair I 2005 Fostering now: messages from research. Jessica Kingsley, London

Sinclair I, Gibbs I 1998 Children's homes: a study in diversity. In: DOH Caring for children away from home – messages from research. Wiley, Chichester

Sinclair I, Gibbs I, Wilson K 2004 Foster carers: why they stay and why they leave. Jessica Kingsley, London

Sinclair I, Wilson K, Gibbs I 2005a Foster placements: why they succeed and why they fail. Jessica Kingsley, London

Sinclair I, Baker C, Wilson K, Gibbs I 2005b Foster children: where they go and how they get on. Jessica Kingsley, London

Sinclair R, Bullock R 2002 Learning from past experience: a review of serious case reviews. DoH, London

Skellington R 1996 'Race' in Britain today, 2nd edn. Open University/Sage, London

Skellington R, Morris P 1992 'Race' in Britain today. Open University/Sage, London

Skinner C 2003 New Labour and family policy. In: Bell M, Wilson K (eds) The practitioner's guide to working with families. Palgrave Macmillan, Basingstoke

Skuse D 1985 Failure to thrive: failure to feed. Community Paediatric Group Newsletter (British Paediatric Association) August:6–7

Sloper P 2004 Facilitators and barriers for co-ordinated multi-agency services. Child: Care, Health and Development 30(6):571–580

Smallbone S 2005 Attachment and insecurity as a predisposing factor for sexually abusive behaviour by young people. In: Calder M (ed) Children and young people who sexually abuse: new theory, research and practice developments. Russell House, Lyme Regis

Smart C, Neale B 1999 Family fragments. Polity Press, Cambridge

Smart C, Neale B, Wade A 2001 The changing experience of childhood, families and divorce. Polity Press, Cambridge

Smedley B 1999 Child protection: facing up to fear. In: Milner P, Carolin B (ed) Time to listen to children: personal and professional communication. Routledge, London, p 112–125

Sobsey D, Varnhagen C 1988 Sexual abuse and exploitation of people with disabilities: a study of the victims. Unpublished paper cited in Westcott H L 1991 Institutional abuse of children – from research to policy – a review. NSPCC, London

Social Exclusion Unit 2000 Young people: towards a national strategy for neighbourhood renewal. Report of Policy Action Team 12. TSO, London

Social Services Committee 1984 Children in care (HC 360). HMSO, London

Social Services Inspectorate 1990 In the interests of children, an inspection of the guardian ad litem and reporting officer service. HMSO, London

Social Services Inspectorate 1995 An analysis of a sample of English services plans. HMSO, London

Social Services Inspectorate 1997a Messages from inspections: responding to families in need. Inspection of assessment, planning and decision-making in family support services. DoH, London

Social Services Inspectorate 1997b Messages from inspections: child protection inspections 1992/1996. DoH, London

Social Services Inspectorate 1998 Circular on adoption. TSO, London

Social Services Inspectorate 2002 Fostering for the future: an inspection of foster care services. DoH, London

Social Work Inspection Agency 2005 An inspection into the care and protection of children in Eilean Siar. Scottish Executive, Edinburgh

Solomon J, George C 1999 Attachment disorganization. Guilford Press, New York

Solomons G, Abel C M, Epsley S 1981 A community development approach to the prevention of institutional and societal child maltreatment. Child Abuse and Neglect 5:135–140

Solum L L, Schaffer M A 2003 Ethical problems experienced by school nurses. Journal of School Nursing 19:330–337

Sonkin D, Martin D, Walker L 1985 The male batterer: a treatment approach. Springer, New York

Soul Kids Campaign 1977 Report of the Steering Group of the Soul Kids Campaign. Association of British Fostering and Adoption Agencies, London

Southall D P, Samuels M P, Golden M H 2003 Classification of child abuse by motive and degree rather than type of injury. Archives of Diseases in Childhood 88:101–104

Speight N 1989 Non-accidental injury. In: Meadow R (ed) ABC of child abuse. BMJ Publishing, London

Spencer N 2003 Parenting programmes. Archives of Disease in Childhood 88:99–100

Spencer N, Baldwin N 2005 Economic, cultural and social contexts of neglect. In: Taylor J, Daniel B (eds) Child neglect: practice issues for health and social care. Jessica Kingsley, London

Spratt T 2000 Decision making by senior social workers at point of first referral. British Journal of Social Work 30:597–618

Spratt T, Callan J 2004 Parents' views on social work interventions in child welfare cases. British Journal of Social Work 34:199–224

Spring J 1987 Cry hard and swim: the story of an incest survivor. Virago, London

Srivastava O P, Fountain R, Ayre P, Stewart J 2003 The graded care profile: a measure of care. In: Calder M C, Hackett S (eds) Assessment in child care: using and developing frameworks for practice. Russell House, Lyme Regis, p 227–246

Srivastava O P, Stewart J, Fountain R, Ayre P 2005 Common operational approach using the 'graded care profile' in cases of neglect. In: Taylor J, Daniel B (eds) Child neglect. Practice issues for health and social care. Jessica Kingsley, London, p 131–146

Stalker K 1990 Share the care. Jessica Kingsley, London

Stanley N, Penhale B, Riordan D, Barbour R S, Holden S 2003 Child protection and mental health services. Interprofessional responses to the needs of mothers. Policy Press, Bristol

Stark C, Paterson B, Henderson T, Kidd B, Godwin M 1997 Counting the dead. Nursing Times 93:34–37

Starr R H 1982 Child abuse and prediction: policy implications. Ballinger, Cambridge, MA

Starr R H 1988 Pre- and perinatal risk and physical abuse. Journal of Reproductive and Infant Psychology 6(3):125–138

Starr R H 1990 The need for child maltreatment research and program evaluation. Journal of Family Violence 5(4):311–319

Statham J 2004 Effective services to support children in special circumstances. Child: Care, Health and Development 30:589–598

Stedman Jones C 1971 Outcast London. Penguin, Harmondsworth

Stein M 1993 The abuses and uses of residential care: surviving childhood adversity. Social Services Press, Dublin

Stein M, Carey K 1986 Leaving care. Blackwell, London

Stepans M B, Thompson C L, Buchanan M L 2002 The role of the nurse on a transdisciplinary early assessment team. Public Health Nursing 19:238–245

Stevenson J 1999 The treatment of the long-term sequelae of child abuse. Journal of Child Psychology and Psychiatry 40(1):89–113

Stevenson O (ed) 1989 Multidisciplinary work in child protection. In: Child abuse: professional practice and public policy. Harvester Wheatsheaf, Hemel Hempstead, ch 8

Stevenson O 1991 Preface. In: CCETSW (ed) The teaching of child care in the Diploma in Social Work: guidance notes for programme planners: improving social work education and training, No. 6. CCETSW, London, p 5–7

Stevenson O 1995 Case conferences in child protection. In: Wilson K, James A (eds) The child protection handbook. Baillière Tindall, London

Stevenson O 1998a Neglected children: issues and dilemmas. Blackwell Science, Oxford

Stevenson O (ed) 1998b Child welfare in the UK. Blackwell Science, Oxford

Stevenson O 1998c Neglect: where now? Some reflections. Child Abuse Review 7:111–115

Stevenson O (ed) 1999 Child welfare in the UK, 1948–1998. Blackwell Science, Oxford

Stevenson O 2003 Safeguarding children: critical factors in success and failure. Keynote paper, BASPCAN Conference, June 2003, University of York

Stevenson O 2005a Child protection and mental health services: interprofessional responses to the needs of mothers [book review]. Child and Family Social Work 10(1):87

Stevenson O 2005b Working together in cases of neglect: key issues. In: Taylor J, Daniel, B (eds) Child neglect. Practice issues for health and social care. Jessica Kingsley, London, p 98–113

Stevenson O (ed) 2005c Interdisciplinary working in child welfare. Child and Family Social Work (Special issue) 10(3)

Stone B 2003 A framework for assessing neglect. In: Calder M C, Hackett S (eds) Assessment in child care: using and developing frameworks for practice. Russell House, Lyme Regis, p 214–226

Stone M 1990 Child protection work: a professional guide. Venture Press, Birmingham

Stone M 1993 Child protection: a model for risk assessment of physical abuse/neglect. Surrey County Council Social Services, Kingston upon Thames

Stratton P 2003 Contemporary families as contexts for development: contributions from systemic family therapy. In: Valsiner J, Connolly K (eds) Handbook of developmental psychology. Sage, New York, p 333–357

Stratton P, Hanks H 1991 Incorporating circularity in defining and classifying child maltreatment. Human Systems 2:181–200

Stratton P, Swaffer R 1988 Maternal causal beliefs for abused and handicapped children. Journal of Reproductive and Infant Psychology 5:201–216

Straus M A 1979 Family patterns and child abuse in a nationally representative American sample. Child Abuse and Neglect 3(1):213–225

Straus M A 1980 A sociological perspective on causes of family violence. In: Green R (ed) Violence and the family. Bould and Westview, New York, p 7–13

Straus M A 1997 Physical assaults by women partners: a major social problem. In: Walsh M R (ed) Women, men and gender: ongoing debates. Yale University Press, New Haven, CT, p 210–221

Straus M A 1999 The controversy over domestic violence by women: a methodological, theoretical and sociology of science analysis. In: Arriaga X B, Oskamp S (eds) Violence in intimate relationships. Sage, Thousand Oaks, CA, p 17–44

Straus M A, Gelles R J 1986 Societal change and change in family violence from 1975 to 1985 as revealed by two national surveys. Journal of Marriage and the Family 48:465–479

Straus M, Gelles R 1987 Family violence, 2nd edn. Sage, London

Straus M A, Smith C 1990 Family patterns and child abuse. In: Straus M A, Gelles R J (eds) Physical violence in American families: risk factors and adaptations to violence in 8,145 families. Transaction Publishers, New Brunswick, NJ, p 245–261

Straus M A, Gelles R J, Steinmetz S K 1988 Behind closed doors: violence in the American family, 2nd edn. Sage, Beverly Hills, CA

Straus M A, Hamby S L, Finkelhor D et al 1998 Identification of child maltreatment with the parent–child conflict tactics scales: development and psychometric data for a national sample of American parents. Child Abuse and Neglect 22(4):249–270

Stuart M, Baines C 2004 Progress on safeguards for children living away from home. Joseph Rowntree Foundation, York

Sullivan J 2002 The spiral of sexual abuse: a conceptual framework for understanding and illustrating the evolution of sexually abusive behaviour. NOTA News 41:17–21

Sullivan P M, Knutson J F 2000 Maltreatment and disabilities: a population-based epidemiological study. Child Abuse and Neglect 24:1257–1274

Summit R 1988 Hidden victims, hidden pain: societal avoidance of child sexual abuse. In: Wyatt G E, Powell G J (eds) Lasting effects in child sexual abuse. Sage, Newbury Park, CA

Sutton C 2000 Child and adolescent behaviour problems: a multi-disciplinary approach to assessment and intervention. BPS Books, Leicester

Sutton C, Utting D, Farrington D 2004 Support from the start. DfES, London

Sweet M A, Appelbaum M I 2004 Is home visiting an effective strategy? A meta-analytic review of home visiting programs for families with young children. Child Development 75(5):1435–1456

Sykes J, Sinclair I, Wilson K, Gibbs I 2002 Kinship and stranger foster care: how do they compare? Adoption and Fostering 26(2):39–48

Sylvester J, Bentovim A, Stratton P, Hanks H 1995 Using spoken attributions to classify abusive families. Child Abuse and Neglect 19:1221–1232

Tang C 2002 Childhood experience of sexual abuse among Hong Kong Chinese college students. Child Abuse and Neglect 26:23–37

Tanner K, Le Riche P 2000 Intentional observation. Exploring transfer in action. In: Cree V E, Macaulay C (eds) Transfer of learning in professional and vocational education. Routledge, London, p 106–118

Tardif M, Auclair N, Jacob M, Carpentier J 2005 Sexual abuse perpetrated by adult and juvenile females. Child Abuse and Neglect 29(2):153–167

Taylor C, Taylor E 1976 Multifactorial causation of malnutrition. In: McClaren D (ed) Nutrition in the community. Wiley, Chichester

Taylor C, White S 2001 Knowledge, truth and reflexivity. The problem of judgement in social work. Journal of Social Work 1(1):37–59

Taylor J 2003 Children and young people accused of child sexual abuse: a study within a community. Journal of Sexual Aggression 9:57–70

Taylor J, Daniel B 1999 Interagency practice in children with nonorganic failure to thrive: is there a gap between health and social care? Child Abuse Review 8:325–338

Taylor J S, Redman S 2004 The smacking controversy continues: what advice should we be giving parents? Journal of Advanced Nursing 46:311–318

Taylor J, Spencer N, Baldwin N 2000 Social, economic and political context of parenting. Archives of Disease in Childhood 8:113–120

Taylor L, Lacey R, Bracken D 1980 In whose best interests? Cobden Trust/Mind, London

TEN (The Education Network) 2004 Every child matters: change for children. TEN Policy Briefing. Online. Available: www.everychildmatters.gov.uk

Tharp R 1991 Cultural diversity and the treatment of children. Journal of Consulting and Clinical Psychology 59(6):799–812

Thistletwaite P 2004 Integrated working: a guide. Online. Available: www.integratedcarenetwork. gov.uk

Thoburn J 1990 Success and failure in permanent family placement. Gower/Avebury, Aldershot

Thoburn J 1991 Permanent family placement and the Children Act 1989: implications for foster carers and social workers. Adoption and Fostering 15(3):15–20

Thoburn J 1994 Child placement: principles and practice, 2nd edn. Arena, Aldershot

Thoburn J 1996 Psychological parenting and child placement. In: Howe D (ed) Attachment and loss in child and family social work. Avebury, Aldershot, p 129–145

Thoburn J 2000 The effects on child mental health of adoption and foster care. In: Gelder M, Lopez-Ibor J J, Andreasen N (eds) New Oxford textbook of psychiatry. Oxford University Press, Oxford

Thoburn J 2001 The good news on children's services. Community Care 11–17 October:36–37

Thoburn J 2002 Adoption and permanence for children who cannot live safely with birth parents or relatives. Quality Protects Research Briefing No. 5. Department of Health research in practice Making Research Count, Dartington

Thoburn J 2003 The risks and rewards of adoption for children in public care. Child and Family Law Quarterly 15(4):391–401

Thoburn J, Murdoch A, O'Brien A 1986 Permanence in child care. Basil Blackwell, Oxford

Thoburn J, Lewis A, Shemmings D 1995 Paternalism or partnership? Family involvement in the child protection process. HMSO, London

Thoburn J, Wilding J, Watson J 2000a Family support in cases of emotional maltreatment and neglect. TSO, London

Thoburn J, Norford L, Rashid S P 2000b Permanent family placement for children of minority ethnic origin. Jessica Kingsley, London

Thoburn J, Chand A, Proctor J 2005 Child welfare services for minority ethnic families: the research reviewed. Jessica Kingsley, London

Thomas C, Beckford V 1999 Adopted children speaking. BAAF, London

Thomas Coram Research Unit 2003 The use of child protection registers. Institute of Education, University of London

Thomas G 1990 Institutional child abuse: the making and prevention of an un-problem. Journal of Child and Youth Care 4(6):1–22

Thomas N 1995 Allegations of child abuse in local authority care. Practice 7(3):35–44

Thomas N 2005 Social work with young people in care: looking after children in theory and practice. Palgrave, London

Thompson N 1997 Anti-discriminatory practice, 2nd edn. Macmillan, Basingstoke

Thompson R 1995 Preventing child maltreatment through social support: a crucial analysis. Sage, Thousand Oaks, CA

Thorpe D 1994 Evaluating child protection. Open University Press, Buckingham

Thorpe D, Bilson A 1998 From protection to concern: child protection careers without apologies. Children and Society 12:373–386

Timmis G 2001 The welfare checklist for children and young people. Seen and Heard 11:45

Timmis G 2005 Being the children's champion: information, consultation and representation. Seen and Heard 15(2):33

Timms J, Thoburn J 2003 Your shout! NSPCC, London

Toch H 1969 Violent men. Aldine, Chicago

Toro P A 1982 Developmental effects of child abuse: a review. Child Abuse and Neglect 6: 423–431

Townsley R, Abbott D, Watson D 2004 Making a difference? Exploring the impact of multi-agency working on disabled children with complex health care needs, their families and the professionals who support them. Policy Press, Bristol

Toynbee P 2003 Hard work: life in low-pay Britain. Bloomsbury, London

Triseliotis J P 1983 Identity and security in adoption and long-term fostering. Adoption and Fostering 7(1):22–23

Triseliotis J P (ed) 1988 Group work in adoption and foster care. Batsford, London

Triseliotis J P, Russell J 1984 Hard to place: the outcomes of adoption and residential care. Heinemann and Gower, London

Triseliotis J P, Sellick C, Short R 1995 Foster care: theory and practice. Batsford, London

Triseliotis J P, Shireman J, Hundleby M 1997 Adoption: theory, policy and practice. Cassell, London

Triseliotis J P, Borland N, Hill M 2000 Delivering foster care. BAAF, London

Trocme N, Wolfe D 2001 Child maltreatment in Canada: selected results from the Canadian Incidence Study of Reported Child Abuse and Neglect. Minister of Public Works and Government Services Canada, Ottawa, Ontario

Trotter R, Ackerman A, Rodman D, Martinez A, Sorvillo F 1983 'Azarcon' and 'Greta': ethnomedical solution to epidemiological mystery. Medical Anthropology Quarterly 14(3):18

Truax C B, Carkhuff R R 1967 Towards effective counselling and psychotherapy. Aldine, Chicago

Tuck V 2000 Links between social deprivation and harm to children. In: Baldwin N (ed) Protecting children: promoting their rights. Whiting and Birch, London

Tunstill J 1997 Implementing the family support clauses in the 1989 Children Act: legislative, professional and organisational obstacles. In: Parton N (ed) Child protection and family support: tensions, contradictions and possibilities. Routledge, London

Tunstill J (ed) 1999 Social services provision for children and young people: answer or problem? In: Children and the state: whose problem? Cassell, London

Tunstill J, Allnock D, Akhurst S, Garbers C 2005 Sure Start local programmes: implications of case study data from the national evaluation of Sure Start. Children and Society 19:158–171

Turner C F, Ku L, Rogers S M et al 1998 Adolescent sexual behaviour, drug use, and violence: increased reporting with computer survey technology. Science 280(5365):867–873

Turney D 2005 Who cares? The role of mothers in cases of child neglect. In: Taylor J, Daniel B (eds) Child neglect: practice issues for health and social care. Jessica Kingsley, London

Tye C, Precey G 1999 Building bridges: the interface between adult mental health and child protection. Child Abuse Review 8(3):164–171

UK Government's written replies to the UN Monitoring Committee on the Rights of the Child (See CRC/C/Resp/12 at www.unhchr.ch/tbs/doc.nsf submitted to the UN Monitoring Committee in August 2002)

UN Committee on Economic, Social and Political Rights 2002 Concluding observations on the Fourth UK Periodic Report to the Committee. Observation 36 at www.unhchr.ch/tbs/doc.nsf

UNCRC 2004 The record of this agreement can be found, and the website address must be exactly followed as set out here at http://daccessdds.un.org/doc/UNDOC/GEN//GO5/401/61/PDF/GO541061.pdf?OpenElement

UNCRC Monitoring Committee on the Rights of the Child 1995 Concluding observations 8th session, 15 February 1995. UNCRC/C/15/Add.34

UNCRC Monitoring Committee on the Rights of the Child 2002 Concluding observations 31st session, 4 October 2002. UNCRC/C/15/Add.188/paragraph 16

UNICEF 2003 Child maltreatment deaths in rich nations. Innocenti Report Card No. 5. UNICEF Innocenti Research Centre, Florence

UNICEF 2005 Children in residential institutions vulnerable to abuse. Press release 31st May 2005 Online. Available: www.unicef.org.uk/press/news_detail.asp?news_id=451

United Nations 1989 UN convention on the rights of the child. United Nations, New York

United Nations 2005 Ending legalised violence against children: Report for Europe and Central Asia Regional Consultation, Ljubljana, Slovenia. UN Secretary General's study on violence against children. United Nations, Geneva

University of East Anglia 2005 Realising children's trust arrangements. National Evaluation of Children's Trusts Phase 1 Report. In association with the National Children's Bureau. Research Report RR682. DfES Publications, Nottingham

US Department of Health and Human Services 1988 Study findings. Study of national incidence and prevalence of child abuse and neglect. National Center on Child Abuse and Neglect, Washington, DC

US Department of Health and Human Services 1996 The Third National Incidence Study of child abuse and neglect (NIS-3). National Center on Child Abuse and Neglect, Washington

US Department of Health and Human Services, Administration on Children, Youth and Families 2005 Child maltreatment 2003. US Government Printing Office, Washington, DC

Utting D (ed) 1998 Children's services: now and in the future. National Children's Bureau, London

Utting W 1991 Children in the public care: a review of residential care. Social Services Inspectorate study. HMSO, London

Utting W 1992 Children in the public care. HMSO, London

Utting W, Department of Health, Welsh Office 1997 People like us: the report of the review of the safeguards for children living away from home. TSO, London

Van der Kolk B A 1994 The body keeps the score: memory and the emerging psychobiology of post traumatic stress. Harvard Review of Psychiatry 1:253–265

Van der Kolk B A, Fisler R 1995 Dissociation and the fragmentary nature of traumatic memories: overview and exploratory study. Journal of Traumatic Stress 8:505–525

Van der Kolk B A, McFarlane A C, Weisaeth L 1996a Traumatic stress: the effects of overwhelming experiences on mind, body and society. Guilford Press, London

Van der Kolk B A, Pelcovitz D, Roth S, Mandel F S, McFarlane A, Herman J L 1996b Dissociation, somatization, and affect dysregulation: the complexity of adaptation of trauma. American Journal of Psychiatry 153(Suppl):83–93

Van Ijzendoorn M H 1995 Adult attachment representations, parental responsiveness, and infant attachment: a meta-analysis on the predictive validity of the adult attachment interview. Psychological Bulletin 117:387–403

VanFleet R, Ryan S D, Smith S K 2005 Filial therapy: a critical review. In: Reddy L A, Files-Hall T M, Schaefer C E (eds) Empirically based play interventions for children. American Psychological Association, Washington, DC, p 241–264

Verity P, Nixon S 1995 Allegations against foster families: survey results. Foster Care 83:13–16

Vetere A, Cooper J 2005 The effects of domestic violence: trauma, resilience and breaking the cycle of violence. In: Newnes C, Radcliffe N (eds) Making and breaking children's lives. PCCS Books, Ross-on-Wye

Vizard E 1993 Interviewing sexually abused children. In: Hobbs C, Wynne J (eds) Baillière's clinical paediatrics. Baillière Tindall, London

Vizard E, Monck E, Misch P 1995 Child and adolescent sex abuse perpetrators: a review of the research literature. Journal of Child Psychology and Psychiatry 5:731–756

Wade J, Biehal N, Clayden J, Stein M 1998 Going missing: young people absent from care. Wiley, Chichester

Walker M, Hill M, Triseliotis J 2002 Testing the limits of foster care: fostering as an alternative to secure accommodation. BAAF, London

Wall N 1999 Concurrent planning: a judicial perspective. Child and Family Law Quarterly 11:97–108

Walsh F 1996 The concept of family resilience: crisis and challenge. Family Process 35:261–281

Ward H 2001 The developmental needs of children: implications for assessment. In: Horwath J (ed) The child's world: assessing children in need. Jessica Kingsley, London, p 167–179

Ward H, Munro E, Dearden C, Nicholson D 2003 Outcomes for looked after children: life pathways and decision making for very young children in care or accommodation. Centre for Child and Family Research, Loughborough.

Ward L 2005 Sex advice for teenagers 'must stay confidential'. Guardian 19 October

Ward T, Stewart C 2003 Good lives and the rehabilitation of sex offenders. In: Ward T, Laws D R, Hudson S (eds) Sexual deviance: issues and controversies. Sage, Thousand Oaks, CA

Ward T, Polaschek D, Beech A 2006 Theories of sexual offending. Wiley, Chichester

Wardhaugh J, Wilding P 1993 Towards an explanation of the corruption of care. Critical Social Policy 37:4–31

Warken W J, Rosenbaum A, Fletcher K E, Hoge S K, Adelman S A 1994 Head injured males: a population at risk for relationship aggression. Violence and Victims 9:153–166

Warner J 2003 An initial assessment of the extent to which risk factors, frequently identified in research, are taken into account when assessing risk in child protection cases. Journal of Social Work 3:339–363

Warner M 2000 Person-centred therapy at the difficult edge: a developmentally based model of fragile and dissociated process. In: Mearns D, Thorne B (eds) Person-centred therapy today. Sage, London, p 144–171

Waterhouse R 2000 Lost in care: report of the Tribunal of Inquiry into the abuse of children in care in the former county council areas of Gwynedd and Clwyd since 1974. TSO, London

Waterhouse S 1997 The organisation of fostering services. NFCA, London

Waterston T 2005 A general paediatrician's practice in children's rights. Archives of Disease in Childhood 90:178–181

Waterston T, Mann N 2005 Children's rights. Archives of Disease in Childhood 90:171

Watkins B, Bentovim A 1992 The sexual abuse of male children and adolescents: a review of current research. Journal of Child Psychology and Psychiatry 33(1):197–248

Wattam C 1992 Making a case in child protection. Longman, Loughborough

Wattam C 1999 The prevention of child abuse. Children and Society 13:317–329

Webster-Stratton C 1990 Stress: a potential disruptor of parent perceptions and family interactions. Journal of Clinical Child Psychology 19:302–312

Webster-Stratton C 1999 Researching the impact of parent training programmes on child conduct problems. In: Lloyd E (ed) Parenting matters: what works in parenting education? Barnardo's, Barkingside, Ilford

Webster-Stratton C, Herbert M 1994 Troubled families – problem children. Wiley, Chichester

Wedge P, Mantle G 1991 Sibling groups and social work. Avebury, Aldershot

Weinrott M, Saylor M 1991 Self-report of crimes committed by sex offenders. Journal of Interpersonal Violence 6(3):286

Welsh Assembly 2006 Working together to safeguard children – a guide to inter-agency working to safeguard and promote the welfare of children. Welsh Assembly Government, Cardiff. Online. Available: http://new.wales.gov.uk/?lang=en

West J 1996 Child centred play therapy, 2nd edn. Arnold, London

Westcott H 1991 The abuse of disabled children: a review of the literature. Child: Care, Health and Development 17:243–258

Westcott H L 1991b Institutional abuse of children – from research to policy – a review. NSPCC, London

Westcott H 1993 Abuse of children and adults with disabilities. NSPCC, London

Westcott H 1994 Abuse of children and adults who are disabled. In: French S (ed) On equal terms: working with disabled people. Butterworth-Heinemann, Oxford

Westcott H 1999 Communication. In: Parton N, Wattam C (eds) Child sexual abuse: responding to the experiences of children. Wiley, Chichester

Westcott H L, Clement M 1992 Experience of child abuse in residential care and educational placements: results of a survey. NSPCC, London

Westcott H, Cross M 1996 This far and no further: towards ending the abuse of disabled children. Venture Press, Birmingham

Wheal A (ed) 2005 The RHP companion to foster care, 2nd edn. Russell House, Lyme Regis

Whitaker D, Archer L, Hicks L 1998 Working in children's homes: challenges and complexities. In: DOH Caring for children away from home – messages from research. Wiley, Chichester

White S, Featherstone B 2005 Communicating misunderstandings: multi-agency work as social practice. Child and Family Social Work 10:207–216

Whittaker J K, Maluccio A N 2002 Rethinking 'child placement': a reflective essay. Social Services Review 76(1):108–134

Wilcox R 1991 Family decision-making: family group conferences: practitioners' views. Practitioners Publishing, Lower Hutt, New Zealand

Wilczynski A 1997 Child homicide. Greenwich Medical Media, London

Wilkinson A 1982 Children who come into care in Tower Hamlets. London Borough of Tower Hamlets, London

Wilkinson R G 1994 Unfair shares: the effects of widening income differences on the welfare of the young. Barnardo's, London

Williams A, Morris J 2003 Child protection and disabled children at residential schools. In: It doesn't happen to disabled children. NSPCC, London

Williams F 1995 Social policy: a critical introduction. Polity Press, London

Williams F 1999 Good enough principles for welfare. Journal of Social Policy 28(4):667–689

Williams F 2001 In and beyond New Labour: towards a new political ethics of care. Critical Social Policy 21(4):467–494

Williams L M 1994 Recall of childhood trauma: a prospective study of women's memories of child sexual abuse. Journal of Consulting and Clinical Psychology 62:1167–1176

Williams L M 1995 Recovered memories of abuse in women with documented child sexual victimization histories. Journal of Traumatic Stress 8:649–673

Wilson E 1980 Women and the welfare state. Tavistock, London

Wilson K, James A 1995 The child protection handbook. Baillière Tindall, London

Wilson K, Ryan V 1994 Working with the sexually abused child: the use of non-directive play therapy and family therapy. Journal of Social Work Practice 8(1):71–78

Wilson K, Ryan V 2002 Play therapy with emotionally damaged adolescents. Emotional and Behavioural Difficulties 7(3):178–192

Wilson K, Ryan V 2005 Play therapy: a non-directive approach for children and adolescents, 2nd edn. Elsevier, Edinburgh

Wilson K, Sinclair I 2004 Contact in foster care: some dilemmas and opportunities. In: Neil E, Howe D (eds) Contact in adoption and permanent foster care. BAAF, London

Wilson K, Kendrick P, Ryan V 1992 Play therapy: a non-directive approach for children and adolescents. Baillière Tindall, London

Wilson K, Sinclair I, Taylor C, Pithouse A, Sellick C 2004 Fostering success: an exploration of the literature on foster care. Knowledge Review No. 5. Social Care Institute of Excellence, London

Wind T W, Silvern L 1992 Type and extent of child abuse as predictors of adult functioning. Journal of Family Violence 7(4):261–281

Winnicott C 1964 Child care and social work: a collection of papers written between 1954 and 1962. Codicote, Welwyn

Winnicott C 1986 Face to face with children. In: British Agencies for Adoption and Fostering (eds) Working with children. BAAF, London

Wissow L S 1990 Child advocacy for the clinician – an approach to child abuse and neglect. Williams and Wilkins, Baltimore

Wolf S C 1985 A multi-factor model of deviant sexuality. Victimology 10:359–374

Wolfe D A 1985 Child abuse parents. An empirical review and analysis. Psychological Bulletin 97:461–482

Wolfe D A, Fairbank J, Kelly J A, Bradlyn A S 1983 Child abusive parents and physiological responses to stressful and non-stressful behaviour in children. Behavioural Assessment 5:363–371

Wolff S 1996 Childhood psychotherapy. In: Block S (ed) An introduction to the psychotherapies, 3rd edn. Oxford University Press, Oxford, p 261–293

World Health Organization 1999 Report of the consultation on child abuse prevention. WHO, Geneva

Wright C M 2005 What is weight faltering ('failure to thrive') and when does it become a child protection issue? In: Taylor J, Daniel B (eds) Child neglect: practice issues for health and social care. Jessica Kingsley, London, p 166–185

Wright C M, Waterston A 1994 How not to succeed with weight screening despite really trying. Journal of Epidemiology and Community Health 45:502

Wright M O, Fopma-Loy J, Fischer S 2005 Multidimensional assessment of resilience in mothers who are child sexual abuse survivors. Child Abuse and Neglect 29(10):1173–1193

Wrobel G, Grotevant H, Berge J, Mendenhall T, McRoy R 2003 Contact in adoption: the experience of adoptive families in the USA. Adoption and Fostering 27(1):57–67

Wulczyn F, Kogan J, Harden B J 2003 Placement stability and movement trajectories. Social Service Review 77(2):212–236

Wyatt G E, Powell G J 1988 Lasting effects of child sexual abuse. Sage, Newbury Park, CA

Wyre R 1991 Working with sex offenders. In: Wilson K (ed) Child protection: helping or harming. Papers in Social Policy and Professional Studies, No. 15. University of Hull, Hull

Wyre R 1996 The mind of the paedophile. In: Bibby P C (ed) Organised abuse – the current debate. Arena/Ashgate, Aldershot

Yang S 2005 Family patterns, attitudes and behaviour in relation to the upbringing of children in South Korea: the social construction of child abuse. Doctoral Thesis, University of Nottingham

Yeatman G W, Shaw C, Barlow M J, Bartlett G 1976 Pseudobattering in Vietnamese children. Pediatrics 58(4):616–618

Yelloly M 1980 Social work theory and psychoanalysis. Van Nostrand Reinhold, New York

Yoshikawa H 1994 Prevention as cumulative protection: effects of early family support and education on chronic delinquency and its risks. Psychological Bulletin 115:28–54

Youth Justice Board 2003 Parenting Reader, Professional Certificate in Effective Practice. Youth Justice Board, London

Youth Justice Board 2005 Youth Justice Annual Statistics 2003/04: Youth Justice Board, London. Online. Available: www.youth-justice-board.gov.uk

Zeanah C H, Zeanah P D 1989 Intergenerational transmission of maltreatment: insights from attachment theory and research. Psychiatry 52:177–196

Zellman G L 1990 Child abuse reporting and failure to report among mandated reporters: prevalence, incidence and reasons. Journal of Interpersonal Violence 5:3–22

Zimrin H 1986 A profile of survival. Child Abuse and Neglect 10(3):339–349

Index